MEMMLER'S

The Human Body in Health and Disease

11TH EDITION

MEMMLER'S
The Human Body in Health and Disease

11TH EDITION

Barbara Janson Cohen

Jason James Taylor

(contributor)

Wolters Kluwer | Lippincott Williams & Wilkins
Health

Philadelphia · Baltimore · New York · London
Buenos Aires · Hong Kong · Sydney · Tokyo

Senior Acquisitions Editor: David Troy
Developmental Editor: Dana Knighten
Managing Editor: Renee Thomas
Marketing Manager: Allison Noplock
Managing Editor, Production: Eve Malakoff-Klein
Designer: Doug Smock
Artist: Dragonfly Media Group
Compositor: Maryland Composition, Inc.
Printer: R.R. Donnelley

11th Edition
Copyright © 2009, 2005 Lippincott Williams & Wilkins, a Wolters Kluwer business.

351 West Camden Street   530 Walnut Street
Baltimore, MD 21201   Philadelphia, PA 19106

Printed in China

9 8 7 6 5 4 3 2 1

Library of Congress Cataloging-in-Publication Data

Cohen, Barbara J.
  Memmler's the human body in health and disease. — 11th ed. / Barbara Janson Cohen, Jason James Taylor.
    p. ; cm.
  Includes bibliographical references and index.
  ISBN 978-0-7817-6577-0 – 978-0-7817-9073-4 (pbk.)
  1. Human physiology. 2. Physiology, Pathological. 3. Human anatomy. I. Taylor, Jason J. II. Memmler, Ruth Lundeen. III. Title. IV. Title: Human body in health and disease.
  [DNLM: 1. Physiology. 2. Anatomy. 3. Pathology. QT 104 C678m 2009]
  QP34.5.M48 2009
  612--dc22

                              2008013977

DISCLAIMER

Care has been taken to confirm the accuracy of the information present and to describe generally accepted practices. However, the authors, editors, and publisher are not responsible for errors or omissions or for any consequences from application of the information in this book and make no warranty, expressed or implied, with respect to the currency, completeness, or accuracy of the contents of the publication. Application of this information in a particular situation remains the professional responsibility of the practitioner; the clinical treatments described and recommended may not be considered absolute and universal recommendations.

The authors, editors, and publisher have exerted every effort to ensure that drug selection and dosage set forth in this text are in accordance with the current recommendations and practice at the time of publication. However, in view of ongoing research, changes in government regulations, and the constant flow of information relating to drug therapy and drug reactions, the reader is urged to check the package insert for each drug for any change in indications and dosage and for added warnings and precautions. This is particularly important when the recommended agent is a new or infrequently employed drug.

Some drugs and medical devices presented in this publication have Food and Drug Administration (FDA) clearance for limited use in restricted research settings. It is the responsibility of the health care provider to ascertain the FDA status of each drug or device planned for use in their clinical practice.

To purchase additional copies of this book, call our customer service department at (800) 638-3030 or fax orders to (301) 223-2320. International customers should call (301) 223-2300.

Visit Lippincott Williams & Wilkins on the Internet: http://www.lww.com. Lippincott Williams & Wilkins customer service representatives are available from 8:30 am to 6:00 pm, EST.

Preface

Memmler's *The Human Body in Health and Disease* is a textbook for introductory-level health professions and nursing students who need a basic understanding of anatomy and physiology, the interrelationships between structure and function, and the effects of disease on body systems.

Like preceding editions, the 11th edition remains true to Ruth Memmler's original vision. Designed for health professions and nursing students, the features and content specifically meet the needs of those who may be starting their health career preparation with little or no science background. This book's primary goals are:

- To provide the essential knowledge of human anatomy, physiology, and the effects of disease at an ideal level of detail and in language that is clear and understandable.

- To illustrate the concepts discussed with anatomic art that depicts the appropriate level of detail with accuracy, simplicity, and elegance and that is integrated seamlessly with the narrative.

- To incorporate the most recent scientific findings into the fundamental material on which Ruth Memmler's classic text is based.

- To include pedagogy designed to enhance interest in and understanding of the concepts presented.

- To teach the basic anatomic and medical terminology used in healthcare settings, preparing students to function efficiently in their chosen health career.

- To present an integrated teaching-learning package that includes all of the elements necessary for a successful learning experience.

This revision is the direct result of in-depth market feedback solicited to tell us what instructors and students at this level most need. We listened carefully to the feedback, and the results we obtained are integrated into many features of this book and into the ancillary package accompanying it. The text itself has been revised and updated where needed to improve organization of the material and to reflect current scientific thought. Because visual learning devices are so important to students at this level, this edition includes a new appendix with a series of dissection photographs. It also retains its extensive art program with updated versions of figures from previous editions. These features appear in an all-new design that makes the content more user-friendly and accessible than ever. The new ancillary package includes the innovative PASSport to Success for students as well as a com-

prehensive package of instructor resources designed to provide instructors with maximum flexibility and efficiency.

Organization and Structure

Like previous editions, the 11th edition uses a body systems approach to the study of the normal human body and how disease affects it. The book is divided into seven units, grouping related information and body systems together as follows:

- Unit I, The Body as a Whole (Chapters 1–4), focuses on the body's organization, basic chemistry needed to understand body functions, cells and their functions, and tissues, glands, and membranes.

- Unit II, Disease and the First Line of Defense (Chapters 5 and 6), presents information on disease, organisms that produce disease, and the integumentary system, which is the body's first line of defense against injury and disease.

- Unit III, Movement and Support (Chapters 7 and 8), includes the skeletal and muscular systems.

- Unit IV, Coordination and Control (Chapters 9–12), focuses on the nervous system, the sensory system, and the endocrine system.

- Unit V, Circulation and Body Defense (Chapters 13–17), includes the blood, the heart and heart disease, blood vessels and circulation, the lymphatic system, and the immune system.

- Unit VI, Energy: Supply and Use (Chapters 18–22), includes the respiratory system; the digestive system; metabolism, nutrition, and temperature control; body fluids; and the urinary system.

- Unit VII, Perpetuation of Life (Chapters 23–25), covers the male and female reproductive systems, development and birth, and heredity and hereditary diseases.

The main Glossary defines the chapters' boldfaced terms. An additional Glossary of Word Parts is a reference tool that not only teaches basic medical and anatomic terminology but also helps students learn to recognize unfamiliar terms. Appendices include a variety of supplementary information that students will find useful as they work with the text, including the new dissection photograph appendix (Appendix 7) and answers to the Chapter Checkpoint questions and Zooming In illustration questions (Appendix 6) that are found in every chapter.

Pedagogic Features

Every chapter contains pedagogy that has been designed with the health professions and nursing student in mind

- **Learning Outcomes:** Chapter objectives on the first page of every chapter help the student organize and prioritize learning

- **Selected Key Terms:** List that accompanies the Learning Outcomes presents the most important terms covered in the chapter

- **Disease in Context (NEW to this edition):** Brief chapter-opening stories based on medical cases draw readers in by highlighting information in the chapters and showing how disease may affect the body's state of internal balance.

- **Chapter Checkpoints:** Brief questions at the end of main sections test and reinforce the student's recall of key information in that section. Answers are in Appendix 6.

- **"Zooming In" questions:** Questions with the figure legends test and reinforce the student's understanding of concepts depicted in the illustration. They are set in red to increase their visibility. Answers are in Appendix 6.

- **Phonetic pronunciations:** Easy-to-learn phonetic pronunciations are spelled out in the narrative, appearing in parentheses directly following many terms—no need for students to understand dictionary-style diacritical marks. (See the "Guide to Pronunciation" below.)

- **Special interest boxes:** Each chapter contains three special interest boxes focusing on topics that augment chapter content. The book includes five kinds of boxes altogether:

  - > **Disease in Context Revisited (NEW to this edition):** Boxes that trace the outcome of the medical story that opens each chapter and show how the cases relate to material in the chapter and to others in the book.

  - > **A Closer Look:** Provide additional in-depth scientific detail on topics in or related to the chapter.

  - > **Clinical Perspective:** Focus on diseases and disorders relevant to the chapter, exploring what happens to the body when the normal structure-function relationship breaks down.

  - > **Hot Topic:** Focus on current trends and research, reinforcing the link between anatomy and physiology and related news coverage that students may have seen.

  - > **Health Maintenance:** Offer supplementary information on health and wellness issues.

- **Figures:** The art program includes full-color anatomic line art, some new or revised, with a level of detail that matches that of the narrative. Photomicrographs, radiographs, and other scans give students a preview of what they might see in real-world healthcare settings. Supplementary figures are available on the companion website as well as on the Student and Instructor Resource DVD-ROMs.

- **Tables:** The numerous tables in this edition summarize key concepts and information in an easy-to-review form. Additional summary tables are available on the companion website as well as on the Student and Instructor Resource DVD-ROMs.

- **Color figure and table numbers:** Figure and table numbers appear in color in the narrative, helping students quickly find their place after stopping to look at an illustration or table. Figure callouts appear in blue type, and table callouts, in red.

- **Word Anatomy:** This chart defines and illustrates the various word parts that appear in terms within the chapter. The prefixes, roots, and suffixes presented are grouped according to chapter headings so that students can find the relevant text. This learning tool helps students build vocabulary and promotes understanding of even unfamiliar terms based on a knowledge of common word parts.

- **Summary:** Outline-format summary provides a concise overview of chapter content, aiding in study and test preparation.

- **Questions for Study and Review:** Study questions have been thoroughly revised and organized hierarchically into three levels. (Note that answers appear on the Instructor's Resource DVD-Rom in the Instructor's Manual as well as on the Instructor's companion website):

  - > **Building Understanding:** Includes fill-in-the-blank, matching, and multiple choice questions that test factual recall.

  - > **Understanding Concepts:** Includes short-answer questions (define, describe, compare/contrast) that test and reinforce understanding of concepts.

  - > **Conceptual Thinking:** : Includes short-essay questions that promote critical thinking skills. New in this edition are thought questions related to the Disease in Context case stories.

PASSport to Success for Students

 Look for this icon throughout the book for pertinent supplementary material on the companion website and student resource CD

The PASSport to Success is a practical system that lets students learn faster, remember more, and achieve success. Students discover their unique learning styles—visual, auditory, or kinesthetic—with a simple online assessment, then choose from a wealth of resources for each learning style including animations, 11 different types of online learning activities, an audio glossary, and other supplemental materials such as health professions career information, additional summary tables, additional images, study and test-taking tips, and a searchable online version of the text. Throughout the textbook, the graphic icon shown above alerts students to pertinent supplementary material.

The PASSport to Success is available on the DVD-Rom bound into this textbook as well as on the book's companion website at http://thePoint.lww.com/Memmler HumanBody11e. See the inside front cover of this text for the passcode you will need to gain access to the website, and see pages ix–xix for all details about the PASSport to Success and a complete listing of student resources.

Instructor Ancillary Package

All instructor resources are available to approved adopting instructors online at http://thePoint.lww.com/Memmler HumanBody11e as well as on the Instructor Resource DVD-Rom:

- **Print Instructor's Manual** includes the Instructor Resource DVD-Rom, and is also available in PDF format online.

- **Using the PASSport to Success in Your Course** provides practical tips for integrating this innovative approach.

- **Brownstone Test Generator** allows you to create customized exams from a bank of questions.

- **PowerPoint Presentations** include multiple choice and true/false questions for use with Student Response System technology.

- **Image Bank** includes labels-on and labels-off options.

- **Lesson Plans** are organized around the learning objectives and include lecture notes, in-class activities, and assignments, including student activities from the PASSport to Success.

- **Answers to Study Guide Questions** are the instructor's companions to the print student Study Guide.

- **Answers to Questions for Study and Review** match up with the quiz material found at the end of each chapter in the textbook.

- **Strategies for Effective Teaching** provide sound, tried-and-true advice for successful instruction.

- **LiveAdvise Tutoring Service** is available for instructors as well as students.

- **WebCT and Blackboard-ready Cartridge** allows you to integrate the ancillary materials into learning management systems.

Instructors also have access to all student ancillary assets, including the PASSport to Success, via thePoint website.

Guide to Pronunciation

The stressed syllable in each word is shown with capital letters. The vowel pronunciations are as follows:

Any vowel at the end of a syllable is given a long sound, as follows:

a as in say
e as in be
i as in nice
o as in go
u as in true

A vowel followed by a consonant and the letter e (as in rate) also is given a long pronunciation.

Any vowel followed by a consonant receives a short pronunciation, as follows:

a as in absent
e as in end
i as in bin
o as in not
u as in up

Summary

The 11th edition of *Memmler's The Human Body in Health and Disease* builds on the successes of the previous ten editions by offering clear, concise narrative into which accurate, aesthetically pleasing anatomic art has been woven. We have made every effort to respond thoughtfully and thoroughly to reviewers' and instructors' comments, offering the ideal level of detail for students preparing for a career in the health professions and nursing, the pedagogic features that best support it, and with the PASSport to Success, providing students with an integrated system for understanding and using their unique learning styles—and ultimately succeeding in the course. We hope you will agree that the 11th edition of *Memmler's* suits your educational needs.

Introducing... **PASSport** to **Success**

Succeed in anatomy and physiology with easy-to-use, multimedia tools that are tailored to your unique learning style.

Anatomy & Physiology may be the toughest course you ever *ace.*

You've probably heard horror stories from other students about learning A&P.

"It's challenging."
"Too much information, not enough time."
"Definitely the hardest class in the program."

It's true – anatomy and physiology is a tough subject. You will need to understand and remember the essentials of how the human body works – the organs, the systems, and the processes. Grasping this material is the foundation of your success, because you will use what you learn in this class throughout your coursework and your career.

There is no need to feel overwhelmed. You will succeed. Because you're about to discover something very important about yourself: your unique learning style.

How do you learn best? By seeing? By hearing? Or by doing?

Different people learn in different ways. Some students learn by reading. Others take in new information by listening to their instructors. You may prefer to write down notes. A simple self-assessment can tell you whether you're a visual, auditory, or kinesthetic learner.

When you understand the way that you process information most effectively, you can choose resources that fit your learning style.

The PASSport to Success is a practical system that lets you **learn faster, remember more, and achieve success**.

**Your PASSport to Success begins now.
Turn the page for a snapshot of your journey!**

→ → →

PASSport to Success

USE YOUR TIME EFFECTIVELY

> Icons in the textbook, on the website, and on the CD-ROM guide you to visual, auditory and kinesthetic activities that will help you learn and succeed.

ACHIEVE SUCCESS!

> Ace the exam and pass the course!

Turn the page to begin your tour!

→ → →

UNDERSTAND THE JOURNEY AHEAD

Your journey begins with your textbook, *Memmler's The Human Body in Health and Disease*. Newly updated and fully illustrated, this easy-to-use textbook is filled with icons that guide you to resources and activities that are designed for your

thePoint
Where Teaching, Learning, & Technology Click

Provides flexible learning solutions and resources for students and faculty using
Memmler's The Human Body in Health and Disease, 11th Edition

PASSport to Success resources for students:
- More than 25 Animations
- Printable Learning Styles Report
- LiveAdvise Online Student Tutoring
- Chapter Pre-Quizzes
- Audio Glossary
- More than 200 Learning Activities
- And More!

Tools to make instructors' jobs easier*:
- Test Generator
- Lesson Plans
- PASSport to Success Pre-Test
- Image Bank
- PowerPoint Slides
- And More!

Log on today!
Visit **http://thepoint.lww.com/MemmlerHumanBody11e** to learn more about **thePoint™** and the resources available. Use the code provided below to access the student resources.

http://thepoint.lww.com/MemmlerHumanBody11e

SCRATCH OFF BELOW

Note: Book cannot be returned once panel is scratched off.

Wolters Kluwer Health | Lippincott Williams & Wilkins

*The faculty resources are restricted to adopters of the text. Adopters have to be approved before accessing the faculty resources.

Inside the front cover of your textbook, you'll find your **personal access code**. Use it to log on to *thePoint* – the companion website for this textbook. On the website, you can search and sort learning activities by learning style and choose the ones that will help you understand the material quickly and efficiently.

Every chapter begins with a set of **Learning Outcomes** that explain what you need to learn, so you can focus your study time on the most important material.

Each chapter begins with **Disease in Context**, an interesting case story that uses a familiar, real-life scenario to illustrate key concepts in anatomy and physiology. Later in the chapter, the case story is revisited in more detail—improving your understanding and helping you remember the information.

Look for the **PASSport to Success** symbol throughout your textbook to locate additional resources and exercises that are designed for your learning style.

CHAPTER

16

The Lymphatic System and Lymphoid Tissue

Learning Outcomes

After careful study of this chapter, you should be able to:

1. Define disease and list seven categories of disease
2. List seven predisposing cause of disease
3. Define terminology used in describing and treating disease
4. Define complementary and alternative medicine; cite several alternative or complementary fields of practice
5. Explain methods by which microorganisms can be transmitted from one host to another
6. List four types of organisms studied in microbiology and give the characteristics of each
7. List some diseases caused by each type of microorganism
8. Define normal flora and explain the value of the normal flora
9. Describe the three types of bacteria according to shape
10. List several diseases in humans caused by worms
11. Give some reasons for the emergence and spread of microorganisms today
12. Describe several public health measures taken to prevent the spread of disease
13. Differentiate sterilization, disinfection, and antisepsis
14. Describe techniques included as part of body substance precautions
15. List some antimicrobial agents and describe how they work
16. Describe several methods used to identify microorganisms in the laboratory
17. Show how word parts are used to build words related to disease (see Word Anatomy at the end of the chapter)

Selected Key Terms

The following terms and other boldface terms in the chapter are defined in the Glossary:

acute
antisepsis
asepsis
chronic
diagnosis
disease
disinfection
epidemic
etiology
helminth
microorganism
nosocomial infection
opportunistic infection
pathogen
pathophysiology
prion
prognosis
sign
spore
sterilization
symptom
syndrome
systemic
therapy
toxin
vector

PASSport to Success

Visit thePoint or see the Student Resource CD in the back of this book for definitions and pronunciations of key terms as well as a pretest for this chapter

---

Disease in Context

Maria's Case: When Pathogens Attack

The man sharing the elevator with Maria Sanchez looked terrible — watery eyes, runny nose, and a sickly, run-down appearance. As the elevator opened and the man stepped toward the door, he let out a loud sneeze. "Pardon me," he said, as the elevator closed behind him. If I was that sick, I'd stay in bed, Maria thought. Maria didn't know it yet, but soon she would be.

The passenger left something behind when he exited the elevator. Microscopic droplets of mucus and water from his sneeze floated in the air. Inside each droplet were thousands of microorganisms, called viruses, capable of making Maria very sick. She inhaled several of these germ laden droplets into her respiratory system as she waited for the elevator to reach her floor. Maria exited the elevator unaware that her body had been invaded.

Maria's warm, moist respiratory tract was a perfect environment for this microorganism. When a virus landed on the epithelial tissue lining her throat, protein spikes protruding from its surface fit snugly into receptors on an epithelial cell, stimulating endocytosis of the virus. Having successfully, the virus was inside the cell and ready to begin the second phase of its attack!

Shortly after entering the cell, the virus released its RNA, which was then transported into the cell's nucleus. Unable to recognize the viral RNA as foreign, the nucleus transcribed it into viral messenger RNA. Returning to the cytoplasm, this new RNA was translated into viral proteins at the ribosomes. Some of these proteins were combined with viral RNA to make new viruses. Others took over the machinery of the host cell to make more viral components.

Since entering the epithelial cell about 24 hours ago, the virus had successfully hijacked cellular RNA and protein synthesis. The cell had been turned into a virus-making factory! With the cell

nearly exhausted, the new viruses that filled its cytoplasm exited to infect new hosts. Although finally free of the pathogen, the cell had no more resources left and died. Maria Sanchez' body had been invaded by the influenza virus. In this chapter we'll learn more about viruses as well as other disease-producing organisms. Later in the case, we'll see how Maria's body is coping with its unwanted visitors.

Maria Sanchez' body has been invaded by the influenza virus. In this chapter, we'll learn more about viruses as well as other disease-producing organisms. Later in the case, we'll see how Maria's body is coping with its unwanted visitors.

Maria's warm, moist respiratory tract was a perfect environment for this microorganism. When a virus landed on the epithelial tissue lining her throat, protein spikes protruding from its surface fit snugly into receptors on an epithelial cell, stimulating endocytosis of the virus. Having successfully "picked the lock" on the cell's plasma membrane, the virus was inside the cell and ready to begin the second phase of its attack!

Maria Sanchez' body has been invaded by the influenza virus. In this chapter, we'll learn more about viruses as well as other disease-producing organisms. Later in the case, we'll see how Maria's body is coping with its unwanted visitors.

Shortly after entering the cell, the virus released its RNA, which was then transported into the cell's nucleus. Unable to recognize the viral RNA as foreign, the nucleus transcribed it into viral messenger RNA. Returning to the cytoplasm, this new RNA was translated into viral proteins at the ribosomes. Some of these proteins were combined with viral RNA to make new viruses. Others took over the machinery of the host cell to make more viral components.

DISCOVER YOUR LEARNING STYLE

People learn in different ways. If you like to study animations, illustrations, and diagrams, you may be a visual learner. If you like to sound out new words or discuss material with other students, you may be an auditory learner. If you take a lot of notes during class and benefit from hands-on learning activities, you're probably a kinesthetic learner.

Most people have both a primary and a secondary learning style – and the PASSport to Success helps you identify both! Once you know how you learn best, you can choose learning activities that will help you master new material more efficiently.

 Visual

 Auditory

 Kinesthetic

Take the Learning Styles Assessment

Discovering your learning style is easy – and fun! Here's how to begin:

1. Scratch off the personal access code inside the front cover of your textbook.

2. Log on to http://thePoint.lww.com/MemmlerHumanBody11e.

3. Click on "Student Resources" and then "PASSport to Success."

4. Once you are on the PASSport site, click on "MyPowerLearning."

5. Take the online self-assessment. *(Don't worry – There are no wrong answers!)*

Read your custom report

Identifying your learning style is the first step to your academic success. In fact, many students say, "If I had known this in high school, my grades would have been so much better!" Your personal learning styles report not only reveals your primary and secondary learning styles, it also gives you tips and ideas to make the most of the resources that you'll find in the PASSport to Success.

USE YOUR TIME EFFECTIVELY

Anatomy and physiology is a challenge for many students, because there is so much new material to learn. The PASSport to Success will help you make the most of your study time, because every chapter in the book, *thePoint* website, the CD-ROM and the Study Guide include resources tailored to your learning style.

The PASSport symbol in the textbook will guide you to exercises and resources on *thePoint* website or the CD-ROM that are coded according to your learning style.

Box 3-2   **Hot Topics**

Proteomics: So Many Proteins, So Few Genes

To build the many different proteins that make up the body, cells rely on instructions encoded in the chromosomes' genes. Collectively, all the different genes on all the chromosomes make up the genome. Genes contain the instructions for making proteins, while the proteins themselves perform the body's functions.

Scientists are now studying the human proteome—all the proteins that can be expressed in a cell—to help them understand the proteins' structure and function. Unlike the genome, the proteome changes as the cell's activities and needs change. In 2003, after a decade of intense scientific activity, investigators mapped the entire human genome and realized that it contained only 35,000 genes, far fewer than initially expected. How could this relatively small number of genes code for several million proteins? They concluded that genes were not the whole story.

Gene transcription is only the b[...] thesis. In response to cell conditi[...] newly transcribed mRNA into sever[...] ribosome can use to build a differ[...] protein is built, enzymes can furthe[...] strands to produce several more c[...] molecules help the newly formed p[...] cise shapes and interact with each [...] more variations. Thus, while a gene[...] protein, modifications after gene tr[...] many more unique proteins. There [...] about the proteome, but scientist[...] search will lead to new techniques [...] ing disease.

hours spends only about one hour in mitosis and the remaining time in interphase.

CHECKPOINT 3-10 ➤ What must happen to the DNA in a cell before mitosis can occur? During what stage in the life of a cell does this occur?

PASSport to Success — Visit *thePoint* or see the Student Resource CD in the back of this book for a photomicrograph of a replicated chromosome.

Stages of Mitosis

Although mitosis is a continuous process, distinct changes can be seen in the dividing cell at four stages (Fig. 3-9).

- In **prophase** (PRO-faze), the doubled strands of DNA return to their tightly wound spiral organization and become visible under the microscope as dark, thread-like chromosomes. The nucleolus and the nuclear membrane begin to disappear. In the cytoplasm, the two centrioles move toward opposite ends of the cell and a spindle-shaped structure made of thin fibers begins to form between them.

- In **metaphase** (MET-ah-faze), the chromosomes line up across the center (equator) of the cell attached to the spindle fibers.

- As mitosis continues into t[...] membrane appears around [...] chromosomes, forming two [...]

Also during telophase, the p[...] off to divide the cell. The midsec[...] eas becomes progressively smal[...] splits in two. There are now tw[...] cells, each with exactly the same [...] as was present in the parent ce[...] cells, skeletal muscle cells for ex[...] not divide following nuclear d[...] multiple mitoses, is a giant single[...] This pattern is extremely rare in [...]

During mitosis, all the organ[...] for the division process, tempor[...] cell divides, these organelles re[...] cell. Also at this time, the centr[...] preparation for the next cell divis[...]

Body cells differ in the rate [...] Some, such as nerve cells and mu[...] some point in development and [...] die. They remain in interphase. C[...] sperm cells, and skin cells, multip[...] destroyed by injury, disease, o[...] Cells that multiply slowly may be [...] tissue is injured, as in repair of a [...]

Immature cells that retain th[...] ture when necessary are known [...]

Whether you are a visual, auditory, or kinesthetic learner, you'll find plenty of activities that will help you absorb new information in ways that fit your learning style.

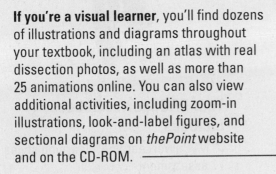

If you're a visual learner, you'll find dozens of illustrations and diagrams throughout your textbook, including an atlas with real dissection photos, as well as more than 25 animations online. You can also view additional activities, including zoom-in illustrations, look-and-label figures, and sectional diagrams on *thePoint* website and on the CD-ROM.

If you're a kinesthetic learner, you get more out of learning activities that let you work with your hands. As you go through your textbook, take notes and actively trace diagrams to take advantage of your touch-learning abilities. You'll also benefit from anatomy puzzles, exercises, and self-quizzes on *thePoint* website and the CD-ROM, as well as writing exercises and a look-and-label coloring atlas in the Study Guide.

If you're an auditory learner, you may find it helpful to read aloud from your textbook. You'll benefit from in-class lectures and discussions about the material with your fellow students. In addition, you'll find audio flash cards, word anatomy exercises, and other resources on *thePoint* website and on the CD-ROM.

Knowing how you learn best will help you succeed in this course, throughout your professional training, and in your chosen career.

Start using your PASSport to Success now to ace anatomy and physiology:

1. Scratch off the personal access code inside the front cover of your textbook.

2. Use your code to log onto http://thePoint.lww.com/MemmlerHumanBody11e.

3. Click on "Student Resources" and then "PASSport to Success."

4. Click on "MyPowerLearning" to take the learning styles assessment.

5. Print and read your personal learning styles report.

6. Look for the PASSport to Success symbol throughout your textbook, which alerts you to resources and activities on *thePoint* website and on the CD-ROM.

7. Search and sort PASSport to Success activities by learning style to choose the most effective way for you to learn the material.

Learn more efficiently and more effectively, ace the exam and pass the course!

Your PASSport to Success includes:

✓ MyPowerLearning™ learning styles assessment
✓ Printable learning style report
✓ LiveAdvise one-to-one online student tutoring
✓ Chapter pre-quizzes
✓ More than 25 animations
✓ 11 different types of learning activities on *thePoint* website and your CD-ROM:
   • Multiple Choice
   • True or False?
   • Key Terms Categories
   • Fill-in-the-Blank
   • Look & Label
   • Audio Flash Cards
   • Word Anatomy
   • Piece It Together
   • Zooming In
   • Listen & Label
   • Body Building
✓ Audio glossary
✓ Supplementary images and tables
✓ Study and test-taking tips
✓ Career information boxes
✓ Answers to the textbook's Questions for Study and Review

Reviewers

We gratefully acknowledge the generous contributions of the reviewers whose names appear in the list that follows.

Kelsey Abrams
Student
Heritage High School
Littleton, Colorado

Diana Alagna
Instructor
Branford Hall Career Institute
Southington, Connecticut

Martin Alenduff
Instructor
Ivy Technical Community College
Columbus, Indiana

Christine Alger
Professor
SUNY at Stony Brook
Stony Brook, New York

Fara Amsalem
Instructor
International College
Naples, Florida

Darryl Anderson, MD
Medical Director
Medical Assisting Program
Plaza College
Jackson Heights, New York

Marty Arnson
Instructor
Gwinnett Area Technical Institute
Lawrenceville, Georgia

Judith Aronow
Instructor
Vermont Technical College
Randolph Center, Vermont

Dr. Joseph H. Balatbat
Vice-President of Academics Affairs
Sanford-Brown Institute
New York, New York

Gail A. Balser RN, BSN, MSN
Practical Nurse Instructor
Travias Career Center
Lakeland, Florida

Kristen Blake-Bruzzini, PhD
Assistant Professor of Biology
College of Arts and Sciences
Maryville University
St. Louis, Missouri

Lynn Bolin
Instructor
Ohio Institute of Health Careers
Columbus, Ohio

Jackie Brittingham
Professor
Simpson College
Indianola, Iowa

Brendalyn Browner, RN, MSN
Assistant Department Chair, Nursing
Associate Professor
Georgia Perimeter College
Dunwoody, Georgia

Sheila Burcham
Instructor
Northwest Mississippi Community College
Senatobia, Mississippi

Naomi E. W. Carroll, PhD, RN
Professor, Health Information Technology
Austin Community College
Austin, Texas

Marianne Ciotti
Instructor
Lehigh Carbon Community College
Schnecksville, Pennsylvania

Sharon A. Coffey
Instructor
Huston Community College
Huston, Texas

W. Wade Cooper
Instructor
Shelton State Community College
Tuscaloosa, Alabama

Janie Corbitt, MLS, RN
Instructor, Allied Health Core
Central Georgia Technical College
Milledgeville, Georgia

Sarah Crum
Student
Lansdale School of Business
North Wales, Pennsylvania

Rachel J. Diehl, NR-CMA
Associate in Specialized Business Degree
Allied Health, Medical Assistant
Lansdale School of Business
North Wales, Pennsylvania

Georgiann Dudek
Instructor
Erie 2-Chautauqua-Cattaraugus BOCES
Angola, New York

Jason Egginton
Instructor
Sister Rosalind Schools and Clinics of
    Massage
St. Paul, Minnesota

Peter Embriano
Instructor
Fox Institute
West Hartford, Connecticut

Paul Enns, RN, BScN
Instructor
Assiniboine Community College
Brandon, Manitoba, Canada

Pamela A. Eugene, BAS, LRT, (R)
Associate Professor Health Sciences
Allied Health Division
Delgado Community College
New Orleans, Lousiana

Y. Everett
Student
Orlando Tech
Orlando, Florida

Janice H. Fortenberry, BS, MCS
Instructor of Human Anatomy and
    Physiology I and II
Science Division
Copiah-Lincoln Community College
Wesson, Mississippi

Rita Fulton, MS, MEd
Professor of Biology
Health Department
Belmont Technical College
St. Clairsville, Ohio

Carmen Gallien
Instructor
Louisiana Technical College
Louisiana

Mary Sue Gamroth
Instructor
Georgian College
Barrie, Ontario, Canada

David Gantt
Instructor
Georgia Campus - Philadelphia College
   of Osteopathic Medicine
Suwanne, Georgia

Rosalind Giles-Pereira, RN, BSN
Instructor
School of Health and Human Services
Camosun College
Victoria, British Columbia, Canada

Candace Gioia
Instructor
Pinellas Technical Education Center
Clearwater, Florida

Meredyth Given
Instructor
Pearl River Community College
Poplarville, Mississippi

Sabina Grigoryan
Student Practical Nurse
Nova Scotia Community College
Halifax, Nova Scotia, Canada

Michael J. Harman MS
Professor of Biology
Lone Star College - North Harris
Houston, Texas

William Havins
Instructor
Albuquerque Technical Vocational
   Institue
Albuquerque, New Mexico

Ann Henninger, PhD
Professor of Biology
Wartburg College
Waverly, Iowa

Liz Hoffman, MA Ed, CMA, (AAMA)
   CPT, (ASPT)
Associate Dean of Health Science
Baker College of Clinton Township
Clinton Township, Michigan

Kathleen Holbrook, CMT
Director/Instructor
Andrews & Holbrook Training Corp.
Latham, New York

Ladeen Hubbell
Instructor
Pearl River Community College
Poplarville, Mississippi

Atanas Ignatov, PhD
Associate Professor
Logan College of Chiropractic
Chesterfield, Missouri

Shakila Jalili
Practical Nursing student year 1
Akerley Campus, Nova Scotia
   Community College
Dartmouth, Nova Scotia, Canada

Linda M. Johnson, RN, MSN, MS
Nursing Instructor
City College of San Francisco
San Francisco, California

Ethel M. Jones, RN, EdS, DSN
Nursing Educator
H. Councill Trenholm State Technical
   College
Montgomery, Alabama

Jackie Jones
Instructor
Delgado Community College - City Park
New Orleans, Louisiana

Marie Kelley
Professor
Our Lady of the Lake College
Baton Rogue, Louisiana

Beverly Kirk
Instructor
Northeast Mississippi Community College
Booneville, Mississippi

Tom Kober
Instructor
Cincinnati State Technical and Community
   College
Cincinnati, Ohio

Megan Kowalski
Instructor
Northwest Business College - Chicago
Chicago, Illinois

Matthew A. Kreitzer, PhD
Associate Professor of Biology
Division of Natural Science and
   Mathematics
Indiana Wesleyan University
Marion, Indiana

Laura Latoza
Student
Orlando Tech
Orlando, Florida

Celinda Kay Leach
Division Chair for the School of Health
   Sciences
Ivy Tech Community College
Bloomington, Indiana

John J. Lepri, PhD
Associate Professor of Biology
The University of North Carolina at
   Greensboro
Greensboro, North Carolina

Connie Lieseke, CMA (AAMA), PBT,
   MLT(ASCP)
Medical Assisting Program Coordinator
Olympic College
Bremerton, Washington

Heather Longaphy
Student
Akerley Campus, Nova Scotia
   Community College
Dartmouth, Nova Scotia, Canada

Samuel T. Lopez, DPT
Associate Professor of Exercise Science
University of Nebraska at Kearney
Kearney, Nebraska

Charlene Mac Donnell
Student
Nova Scotia Community College
Dartmouth, Nova Scotia, Canada

Claire Maday-Travis
Instructor
The Salter School
Worcester, Massachusetts

Christel Marschall
Professor
Science Department
Lansing Community College
Lansing, Michigan

Wilsetta McClain
Department Chair
Coding and Phlebotomy
Baker College
Auburn Hills, Michigan

Katherine McCulloch
Instructor
Lincoln Technical Institute
Mount Laurel/Edison, New Jersey

Leanne McKinzey
Student
Centennial College
Toronto, Ontario, Canada

Nonna Morozova
Instructor
ASA College
Brooklyn/Manhattan, New York

Cora Newcomb, GCHE, ABD, MEd,
   PhD candidate
Professor
Medical Assistant Division
Technical College of the Lowcountry
Beaufort, South Carolina

David Newton
Professor
Dalton State College
Dalton, Georgia

Brian Nichols
Instructor
Lane Community College
Eugene, Oregon

Amy Obringer, PhD
Associate Professor of Biology
University of Saint Francis
Fort Wayne, Indiana

Eva Oltman, MEd, CPC, CMA
Professor/Division Chair of Allied Health
Jefferson Community and Technical College
Louisville, Kentucky

Stephen W. Perry, MS, MAR
Assistant Professor of Biology
Liberty University
Lynchburg, Virginia

Jennifer Pitcher
Student
Centennial College
Toronto, Ontario, Canada

Roberta L. Pohlman, PhD
Associate Professor of Biology
College of Science and Math
Wright State University
Dayton, Ohio

Merle D. Potter, NREMTP
EMS Educator/Flight Paramedic
Wyoming Medical Center/Wyoming Life
    Flight
Casper, Wyoming

Angela Powell
Student
Nova Scotia Community College
Dartmouth, Nova Scotia, Canada

Portia Resnick
Instructor
Somerset School of Massage Therapy
Piscataway, New Jersey

Holly Ressetar, PhD
Medical Course Coordinator
Department of Neurobiology and Anatomy
West Virginia University School of Medicine
Morgantown, West Virginia

Marshall Robb
Professor
William Woods University
Jefferson City/Columbia, Missouri

Kathy Sargent
Instructor
Ivy Tech Community College
Indianapolis, Indiana

Jenny Sarkovski
Student
Centennial College
Toronto, Ontario, Canada

Linda Scarborough, RN, CMA (AAMA),
    CPC, MSHA
Healthcare Management Technology
    Instructor
Lanier Technical College
Oakwood, Georgia

Rebecca Scheid
Instructor
Community College of Spokane
Spokane, Washington

Lorissa A. Sickmiller, BS, LMT,
    NCTMB
Instructor, Anatomy & Physiology
Institute of Therapeutic Massage
Ottawa, Ohio

Anne Simko, RN, BSN, MS
Department Head - LPN Program
Eli Whitney Technical School
Hamden, Connecticut

Alyssa Simonis
Student
Lansdale School of Business
North Wales, Pennsylvania

Richard Sims, MS
Adjunct Instructor of Biology
Jones County Jr. College
Ellisville, Mississippi

Doug Sizemore
Instructor
Bevill State Community College
Jasper, Alabama

Mitzie L. Sowell, PhD
Instructor
Pensacola Junior College
Pensacola, Florida

Amanda Smyth
Student
Lansdale School of Business
North Wales, Pennsylvania

Nita Stika, PhD, ABD
Professor
Concordia University Wisconsin
Mequon, Wisconsin

Kimberly Stone
Instructor
Heritage College
Denver, Colorado

Aleta Sullivan, PhD
Professor of Biology
Science, Mathematics and Business
    Department
Pearl River Community College
Poplarville, Mississippi

Eric L. Sun, PhD
Associate Dean and Professor of Biology
School of Arts and Sciences
Macon State College
Macon, Georgia

Tamara Thell
Instructor
Anoka Technical College
Anoka, Minnesota

Pamela Thinesen, MS
Biology Faculty
Century College
White Bear Lake, Minnesota

Anne Tiemann RN, MS
Associate Professor and Program Chair
Massage Therapy and Medical Assisting
McIntosh College
Dover, New Hampshire

Sandi Tschritter, BA, CPhT
Director, Pharmacy Technician Program
Spokane Community College
Spokane, Washington

Laura Travis
Instructor
Tennessee Technology Center at
    Dickson
Dickson, Tennessee

Judy K. Ward CMA(AAMA), PBT(ASCP),
    EMT-P
Medical Assisting Program Chair
School of Health Sciences
Ivy Tech Community College
Indianapolis, Indiana

Jamey Watson
Instructor
Lanier Technical College
Oakwood, Georgia

Henry C. Wormser, PhD
Professor of Medicinal Chemistry
Wayne State University
Eugene Applebaum College of Pharmacy
    and Health Sciences
Detroit, Michigan

Omyra M Vega, NRCMA
Associates in Allied Health
Lansdale School of Business
North Wales, Pennsylvania

Acknowledgments

It's on this page that I get to thank the many talented people who have helped in the preparation of this 11th edition of *Memmler's The Human Body in Health and Disease*. David Troy, Senior Acquisitions Editor, and Renee Thomas, Managing Editor, at Lippincott Williams and Wilkins, have guided this project with great dedication and skill from start to finish. Jason Taylor reviewed the entire manuscript and gave me much good advice on content and organization. He also wrote the Disease in Context case stories that enliven each chapter and unify the text. Kerry Hull reviewed the manuscript with a great eye for detail and a willingness to discuss any issue with us for as long as needed to reach a decision. Kerry also prepared the Study Guide and the Instructor's Manual with the aid of Molly Ward, Project Manager. Jennifer Clements, as always, advised on the art program and managed the electronic art files, helping to find illustrations when necessary.

My thanks to all the many reviewers, listed separately, who made such valuable and detailed comments on the text. Their insights and advice truly guided every aspect of this new edition.

Once again, thanks to Craig Durant and Dragonfly Media Group for executing any revisions needed to their brilliant drawings.

And as always, thanks to my husband Matthew, currently an instructor in anatomy and physiology, for his advice on and contributions to the text.

Barbara Janson Cohen

Brief Contents

Contents

UNIT I

The Body as a Whole

This unit presents the basic levels of organization within the human body. Included is a description of the smallest units of life, called cells. Similar cells are grouped together as tissues, which are combined to form organs. Organs, in turn, work together in the various body systems, which together satisfy the needs of the entire organism. A short survey of chemistry, which deals with the composition of all matter and is important for the understanding of human physiology, is incorporated into this unit. These chapters prepare the student for the more detailed study of individual body systems in the units that follow.

Organization of the Human Body

Learning Outcomes

After careful study of this chapter, you should be able to:

1. Define the terms *anatomy*, *physiology*, and *pathology*
2. Describe the organization of the body from chemicals to the whole organism
3. List 11 body systems and give the general function of each
4. Define *metabolism* and name the two phases of metabolism
5. Briefly explain the role of ATP in the body
6. Differentiate between extracellular and intracellular fluids
7. Define and give examples of homeostasis
8. Compare negative feedback and positive feedback
9. List and define the main directional terms for the body
10. List and define the three planes of division of the body
11. Name the subdivisions of the dorsal and ventral cavities
12. Name and locate the subdivisions of the abdomen
13. Name the basic units of length, weight, and volume in the metric system
14. Define the metric prefixes *kilo-*, *centi-*, *milli-*, and *micro-*
15. Show how word parts are used to build words related to the body's organization (see Word Anatomy at the end of the chapter)

Selected Key Terms

The following terms and other boldface terms in the chapter are defined in the Glossary

anabolism
anatomy
ATP
catabolism
cell
disease
dissect
feedback
gram
homeostasis
liter
metabolism
meter
organ
pathology
physiology
system
tissue

PASSport to Success

Visit *thePoint* or see the Student Resource CD in the back of this book for definitions and pronunciations of key terms as well as a pretest for this chapter.

Disease in Context

► Mike's Case: Emergency Care and Homeostatic Imbalance

"Location—Belle Grove Road. Single MVA. Male. Early 20s. Fire and police on scene," crackled the radio. "Medic 12. Respond channel 2."

"Medic 12 responding. En route to Belle Grove Road," Ed radioed back, while his partner, Samantha, flipped the switch for the lights and siren and hit the accelerator. The ambulance sped forward, weaving its way through traffic toward the car accident. When they arrived at the scene, police officers were directing traffic and a fire crew was at work on the vehicle. Samantha maneuvered the ambulance into position just as the crew breached the door of the crumpled minivan. Samantha and Ed grabbed their trauma bags and approached the wreck.

Ed bent down toward the injured man. "My name is Ed. I'm a paramedic. My partner and I are here to help you. I'm going to take a quick look at you, and then we're going to get you out of here."

Samantha inspected the vehicle. "Looks like the impact sent him up and over the steering wheel. Guessing from the cracked windshield, he may have a head injury. The steering column is bent, so I wouldn't rule out thorax or abdomen either."

"That fits with my initial assessment," replied Ed. "Patient's name is Mike. He's got forehead lacerations and he's disoriented. Chest seems fine, but his abdominal cavity could be a problem. There is significant bruising across the left lumbar and umbilical regions—probably from the steering wheel. When I palpated his upper left quadrant, it caused him considerable pain."

Samantha and Ed carefully immobilized Mike's cervical spine and, with the help of the fire crew, transferred him to a stretcher. Samantha started an IV of saline while Ed performed a detailed physical examination beginning cranially and working caudally. Mike's blood pressure was very low and his heart rate was very high—both signs of a cardiovascular emergency. In addition, he had become unresponsive to Ed's questions.

Ed shared his findings with Samantha while she placed an oxygen mask on Mike's nose and mouth. "He's hypotensive and has tachycardia. With the pain he reported earlier, signs are pointing to intraabdominal hemorrhage. We've got to get him to the trauma center right now."

Ed depends on his understanding of anatomy and physiology to help his patient and communicate with his partner. He suspects that Mike is bleeding internally, and that his heart is working hard to compensate for the drastic decrease in blood pressure. As we will see later, this homeostatic crisis must be reversed, or Mike's body systems will fail.

tudies of the normal structure and functions of the body are the basis for all medical sciences. It is only from understanding the normal that one can analyze what is going wrong in cases of disease. These studies give one an appreciation for the design and balance of the human body and for living organisms in general.

Studies of the Human Body

The scientific term for the study of body structure is **anatomy** (ah-NAT-o-me). The *–tomy* part of this word in Latin means "cutting," because a fundamental way to learn about the human body is to cut it apart, or **dissect** (dis-sekt) it. **Physiology** (fiz-e-OL-o-je) is the term for the study of how the body functions, and is based on a Latin term meaning "nature." Anatomy and physiology are closely related—that is, structure and function are intertwined. The stomach, for example, has a pouch-like shape because it stores food during digestion. The cells in the lining of the stomach are tightly packed to prevent strong digestive juices from harming underlying tissue. Anything that upsets the normal structure or working of the body is considered a **disease** and is studied as the science of **pathology** (pah-THOL-o-je).

Levels of Organization

All living things are organized from very simple levels to more complex levels (Fig. 1-1). Living matter is derived from simple chemicals. These chemicals are formed into the complex substances that make living **cells**—the basic units of all life. Specialized groups of cells form **tissues,** and tissues may function together as **organs.** Organs working together for the same general purpose make up the body **systems.** All of the systems work together to maintain the body as a whole organism.

CHECKPOINT 1-1 ➤ In studying the human body, one may concentrate on its structure or its function. What are these two studies called?

Body Systems

Most studies of the human body are organized according to the individual systems, as listed below, grouped according to their general functions.

- Protection, support, and movement
  - > The **integumentary** (in-teg-u-MEN-tar-e) **system.** The word *integument* (in-TEG-u-ment) means skin. The skin with its associated structures is considered a separate body system. The structures associated with the skin include the hair, the nails, and the sweat and oil glands.

Figure 1-1 **Levels of organization.** The organ shown is the stomach, which is part of the digestive system.

- > The **skeletal system.** The basic framework of the body is a system of 206 bones and the joints between them, collectively known as the **skeleton.**
  - > The **muscular system.** The muscles in this system are attached to the bones and produce movement of the skeleton. These skeletal muscles also give the

body structure, protect organs, and maintain posture. The two other types of muscles are smooth muscle, present in the walls of body organs, such as the stomach and intestine, and cardiac muscle, which makes up the wall of the heart.

- Coordination and control
  - > The **nervous system.** The brain, the spinal cord, and the nerves make up this complex system by which the body is controlled and coordinated. The special sense organs (the eyes, ears, taste buds, and organs of smell), together with the receptors for pain, touch, and other generalized senses, receive stimuli from the outside world. These stimuli are converted into impulses that are transmitted to the brain. The brain directs the body's responses to these outside stimuli and also to stimuli that originate internally. Such higher functions as memory and reasoning also occur in the brain.
  - > The **endocrine** (EN-do-krin) **system.** The scattered organs known as endocrine glands are grouped together because they share a similar function. All produce special substances called hormones, which regulate such body activities as growth, food utilization within the cells, and reproduction. Examples of endocrine glands are the thyroid, pituitary, and adrenal glands.
- Circulation
  - > The **cardiovascular system.** The heart and blood vessels make up the system that pumps blood to all the body tissues, bringing with it nutrients, oxygen, and other needed substances. This system then carries waste materials away from the tissues to points where they can be eliminated.
  - > The **lymphatic system.** Lymphatic vessels assist in circulation by bringing fluids from the tissues back to the blood. Lymphatic organs, such as the tonsils, thymus gland, and spleen, play a role in immunity, protecting against disease. The lymphatic system also aids in the absorption of digested fats through special vessels in the intestine. The fluid that circulates in the lymphatic system is called lymph. The lymphatic and cardiovascular systems together make up the circulatory system.
- Nutrition and fluid balance
  - > The **respiratory system.** This system includes the lungs and the passages leading to and from the lungs. The respiratory system's purpose is to take in air and conduct it to the areas designed for gas exchange. Oxygen passes from the air into the blood and is carried to all tissues by the cardiovascular system. In like manner, carbon dioxide, a gaseous waste product, is taken by the circulation from the tissues back to the lungs to be expelled.
  - > The **digestive system.** This system is composed of all the organs that are involved with taking in nu-

trients (foods), converting them into a form that body cells can use, and absorbing them into the circulation. Organs of the digestive system include the mouth, esophagus, stomach, intestine, liver, and pancreas.

- > The **urinary system.** The chief purpose of the urinary system is to rid the body of waste products and excess water. This system's main components are the kidneys, the ureters, the bladder, and the urethra. (Note that some waste products are also eliminated by the digestive and respiratory systems and by the skin.)
- Production of offspring
  - > The **reproductive system.** This system includes the external sex organs and all related internal structures that are concerned with the production of offspring.

The number of systems may vary in different lists. Some, for example, show the sensory system as separate from the nervous system. Others have a separate entry for the immune system, which protects the body from foreign matter and invading organisms. The immune system is identified by its function rather than its structure and includes elements of both the cardiovascular and lymphatic systems. Bear in mind that even though the systems are studied as separate units, they are interrelated and must cooperate to maintain health.

PASSport to Success
Visit **thePoint** or see the Student Resource CD in the back of this book for a chart summarizing the body systems and their functions.

Metabolism and Its Regulation

All the life-sustaining reactions that occur within the body systems together make up **metabolism** (meh-TAB-o-lizm). Metabolism can be divided into two types of activities:

- In **catabolism** (kah-TAB-o-lizm), complex substances are broken down into simpler compounds (Fig. 1-2). The breakdown of food yields simple chemical building blocks and energy to power cellular activities.
- In **anabolism** (ah-NAB-o-lizm), simple compounds are used to manufacture materials needed for growth, function, and repair of tissues. Anabolism is the building phase of metabolism.

The energy obtained from the breakdown of nutrients is used to form a compound often described as the cell's "energy currency." It has the long name of **adenosine triphosphate** (ah-DEN-o-sene tri-FOS-fate), but is commonly abbreviated ATP. Chapter 20 has more information on metabolism and ATP.

Figure 1-2 **Metabolism.** In catabolism substances are broken down into their building blocks. In anabolism simple components are built into more complex substances.

Homeostasis

Normal body function maintains a state of internal balance, an important characteristic of all living things. Such conditions as body temperature, the composition of body fluids, heart rate, respiration rate, and blood pressure must be kept within set limits to maintain health. (See Box 1-1, Homeostatic Imbalance: When Feedback Fails.) This steady state within the organism is called **homeostasis** (home-o-STA-sis), which literally means "staying (stasis) the same (homeo)."

FLUID BALANCE Our bodies are composed of large amounts of fluids. The amount and composition of these fluids must be regulated at all times. One type of fluid bathes the cells, carries nutrient substances to and from the cells, and transports the nutrients into and out of the cells. This type is called **extracellular fluid** because it includes all body fluids outside the cells. Examples of extracellular fluids are blood, lymph, and the fluid between the cells in tissues. A second type of fluid, **intracellular fluid**, is contained within the cells. Extracellular and intracellular fluids account for about 60% of an adult's weight. Body fluids are discussed in more detail in Chapter 21.

FEEDBACK The main method for maintaining homeostasis is **feedback**, a control system based on information returning to a source. We are all accustomed to getting feedback about the results of our actions and using that information to regulate our behavior. Grades on tests and assignments, for example, may inspire us to work harder if they're not so great or "keep up the good work" if they are good.

Most feedback systems keep body conditions within a set normal range by reversing any upward or downward shift. This form of feedback is called **negative feedback**, because actions are reversed. A familiar example of negative feedback is the thermostat in a house (Fig. 1-3). When the house temperature falls, the thermostat triggers the furnace to turn on and increase the temperature; when the house temperature reaches an upper limit, the furnace is shut off. In the body, a center in the brain detects changes in temperature and starts mechanisms for cooling or

Box 1-1   **Clinical Perspectives**

Homeostatic Imbalance: When Feedback Fails

Each body structure contributes in some way to homeostasis, often through feedback mechanisms. The nervous and endocrine systems are particularly important in feedback. The nervous system's electrical signals react quickly to changes in homeostasis, while the endocrine system's chemical signals (hormones) react more slowly but over a longer time. Often both systems work together to maintain homeostasis.

As long as feedback keeps conditions within normal limits, the body remains healthy, but if feedback cannot maintain these conditions, the body enters a state of *homeostatic imbalance*. Moderate imbalance causes illness and disease, while severe imbalance causes death. At some level, all illnesses and diseases can be linked to homeostatic imbalance.

For example, feedback mechanisms closely monitor and maintain normal blood pressure. When blood pressure rises, negative feedback mechanisms lower it to normal limits. If these mechanisms fail, *hypertension* (high blood pressure) de-

velops. Hypertension further damages the cardiovascular system and, if untreated, may lead to death. With mild hypertension, lifestyle changes in diet, exercise, and stress management may lower blood pressure sufficiently, whereas severe hypertension often requires drug therapy. The various types of antihypertensive medication all help negative feedback mechanisms lower blood pressure.

Feedback mechanisms also regulate body temperature. When body temperature falls, negative feedback mechanisms raise it back to normal limits, but if these mechanisms fail and body temperature continues to drop, *hypothermia* develops. Its main effects are uncontrolled shivering, lack of coordination, decreased heart and respiratory rates, and, if left untreated, death. Cardiac surgeons use hypothermia to their advantage during open heart surgery. Cooling the body slows the heart and decreases its blood flow, helping to create a motionless and bloodless surgical field.

Figure 1-3   **Negative feedback.** A home thermostat illustrates how this type of feedback keeps temperature within a set range.

Figure 1-5   **Negative feedback in the endocrine system.** Glucose utilization regulates insulin production by means of negative feedback.

warming if the temperature is above or below the average set point of 37°C (98.6°F) (Fig. 1-4).

As another example, when glucose (a sugar) increases in the blood, the pancreas secretes insulin, which causes body cells to use more glucose. Increased uptake of glucose and the subsequent drop in blood sugar level serve as a signal to the pancreas to reduce insulin secretion (Fig. 1-5). As a result of insulin's action, the secretion of insulin is reversed. This type of self-regulating feedback loop is used in the endocrine system to maintain proper levels of hormones, as described in Chapter 12.

A few activities involve **positive feedback,** in which a given action promotes more of the same. The process of childbirth illustrates positive feedback. As the contractions of labor begin, the muscles of the uterus are stretched. The stretching sends nervous signals to the pituitary gland to release the hormone oxytocin into the blood. This hormone stimulates further contractions of the uterus. As contractions increase in force, the uterine muscles are stretched even more, causing further release of oxytocin. The escalating contractions and hormone release continue until the baby is born. In positive feedback, activity continues until the stimulus is removed or some outside force interrupts the activity. Positive and negative feedback are compared in Figure 1-6.

Visit **thePoint** or see the Student Resource CD in the back of this book to view an animation on feedback.

The Effects of Aging

With age, changes occur gradually in all body systems. Some of these changes, such as wrinkles and gray hair, are obvious. Others, such as decreased kidney function, loss of bone mass, and formation of deposits within blood vessels, are not visible. However, they may make a person more subject to injury and disease. Changes due to aging will be described in chapters on the body systems.

Figure 1-4   **Negative feedback and body temperature.** Body temperature is kept at a set point of 37°C by negative feedback acting on a center in the brain.

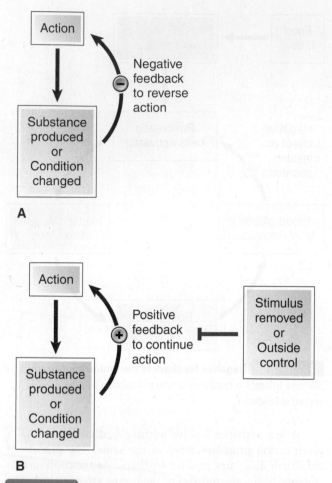

A

B

Figure 1-6 **Comparison of positive and negative feedback.** **(A)** In negative feedback, the result of an action reverses the action. **(B)** In positive feedback, the result of an action stimulates further action. Positive feedback continues until the stimulus is removed or an outside force stops the cycle.

CHECKPOINT **1-2** ➤ Metabolism is divided into a breakdown phase and a building phase. What are these two phases called?

CHECKPOINT **1-3** ➤ What type of system is used primarily to maintain homeostasis?

Directions in the Body

Because it would be awkward and inaccurate to speak of bandaging the "southwest part" of the chest, a number of terms are used universally to designate body positions and directions. For consistency, all descriptions assume that the body is in the **anatomic position.** In this posture, the subject is standing upright with face front, arms at the sides with palms forward, and feet parallel, as shown in Figure 1-7.

Figure 1-7 **Directional terms.** [**ZOOMING IN** ➤ What is the scientific name for the position in which the figures are standing?]

Directional Terms

The main terms for describing directions in the body are as follows (see Fig. 1-7):

- **Superior** is a term meaning above, or in a higher position. Its opposite, **inferior,** means below, or lower. The heart, for example, is superior to the intestine.

- **Ventral** and **anterior** have the same meaning in humans: located toward the belly surface or front of the body. Their corresponding opposites, **dorsal** and **posterior,** refer to locations nearer the back.

- **Cranial** means nearer to the head. **Caudal** means nearer to the sacral region of the spinal column (i.e., where the tail is located in lower animals), or, in humans, in an inferior direction.

- **Medial** means nearer to an imaginary plane that passes through the midline of the body, dividing it into left and right portions. **Lateral**, its opposite, means farther away from the midline, toward the side.

■ **Proximal** means nearer the origin of a structure; **distal**, farther from that point. For example, the part of your thumb where it joins your hand is its proximal region; the tip of the thumb is its distal region.

Planes of Division

To visualize the various internal structures in relation to each other, anatomists can divide the body along three planes, each of which is a cut through the body in a different direction (Fig. 1-8).

■ The **frontal plane**. If the cut were made in line with the ears and then down the middle of the body, you would see an anterior, or ventral (front), section and a posterior, or dorsal (back), section. Another name for this plane is *coronal plane*.

■ The **sagittal** (SAJ-ih-tal) **plane**. If you were to cut the body in two from front to back, separating it into right and left portions, the sections you would see would be sagittal sections. A cut exactly down the midline of the body, separating it into equal right and left halves, is a **midsagittal** section.

■ The **transverse plane**. If the cut were made horizontally, across the other two planes, it would divide the body

into a superior (upper) part and an inferior (lower) part. A transverse plane is also called a *horizontal plane*.

TISSUE SECTIONS Some additional terms are used to describe sections (cuts) of tissues, as used to prepare them for study under the microscope (Fig. 1-9). A cross section (see figure) is a cut made perpendicular to the long axis of an organ, such as a cut made across a banana to give a small round slice. A longitudinal section is made parallel to the long axis, as in cutting a banana from tip to tip to make a slice for a banana split. An oblique section is made at an angle. The type of section used will determine what is seen under the microscope, as shown with a blood vessel in Figure 1-9.

These same terms are used for images taken by techniques such as computed tomography (CT) or magnetic resonance imaging (MRI). (See Box 1-2, Medical Imaging: Seeing Without Making a Cut.) In imaging studies, the term cross-section is used more generally to mean any two-dimensional view of an internal structure obtained by imaging, as shown in Figure 1-10.

CHECKPOINT 1-4 ➤ What are the three planes in which the body can be cut? What kind of a plane divides the body into two equal halves?

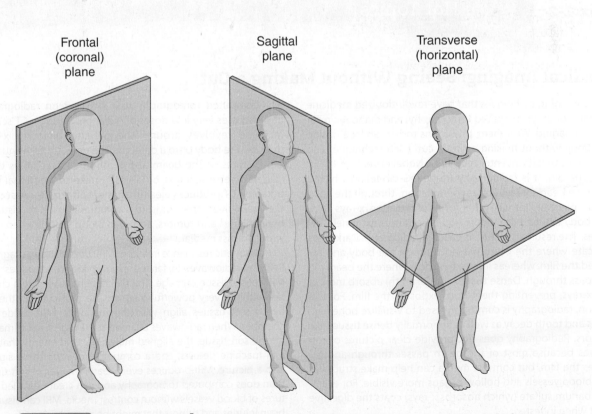

Frontal (coronal) plane

Sagittal plane

Transverse (horizontal) plane

Figure 1-8 **Planes of division.** [**ZOOMING IN** ➤ Which plane divides the body into superior and inferior parts? Which plane divides the body into anterior and posterior parts?]

Cross section   Longitudinal section   Oblique section

Figure 1-9 **Tissue sections.**

Body Cavities

Internally, the body is divided into a few large spaces, or **cavities**, which contain the organs. The two main cavities are the **dorsal cavity** and **ventral cavity** (Fig. 1-11).

Dorsal Cavity

The dorsal body cavity has two subdivisions: the **cranial cavity**, containing the brain, and the **spinal cavity (canal)**, enclosing the spinal cord. These two areas form one continuous space.

Ventral Cavity

The ventral cavity is much larger than the dorsal cavity. It has two main subdivisions, which are separated by the **diaphragm** (DI-ah-fram), a muscle used in breathing. The **thoracic** (tho-RAS-ik) **cavity** is located superior to (above) the diaphragm. Its contents include the heart, the lungs, and the large blood vessels that join the heart. The heart is contained in the pericardial cavity, formed by the pericardial sac; the lungs are in the pleural cavity, formed by the pleurae, the membranes that enclose the lungs (Fig. 1-12). The **mediastinum** (me-de-as-TI-num) is the space between the lungs, including the organs and vessels contained in that space.

Box 1-2   Hot Topics

Medical Imaging: Seeing Without Making a Cut

Three imaging techniques that have revolutionized medicine are radiography, computed tomography, and magnetic resonance imaging. With them, physicians today can "see" inside the body without making a single cut. Each technique is so important that its inventor received a Nobel Prize.

The oldest is radiography (ra-de-OG-rah-fe), in which a machine beams x-rays (a form of radiation) through the body onto a piece of film. Like other forms of radiation, x-rays damage body tissues, but modern equipment uses extremely low doses. The resulting picture is called a radiograph. Dark areas indicate where the beam passed through the body and exposed the film, whereas light areas show where the beam did not pass through. Dense tissues (bone, teeth) absorb most of the x-rays, preventing them from exposing the film. For this reason, radiography is commonly used to visualize bone fractures and tooth decay as well as abnormally dense tissues like tumors. Radiography does not provide clear pictures of soft tissues because most of the beam passes through and exposes the film, but contrast media can help make structures like blood vessels and hollow organs more visible. For example, barium sulfate (which absorbs x-rays) coats the digestive tract when ingested.

Computed tomography (CT) is based on radiography and also uses very low doses of radiation. During a CT scan, a machine revolves around the patient, beaming x-rays through the body onto a detector. The detector takes numerous pictures of the beam and a computer assembles them into transverse sections, or "slices." Unlike conventional radiography, CT produces clear images of soft structures such as the brain, liver, and lungs. It is commonly used to visualize brain injuries and tumors, and even blood vessels when used with contrast media.

Magnetic resonance imaging (MRI) uses a strong magnetic field and radiowaves. So far, there is no evidence to suggest that MRI causes tissue damage. The MRI patient lies inside a chamber within a very powerful magnet. The molecules in the patient's soft tissues align with the magnetic field inside the chamber. When radiowaves beamed at the region to be imaged hit the soft tissue, the aligned molecules emit energy that the MRI machine detects, and a computer converts these signals into a picture. MRI produces even clearer images of soft tissue than does computed tomography and can create detailed pictures of blood vessels without contrast media. MRI can visualize brain injuries and tumors that might be missed using CT.

Right portal vein (to liver)
Diaphragm

Contrast medium in stomach
Main portal vein (to liver)
Inferior vena cava (vein)
Aorta
Spleen
Vertebra of spine
Ribs

A

Left breast
Portal veins (to liver)
Hepatic veins (from liver)

Liver

Stomach
Inferior vena cava (vein)
Spleen
Aorta
Vertebra of spine
Spinal cord

B

Figure 1-10 **Cross-sections in imaging.** Images taken across the body through the liver and spleen by **(A)** computed tomography (CT) and **(B)** magnetic resonance imaging (MRI). (Reprinted with permission from Erkonen WE. *Radiology 101: Basics and Fundamentals of Imaging.* Philadelphia: Lippincott Williams & Wilkins, 1998.)

The **abdominopelvic** (ab-dom-ih-no-PEL-vik) **cavity** (see Fig. 1-11) is located inferior to (below) the diaphragm. This space is further subdivided into two regions. The superior portion, the **abdominal cavity**, contains the stomach, most of the intestine, the liver, the gallbladder, the pancreas, and the spleen. The inferior portion, set off by an imaginary line across the top of the hip bones, is the **pelvic cavity**. This cavity contains the urinary bladder, the rectum, and the internal parts of the reproductive system. See Appendix 7, Dissection Atlas, for a dissection photograph showing organs of the ventral cavity.

CHECKPOINT 1-5 ➤ There are two main body cavities, one posterior and one anterior. Name these two cavities.

REGIONS OF THE ABDOMEN It is helpful to divide the abdomen for examination and reference into nine regions (Fig. 1-13).

The three central regions, from superior to inferior, are:

- the **epigastric** (ep-ih-GAS-trik) **region,** located just inferior to the breastbone
- the **umbilical** (um-BIL-ih-kal) **region** around the umbilicus (um-BIL-ih-kus), commonly called the *navel*
- the **hypogastric** (hi-po-GAS-trik) **region,** the most inferior of all the midline regions

The regions on the right and left, from superior to inferior, are:

- the **hypochondriac** (hi-po-KON-dre-ak) **regions,** just inferior to the ribs
- the **lumbar regions,** which are on a level with the lumbar regions of the spine

CHECKPOINT 1-6 ➤ Name the three central regions and the three left and right lateral regions of the abdomen.

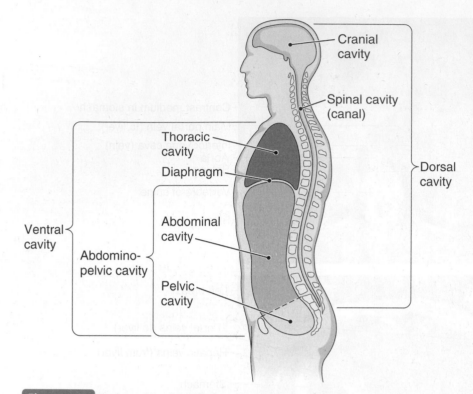

Figure 1-11 **Body cavities, lateral view.** Shown are the dorsal and ventral cavities with their subdivisions. **[ZOOMING IN ➤** What cavity contains the diaphragm? **]**

- the iliac, or **inguinal** (IN-gwih-nal), **regions**, named for the upper crest of the hipbone and the groin region, respectively

A simpler but less precise division into four quadrants is sometimes used. These regions are the right upper quadrant (RUQ), left upper quadrant (LUQ), right lower quadrant (RLQ), and left lower quadrant (LLQ) (Fig. 1-14).

PASSport to Success

Visit *thePoint* or see the Student Resource CD in the back of this book for photographic versions of Figures 1-13 and 1-14, a list of the organs in each quadrant, and figures naming other body regions. Also see the Health Professions box, Health Information Technicians, for description of a profession that uses anatomic, physiologic, and medical terms.

The Metric System

Now that we have set the stage for further study of the body's structure and

function, we should take a look at the metric system, because this system is used for all scientific measurements. The drug industry and the healthcare industry already have converted to the metric system, so anyone who plans a career in healthcare should be acquainted with metrics.

The metric system is like the monetary system in the United States. Both are decimal systems based on multiples of the number 10. One hundred cents equal 1 dollar; 100 centimeters equal 1 meter. Each multiple in the decimal system is indicated by a prefix:

kilo = 1,000
centi = 1/100
milli = 1/1,000
micro = 1/1,000,000

Units of Length

The basic unit of length in the metric system is the **meter** (m). Using the prefixes above, 1 kilometer is equal to 1,000 meters. A centimeter is 1/100 of a meter; stated another way, there are 100 centimeters in 1 meter. The United States has not changed over to the metric system, as was once expected. Often, measurements on packages, bottles, and yard goods are now given according to both scales. In this text, equivalents in the more familiar units of inches and feet are included along with the metric units for comparison. There are 2.5 centimeters (cm) or 25 millimeters (mm) in 1 inch, as shown in Figure 1-15. Some equivalents that may help

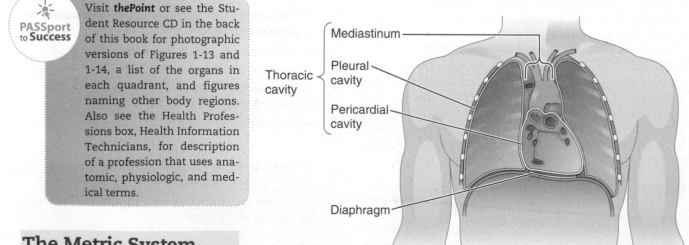

Figure 1-12 **The thoracic cavity.** Shown are the pericardial cavity, which contains the heart, and the pleural cavity, which contains the lungs.

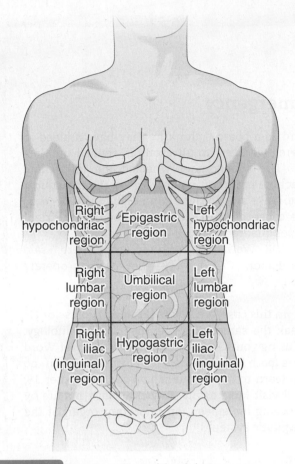

Figure 1-13 The nine regions of the abdomen.

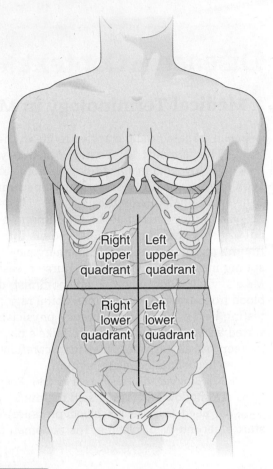

Figure 1-14 **Quadrants of the abdomen.** The organs within each quadrant are shown.

you to appreciate the size of various body parts are as follows:

    1 mm = 0.04 inch, or 1 inch = 25 mm
    1 cm = 0.4 inch, or 1 inch = 2.5 cm
    1 m = 3.3 feet, or 1 foot = 30 cm

Units of Weight

The same prefixes used for linear measurements are used for weights and volumes. The **gram** (g) is the basic unit of weight. Thirty grams are about equal to 1 ounce and 1 kilogram to 2.2 pounds. Drug dosages are usually stated in grams or milligrams. One thousand milligrams equal 1 gram; a 500-milligram (mg) dose would be the equivalent of 0.5 gram (g), and 250 mg is equal to 0.25 g.

Units of Volume

The dosages of liquid medications are given in units of volume. The basic metric measurement for volume is the **liter** (L) (LE-ter). There are 1,000 milliliters (mL) in a liter. A liter is slightly greater than a quart, a liter being equal to 1.06 quarts. For smaller quantities, the milliliter is used most of the time. There are 5 mL in a teaspoon and 15 mL in a tablespoon. A fluid ounce contains 30 mL.

Temperature

The Celsius (centigrade) temperature scale, now in use by most countries and by scientists in this country, is discussed in Chapter 20.

A chart of all the common metric measurements and their equivalents is shown in Appendix 1. A Celsius-Fahrenheit temperature conversion scale appears in Appendix 2.

CHECKPOINT **1-7** ➤ Name the basic units of length, weight, and volume in the metric system.

Figure 1-15 **Comparison of centimeters and inches.**

Disease in Context revisited

➤ Medical Terminology in Mike's Emergency

The dispatch radio crackled to life in the ER. "This is medic 12. We have Mike. 21 years old. Involved in a head-on collision. Patient is on oxygen and an IV of normal saline running wide open. ETA is 15 minutes."

When they arrived at the ER, Samantha and Ed wheeled their unconscious patient into the trauma room. Immediately, the emergency team sprang into action. The trauma nurse measured Mike's vital signs while a phlebotomist drew blood from a vein in Mike's antecubital region for testing in the lab. The emergency physician inserted an endotracheal tube into Mike's pharynx to keep his airway open, and then carefully examined his abdominopelvic cavity.

"BP is 80 over 40. Heart rate is 146. Respirations are shallow and rapid," said the nurse.

"We need to raise his blood pressure—let's start a second IV of plasma. His abdomen is as hard as a board. I think he may have a bleed in there—we need an ultrasound," replied the doctor. The sonographer wheeled the ultrasound machine into position and placed the transducer onto Mike's abdomen. Immediately, she located the cause of Mike's trauma—blood in the right upper quadrant.

"OK. We have a ruptured spleen here," said the doctor. "Call surgery—they need to operate right now."

In this case, we saw that health professionals speak the same language: medical terminology. By using your Glossary and the Glossary of Word Parts (both found at the back of this text), you too can learn to speak this language. In Chapter 16, we'll visit Mike again as doctors save his life by removing his spleen, an important organ of the lymphatic system.

PASSport to Success Interested in some of the health professions featured in this Disease in Context? Visit *thePoint* or see the Student Resource CD in the back of this book for more information on careers in the health professions.

Word Anatomy

Medical terms are built from standardized word parts (prefixes, roots, and suffixes). Learning the meanings of these parts can help you remember words and interpret unfamiliar terms.

WORD PART	MEANING	EXAMPLE
Studies of the Human Body		
-tomy	cutting, incision of	*Anatomy* can be revealed by making incisions in the body.
dis-	apart, away from	To *dissect* is to cut apart.
physi/o	nature, physical	*Physiology* is the study of how the body functions.
path/o	disease	*Pathology* is the study of disease.

WORD PART	MEANING	EXAMPLE
Body Systems		*Catabolism* is the breakdown of complex substances into simpler ones.
cata-	down	
ana-	upward, again, back	*Anabolism* is the building up of simple compounds into more complex substances.
home/o-	same	*Homeostasis* is the steady state (sameness) within an organism.
stat	stand, stoppage, constancy	In *homeostasis*, "-stasis" refers to constancy.

Summary

I. STUDIES OF THE HUMAN BODY
  A. Anatomy—study of structure
  B. Physiology—study of function
  C. Pathology—study of disease
  D. Levels of organization—chemicals, cell, tissue, organ, organ system, whole organism

II. BODY SYSTEMS
  A. Integumentary system—skin and associated structures
  B. Skeletal system—support
  C. Muscular system—movement
  D. Nervous system—reception of stimuli and control of responses
  E. Endocrine system—production of hormones for regulation of growth, metabolism, and reproduction
  F. Cardiovascular system—movement of blood for transport
  G. Lymphatic system—aids in circulation, immunity, and absorption of digested fats
  H. Respiratory system—intake of oxygen and release of carbon dioxide
  I. Digestive system—intake, breakdown, and absorption of nutrients
  J. Urinary system—elimination of waste and water
  K. Reproductive system—production of offspring

III. METABOLISM AND ITS REGULATION
  A. Metabolism—all the chemical reactions needed to sustain life
    1. Catabolism—breakdown of complex substances into simpler substances; release of energy from nutrients
      a. ATP (adenosine triphosphate)—energy compound of cells
    2. Anabolism—building of body materials
  B. Homeostasis—steady state of body conditions
    1. Fluid balance
      a. Extracellular fluid—outside the cells
      b. Intracellular fluid—inside the cells
    2. Feedback—regulation by return of information within a system

      a. Negative feedback—reverses an action
      b. Positive feedback—promotes continued activity
  C. Effects of aging—changes in all systems

IV. DIRECTIONS IN THE BODY
  A. Anatomic position—upright, palms forward, face front, feet parallel
  B. Directional terms
    1. Superior—above or higher; inferior—below or lower
    2. Ventral (anterior)—toward belly or front surface; dorsal (posterior)—nearer to back surface
    3. Cranial—nearer to head; caudal—nearer to sacrum
    4. Medial—toward midline; lateral—toward side
    5. Proximal—nearer to point of origin; distal—farther from point of origin
  C. Planes of division
    1. Body divisions
      a. Sagittal—from front to back, dividing the body into left and right parts
        (1) Midsagittal—exactly down the midline
      b. Frontal (coronal)—from left to right, dividing the body into anterior and posterior parts
      c. Transverse—horizontally, dividing the body into superior and inferior parts
    2. Tissue sections
      a. Cross-section—perpendicular to long axis
      b. Transverse section—parallel to long axis
      c. Oblique section—at an angle

V. BODY CAVITIES
  A. Dorsal cavity—contains cranial and spinal cavities for brain and spinal cord
  B. Ventral cavity
    1. Thoracic—chest cavity
      a. Divided from abdominal cavity by diaphragm
      b. Contains heart and lungs

c. Mediastinum—space between lungs and the organs contained in that space
2. Abdominopelvic
   a. Abdominal—upper region containing stomach, most of intestine, pancreas, liver, spleen, and others
   b. Pelvic—lower region containing reproductive organs, urinary bladder, and rectum
   c. Nine regions of the abdomen
      (1) Central—epigastric, umbilical, hypogastric
      (2) Lateral (right and left)—hypochondriac, lumbar, iliac (inguinal)

d. Quadrants—abdomen divided into four regions
VI. **THE METRIC SYSTEM**—Based on multiples of 10
   A. Prefixes—indicate multiples of 10
      1. Kilo—1,000 times
      2. Centi—1/100th (0.01)
      3. Milli—1/1,000th (0.001)
      4. Micro—1/1,000,000 (0.000001)
   B. Units of length—meter is basic unit
   C. Units of weight—gram is basic unit
   D. Units of volume—liter is basic unit
   E. Temperature—measured in Celsius (centigrade) scale

Questions for Study and Review

BUILDING UNDERSTANDING

Fill in the blanks

1. Tissues may function together as _____.
2. Glands that produce hormones belong to the _____ system.
3. The eyes are located _____ to the nose.
4. Normal body function maintains a state of internal balance called _____.
5. The basic unit of volume in the metric system is the _____.

Matching > Match each numbered item with the most closely related lettered item.

___ 6. One of two systems that control and coordinate other systems
___ 7. The system that brings needed substances to the body tissues
___ 8. The system that converts foods into a form that body cells can use
___ 9. The cavity that contains the liver
___ 10. The cavity that contains the urinary bladder

a. nervous system
b. abdominal cavity
c. cardiovascular system
d. pelvic cavity
e. digestive system

Multiple Choice

___ 11. The study of normal body structure is
   a. homeostasis
   b. anatomy
   c. physiology
   d. pathology

___ 12. Fluids contained within cells are described as
   a. intracellular
   b. ventral
   c. extracellular
   d. dorsal

___ 13. A type of feedback in which a given action promotes more of the same is called
   a. homeostasis
   b. biofeedback
   c. positive feedback
   d. negative feedback

___ 14. The cavity that contains the mediastinum is the
   a. dorsal
   b. ventral
   c. abdominal
   d. pelvic

___ 15. The foot is located _____ to the knee.
   a. superior
   b. inferior
   c. proximal
   d. distal

UNDERSTANDING CONCEPTS

16. Compare and contrast the studies of anatomy and physiology. Would it be wise to study one without the other?

17. List in sequence the levels of organization in the body from simplest to most complex. Give an example for each level.

18. Compare and contrast the anatomy and physiology of the nervous system with that of the endocrine system.

19. What is ATP? What type of metabolic activity releases the energy used to make ATP?

20. Compare and contrast intracellular and extracellular fluids.

21. Explain how an internal state of balance is maintained in the body.

22. List the subdivisions of the dorsal and ventral cavities. Name some organs found in each subdivision.

CONCEPTUAL THINKING

23. The human body is organized from very simple levels to more complex levels. With this in mind, describe why a disease at the chemical level can have an effect on organ system function.

24. In Mike's case, the paramedics and the emergency doctor suspected that Mike's hypotension and tachycardia both resulted from intraabdominal hemorrhage. Using your understanding of negative feedback, discuss why Mike's heart rate increased when his blood pressure decreased.

25. In Mike's case, the paramedics and emergency team injected several liters of saline and blood plasma into

Mike's cardiovascular system. How might the addition of IV fluids stabilize Mike's blood pressure?

26. In Mike's case, the paramedics discovered bruising of the skin over Mike's left lumbar region and umbilical region. Mike also reported considerable pain in his upper left quadrant. Locate these regions on your own body and explain why it is important for health professionals to use medical terminology when describing the human body.

CHAPTER 2

Chemistry, Matter, and Life

Learning Outcomes

After careful study of this chapter, you should be able to:

1. Define an element
2. Describe the structure of an atom
3. Differentiate between molecules and compounds
4. Explain why water is so important to the body
5. Define *mixture*; list the three types of mixtures and give two examples of each
6. Differentiate between ionic and covalent bonds
7. Define an electrolyte
8. Define the terms *acid*, *base*, and *salt*
9. Explain how the numbers on the pH scale relate to acidity and basicity (alkalinity)
10. Define *buffer* and explain why buffers are important in the body
11. Define *radioactivity* and cite several examples of how radioactive substances are used in medicine
12. List three characteristics of organic compounds
13. Name the three main types of organic compounds and the building blocks of each
14. Define *enzyme*; describe how enzymes work
15. Show how word parts are used to build words related to chemistry, matter, and life (see Word Anatomy at the end of the chapter)

PASSport to Success

Visit *thePoint* or see the Student Resource CD in the back of this book for definitions and pronunciations of key terms as well as a pretest for this chapter.

Disease in Context

➤ Margaret's Case: Chemistry's Role in Health Science

"Ugghh," sighed Angela as she pulled into her parking spot. The heat wave was into its second week and she was getting tired of it. It was beginning to take its toll on the city too, especially on its young and old inhabitants. As Angela walked toward the hospital she thought back to yesterday's ICU shift. One particular elderly patient stood out in Angela's mind, probably because she reminded the nurse of her own grandmother.

The patient, Margaret Ringland, a 78-year-old widow, lived alone in her apartment on New York's Upper East Side. Yesterday, her niece, who comes every Monday to drop off some groceries, found Margaret collapsed on the floor, weak and confused. Her niece called 911, and Margaret was rushed to the emergency room. According to her medical chart, Margaret presented with flushed dry skin, a sticky oral cavity, and a furrowed tongue. She was confused and disoriented. She also had hypotension (low blood pressure) and tachycardia (an elevated heart rate). All were classic signs of dehydration, a severe deficiency of water. Without water, a compound composed of two hydrogen atoms covalently bonded to an oxygen atom (H_2O), Margaret's body was unable to perform essential metabolic processes and her tissues and organs were not in homeostatic balance. The central nervous system is particularly sensitive to changes in water volume, which accounted for Margaret's neurologic symptoms.

Although it was difficult to get a blood sample from Margaret's flattened veins, her blood work confirmed the initial diagnosis. Margaret's electrolyte levels were out of balance—especially her blood's sodium ion concentration, which was much too high, a condition called hypernatremia. Margaret's hematocrit was also higher than normal—a sign that the volume of water in her blood was too low. This decrease in blood volume was having serious consequences for her cardiovascular system. Margaret's blood pressure had dropped, which forced her heart to beat faster to ensure proper delivery of blood to her tissues.

The emergency team started an IV line in Margaret's antebrachium. An aqueous solution of 5% dextrose (another name for the carbohydrate monosaccharide called glucose) was delivered through the IV at a rate of 500 mL per hour. A catheter was also inserted into Margaret's urethra to allow for drainage of urine from her urinary bladder. Once stabilized, Margaret was moved to ICU for recovery.

Angela depends on her knowledge of chemistry to make sense of the signs and symptoms she observes in her patients. As you read Chapter 2, keep in mind that a firm understanding of the chemistry presented in this chapter will help you understand the anatomy and physiology of the cells, tissues, and organ systems discussed in subsequent chapters.

reater understanding of living organisms has come to us through **chemistry**, the science that deals with the composition and properties of matter. Knowledge of chemistry and chemical changes helps us understand the normal and abnormal functioning of the body. The digestion of food in the intestinal tract, the production of urine by the kidneys, the regulation of breathing, and all other body activities involve the principles of chemistry. The many drugs used to treat diseases are chemicals. Chemistry is used for the development of drugs and for an understanding of their actions in the body.

To provide some insights into the importance of chemistry in the life sciences, this chapter briefly describes elements, atoms and molecules, compounds, and mixtures, which are fundamental forms of matter.

Elements

Matter is anything that takes up space, that is, the materials from which all of the universe is made. Elements are the substances that make up all matter. The food we eat, the atmosphere, water—everything around us, everything we can see and touch—is made of elements. There are 92 naturally occurring elements. (Twenty additional elements have been created in the laboratory.) Examples of elements include various gases, such as hydrogen, oxygen, and nitrogen; liquids, such as mercury used in barometers and other scientific instruments; and many solids, such as iron, aluminum, gold, silver, and zinc. Graphite (the so-called "lead" in a pencil), coal, charcoal, and diamonds are different forms of the element carbon.

Elements can be identified by their names or their chemical symbols, which are abbreviations of the modern or Latin names of the elements. Each element is also identified by its own number, which is based on the structure of its subunits, or atoms. The periodic table is a chart used by chemists to organize and describe the elements. Appendix 3 shows the periodic table and gives some information about how it is used. Table 2-1 lists some elements found in the human body along with their functions.

Atoms

The subunits of elements are **atoms**. These are the smallest complete units of matter. They cannot be broken down or changed into another form by ordinary chemical and physical means. These subunits are so small that millions of them could fit on the sharpened end of a pencil.

ATOMIC STRUCTURE Despite the fact that the atom is such a tiny particle, it has been carefully studied and has been found to have a definite structure. At the center of the atom is a nucleus, which contains positively charged electrical particles called **protons** (PRO-tonz) and noncharged particles called **neutrons** (NU-tronz). Together, the protons and neutrons contribute nearly all of the atom's weight.

In orbit outside the nucleus are **electrons** (e-LEK-tronz) (Fig. 2-1). These nearly weightless particles are negatively charged. It is the electrons that determine how the atom will react chemically. The protons and electrons of an atom always are equal in number, so that the atom as a whole is electrically neutral.

The **atomic number** of an element is equal to the number of protons that are present in the nucleus of each of its atoms. Because the number of protons is equal to the number of electrons, the atomic number also represents the

Table 2-1	Some Common Chemical Elements*	
Name	Symbol	Function
Oxygen	O	Part of water; needed to metabolize nutrients for energy
Carbon	C	Basis of all organic compounds; in carbon dioxide, the waste gas of metabolism
Hydrogen	H	Part of water; participates in energy metabolism, acid–base balance
Nitrogen	N	Present in all proteins, ATP (the energy compound), and nucleic acids (DNA and RNA)
Calcium	Ca	Builds bones and teeth; needed for muscle contraction, nerve impulse conduction, and blood clotting
Phosphorus	P	Active ingredient in the energy-storing compound ATP; builds bones and teeth; in cell membranes and nucleic acids
Potassium	K	Nerve impulse conduction; muscle contraction; water balance and acid–base balance
Sulfur	S	Part of many proteins
Sodium	Na	Active in water balance, nerve impulse conduction, and muscle contraction
Chlorine	Cl	Active in water balance and acid–base balance; found in stomach acid
Iron	Fe	Part of hemoglobin, the compound that carries oxygen in red blood cells

* The elements are listed in decreasing order by weight in the body.

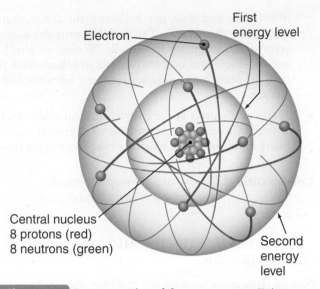

First
energy level

Electron

Central nucleus
8 protons (red)
8 neutrons (green)

Second
energy
level

Figure 2-1 **Representation of the oxygen atom.** Eight protons and eight neutrons are tightly bound in the central nucleus. The eight electrons are in orbit around the nucleus, two at the first energy level and six at the second. **[ZOOMING IN ➤** How does the number of protons in this atom compare with the number of electrons? **]**

number of electrons whirling around the nucleus. Each element has a specific atomic number. No two elements share the same number. In Periodic Table of the Elements (see Appendix 3), the atomic number is located at the top of the box for each element.

The positively charged protons keep the negatively charged electrons in orbit around the nucleus by means of the opposite charges on the particles. Positively (+) charged protons attract negatively (−) charged electrons.

CHECKPOINT 2-1 ➤ What are atoms?

CHECKPOINT 2-2 ➤ What are three types of particles found in atoms?

ENERGY LEVELS An atom's electrons orbit at specific distances from the nucleus in regions called energy levels. The first energy level, the one closest to the nucleus, can hold only two electrons. The second energy level, the next in distance away from the nucleus, can hold eight electrons. More distant energy levels can hold more than eight electrons, but they are stable (nonreactive) when they have eight.

The electrons in the energy level farthest away from the nucleus give the atom its chemical characteristics. If the outermost energy level has more than four electrons but less than its capacity of eight, the atom normally completes this level by gaining electrons. In the process, it becomes negatively charged, because it has more electrons than protons. The oxygen atom illustrated in Figure 2-1 has six electrons in its second, or outermost, level. When oxygen enters into chemical reactions, it gains two electrons, as when it reacts with hydrogen to form water (Fig. 2-2). The oxygen atom then has two more electrons than protons. If the outermost

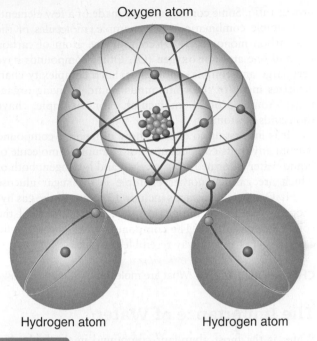

Oxygen atom

Hydrogen atom   Hydrogen atom

Figure 2-2 **Formation of water.** When oxygen reacts, two electrons are needed to complete the outermost energy level, as shown in this reaction with hydrogen to form water. **[ZOOMING IN ➤** How many hydrogen atoms bond with an oxygen atom to form water? **]**

energy level has fewer than four electrons, the atom normally loses those electrons. In so doing, it becomes positively charged, because it now has more protons than electrons.

The number of electrons lost or gained by atoms of an element in chemical reactions is known as the **valence** of that element (from a Latin word that means "strength"). The outermost energy level, which determines the combining properties of the element, is the valence level. Valence is reported as a number with a + or − to indicate whether electrons are lost or gained in chemical reactions. Remember that electrons carry a negative charge, so when an atom gains electrons it becomes negatively charged and when an atom loses electrons it becomes positively charged. For example, the valence of oxygen, which gains two electrons in chemical reactions, is shown as O^{2-}.

Molecules and Compounds

A **molecule** (MOL-eh-kule) is formed when two or more atoms unite on the basis of their electron structures. A molecule can be made of like atoms—the oxygen molecule is made of two identical atoms—but more often a molecule is made of atoms of two or more different elements. For example, a molecule of water (H_2O) contains one atom of oxygen (O) and two atoms of hydrogen (H) (see Fig. 2-2).

Substances composed of two or more different elements are called **compounds.** Molecules are the smallest subunits of a compound. Each molecule of a compound contains the elements that make up that compound in the proper ratio. Some compounds are made of a few elements in a simple combination. For example, molecules of the gas carbon monoxide (CO) contain one atom of carbon (C) and one atom of oxygen (O). Other compounds have very large and complex molecules. Such complexity characterizes many of the compounds found in living organisms. Some protein molecules, for example, have thousands of atoms.

It is interesting to observe how different a compound is from any of its constituents. For example, a molecule of liquid water is formed from oxygen and hydrogen, both of which are gases. Another example is the sugar glucose ($C_6H_{12}O_6$). Its constituents include 12 atoms of the gas hydrogen, 6 atoms of the gas oxygen, and 6 atoms of the solid element carbon. The component gases and the solid carbon do not in any way resemble the glucose.

CHECKPOINT 2-3 ➤ What are molecules?

The Importance of Water

Water is the most abundant compound in the body. No plant or animal, including the human, can live very long without it. Water is of critical importance in all physiological processes in body tissues. A deficiency of water, or dehydration (de-hi-DRA-shun), can be a serious threat to health. Water carries substances to and from the cells and makes possible the essential processes of absorption, exchange, secretion, and excretion. What are some of the properties of water that make it such an ideal medium for living cells?

■ Water can dissolve many different substances in large amounts. For this reason, it is called the **universal solvent**. Many of the body's necessary materials, such as gases, minerals, and nutrients, dissolve in water to be carried from place to place. Substances, such as salts, that mix with or dissolve in water are described as *hydrophilic* ("water-loving"); those, such as fats, that repel and do not dissolve in water are described as *hydrophobic* ("water-fearing").

■ Water is stable as a liquid at ordinary temperatures. Water does not freeze until the temperature drops to 0°C (32°F) and does not boil until the temperature reaches 100°C (212°F). This stability provides a constant environment for living cells. Water can also be used to distribute heat throughout the body and to cool the body by evaporation of sweat from the body surface.

■ Water participates in the body's chemical reactions. It is needed directly in the process of digestion and in many of the metabolic reactions that occur in the cells.

CHECKPOINT 2-4 ➤ What is the most abundant compound in the body?

Mixtures: Solutions and Suspensions

Not all elements or compounds combine chemically when brought together. The air we breathe every day is a mixture of gases, largely nitrogen, oxygen, and carbon dioxide, along with smaller percentages of other substances. The constituents in the air maintain their identity, although the proportions of each may vary. Blood plasma is also a mixture in which the various components maintain their identity. The many valuable compounds in the plasma remain separate entities with their own properties. Such combinations are called **mixtures**—blends of two or more substances (Table 2-2).

A mixture formed when one substance dissolves in another is called a **solution**. One example is salt water. In a solution, the component substances cannot be distinguished from each other and remain evenly distributed throughout; that is, the mixture is homogeneous (ho-mo-JE-ne-us). The dissolving substance, which in the body is water, is the **solvent**. The substance dissolved, salt in the case of salt water, is the **solute**. An **aqueous** (A-kwe-us) **solution** is one in which water is the solvent. Aqueous solutions of glucose, salts, or both of these together are used for intravenous fluid treatments.

In some mixtures, the substance distributed in the background material is not dissolved and will settle out unless the mixture is constantly shaken. This type of nonuniform, or heterogeneous (het-er-o-JE-ne-us), mixture is

Table 2-2	Mixtures	
Type	**Definition**	**Example**
Solution	Homogeneous mixture formed when one substance (solute) dissolves in another (solvent)	Table salt (NaCl) dissolved in water; table sugar (sucrose) dissolved in water
Suspension	Heterogeneous mixture in which one substance is dispersed in another but will settle out unless constantly mixed	Red blood cells in blood plasma; milk of magnesia
Colloid	Heterogeneous mixture in which the suspended material remains evenly distributed based on the small size and opposing charges of the particles	Blood plasma; cytosol

called a **suspension**. The particles in a suspension are separate from the material in which they are dispersed, and they settle out because they are large and heavy. Examples of suspensions are milk of magnesia, finger paints, and, in the body, red blood cells suspended in blood plasma.

One other type of mixture is important in body function. Some organic compounds form **colloids**, in which the molecules do not dissolve yet remain evenly distributed in the suspending material. The particles have electrical charges that repel each other, and the molecules are small enough to stay in suspension. The fluid that fills the cells (cytosol) is a colloidal suspension, as is blood plasma.

Many mixtures are complex, with properties of solutions, suspensions, and colloidal suspensions. Blood plasma has dissolved compounds, making it a solution. The red blood cells and other formed elements give blood the property of a suspension. The proteins in the plasma give it the property of a colloidal suspension. Chocolate milk also has all three properties.

CHECKPOINT 2-5 ➤ Both solutions and suspensions are types of mixtures. What is the difference between them?

Chemical Bonds

When discussing the structure of the atom, we mentioned the positively charged (+) protons that are located in the nucleus and the equal number of orbiting negatively charged (−) electrons that neutralize the protons (Fig. 2-3A). Atoms interact, however, to reach a stable number of electrons in the outermost energy level. These chemical interactions alter the neutrality of the atoms and also form a bond between them. In chemical reactions, electrons may be transferred from one atom to another or may be shared between atoms.

Ionic Bonds

When electrons are transferred from one atom to another, the type of bond formed is called an **ionic** (i-ON-ik) **bond**. The sodium atom, for example, tends to lose the single electron in its outermost shell (Fig. 2-3B), leaving an outermost shell with a stable number of electrons (8). Removal of a single electron from the sodium atom leaves one more proton than electrons, and the atom then has a single net positive charge. The sodium atom in this form is symbolized as Na^+. An atom or group of atoms with a positive or negative charge is called an **ion** (I-on). Any ion that is positively charged is a **cation** (CAT-i-on).

Alternately, atoms can gain electrons so that there are more electrons than protons. Chlorine, which has seven electrons in its outermost energy level, tends to gain one electron to fill the level to its capacity. Such an atom of chlorine is negatively charged (Cl^-) (see Fig. 2-3B). (Chemists refer to this charged form of chlorine as *chloride*.) Any negatively charged ion is an **anion** (AN-i-on).

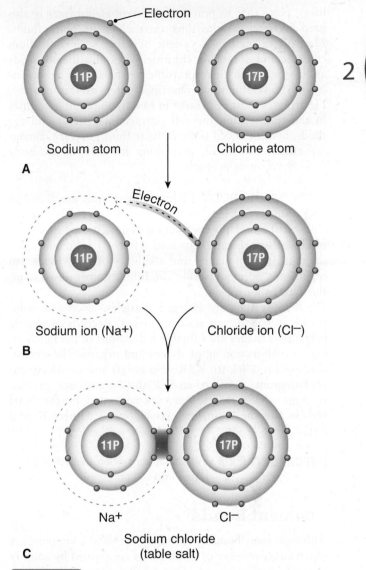

Figure 2-3 **Ionic bonding. (A)** A sodium atom has 11 protons and 11 electrons. A chlorine atom has 17 protons and 17 electrons. **(B)** A sodium atom gives up one electron to a chlorine atom in forming an ionic bond. The sodium atom now has 11 protons and 10 electrons, resulting in a positive charge of one. The chlorine becomes negatively charged by one, with 17 protons and 18 electrons. **(C)** The sodium ion (Na^+) is attracted to the chloride ion (Cl^-), forming the compound sodium chloride (table salt).

Let us imagine a sodium atom coming in contact with a chlorine atom. The chlorine atom gains an electron from the sodium atom, forming an ionic bond. The two newly formed ions (Na^+ and Cl^-), because of their opposite charges, attract each other to produce the compound sodium chloride, ordinary table salt (Fig. 2-3C).

ELECTROLYTES Ionically bonded substances, when they go into solution, separate into charged particles. Compounds formed by ionic bonds that release ions when they are in solution are called **electrolytes** (e-LEK-trolites). Note that in practice, the term *electrolytes* is also used to refer to the ions themselves in body fluids. Electrolytes include a variety of salts, such as sodium chloride and potassium chloride. They also include acids and bases, which are responsible for the acidity or alkalinity of body fluids, as described later in this chapter. Electrolytes must be present in exactly the right quantities in the fluid within the cell (intracellular fluid) and the fluid outside the cell (extracellular fluid), or very damaging effects will result, preventing the cells in the body from functioning properly.

IONS IN THE BODY Many different ions are found in body fluids. Calcium ions (Ca^{2+}) are necessary for the clotting of blood, the contraction of muscle, and the health of bone tissue. Bicarbonate ions (HCO_3^-) are required for the regulation of acidity and alkalinity of body fluids. An organism's normally stable condition, homeostasis, is influenced by ions.

Because ions are charged particles, electrolyte solutions can conduct an electric current. Records of electric currents in tissues are valuable indications of the functioning or malfunctioning of tissues and organs. The **electrocardiogram** (e-lek-tro-KAR-de-o-gram) and the **electroencephalogram** (e-lek-tro-en-SEF-ah-lo-gram) are graphic tracings of the electric currents generated by the heart muscle and the brain, respectively (see Chapters 10 and 14).

CHECKPOINT 2-6 ➤ What happens when an electrolyte goes into solution?

Covalent Bonds

Although ionic bonds form many chemical compounds, a much larger number of compounds are formed by another type of chemical bond. This bond involves not the exchange of electrons but a sharing of electrons between the atoms in the molecule and is called a **covalent bond**. This name comes from the prefix *co-*, meaning "together," and *valence*, referring to the electrons involved in chemical reactions between atoms. In a covalently bonded molecule, the valence electrons orbit around both of the atoms, making both of them stable. Covalent bonds may involve the sharing of one, two, or three pairs of electrons between atoms.

In some covalently bonded molecules, the electrons are equally shared, as in the case of a hydrogen molecule (H_2) and other molecules composed of identical atoms (Fig. 2-4). Electrons may also be shared equally in some molecules composed of different atoms, methane (CH_4), for example. If electrons are equally shared in forming a molecule, the electrical charges are evenly distributed around the atoms and the bond is described as a *nonpolar covalent bond*. That is, no part of the molecule is more negative or positive than any other part. More commonly, the electrons are held closer to one atom than the other, as in the case of water (H_2O), shown in

Hydrogen molecule (H₂)

Figure 2-4 **A nonpolar covalent bond.** The electrons involved in the bonding of a hydrogen molecule are equally shared between the two atoms of hydrogen. The electrons orbit evenly around the two. **[ZOOMING IN ➤** How many electrons are needed to complete the energy level of each hydrogen atom? **]**

Figure 2-2. In a water molecule, the shared electrons are actually closer to the oxygen at any one time, making that region of the molecule more negative. Such bonds are called *polar covalent bonds*, because one part of the molecule is more negative and one part is more positive at any one time.

Anyone studying biological chemistry (biochemistry) is interested in covalent bonding because carbon, the element that is the basis of organic chemistry, forms covalent bonds with a wide variety of different elements. Thus, the compounds that are characteristic of living things are covalently bonded compounds. For a description of another type of bond, see Box 2-1, Hydrogen Bonds: Strength in Numbers.

CHECKPOINT 2-7 ➤ How is a covalent bond formed?

Compounds: Acids, Bases, and Salts

An **acid** is a chemical substance capable of donating a hydrogen ion (H^+) to another substance. A common example is hydrochloric acid, the acid found in stomach juices:

$$HCl \rightarrow H^+ + Cl^-$$
(hydrochloric acid)   (hydrogen ion)   (chloride ion)

A **base** is a chemical substance, usually containing a hydroxide ion (OH^-), that can accept a hydrogen ion. A base is also called an alkali (AL-kah-li). Sodium hydroxide, which releases hydroxide ion in solution, is an example of a base:

$$NaOH \rightarrow Na^+ + OH^-$$
(sodium hydroxide)   (sodium ion)   (hydroxide ion)

A reaction between an acid and a base produces a **salt**, such as sodium chloride:

$$HCl + NaOH \rightarrow NaCl + H_2O$$

The pH Scale

The greater the concentration of hydrogen ions in a solution, the greater the acidity of that solution. The greater the concentration of hydroxide ion (OH^-), the greater the basicity (alkalinity) of the solution. Based on changes in the

Box 2-1 A Closer Look

Hydrogen Bonds: Strength in Numbers

In contrast to ionic and covalent bonds, which hold atoms together, hydrogen bonds hold molecules together. Hydrogen bonds are much weaker than ionic or covalent bonds—in fact, they are more like "attractions" between molecules. While ionic and covalent bonds rely on electron transfer or sharing, hydrogen bonds form bridges between two molecules. A hydrogen bond forms when a slightly positive hydrogen atom in one molecule is attracted to a slightly negative atom in another molecule. Even though a single hydrogen bond is weak, many hydrogen bonds between two molecules can be strong.

Hydrogen bonds hold water molecules together, with the slightly positive hydrogen atom in one molecule attracted to a slightly negative oxygen atom in another. Many of water's unique properties come from its ability to form hydrogen bonds. For example, hydrogen bonds keep water liquid over a wide range of temperatures, which provides a constant environment for body cells.

Hydrogen bonds form not only between molecules but also within large molecules. Hydrogen bonds between regions of the same molecule cause it to fold and coil into a specific shape, as in the process that creates the precise three-dimensional structure of proteins. Because a protein's structure determines its function in the body, hydrogen bonds are essential to protein activity.

Hydrogen bonds. The bonds shown here are holding water molecules together.

balance of ions in solution, as the concentration of hydrogen ions increases, the concentration of hydroxide ions decreases. Conversely, as the concentration of hydroxide ions increases, the concentration of hydrogen ions decreases.

Acidity and alkalinity are indicated by pH units, which represent the relative concentrations of hydrogen and hydroxide ions in a solution. The pH units are listed on a scale from 0 to 14, with 0 being the most acidic and 14 being the most basic (Fig. 2-5). A pH of 7.0 is neutral. At pH 7.0 the solution has an equal number of hydrogen and hydroxide ions. Pure water has a pH of 7.0. Solutions that measure less than 7.0 are acidic; those that measure above 7.0 are alkaline (basic).

Because the pH scale is based on multiples of 10, each pH unit on the scale represents a 10-fold change in the number of hydrogen and hydroxide ions present. A solution registering 5.0 on the scale has 10 times the number of hydrogen ions as a solution that registers 6.0. The pH 5.0 solution also has one-tenth the number of hydroxide ions as the solution of pH 6.0. A solution registering 9.0 has one-tenth the number of hydrogen ions and 10 times the number of hydroxide ions as one registering 8.0. Thus, the lower the pH reading, the greater is the acidity, and the higher the pH, the greater is the alkalinity.

Blood and other body fluids are close to neutral but are slightly on the alkaline side, with a pH range of 7.35 to 7.45. Urine averages pH 6.0 but may range from 4.6 to 8.0 depending on body conditions and diet. Figure 2-5 shows the pH of some other common substances.

Because body fluids are on the alkaline side of neutral, the body may be in a relatively acidic state even if the pH does not drop below 7.0. For example, if the pH falls below 7.35 but is still greater than 7.0, one is described as being in an acidic state known as *acidosis*. Thus, within this narrow range, physiologic acidity differs from acidity as defined by the pH scale.

An increase in pH to readings greater than 7.45 is termed *alkalosis*. Any shifts in pH to readings above or below the normal range can be dangerous, even fatal.

Buffers

If a person is to remain healthy, a delicate balance must exist within the narrow limits of acidity and alkalinity of body fluids. This balanced chemical state is maintained in large part by **buffers**. Chemicals that serve as buffers form a system that prevents sharp changes in hydrogen ion concentration and thus maintains a relatively constant pH. Buffers are important in maintaining stability in the pH of body fluids. More information about body fluids, pH, and buffers can be found in Chapter 21.

Increasing acidity
H⁺ > OH⁻

Increasing basicity (alkalinity)
OH⁻ > H⁺

Figure 2-5 **The pH scale.** Degree of acidity or alkalinity is shown in pH units. This scale also shows the pH of some common substances. **[ZOOMING IN ➤** What happens to the amount of hydroxide ion (OH⁻) present in a solution when the amount of hydrogen ion (H⁺) increases? **]**

CHECKPOINT 2-8 ➤ The pH scale is used to measure acidity and alkalinity of fluids. What number is neutral on the pH scale? What kind of compound measures lower than this number? Higher?

CHECKPOINT 2-9 ➤ What is a buffer?

Isotopes and Radioactivity

Elements may exist in several forms, each of which is called an **isotope** (I-so-tope). These forms are alike in their numbers of protons and electrons, but differ in their atomic weights because of differing numbers of neutrons in the nucleus. The most common form of oxygen, for example, has eight protons and eight neutrons in the nucleus, giving the atom an atomic weight of 16 atomic mass units (amu). But there are some isotopes of oxygen with only 6 or 7 neutrons in the nucleus and others with 9 to 11 neutrons. The isotopes of oxygen thus range in weight from 14 to 19 amu.

Some isotopes are stable and maintain constant characteristics. Others disintegrate (fall apart) and give off rays of atomic particles. Such isotopes are said to be **radioactive**. Radioactive elements may occur naturally, as is the case with isotopes of the very heavy elements radium and uranium. Others may be produced artificially by placing the atoms of lighter, nonradioactive elements in accelerators that smash their nuclei together.

Use of Radioactive Isotopes

The rays given off by some radioactive elements, also called *radioisotopes*, are used in the treatment of cancer because they have the ability to penetrate and destroy tissues. Radiation therapy is often given by means of machines that are able to release tumor-destroying particles. The sensitivity of the younger, dividing cells in a growing cancer allows selective destruction of these abnormal cells with minimal damage to normal tissues. Modern radiation instruments produce tremendous amounts of energy (in the multimillion electron-volt range) and yet can destroy deep-seated cancers without causing serious skin reactions.

In radiation treatment, a radioactive isotope, such as cobalt 60, is sealed in a stainless steel cylinder and mounted on an arm or crane. Beams of radioactivity are then directed through a porthole to the area to be treated. Implants containing radioactive isotopes in the form of needles, seeds, or tubes also are widely used in the treatment of different types of cancer.

In addition to its therapeutic values, irradiation is extensively used in diagnosis. X-rays penetrate tissues and produce an image of their interior on a photographic plate. Radioactive iodine and other "tracers" taken orally or injected into the bloodstream are used to diagnose abnormalities of certain body organs, such as the thyroid gland (see Box 2-2, Radioactive Tracers: Medicine Goes Nuclear). Rigid precautions must be followed by healthcare personnel to protect themselves and the patient when using radiation in diagnosis or therapy because the rays can destroy both healthy and diseased tissues.

CHECKPOINT 2-10 ➤ Some isotopes are stable; others break down to give off atomic particles. What word is used to describe isotopes that give off radiation?

Chemistry of Living Matter

Of the 92 elements that exist in nature, only 26 have been found in living organisms. Most of these are elements that are light in weight. Not all are present in large quantity. Hydrogen, oxygen, carbon, and nitrogen are the elements that make up about 96% of body weight (Fig. 2-6). Nine additional elements—calcium, sodium, potassium, phosphorus, sulfur, chlorine, magnesium, iron, and iodine—make up most of the remaining 4% of the body's elements. The remaining 13, including zinc, selenium, copper,

Box 2-2   Hot Topics

Radioactive Tracers: Medicine Goes Nuclear

Like radiography, computed tomography (CT), and magnetic resonance imaging (MRI), **nuclear medicine imaging** (NMI) offers a noninvasive way to look inside the body. An excellent diagnostic tool, NMI shows not only structural details but also provides information about body function. NMI can diagnose cancer, stroke, and heart disease earlier than techniques that provide only structural information.

NMI uses **radiotracers**, radioactive substances that specific organs absorb. For example, radioactive iodine is used to image the thyroid gland, which absorbs more iodine than any other organ. After a patient ingests, inhales, or is injected with a radiotracer, a device called a gamma camera detects the radiotracer in the organ under study and produces a picture, which is used in making a diagnosis. Radiotracers are broken down and eliminated through urine or feces, so they leave the body quickly. A patient's exposure to radiation in NMI is usually considerably lower than with x-ray or CT scan.

Three NMI techniques are **positron emission tomography** (PET), **bone scanning**, and the **thallium stress test**. PET is often used to evaluate brain activity by measuring the brain's use of radioactive glucose. PET scans can reveal brain tumors because tumor cells are often more metabolically active than normal cells and thus absorb more radiotracer. Bone scanning detects radiation from a radiotracer absorbed by bone tissue with an abnormally high metabolic rate, such as a bone tumor. The thallium stress test is used to diagnose heart disease. A nuclear medicine technologist injects the patient with radioactive thallium, and a gamma camera images the heart during exercise and then rest. When compared, the two sets of images help to evaluate blood flow to the working, or "stressed," heart.

cobalt, chromium, and others, are present in extremely small (trace) amounts totaling about 0.1% of body weight.

Organic Compounds

The chemical compounds that characterize living things are called **organic compounds**. All of these contain the element **carbon**. Because carbon can combine with a variety of different elements and can even bond to other carbon atoms to form long chains, most organic compounds consist of large, complex molecules. The starch found in potatoes, the fat in tissues, hormones, and many drugs are examples of organic compounds. These large molecules are often formed from simpler molecules called *building blocks*, which bond together in long chains.

The main types of organic compounds are carbohydrates, lipids, and proteins. (Another category, the nucleic acids, which are important in cellular functions, are discussed in Chapter 3.) All of these organic compounds contain carbon, hydrogen, and oxygen as their main ingredients.

Carbohydrates, lipids, and proteins, in addition to minerals and vitamins, must be taken in as part of a normal diet. These compounds are discussed further in Chapters 19 and 20.

CHECKPOINT 2-11 ➤ Where are organic compounds found?

CHECKPOINT 2-12 ➤ What element is the basis of organic chemistry?

CARBOHYDRATES The basic units of carbohydrates are simple sugars, or **monosaccharides** (mon-o-SAK-ah-rides) (Fig. 2-7A). **Glu-cose** (GLU-kose), a simple sugar that circulates in the blood as a nutrient for cells, is an example of a monosaccharide. Two simple sugars may be linked together to form a **disaccharide** (Fig. 2-7B), as represented by sucrose, or table sugar. More complex carbohydrates, or **polysaccharides** (Fig. 2-7C), consist of many simple sugars linked together with multiple side chains. Examples of polysaccharides are starch, which is manufactured in plant cells, and **glycogen** (GLI-ko-jen), a storage form of glucose found in liver cells and skeletal muscle cells. Carbohydrates in the form of sugars and starches are important dietary sources of energy.

Oxygen 65%

Carbon 18.5%

Hydrogen 9.5%
Nitrogen 3%
Other 4%

Figure 2-6 The body's chemical composition by weight.

A Monosaccharide

B Disaccharide

C Polysaccharide

Figure 2-7 **Examples of carbohydrates.** A monosaccharide (**A**) is a simple sugar. A disaccharide (**B**) consists of two simple sugars linked together, whereas a polysaccharide (**C**) consists of many simple sugars linked together in chains. [**ZOOMING IN** ➤ What are the building blocks of disaccharides and polysaccharides?]

LIPIDS Lipids are a class of organic compounds mainly found in the body as **fat**. Fats insulate the body and protect internal organs. In addition, fats are the main form in which energy is stored.

Simple fats are made from a substance called **glycerol** (GLIS-er-ol), commonly known as glycerin, in combination with fatty acids (Fig. 2-8A). One fatty acid is attached to each of the three carbon atoms in glycerol, so simple fats are described as **triglycerides** (tri-GLIS-er-ides). **Phospholipids** (fos-fo-LIP-ids) are complex lipids containing the element phosphorus. Among other functions, phospholipids make up a major part of the membrane around living cells. **Steroids** are lipids that contain rings of carbon atoms. They include **cholesterol** (ko-LES-ter-ol), another component of cell membranes (Fig. 2-8B); the steroid hormones, such as cortisol, produced by the adrenal gland; and the sex hormones, such as testosterone, produced by the testes, and estrogen and progesterone, produced by the ovaries.

PROTEINS All **proteins** (PRO-tenes) contain, in addition to carbon, hydrogen, and oxygen, the element **nitrogen** (NI-tro-jen). They may also contain sulfur or phosphorus. Proteins are the body's structural materials, found in muscle, bone, and connective tissue. They also make up the

pigments that give hair, eyes, and skin their color. It is protein that makes each individual physically distinct from others.

Proteins are composed of building blocks called **amino** (ah-ME-no) **acids** (Fig. 2-9A). Although there are only about 20 different amino acids found in the body, a vast number of proteins can be made by linking them together in different sized molecules and in different combinations.

Each amino acid contains an acid group (COOH) and an amino group (NH_2), the part of the molecule that has the nitrogen. Many amino acids link together to form a polypeptide, which is then arranged into a particular shape. The polypeptide chain is coiled into a helix and may then be pleated or folded back on itself. Several chains also may be folded together (see Fig. 2-9B). The overall shape of a protein is important to its function, as can be seen in the activity of enzymes.

CHECKPOINT **2-13** ➤ What are the three main categories of organic compounds?

ENZYMES Enzymes (EN-zimes) are proteins that are essential for metabolism. They serve as **catalysts** in the hundreds of reactions that take place within cells. Without

Glycerol

A **Triglyceride (a simple fat)**

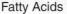

B **Cholesterol (a steroid)**

Figure 2-8 **Lipids. (A)** A triglyceride, a simple fat, contains glycerol combined with three fatty acids. **(B)** Cholesterol is a type of steroid, a lipid that contains rings of carbon atoms. [**ZOOMING IN** ➤ How many carbon atoms are in glycerol?]

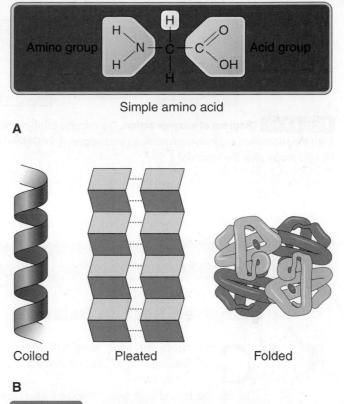

Simple amino acid

A

Coiled   Pleated   Folded

B

Figure 2-9 **Proteins. (A)** Amino acids are the building blocks of proteins. **(B)** Some shapes of proteins. [**ZOOMING IN** ➤ What part of an amino acid contains nitrogen?]

needed in very small amounts. Many of the vitamins and minerals required in the diet are parts of enzymes.

An enzyme's shape is important in its action. Its form must match the shape of the substrate or substrates the enzyme combines with in much the same way as a key fits a lock. This so-called "lock-and-key" mechanism is illustrated in Figure 2-10. Harsh conditions, such as extremes of temperature or pH, can alter an enzyme's shape and stop its action. The alteration of any protein so that it can no longer function is termed **denaturation**. Such an event is always harmful to the cells.

You can usually recognize the names of enzymes because, with few exceptions, they end with the suffix *-ase*. Examples are lipase, protease, and oxidase. The first part of the name usually refers to the substance acted on or the type of reaction in which the enzyme is involved.

CHECKPOINT 2-14 ➤ Enzymes are proteins that act as catalysts. What is a catalyst?

PASSport to Success — Visit ***thePoint*** or see the Student Resource CD in the back of this book to view an animation on enzymes. In addition, the Health Professions box, Pharmacists and Pharmacy Technicians, describes some professions that require knowledge of chemistry.

these catalysts, which increase the speed of chemical reactions, metabolism would not occur at a fast enough rate to sustain life. Because each enzyme works only on a specific substance, or **substrate**, and does only one specific chemical job, many different enzymes are needed. Like all catalysts, enzymes take part in reactions only temporarily; they are not used up or changed by the reaction. Therefore, they are

Figure 2-10 **Diagram of enzyme action.** The enzyme combines with substrate 1 (S_1) and substrate 2 (S_2). Once a new product is formed from the substrates, the enzyme is released unchanged. [**ZOOMING IN >** How does the shape of the enzyme before the reaction compare with its shape after the reaction?]

Disease in Context revisited

➤ Margaret: Back in Balance

"Good morning, Mrs. Ringland. How are you feeling today?" asked Angela.

"Much better, thank you," replied Margaret. "I'm so grateful that my niece found me when she did."

"I'm glad, too," said Angela. "With the heat wave we're having, dehydration can become a very serious problem. Older adults are particularly at risk of dehydration because with age there usually is a decrease in muscle protein, which contains a lot of water, and a relative increase in body fat, which does not. So, older adults don't have as much water reserve as younger adults. But," Angela continued as she flipped through Margaret's chart, "It looks like you are well on your way to a full recovery. Your electrolytes are back in balance. Your blood pressure is back to normal and your heart rate is good too. Your increased urine output tells me that your other organs are recovering as well."

"Does that mean I can get rid of this IV?" asked Margaret.

"Well, I'll check with your doctor first," replied Angela, "But, when you do have the IV removed, you will need to make sure that you drink plenty of fluids."

It was the end of another long shift and Angela was at her locker, changing into a pair of shorts and a T-shirt. As she closed her locker she thought of Margaret once again. It always amazed her that chemistry could have such a huge impact on the body as a whole. She grabbed her water bottle, took a long sip, and headed out into the scorching heat.

In this case, we see that health professionals require a background in chemistry to understand how the body works—when healthy and when not. As you learn more about the human body, consider referring back to this chapter when necessary. For more information about the elements that make up every single molecule within the body, see Appendix 3: Periodic Table of the Elements at the back of this book.

Word Anatomy

Medical terms are built from standardized word parts (prefixes, roots, and suffixes). Learning the meanings of these parts can help you remember words and interpret unfamiliar terms.

WORD PART	MEANING	EXAMPLE
Molecules and Compounds		
hydr/o	water	*Dehydration* is a deficiency of water.
phil	to like	*Hydrophilic* substances "like" water—they mix with or dissolve in it.
-phobia	fear	*Hydrophobic* substances "fear" water—they repel and do not dissolve in it.
hom/o-	same	*Homogeneous* mixtures are the same throughout.
heter/o-	different	*Heterogeneous* solutions are different (not uniform) throughout.
aqu/e	water	In an *aqueous* solution, water is the solvent.
Chemical Bonds		
co-	together	*Covalent* bonds form when atoms share electrons.
Chemistry of Living Matter		
sacchar/o	sugar	A *monosaccharide* consists of one simple sugar.
mon/o-	one	In *monosaccharide*, "mono-" refers to one.
di-	twice, double	A *disaccharide* consists of two simple sugars.
poly-	many	A *polysaccharide* consists of many simple sugars.
glyc/o	sugar, glucose, sweet	*Glycogen* is a storage form of glucose. It breaks down to release (generate) glucose.
tri-	three	*Triglycerides* have one fatty acid attached to each of three carbon atoms.
de-	remove	*Denaturation* of a protein removes its ability to function (changes its nature).
-ase	suffix used in naming enzymes	A *lipase* is an enzyme that acts on lipids.

Summary

I. **ELEMENTS**—Substances from which all matter is made
   A. Atoms—subunits of elements
      1. Atomic structure
         a. Protons—positively charged particles in the nucleus
         b. Neutrons—noncharged particles in the nucleus
         c. Electrons—negatively charged particles in energy levels around the nucleus
      2. Energy levels—orbits that hold electrons at specific distances from the nucleus
         a. Valence—number of electrons lost or gained in chemical reactions

II. **MOLECULES AND COMPOUNDS**
   A. Molecules—combinations of two or more atoms
   B. Compounds—substances composed of different elements
   C. The importance of water—solvent; stable; essential for metabolism
   D. Mixtures: solutions and suspensions
      1. Mixtures—blend of two or more substances
      2. Solution—substance (solute) remains evenly distributed in solvent (e.g., salt in water); homogeneous

3. Suspension—material settles out of mixture on standing (e.g., red cells in blood plasma); heterogeneous

4. Colloid—particles do not dissolve but remain suspended (e.g., cytosol)

III. **CHEMICAL BONDS**

A. Ionic bonds—formed by transfer of electrons from one atom to another

1. Electrolytes
   a. Ionically bonded substances
   b. Separate in solution into charged particles (ions); cation positive and anion negative
   c. Conduct electric current
2. Ions in body fluids important for proper function

B. Covalent bonds—formed by sharing of electrons between atoms

1. Nonpolar—equal sharing of electrons (e.g., hydrogen gas, H_2)
2. Polar—unequal sharing of electrons (e.g., water, H_2O)

IV. **COMPOUNDS: ACIDS, BASES AND SALTS**

A. Acids—donate hydrogen ions

B. Bases—accept hydrogen ions

C. Salts—formed by reaction between acid and base

D. The pH scale

1. Measure of acidity or alkalinity of a solution
2. Scale goes from 0 to 14
   a. 7 is neutral; below 7 is acidic; above 7 is alkaline (basic)

E. Buffer—maintains constant pH of a solution

V. **ISOTOPES AND RADIOACTIVITY**

A. Isotopes—forms of an element that differ in atomic weights (number of neutrons)

1. Radioactive isotope gives off rays of atomic particles

B. Use of radioactive isotopes

2. Cancer therapy
3. Diagnosis—tracers, x-rays

VI. **CHEMISTRY OF LIVING MATTER**

A. Organic compounds—all contain carbon

1. Carbohydrates (e.g., sugars, starches); made of simple sugars (monosaccharides)
2. Lipids (e.g., fats, steroids); fats made of glycerol and fatty acids
3. Proteins (e.g., structural materials, enzymes); made of amino acids
   a. Enzymes—organic catalysts

Questions for Study and Review

BUILDING UNDERSTANDING

Fill in the blanks

1. The basic units of elements are _____.
2. The atomic number is the number of_____ in an atom's nucleus.
3. A mixture of solute dissolved in solvent is called a(n) _____.
4. Blood has a pH of 7.35 to 7.45. Gastric juice has a pH of about 2.0. The more alkaline fluid is _____.
5. Proteins that catalyze metabolic reactions are called _____.

Matching > Match each numbered item with the most closely related lettered item.

___ **6.** A simple carbohydrate such as glucose

___ **7.** A complex carbohydrate such as glycogen

___ **8.** An important component of cell membranes

___ **9.** A hormone such as estrogen

___ **10.** The basic building block of protein

a. polysaccharide

b. phospholipid

c. steroid

d. amino acid

e. monosaccharide

Multiple Choice

___ **11.** Red blood cells "floating" in plasma are an example of a mixture called a
  a. compound
  b. suspension
  c. colloid
  d. solution

___ **12.** The most abundant compound in the body is
  a. carbohydrate
  b. protein
  c. lipid
  d. water

2

___ **13.** A compound that releases ions when it is in solution
is called a(n)

  a. solvent
  b. electrolyte
  c. anion
  d. colloid

___ **14.** A chemical capable of donating hydrogen ions to
other substances is called a(n)

  a. acid
  b. base
  c. salt
  d. catalyst

___ **15.** Organic compounds always contain the element

  a. oxygen
  b. carbon
  c. nitrogen
  d. phosphorus

UNDERSTANDING CONCEPTS

16. Compare and contrast the following terms:

  a. element and atom
  b. molecule and compound
  c. proton, neutron, and electron
  d. anion and cation
  e. ionic bond and covalent bond
  f. acid and base

17. What are some of the properties of water that make it an
ideal medium for living cells?

18. Explain the importance of ions in the structure and function of the human body.

19. What is pH? Discuss the role of buffers in maintaining
pH homeostasis in the body.

20. Compare and contrast carbohydrates and proteins.

21. Describe three different types of lipid.

22. Define the term *enzyme* and discuss the relationship
between enzyme structure and enzyme function.

CONCEPTUAL THINKING

23. Based on your understanding of strong acids and bases,
why does the body have to be kept at a close-to-neutral
pH?

24. Why do we need enzymes, when usually heat is used to
speed up chemical reactions?

25. In Margaret's case, she was hypotensive when she arrived
at the hospital. Explain the link between dehydration and
low blood pressure.

26. In Margaret's case, an aqueous solution of 5% dextrose
was used to rehydrate her. Name the solution's solute
and solvent.

CHAPTER 3

Cells and Their Functions

Learning Outcomes

After careful study of this chapter, you should be able to:

1. List three types of microscopes used to study cells
2. Describe the function and composition of the plasma membrane
3. Describe the cytoplasm of the cell, including the name and function of the main organelles
4. Describe the composition, location, and function of the DNA in the cell
5. Compare the function of three types of RNA in the cells
6. Explain briefly how cells make proteins
7. Name and briefly describe the stages in mitosis
8. Define eight methods by which substances enter and leave cells
9. Explain what will happen if cells are placed in solutions with concentrations the same as or different from those of the cell fluids
10. Define *cancer*
11. List several risk factors for cancer
12. Show how word parts are used to build words related to cells and their functions (see Word Anatomy at the end of the chapter)

Disease
in Context

> ## Jim's Case: Heart Disease from a Cell's Perspective

The buzzer sounded, signaling the end of the third quarter, and the Legal Eagles trailed by 10 points. Jim slammed the basketball down with disgust—he wasn't about to lose to a bunch of accountants. As usual, he'd have to step up his game to make up for the rest of the team.

Jim's attitude on the basketball court reflected his approach off the court. He worked long hours and had little patience for anyone who did not keep up with his grueling pace. By some accounts, Jim was a success—he was a partner in a large downtown law firm, he owned a big house, and he drove a fast car. However, his success came at a heavy cost. Jim's body wasn't keeping up with his lifestyle. He was overweight, out of shape, and had high blood pressure. The extra blood vessels needed to feed Jim's fat cells (called adipocytes) required his heart to pump harder to force blood through them. Since most cardiac muscle cells lack the ability to replicate themselves (a process called mitosis), they responded by synthesizing more contractile proteins. This allowed his cardiac muscle to contract with more force, but also resulted in thickening of the heart walls, which, in the long run, had actually decreased the efficiency of his heart.

Hypertension wasn't the only problem with Jim's cardiovascular system. Cholesterol from Jim's lipid-rich diet formed growths, called plaques, in the walls of many of his blood vessels. In his heart, fatty plaques bulged into the lumens of the coronary arteries, obstructing blood flow to his cardiac muscle cells. Over the years, Jim's coronary arteries compensated for his heart's lack of oxygen and nutrients by growing new vessel branches around the blockages—natural bypasses, made possible by mitosis, which reestablished blood flow to the muscle cells. At the best of times, Jim's heart received just enough oxygen and nutrients to pump adequate amounts of blood to his body's cells. Playing in the basketball game today, Jim had placed an unusually high demand on his heart, and it was having a difficult time keeping up.

The buzzer sounded again, signaling the start of the fourth quarter. With great effort, Jim won the jump ball, and his team began to move toward their opponents' basket. Jim was left behind at center court when he crumpled to the ground, clutching his chest, his cardiovascular system unable to meet the demands of his cardiac muscle. Jim was having a heart attack.

As we will see later, oxygen deficiency caused irreparable damage to Jim's cardiac muscle cells. When reading Chapter 3, keep in mind that events at the cellular level have ramifications for the structure and function of tissues, organs, and even the whole body.

The Role of Cells

The **cell** (sel) is the basic unit of all life. It is the simplest structure that shows all the characteristics of life, including organization, metabolism, responsiveness, homeostasis, growth, and reproduction. In fact, it is possible for a single cell to live independently of other cells. Examples of some free-living cells are microscopic organisms such as protozoa and bacteria, some of which produce disease. In a multicellular organism, cells make up all tissues. All the activities of the human body, which is composed of trillions of cells, result from the activities of individual cells. Cells produce all the materials manufactured within the body. The study of cells is **cytology** (si-TOL-o-je).

Figure 3-1 **Cilia photographed under three different microscopes. (A)** Cilia (hairlike projections) in cells lining the trachea under the highest magnification of a compound light microscope (1,000×). **(B)** Cilia in the bronchial lining viewed with a transmission electron microscope (TEM). Internal components are visible at this much higher magnification. **(C)** Cilia on cells lining an oviduct as seen with a scanning electron microscope (SEM) (7,000×). A three-dimensional view can be seen. (A, Reprinted with permission from Cormack DH. *Essential Histology*, 2nd ed. Philadelphia: Lippincott Williams & Wilkins, 2001; B, Reprinted with permission from Quinton P, Martinez R, eds. *Fluid and Electrolyte Transport in Exocrine Glands in Cystic Fibrosis.* San Francisco: San Francisco Press, 1982; C, Reprinted with permission from Hafez ESE. *Scanning Electron Microscopic Atlas of Mammalian Reproduction.* Tokyo: Igaku Shoin, 1975.) [**ZOOMING IN** ➤ Which microscope shows the most internal structure of the cilia? Which shows the cilia in three dimensions?]

Visit **thePoint** or see the Student Resource CD in the back of this book for information on careers in cytotechnology, the clinical laboratory study of cells.

CHECKPOINT **3-1** ➤ The cell is the basic unit of life. What characteristics of life does it show?

common to most animal cells. Table 3-1 summarizes information about the main cell parts.

CHECKPOINT **3-2** ➤ Name three types of microscopes.

Visit **thePoint** or see the Student Resource CD in the back of this book to view electron microscope pictures of the cell.

Microscopes

The outlines of cells were first seen in dried plant tissue almost 350 years ago. Study of their internal structure, however, depended on improvements in the design of the **microscope**, a magnifying instrument needed to examine structures not visible with the naked eye. The single-lens microscope used in the late 17th century was later replaced by the **compound light microscope** most commonly used in laboratories today. This instrument, which can magnify an object up to 1,000 times, has two lenses and uses visible light for illumination. A much more powerful microscope, the **transmission electron microscope (TEM)**, uses an electron beam in place of visible light and can magnify an image up to 1 million times. Another type of microscope, the **scanning electron microscope (SEM)**, does not magnify as much (100,000×) and shows only surface features, but gives a three-dimensional view of an object. Figure 3-1 shows some cell structures viewed with each of these types of microscopes. The structures are cilia—short, hairlike projections from the cell that move nearby fluids. The metric unit used for microscopic measurements is the **micrometer** (MI-kro-me-ter), formerly called a micron. This unit is 1/1,000 of a millimeter and is symbolized with the Greek letter mu (μ), as μm.

Before scientists can examine cells and tissues under a microscope, they must usually color them with special dyes called **stains** to aid in viewing. These stains produce the variety of colors seen in pictures of cells and tissues taken under a microscope.

Cell Structure

Just as people may look different but still have certain features in common—two eyes, a nose, and a mouth, for example—all cells share certain characteristics. Refer to Figure 3-2 as we describe some of the parts that are

Plasma Membrane

The outer limit of the cell is the **plasma membrane**, formerly called the *cell membrane* (Fig. 3-3). The plasma membrane not only encloses the cell contents but also participates in many cellular activities, such as growth, reproduction, and interactions between cells, and is especially important in regulating what can enter and leave the cell. The main substance of this membrane is a double layer of lipid molecules, described as a bilayer. Because these lipids contain the element phosphorus, they are called **phospholipids**. Some molecules of cholesterol, another type of lipid, are located between the phospholipids. Cholesterol strengthens the membrane.

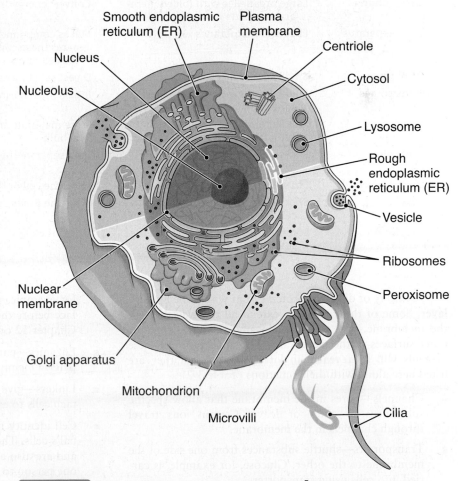

Figure 3-2 **A generalized animal cell, sectional view.** [ZOOMING IN ➤ What is attached to the ER to make it look rough? What is the liquid part of the cytoplasm called?]

Table 3-1	Cell Parts	
Name	**Description**	**Function**
Plasma membrane	Outer layer of the cell; composed mainly of lipids and proteins	Encloses the cell contents; regulates what enters and leaves the cell; participates in many activities, such as growth, reproduction, and interactions between cells
Microvilli	Short extensions of the cell membrane	Absorb materials into the cell
Nucleus	Large, dark-staining organelle near the center of the cell, composed of DNA and proteins	Contains the chromosomes, the hereditary units that direct all cellular activities
Nucleolus	Small body in the nucleus; composed of RNA, DNA, and protein	Makes ribosomes
Cytoplasm	Colloidal suspension that fills the cell from the nuclear membrane to the plasma membrane	Site of many cellular activities; consists of cytosol and organelles
Cytosol	The fluid portion of the cytoplasm	Surrounds the organelles
Endoplasmic reticulum (ER)	Network of membranes within the cytoplasm. Rough ER has ribosomes attached to it; smooth ER does not.	Rough ER sorts proteins and forms them into more complex compounds; smooth ER is involved with lipid synthesis
Ribosomes	Small bodies free in the cytoplasm or attached to the ER; composed of RNA and protein	Manufacture proteins
Mitochondria	Large organelles with folded membranes inside	Convert energy from nutrients into ATP
Golgi apparatus	Layers of membranes	Makes compounds containing proteins; sorts and prepares these compounds for transport to other parts of the cell or out of the cell
Lysosomes	Small sacs of digestive enzymes	Digest substances within the cell
Peroxisomes	Membrane-enclosed organelles containing enzymes	Break down harmful substances
Vesicles	Small membrane-bound sacs in the cytoplasm	Store materials and move materials into or out of the cell in bulk
Centrioles	Rod-shaped bodies (usually two) near the nucleus	Help separate the chromosomes during cell division
Surface projections	Structures that extend from the cell	Move the cell or the fluids around the cell
Cilia	Short, hairlike projections from the cell	Move the fluids around the cell
Flagellum	Long, whiplike extension from the cell	Moves the cell

A variety of different proteins float within the lipid bilayer. Some of these proteins extend all the way through the membrane, and some are located near the inner or outer surfaces of the membrane. The importance of these proteins will be revealed in later chapters, but they are listed here along with their functions (Table 3-2):

- Channels—pores in the membrane that allow specific substances to enter or leave. Certain ions travel through channels in the membrane.

- Transporters—shuttle substances from one side of the membrane to the other. Glucose, for example, is carried into cells using transporters.

- Receptors—points of attachment for materials coming to the cell in the blood or tissue fluid. Some hormones, for example, must attach to receptors on the cell surface before they can act upon the cell, as described in Chapter 12 on the endocrine system.

- Enzymes—participate in reactions occurring at the plasma membrane.

- Linkers—give structure to the membrane and help attach cells to each other.

- Cell identity markers—proteins unique to an individual's cells. These are important in the immune system and are also a factor in transplantation of tissue from one person to another.

Carbohydrates are present in small amounts in the plasma membrane, combined either with proteins (glyco-

Figure 3-3 The plasma membrane. This drawing shows the current concept of its structure. [**ZOOMING IN** ➤ How many layers make up the main substance of the plasma membrane?]

The nucleus is often called the *control center* of the cell because it contains the **chromosomes** (KRO-mo-somes), the threadlike units of heredity that are passed on from parents to their offspring. It is information contained in the chromosomes that governs all cellular activities, as described later in this chapter. Most of the time, the chromosomes are loosely distributed throughout the nucleus, giving that organelle a uniform, dark appearance when stained and examined under a microscope (see Fig. 3-2). When the cell is dividing, however, the chromosomes tighten into their visible threadlike forms.

Within the nucleus is a smaller globule called the **nucleolus** (nu-KLE-o-lus), which means "little nucleus." The job of the nucleolus is to assemble ribosomes, small bodies outside the nucleus that are involved in the manufacture of proteins.

The Cytoplasm

The remaining organelles are part of the **cytoplasm** (SI-to-plazm), the material that fills the cell from the nuclear membrane to the plasma membrane. The liquid part of the cytoplasm is the **cytosol**, a suspension of nutrients, minerals, enzymes, and other specialized materials in water. The main organelles are described here (see Table 3-1).

The **endoplasmic reticulum** (en-do-PLAS-mik re-TIK-u-lum) is a network of membranes located between the nuclear membrane and the plasma membrane. Its name literally means "network" (reticulum) "within the cytoplasm" (endoplasmic), but for ease, it is almost always called simply the **ER**. In some areas, the ER appears to have an even surface and is described as *smooth ER*. This type of ER is involved with the synthesis of lipids. In other areas, the ER has a gritty, uneven surface, causing it to be described as *rough ER*. The texture of rough ER comes from small bodies, called **ribosomes** (RI-bo-somz), attached to its surface. Ribosomes are necessary for the manufacture of proteins, as described later. They may be attached to the ER or be free in the cytoplasm.

proteins) or with lipids (glycolipids). These carbohydrates help cells to recognize each other and to stick together.

In some cells, the plasma membrane is folded out into multiple small projections called microvilli (mi-kro-VIL-li). Microvilli increase the membrane's surface area, allowing for greater absorption of materials from the cell's environment, just as a sponge absorbs water. Microvilli are found on cells that line the small intestine, where they promote absorption of digested foods into the circulation. They are also found on kidney cells, where they reabsorb materials that have been filtered out of the blood.

CHECKPOINT 3-3 ➤ The outer limit of the cell is a complex membrane. What is the main substance of this membrane and what are three types of materials found within the membrane?

The Nucleus

Just as the body has different organs to carry out special functions, the cell contains specialized structures that perform different tasks. These structures are called **organelles,** which means "little organs." The largest of the organelles is the **nucleus** (NU-kle-us).

CHECKPOINT 3-4 ➤ What are cell organelles?

CHECKPOINT 3-5 ➤ Why is the nucleus called the control center of the cell?

PASSport to Success

Visit *thePoint* or see the Student Resource CD in the back of this book to view an animation on the functions of proteins in the plasma membrane.

Table 3-2	Proteins in the Plasma Membrane and Their Functions	
Type of Protein	**Function**	**Illustration**
Channels	Pores in the membrane that allow passage of specific substances, such as ions	
Transporters	Shuttle substances, such as glucose, across the membrane	
Receptors	Allow for attachment of substances, such as hormones, to the membrane	
Enzymes	Participate in reactions at the surface of the membrane	
Linkers	Give structure to the membrane and attach cells to other cells	
Cell identity markers	Proteins unique to a person's cells; important in the immune system and in transplantation of tissue from one person to another	

The **mitochondria** (mi-to-KON-dre-ah) are large organelles that are round or bean-shaped with folded membranes on the inside. Within the mitochondria, the energy from nutrients is converted to energy for the cell in the form of ATP. Mitochondria are the "power plants" of the cell. Active cells, such as muscle cells or sperm cells, need lots of energy and thus have large numbers of mitochondria.

Another organelle in a typical cell is the **Golgi** (GOL-je) **apparatus** (also called Golgi complex), a stack of membranous sacs involved in sorting and modifying proteins and then packaging them for export from the cell.

Several types of organelles appear as small sacs in the cytoplasm. These include **lysosomes** (LI-so-somz), which contain digestive enzymes. Lysosomes remove waste and foreign materials from the cell. They are also involved in destroying old and damaged cells as needed for repair and remodeling of tissue. **Peroxisomes** (per-OK-sih-somz) have enzymes that destroy harmful substances produced in metabolism (see Box 3-1, Lysosomes and Peroxisomes: Cellular Recycling). **Vesicles** (VES-ih-klz) are small, membrane-bound sacs used for storage. They can be used to move materials into or out of the cell, as described later.

Centrioles (SEN-tre-olz) are rod-shaped bodies near the nucleus that function in cell division. They help to organize the cell and divide the cell contents during this process.

Surface Organelles

Some cells have structures projecting from their surface that are used for motion. **Cilia** (SIL-e-ah) are small, hairlike projections that wave, creating movement of the fluids around the cell. For example, cells that line the passageways of the respiratory tract have cilia that move impurities out of the system. Ciliated cells in the female reproductive tract move the egg cell along the oviduct toward the uterus.

A long, whiplike extension from the cell is a **flagellum** (flah-JEL-lum). The only type of cell in the human body that has a flagellum is the male sperm cell. Each human sperm cell has a flagellum that propels it toward the egg in the female reproductive tract.

Cellular Diversity

Although all cells have some fundamental similarities, individual cells may vary widely in size, shape, and composition according to their function. The average cell size is 10 to 15 μm, but cells may range in size from the 7 μm of a red blood cell to the 200 μm or more in the length of a muscle cell.

Cell shape is related to cell function (Fig. 3-4). A neuron (nerve cell) has long fibers that transmit electrical energy from place to place in the nervous system. Cells in surface layers have a modified shape that covers and protects the tissue beneath. Red blood cells are small and round, which lets them slide through tiny blood vessels. They also have a thin outer membrane to allow for passage of gases into and out of the cell. As red blood cells mature, they lose the nucleus and most other organelles, making the greatest possible amount of space available to carry oxygen.

Aside from cilia and flagella, most human cells have all the organelles described above. These may vary in number, however. For example, cells producing lipids have lots of smooth ER. Cells that secrete proteins have lots of ribosomes and a prominent Golgi apparatus. All active cells have lots of mitochondria to manufacture the ATP needed for energy.

CHECKPOINT 3-6 ➤ What are the two types of organelles used for movement, and what do they look like?

Protein Synthesis

Because protein molecules play an indispensable part in the body's structure and function, we need to identify the cellular substances that direct protein production. As noted, the hereditary units that govern the cell are the chromosomes in the nucleus. Each chromosome in turn is divided into multiple subunits, called **genes** (Fig. 3-5). It is the genes that carry the messages for the development of particular inherited characteristics, such as brown eyes,

---

Box 3-1 **Clinical Perspectives**

Lysosomes and Peroxisomes: Cellular Recycling

Two organelles that play a vital role in cellular disposal and recycling are lysosomes and peroxisomes. **Lysosomes** contain enzymes that break down carbohydrates, lipids, proteins, and nucleic acids. These powerful enzymes must be kept within the lysosome because they would digest the cell if they escaped. In a process called **autophagy** (aw-TOF-ah-je), the cell uses lysosomes to safely recycle cellular structures, fusing with and digesting worn out organelles. The digested components then return to the cytoplasm for reuse. Lysosomes also break down foreign material, as when cells known as **phagocytes** (FAG-o-sites) engulf bacteria and then use lysosomes to destroy them. The cell may also use lysosomes to digest itself during **autolysis** (aw-TOL-ih-sis), a normal part of development. Cells that are no longer needed "self-destruct" by releasing lysosomal enzymes into their own cytoplasm.

Peroxisomes are small membranous sacs that resemble lysosomes but contain different kinds of enzymes. They break down toxic substances that may enter the cell, such as drugs and alcohol, but their most important function is to break down free radicals. These substances are byproducts of normal metabolic reactions but can kill the cell if not neutralized by peroxisomes.

Disease may result if either lysosomes or peroxisomes are unable to function. In Tay-Sachs disease, nerve cells' lysosomes lack an enzyme that breaks down certain kinds of lipids. These lipids build up inside the cells, causing malfunction that leads to brain injury, blindness, and death. Disease may also result if lysosomes or peroxisomes function when they should not. Some investigators believe this is the case in autoimmune diseases, in which the body develops an immune response to its own cells. Phagocytes engulf the cells and lysosomes destroy them. In addition, body cells themselves may self-destruct through autolysis. The joint disease rheumatoid arthritis is one such example.

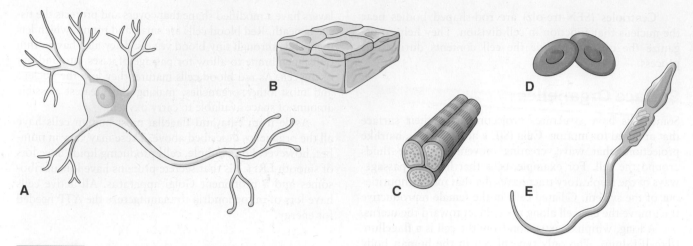

Figure 3-4 **Cellular diversity.** Cells vary in structure according to their functions. **(A)** A neuron has long extensions that pick up and transmit electrical impulses. **(B)** Epithelial cells cover and protect underlying tissue. **(C)** Muscle cells have fibers that produce contraction. **(D)** Red blood cells lose most organelles, which maximizes their oxygen-carrying capacity, and have a small, round shape that lets them slide through blood vessels. **(E)** A sperm cell is small and light and swims with a flagellum. [**ZOOMING IN ➤** Which of the cells shown would best cover a large surface area?]

curly hair, or blood type, and they do so by directing protein manufacture in the cell.

Nucleic Acids: DNA and RNA

Genes are distinct segments of the complex organic chemical that makes up the chromosomes, a substance called **deoxyribonucleic** (de-ok-se-RI-bo-nu-kle-ik) **acid**, or **DNA**. DNA is composed of subunits called **nucleotides** (NU-kle-o-tides) (see Fig. 3-5). A related compound, **ribonucleic**

(RI-bo-nu-kle-ik) **acid**, or **RNA**, which participates in protein synthesis but is not part of the chromosomes, is also composed of nucleotides. There are four different nucleotides in DNA and four in RNA, but only three of these are common to both. Both DNA and RNA have nucleotides containing the components adenine (A), guanine (G), and cytosine (C), but DNA has one nucleotide containing thymine (T), whereas RNA has one containing uracil (U). Table 3-3 compares the structure and function of DNA and RNA.

Figure 3-5 **Subdivisions of a chromosome.** A gene is a distinct region of a chromosome. The entire chromosome is made of DNA. Nucleotides are the building blocks of DNA.

Table 3-3	**Comparison of DNA and RNA**	
	DNA	**RNA**
Location	Almost entirely in the nucleus	Almost entirely in the cytoplasm
Composition	Nucleotides contain adenine (A), guanine (G), cytosine (C), or thymine (T) Sugar: deoxyribose	Nucleotides contain adenine (A), guanine (G), cytosine (C), or uracil (U) Sugar: ribose
Structure	Double-stranded helix formed by nucleotide pairing A-T; G-C	Single strand
Function	Makes up the chromosomes, hereditary units that control all cell activities; divided into genes that carry the nucleotide codes for the manufacture of proteins	Manufacture proteins according to the nucleotide codes carried in the DNA; three types: messenger RNA (mRNA), ribosomal RNA (rRNA), and transfer RNA (tRNA)

Moving one step deeper into the structure of the nucleic acids, each nucleotide is composed of three units:

- A sugar, which in RNA is ribose and in DNA is deoxyribose (that is, a ribose with one less oxygen atom)
- A phosphorus-containing portion, or phosphate
- A nitrogen-containing portion known as a nitrogen base (the A, G, C, T, or U noted above)

The sugar and phosphate alternate to form a long chain to which the nitrogen bases are attached. It is variation in the nitrogen bases that accounts for the differences in the five different nucleotides.

DNA Most of the DNA in the cell is organized into chromosomes within the nucleus (a small amount of DNA is in the mitochondria located in the cytoplasm). Figure 3-6 shows a section of a chromosome and illustrates that the DNA exists as a double strand. Visualizing the complete molecule as a ladder, the sugar and phosphate units of the nucleotides make up the "side rails" of the ladder, and the nitrogen bases project from the side rails to make up the ladder's "steps." The two DNA strands are paired very specifically according to the identity of the nitrogen bases in the nucleotides. The adenine (A) nucleotide always pairs with the thymine (T) nucleotide; the guanine (G) nucleotide always pairs with the cytosine (C) nucleotide. The two strands of DNA are held together by weak bonds (hydrogen bonds; see Box 2-1). The doubled strands then coil into a spiral, giving DNA the descriptive name *double helix*.

The message of the DNA that makes up the individual genes is actually contained in the varying pattern of the four nucleotides along the strand. The nucleotides are like four letters in an alphabet that can be combined in different ways to make a variety of words. The words represent the amino acids used to make proteins, and a long string of words makes up a gene. Each gene thus codes for the building of amino acids into a specific cellular protein. Remember that all enzymes are proteins, and enzymes are

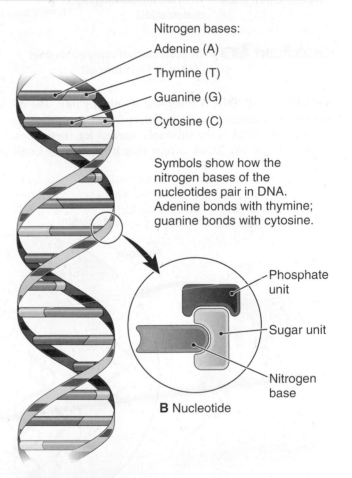

Nitrogen bases:

- Adenine (A)
- Thymine (T)
- Guanine (G)
- Cytosine (C)

Symbols show how the nitrogen bases of the nucleotides pair in DNA. Adenine bonds with thymine; guanine bonds with cytosine.

Phosphate unit

Sugar unit

Nitrogen base

B Nucleotide

A DNA

Figure 3-6 **Structure of DNA. (A)** This schematic representation of a chromosome segment shows the paired nucleic acid strands twisted into a double helix. **(B)** Each structural unit, or nucleotide, consists of a phosphate unit and a sugar unit attached to a nitrogen base. The sugar unit in DNA is deoxyribose. There are four different nucleotides in DNA. Their arrangement "spells out" the genetic instructions that control all activities of the cell. [**ZOOMING IN ➤** Two of the DNA nucleotides (A and G) are larger in size than the other two (T and C). How do the nucleotides pair up with regard to size?]

essential for all cellular reactions. DNA is thus the cell's master blueprint.

In light of observations on cellular diversity, you may wonder how different cells in the body can vary in appearance and function if they all have the same amount and same kind of DNA. The answer to this question is that only portions of the DNA in a given cell are active at any one time. In some cells, regions of the DNA can be switched on and off, under the influence of hormones, for example. However, as cells differentiate during development and become more specialized, regions of the DNA are permanently shut down, leading to the variations in the different cell types. Scientists now realize that the control of DNA action throughout the life of the cell is a very complex matter involving not only the DNA itself but proteins as well.

CHECKPOINT `3-7` ➤ What are the building blocks of nucleic acids?

CHECKPOINT `3-8` ➤ What category of compounds does DNA code for in the cell?

THE ROLE OF RNA A blueprint is only a guide. The information it contains must be interpreted by appropriate actions, and RNA is the substance needed for these steps. RNA is much like DNA except that it exists as a single strand of nucleotides and has the uracil (U) nucleotide instead of the thymine (T) nucleotide. Thus, when RNA pairs up with another molecule of nucleic acid to manufacture proteins, as explained below, adenine (A) bonds with uracil (U) in the RNA instead of thymine (T).

A detailed account of protein synthesis is beyond the scope of this book, but a highly simplified description and illustrations of the process are presented. The process begins with the transfer of information from DNA to RNA in the nucleus, a process known as *transcription* (Fig. 3-7). Before transcription begins, the DNA breaks its weak bonds and uncoils into single strands. Then a matching strand of RNA forms along one of the DNA strands by the process of nucleotide pairing. (For example, if the DNA strand reads CGAT, the corresponding mRNA will read GCUA. (Remember that RNA has U instead of T to bond with A.) When complete, this messenger RNA (mRNA) leaves the nucleus and travels to a ribosome in the cytoplasm (Fig. 3-8). Recall that ribosomes are the site of protein synthesis in the cell.

Ribosomes are composed of an RNA type called ribosomal RNA (rRNA) and also protein. At the ribosomes, the genetic message now contained within mRNA is decoded to build amino acids into the long chains that form proteins, a process termed *translation*. This final step requires a third RNA type, transfer RNA (tRNA), small molecules present in the cytoplasm (see Fig. 3-8).

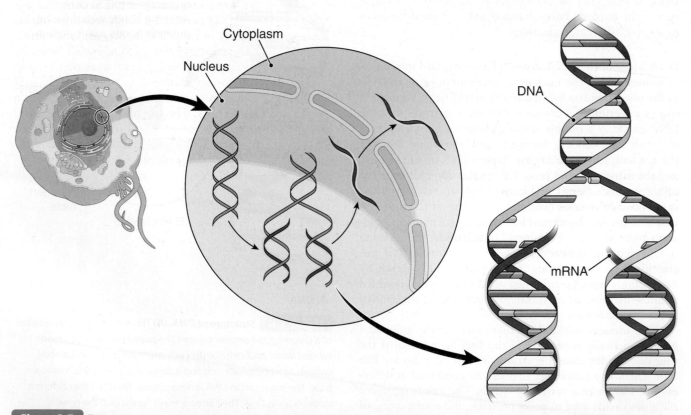

Cytoplasm

Nucleus

DNA

mRNA

Figure 3-7 **Transcription.** In the first step of protein synthesis the DNA code is transcribed into messenger RNA (mRNA) by nucleotide base pairing. An enlarged view of the nucleic acids during transcription shows how mRNA forms according to the nucleotide pattern of the DNA. Note that adenine (A, red) in DNA bonds with uracil (U, brown) in RNA.

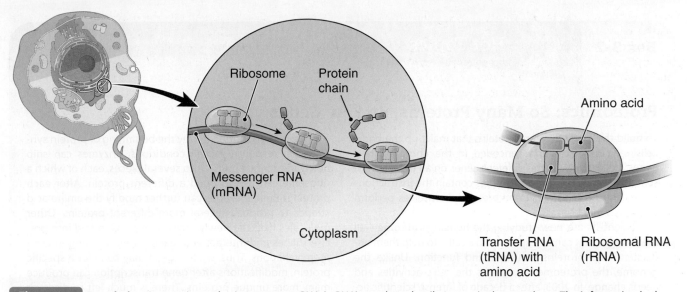

Each transfer RNA carries a specific amino acid that can be added to a protein chain. A nucleotide code on each tRNA determines whether or not its amino acid will be added. After the amino acid chain is formed, it must be coiled and folded into the proper shape for that protein, as noted in Chapter 2. Table 3-4 summarizes information on the different types of RNA. Also see Box 3-2, Proteomics: So Many Proteins, So Few Genes.

CHECKPOINT 3-9 ➤ What three types of RNA are active in protein synthesis?

Cell Division

For growth, repair, and reproduction, cells must multiply to increase their numbers. The cells that form the sex cells (egg and sperm) divide by the process of *meiosis* (mi-O-sis), which cuts the chromosome number in half to prepare for union of the egg and sperm in fertilization. If not for this preliminary reduction, the number of chromosomes in the offspring would constantly double. The process of meiosis is discussed in Chapter 23. All other body cells, known as *somatic cells*, divide by the process of mitosis (mi-TO-sis). In this process, described later, each original parent cell becomes two identical daughter cells.

Before mitosis can occur, the genetic information (DNA) in the parent cell must be replicated (doubled), so that each of the two new daughter cells will receive a complete set of chromosomes. For example, a human cell that divides by mitosis must produce two cells with 46 chromosomes each, the same number of chromosomes that are present in the original parent cell. DNA replicates during **interphase**, the stage in the cell's life between one mitosis and the next. During this phase, DNA uncoils from its double-stranded form, and each strand takes on a matching strand of nucleotides according to the pattern of A-T, G-C pairing. There are now two strands, each identical to the original double helix. The strands are held together at a region called the *centromere* (SEN-tro-mere) until they separate during mitosis. A typical cell lives in interphase for most of its cycle and spends only a relatively short period in mitosis. For example, a cell reproducing every 20

Table 3-4	**RNA**
Types	Function
Messenger RNA (mRNA)	Is built on a strand of DNA in the nucleus and transcribes the nucleotide code; moves to cytoplasm and attaches to a ribosome
Ribosomal RNA (rRNA)	With protein makes up the ribosomes, the sites of protein synthesis in the cytoplasm; involved in the process of translating the genetic message into a protein
Transfer RNA (tRNA)	Works with other forms of RNA to translate the genetic code into protein; each molecule of tRNA carries an amino acid that can be used to build a protein at the ribosome

Box 3-2   Hot Topics

Proteomics: So Many Proteins, So Few Genes

To build the many different proteins that make up the body, cells rely on instructions encoded in the chromosomes' genes. Collectively, all the different genes on all the chromosomes make up the **genome**. Genes contain the instructions for making proteins, while the proteins themselves perform the body's functions.

Scientists are now studying the human **proteome**—all the proteins that can be expressed in a cell—to help them understand the proteins' structure and function. Unlike the genome, the proteome changes as the cell's activities and needs change. In 2003, after a decade of intense scientific activity, investigators mapped the entire human genome and realized that it contained only 35,000 genes, far fewer than initially expected. How could this relatively small number of genes code for several million proteins? They concluded that genes were not the whole story.

Gene transcription is only the beginning of protein synthesis. In response to cell conditions, enzymes can snip newly transcribed mRNA into several pieces, each of which a ribosome can use to build a different protein. After each protein is built, enzymes can further modify the amino acid strands to produce several more different proteins. Other molecules help the newly formed proteins to fold into precise shapes and interact with each other, resulting in even more variations. Thus, while a gene may code for a specific protein, modifications after gene transcription can produce many more unique proteins. There is much left to discover about the proteome, but scientists hope that future research will lead to new techniques for detecting and treating disease.

---

hours spends only about one hour in mitosis and the remaining time in interphase.

CHECKPOINT **3-10** ➤ What must happen to the DNA in a cell before mitosis can occur? During what stage in the life of a cell does this occur?

PASSport to Success   Visit *thePoint* or see the Student Resource CD in the back of this book for a photomicrograph of a replicated chromosome.

Stages of Mitosis

Although mitosis is a continuous process, distinct changes can be seen in the dividing cell at four stages (Fig. 3-9).

- In **prophase** (PRO-faze), the doubled strands of DNA return to their tightly wound spiral organization and become visible under the microscope as dark, threadlike chromosomes. The nucleolus and the nuclear membrane begin to disappear. In the cytoplasm, the two centrioles move toward opposite ends of the cell and a spindle-shaped structure made of thin fibers begins to form between them.

- In **metaphase** (MET-ah-faze), the chromosomes line up across the center (equator) of the cell attached to the spindle fibers.

- In **anaphase** (AN-ah-faze), the centromere splits and the duplicated chromosomes separate and begin to move toward opposite ends of the cell.

- As mitosis continues into **telophase** (TEL-o-faze), a membrane appears around each group of separated chromosomes, forming two new nuclei.

Also during telophase, the plasma membrane pinches off to divide the cell. The midsection between the two areas becomes progressively smaller until, finally, the cell splits in two. There are now two new cells, or daughter cells, each with exactly the same kind and amount of DNA as was present in the parent cell. In just a few types of cells, skeletal muscle cells for example, the cell itself does not divide following nuclear division. The result, after multiple mitoses, is a giant single cell with multiple nuclei. This pattern is extremely rare in human cells.

During mitosis, all the organelles, except those needed for the division process, temporarily disappear. After the cell divides, these organelles reappear in each daughter cell. Also at this time, the centrioles usually replicate in preparation for the next cell division.

Body cells differ in the rate at which they reproduce. Some, such as nerve cells and muscle cells, stop dividing at some point in development and are not replaced if they die. They remain in interphase. Others, such as blood cells, sperm cells, and skin cells, multiply rapidly to replace cells destroyed by injury, disease, or natural wear-and-tear. Cells that multiply slowly may be triggered to divide when tissue is injured, as in repair of a bone fracture.

Immature cells that retain the ability to divide and mature when necessary are known as **stem cells** (see Box 4-1 in Chapter 4). All blood cells, for example, are produced from stem cells in the red bone marrow. Research has been done on stimulating stem cells to divide into various cell

Figure 3-9 **The stages of mitosis.** When it is not dividing, the cell is in interphase. The cell shown is for illustration only. It is not a human cell, which has 46 chromosomes. (Photomicrographs reprinted with permission from Cormack DH. *Essential Histology*, 2nd ed. Philadelphia: Lippincott Williams & Wilkins, 2001.)

[ZOOMING IN ➤ If the original cell shown has 46 chromosomes, how many chromosomes will each new daughter cell have?]

types in the laboratory, but these studies have been controversial. Although it may be possible some day to use such cells to replace cells injured by disease, some people consider these studies unethical.

CHECKPOINT 3-11 ➤ What are the four stages of mitosis?

PASSport to Success — Visit *thePoint* or see the Student Resource CD in the back of this book to view the animation *The Cell Cycle and Mitosis*.

Movement of Substances Across the Plasma Membrane

The plasma membrane serves as a barrier between the cell and its environment. Nevertheless, nutrients, oxygen, and many other substances needed by the cell must be taken in and waste products must be eliminated. Clearly, some substances can be exchanged between the cell and its environment through the plasma membrane. For this reason, the plasma membrane is described at a simple level as **semipermeable** (sem-e-PER-me-ah-bl). It is permeable, or passable, to some molecules but impassable to others. Some particles, proteins for example, are too large to travel through the membrane unaided.

The ability of a substance to travel through the membrane is based on several factors. Molecular size is the main factor that determines passage through the membrane, but solubility and electrical charge are also considerations. Water, a tiny molecule, is usually able to penetrate the membrane with ease. Nutrients, however, must be split into small molecules by digestion so that they can travel through the plasma membrane. For example, digestive enzymes convert sucrose (table sugar) to glucose and fructose, smaller molecules that enter the cell and serve as energy sources.

Various physical processes are involved in exchanges through the plasma membrane. One way of grouping these processes is according to whether they do or do not require cellular energy.

Movement That Does Not Require Cellular Energy

The adjective *passive* describes movement through the plasma membrane that does not require energy output by the cell. Passive mechanisms depend on the internal energy of the moving particles or the application of some outside source of energy. The methods include:

- **Diffusion** is the constant movement of particles from a region of relatively higher concentration to one of lower concentration. Just as couples on a crowded dance floor spread out into all the available space to avoid hitting other dancers, diffusing substances spread throughout their available space until their concentration everywhere is the same—that is, they reach equilibrium (Fig. 3-10). This movement from higher to

Figure 3-10 **Diffusion of a solid in a liquid.** The molecules of the solid tend to spread evenly throughout the liquid as they dissolve.

lower concentrations uses the particles' internal energy and does not require cellular energy, just as a sled will move from the top to the bottom of a snowy hill. The particles are said to follow their *concentration gradient* from higher concentration to lower concentration.

When substances diffuse through a membrane, such as the intact plasma membrane, passage is limited to those particles small enough to pass through spaces between molecules in the membrane, as shown with a large-scale example in Figure 3-11. In the body, soluble materials, such as nutrients, electrolytes, gases, and waste materials, are constantly moving into or out of the cells by diffusion.

■ **Osmosis** (os-MO-sis) is a special type of diffusion. The term applies specifically to the diffusion of water through a semipermeable membrane. The water molecules move, as expected, from an area where there are more of them to an area where there are fewer of them. That is, the solvent (the water molecules) moves from an area of lower *solute* concentration to an area of higher *solute* concentration (Fig. 3-12).

For a physiologist studying water's flow across membranes, as in exchange of fluids through capillaries in the circulation, it is helpful to know the direction in which water will flow and at what rate it will move. A measure of the force driving osmosis is called the *osmotic pressure*. This force can be measured, as illustrated in Figure 3-13, by applying enough pressure to the surface of a liquid to stop the inward flow of water by osmosis. The pressure needed to counteract osmosis is the osmotic pressure. In practice, the term osmotic pressure is used to

describe a solution's tendency to draw water in. This force is directly related to concentration: the higher a solutions' concentration, the greater is its tendency to draw water in.

■ **Filtration** is the passage of water and dissolved materials through a membrane as a result of a mechanical ("pushing") force on one side (Fig. 3-14). One example of filtration in the body is the movement of materials out of the capillaries and into the tissues under the force of blood pressure (see Chapter 15). Another example occurs in the kidneys as materials are filtered out of the blood in the first step of urine formation (see Chapter 22).

■ **Facilitated diffusion** is the movement of materials across the plasma membrane in the direction of the concentration gradient (from higher to lower concentration) but using transporters to move the material at a faster rate (Fig. 3-15). Glucose, the sugar that is the main energy source for cells, moves through the plasma membrane by means of facilitated diffusion.

 PASSport to Success Visit *thePoint* or see the Student Resource CD in the back of this book to view an animation on osmosis and osmotic pressure.

Movement That Requires Cellular Energy

Movement across the membrane that requires energy is describes as *active*. These methods include:

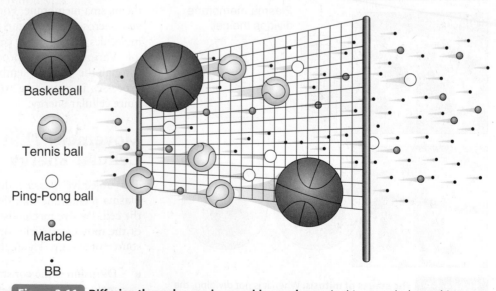

Figure 3-11 **Diffusion through a semipermeable membrane.** In this example, large objects (basketballs, tennis balls) cannot pass through the net, whereas the smaller ones (ping-pong balls, marbles, BBs) can. In the human body, large particles in the blood, such as proteins and blood cells, cannot pass through the walls of the capillaries, whereas small particles, such as nutrients, electrolytes, and gases, can. **[ZOOMING IN ➤** If this picture represented diffusion in the body, what would the net be? **]**

Basketball

Tennis ball

Ping-Pong ball

Marble

BB

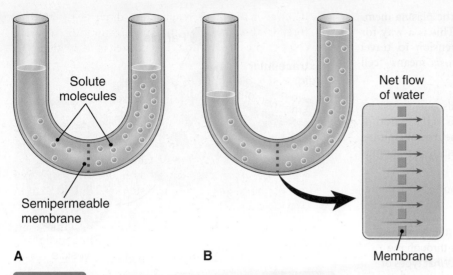

Figure 3-12 **A simple demonstration of osmosis.** Solute molecules are shown in yellow. All of the solvent (blue) is composed of water molecules. **(A)** Two solutions with different concentrations of solute are separated by a semipermeable membrane. Water can flow through the membrane, but the solute cannot. **(B)** Water flows into the more concentrated solution, raising the level of the liquid in that side. **[ZOOMING IN ➤** What would happen in this system if the solute could pass through the membrane? **]**

of a hill requires energy. It also requires proteins in the plasma membrane that act as **transporters** for the particles.

This process of active transport is one important function of the living cellular membrane. The nervous system and muscular system, for example, depend on the active transport of sodium, potassium, and calcium ions for proper function. The kidneys also carry out active transport in regulating the composition of urine. By means of active transport, the cell can take in what it needs from the surrounding fluids and remove materials from the cell. Because the plasma membrane can carry on active transport, the membrane is most accurately described, not as simply semipermeable, but as **selectively permeable.** It regulates what can enter and leave based on the needs of the cell.

There are several active methods for moving large quantities of material into or out of the cell. These methods are grouped together as **bulk transport,** because of the amounts of material moved, or **vesicular transport,** because small sacs, or vesicles, are needed for the processes.

■ **Active transport.** The plasma membrane has the ability to move small solute particles into or out of the cell opposite to the direction in which they would normally flow by diffusion. That is, the membrane moves them against the concentration gradient from an area where they are in relatively lower concentration to an area where they are in higher concentration. Because this movement goes against the natural flow of particles, it requires energy, just as getting a sled to the top

■ **Endocytosis** (en-do-si-TO-sis) is a term that describes the bulk movement of materials into the cell. There are two examples:

> In **phagocytosis** (fag-o-si-TO-sis), relatively large particles are engulfed by the plasma membrane and moved into the cell (Fig. 3-16). Certain white blood cells carry out phagocytosis to rid the body of foreign material and dead cells. Material taken into a cell by phagocytosis is first enclosed in a vesicle made from the plasma membrane and is later destroyed by lysosomes.

PASSport to Success — Visit **thePoint** or see the Student Resource CD in the back of this book for an electron micrograph of pinocytosis.

Figure 3-13 **Osmotic pressure.** Osmotic pressure is the force needed to stop the flow of water by osmosis. Pressure on the surface of the fluid in side B counteracts the osmotic flow of water from side A to side B. **[ZOOMING IN ➤** What would happen to osmotic pressure if the concentration of solute were increased on side B of this system? **]**

Figure 3-14 **Filtration.** A mechanical force pushes a substance through a membrane, although the membrane limits which particles can pass through based on size. The small particles go through the membrane and appear in the filtered solution (filtrate).

> > In **pinocytosis** (pi-no-si-TO-sis), the plasma membrane engulfs droplets of fluid. This is a way for large protein molecules in suspension to travel into the cell. The word *pinocytosis* means "cell drinking."

■ In **exocytosis**, the cell moves materials out in vesicles (Fig. 3-17). One example of exocytosis is the export of neurotransmitters from neurons (neurotransmitters are chemicals that control the activity of the nervous system).

The transport methods described above are summarized in Table 3-5.

CHECKPOINT 3-12 ➤ Substances are constantly moving into and out of cells through the plasma membrane. What types of movement do not require cellular energy and what types of movement do require cellular energy?

How Osmosis Affects Cells

As stated earlier, water usually moves easily through the cell membrane. Therefore, for a normal fluid balance to be maintained, the fluid outside all cells must have the same concentration of dissolved substances (solutes) as the fluids inside the cells (Fig. 3-18). If not, water will move rapidly into or out of the cell by osmosis. Solutions with

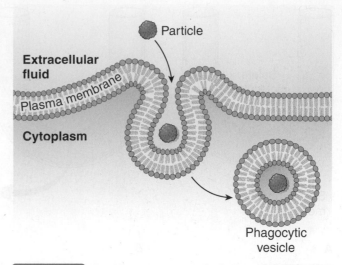

Figure 3-16 **Phagocytosis.** The plasma membrane encloses a particle from the extracellular fluid. The membrane then pinches off, forming a vesicle that carries the particle into the cytoplasm. **[ZOOMING IN ➤** What organelle would likely help to destroy a particle taken in by phagocytosis? **]**

concentrations equal to the concentration of the cytoplasm are described as **isotonic** (i-so-TON-ik). Tissue fluids and blood plasma are isotonic for body cells. Manufactured solutions that are isotonic for the cells and can thus be used to replace body fluids include 0.9% salt, or **normal saline**, and 5% dextrose (glucose).

A solution that is less concentrated than the intracellular fluid is described as **hypotonic**. Based on the principles of osmosis already explained, a cell placed in a hypotonic solution draws water in, swells, and may burst. When a red blood cell draws in water and bursts in this way, the cell is said to undergo **hemolysis** (he-MOL-ih-sis). If a cell is placed in a **hypertonic** solution, which is more concentrated than the cellular fluid, it loses water to the surrounding fluids and shrinks, a process termed **crenation** (kre-NA-shun) (see Fig. 3-18).

Fluid balance is an important facet of homeostasis and must be properly regulated for health. You can figure out in which direction water will move through the plasma membrane if you remember the saying "water follows salt," salt meaning any dissolved material (solute). The total amount and distribution of body fluids is discussed in Chapter 21. Table 3-6 summarizes the effects of different solution concentrations on cells.

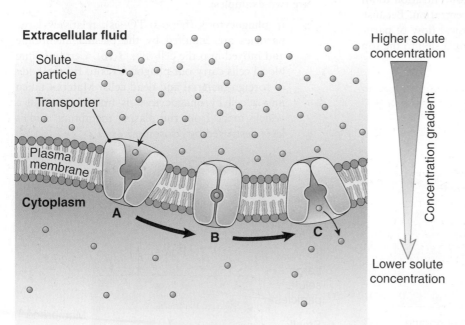

Figure 3-15 **Facilitated diffusion.** Transporters (proteins in the plasma membrane) move solute particles through a membrane from an area of higher concentration to an area of lower concentration. **(A)** A solute particle enters the transporter. **(B)** The transporter changes shape. **(C)** The transporter releases the solute particle on the other side of the membrane. **[ZOOMING IN ➤** How would a change in the number of transporters affect a solute's movement by facilitated diffusion? **]**

Release of stored material

Extracellular fluid

Plasma membrane

Cytoplasm

Vesicle

Fusion with plasma membrane

Stored material

Figure 3-17 **Exocytosis.** A vesicle fuses with the plasma membrane then ruptures and releases its contents.

CHECKPOINT **3-13** ➤ The concentration of fluids in and around the cell is important in homeostasis. What term describes a fluid that is the same concentration as the fluid within the cell (intracellular fluid)? What type of fluid is less concentrated? More concentrated?

Cell Aging

As cells multiply throughout life, changes occur that may lead to their damage and death. Harmful substances known as *free radicals*, produced in the course of normal metabolism, can injure cells unless these materials are destroyed. Chapter 20 covers free radicals in more detail. Lysosomes may deteriorate as they age, releasing enzymes that can harm the cell. Alteration of the genes, or **mutation**, is a natural occurrence in the process of cell division and is increased by exposure to harmful substances and radiation in the environment. Mutations usually harm cells and may lead to cancer.

As a person ages, the overall activity of the body cells slows. One example of this change is the slowing down of repair processes. A bone fracture, for example, takes considerably longer to heal in an old person than in a young person.

Table 3-5	Membrane Transport	
Process	**Definition**	**Example**
Do not require cellular energy (passive)		
Diffusion	Random movement of particles with the concentration gradient (from higher concentration to lower concentration) until they reach equilibrium	Movement of nutrients, electrolytes, gases, wastes, and other soluble materials into and out of the cell
Osmosis	Diffusion of water through a semi-permeable membrane	Movement of water across the plasma membrane
Filtration	Movement of materials through a membrane under mechanical force	Movement of materials out of the blood under the force of blood pressure
Facilitated diffusion	Movement of materials across the plasma membrane along the concentration gradient using transporters to speed the process	Movement of glucose into the cells
Require cellular energy		
Active transport	Movement of materials through the plasma membrane against the concentration gradient using transporters	Transport of ions (e.g., Na^+, K^+, Ca^{2+}) in the nervous system and muscular system
Endocytosis	Transport of bulk amounts of materials into the cell using vesicles	Phagocytosis—intake of large particles, as when white blood cells take in waste materials; also pinocytosis—intake of fluid
Exocytosis	Transport of bulk amounts of materials out of the cell using vesicles	Release of neurotransmitters from neurons

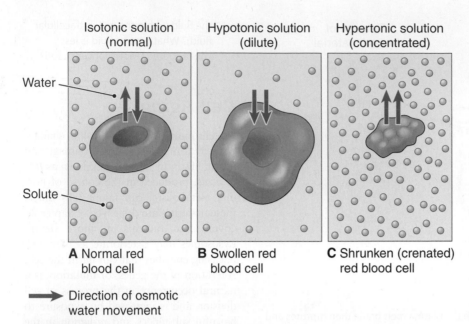

Isotonic solution (normal)   Hypotonic solution (dilute)   Hypertonic solution (concentrated)

Water

Solute

A Normal red blood cell   **B** Swollen red blood cell   **C** Shrunken (crenated) red blood cell

→ Direction of osmotic water movement

Figure 3-18   **The effect of osmosis on cells.** Water moves through a red blood cell membrane in solutions with three different concentrations of solute. **(A)** The isotonic (normal) solution has the same concentration as the cell fluid, and water moves into and out of the cell at the same rate. **(B)** A cell placed in a hypotonic (more dilute) solution draws water in, causing the cell to swell and perhaps undergo hemolysis (bursting). **(C)** The hypertonic (more concentrated) solution draws water out of the cell, causing it to shrink, an effect known as crenation. [**ZOOMING IN ➤** What would happen to red blood cells if blood lost through injury were replaced with pure water?]

One theory on aging holds that cells are preprogrammed to divide only a certain number of times before they die. Support for this idea comes from the fact that cells taken from a young person divide more times when grown in the laboratory than similar cells taken from an older individual. This programmed cell death, known as *apoptosis* (ah-pop-TO-sis), is a natural part of growth and remodeling before birth in the developing embryo. For example, apoptosis removes cells from the embryonic limb buds in the development of fingers and toes. Apoptosis also is needed in repair and remodeling of tissue throughout life. Cells subject to wear and tear regularly undergo

apoptosis and are replaced. For example, the cells lining the digestive tract are removed and replaced every 2 to 3 days. This "cellular suicide" is an orderly, genetically programmed process. The "suicide" genes code for enzymes that destroy the cell quickly without damaging nearby cells. Phagocytes then eliminate the dead cells.

Cells and Cancer

Certain mutations (changes) in a cell's genetic material may cause that cell to reproduce without control. Cells that normally multiply at a fast rate, such as epithelial cells, are more likely than slower-growing cells to undergo such transformations. If these altered cells do not die naturally or get destroyed by the immune system, they will continue to multiply and may spread (metastasize) to other tissues, producing **cancer**. Cancer cells form tumors, which interfere with normal functions, crowding out normal cells and robbing them of nutrients. There is more information on the various types of tumors in Chapter 4.

Cancer Risk Factors

The causes of cancer are complex, involving interactions between cellular factors and the environment. Because cancer may take a long time to develop, it is often difficult to identify its cause or causes. Certain forces increase the chances of developing the disease and are considered risk factors. These include the following:

- **Heredity.** Certain types of cancer occur more frequently in some families than in others, indicating that

Table 3-6	Solutions and Their Effects on Cells		
Type of Solution	**Description**	**Examples**	**Effect on Cells**
Isotonic	Has the same concentration of dissolved substances as the fluid in the cell	0.9% salt (normal saline); 5% dextrose (glucose)	None; cell in equilibrium with its environment
Hypotonic	Has a lower concentration of dissolved substances than the fluid in the cell	Less than 0.9% salt or 5% dextrose	Cell takes in water, swells, and may burst; red blood cell undergoes hemolysis
Hypertonic	Has a higher concentration of dissolved substances than the fluid in the cell	Higher than 0.9% salt or 5% dextrose	Cell will lose water and shrink; cell undergoes crenation

Disease in Context revisited

➤ Jim's Trouble Continues with a Clot

Let's consider what was happening in Jim's body when he overexerted himself on the basketball court: his rapidly beating heart forced blood around a fatty plaque that bulged into the lumen of a coronary artery. Unable to resist the high pressure within the artery, the plaque ruptured and stimulated blood platelets to form a clot in the damaged vessel. Unfortunately for Jim, the clot prevented millions of cardiac muscle cells from receiving oxygen-rich blood. Without oxygen, the cells' mitochondria could not manufacture ATP; without ATP, the contractile proteins in the cells could not shorten. Within minutes, the cardiac muscle cells downstream from the clot stopped contracting, forcing Jim's heart into an irregular rhythm. This alteration dramatically decreased the volume of blood leaving his heart. Brain cells, called neurons, also depend on oxygen to manufacture ATP, and without adequate blood flow, they too began to shut down, causing Jim to lose consciousness.

Inside Jim's oxygen-starved cardiac muscle cells, lack of ATP had other serious consequences. Transporter proteins embedded in the cells' plasma membranes began to shut down. Without these transporters, the cells could not regulate their solute concentration. Quickly, the cells' cytoplasm became hypertonic to the surrounding tissue fluid. Following its osmotic gradient, extracellular water entered the affected cardiac muscle cells, causing them to burst and die. Jim is in big trouble.

In this case, we saw that events within Jim's cardiac muscle cells affected his whole body. Your understanding of cellular structure and function will help you to make sense of the structure and function of tissues, organs, and, ultimately, the entire body. Without immediate help, Jim's chances of survival are low. The case study in Chapter 14, The Heart and Heart Disease, will introduce you to some of the medical techniques that will save Jim's life.

---

there is some inherited predisposition to cancer development.

- **Chemicals.** Certain industrial and environmental chemicals are known to increase the risk of cancer. Any chemical that causes cancer is called a **carcinogen** (kar-SIN-o-jen). The most common carcinogens in our society are those present in cigarette smoke. Carcinogens are also present, both naturally and as additives, in foods. Certain drugs also may be carcinogenic.

- **Ionizing radiation.** Certain types of radiation can produce damage to cellular DNA that may lead to cancer. These include x-rays, rays from radioactive substances, and ultraviolet rays. For example, the ultraviolet rays received from sun exposure are very harmful to the skin.

- **Physical irritation.** Continued irritation, such as the contact of a hot pipe stem on the lip, increases cell division and thus increases the chance of mutation.

- **Diet.** It has been shown that diets high in fats and total calories are associated with an increased occurrence of certain cancers. A general lack of fiber and insufficient amounts of certain fruits and vegetables in the diet can leave one susceptible to cancers of the digestive tract.

- **Viruses** have been implicated in cancers of the liver, the blood (leukemias), lymphatic tissues (lymphomas), and the uterine cervix.

Word Anatomy

Medical terms are built from standardized word parts (prefixes, roots, and suffixes). Learning the meanings of these parts can help you remember words and interpret unfamiliar terms.

WORD PART	MEANING	EXAMPLE
The Role of Cells		
cyt/o	cell	*Cytology* is the study of cells.
Microscopes		
micr/o	small	*Microscopes* are used to view structures too small to see with the naked eye.
Cell Structure		
bi-	two	The lipid *bilayer* is a double layer of lipid molecules.
-some	body	*Ribosomes* are small bodies in the cytoplasm that help make proteins.
chrom/o-	color	*Chromosomes* are small, threadlike bodies that stain darkly with basic dyes.
end/o-	in, within	The *endoplasmic* reticulum is a membranous network within the cytoplasm.
lys/o	loosening, dissolving, separating	*Lysosomes* are small bodies (organelles) with enzymes that dissolve materials (*see also hemolysis*).
Cell Divisions		
inter-	between	*Interphase* is the stage between one cell division (mitosis) and the next.
pro-	before, in front of	*Prophase* is the first stage of mitosis.
meta-	change	*Metaphase* is the second stage of mitosis when the chromosomes change position and line up across the equator.
ana-	upward, back, again	In the *anaphase* stage of mitosis, chromosomes move to opposite sides of the cell.
tel/o-	end	*Telophase* is the last stage of mitosis.
semi-	partial, half	A *semipermeable* membrane lets some molecules pass through but not others.
phag/o	to eat, ingest	In *phagocytosis* the plasma membrane engulfs large particles and moves them into the cell.
pin/o	to drink	In *pinocytosis* the plasma membrane "drinks" (engulfs) droplets of fluid.
ex/o-	outside, out of, away from	In *exocytosis* the cell moves material out in vesicles.
iso-	same, equal	An *isotonic* solution has the same concentration as that of the cytoplasm.
hypo-	deficient, below, beneath	A *hypotonic* solution's concentration is lower than that of the cytoplasm.
hem/o	blood	*Hemolysis* is the destruction of red blood cells.
hyper-	above, over, excessive	A *hypertonic* solution's concentration is higher than that of the cytoplasm.
Cells and Cancer		
carcin/o	cancer, carcinoma	A *carcinogen* is a chemical that causes cancer.
-gen	agent that produces or originates	See preceding example.

Summary

I. **THE ROLE OF CELLS**
   A. Basic unit of life
   B. Show all characteristics of life—organization, metabolism, responsiveness, homeostasis, growth, reproduction

II. **MICROSCOPES**
   A. Types
      1. Compound light microscope
      2. Transmission electron microscope—magnifies up to 1 million times
      3. Scanning electron microscope—gives three-dimensional image
   B. Micrometer—metric unit commonly used for microscopic measurements (μm)
   C. Stains—dyes used to aid in viewing cells under the microscope

III. **CELL STRUCTURE**
   A. Plasma membrane—regulates what enters and leaves cell
      1. Phospholipid bilayer with proteins, carbohydrates, cholesterol
         a. Proteins—channels, transporters, receptors, enzymes, linkers, cell identity markers
   B. Nucleus
      1. Control center of the cell
      2. Contains the chromosomes (units of heredity)
      3. Contains the nucleolus, which manufactures ribosomes
   C. Cytoplasm—colloidal suspension that holds organelles
      1. Cytosol—liquid portion
      2. Organelles—structures that carry out special functions
         a. ER (endoplasmic reticulum), ribosomes, mitochondria, Golgi apparatus, lysosomes, peroxisomes, vesicles, centrioles
         b. Cilia, flagellum—surface organelles used for movement

IV. **PROTEIN SYNTHESIS**
   A. Nucleic acids—DNA and RNA
      1. Composed of nucleotides
         a. Each nucleotide has sugar, phosphate, nitrogen base
         b. Nitrogen bases vary, giving five nucleotides
      2. DNA
         a. Carries the genetic message
         b. Located almost entirely in the nucleus
         c. Composed of nucleotides containing adenine (A), guanine (G), cytosine (C), thymine (T)
         d. Double stranded by pairing of A-T, G-C, and wound into helix

3. The role of RNA
      a. Single strand of nucleotides containing A, G, C, or uracil (U)
      b. Located in the cytoplasm
      c. Translates DNA message into proteins
      d. Three types
         (1) Messenger RNA (mRNA)—transcribes the message of the DNA
         (2) Ribosomal RNA (rRNA)—makes up the ribosomes, the site of protein synthesis
         (3) Transfer RNA (tRNA)—brings amino acids to be made into proteins

V. **CELL DIVISION**
   A. Meiosis—forms the sex cells (egg and sperm)
      1. Divides the chromosome number in half
   B. Mitosis—division of somatic (body) cells
      1. Chromosomes first replicate (double) during interphase
      2. Division of cell into two identical daughter cells
   C. Stages of mitosis—prophase, metaphase, anaphase, telophase

VI. **MOVEMENT OF SUBSTANCES ACROSS THE PLASMA MEMBRANE**
   A. Movement that does not require cellular energy (passive)
      1. Diffusion—molecules move from area of higher concentration to area of lower concentration
      2. Osmosis—diffusion of water through semipermeable membrane
         a. Osmotic pressure—measure of a solution's tendency to draw in water
      3. Filtration—movement of materials through plasma membrane under mechanical force
      4. Facilitated diffusion—movement of materials with aid of transporters in plasma membrane
   B. Movement that requires cellular energy (active)
      1. Active transport
         a. Movement of solute particles from area of lower concentration to area of higher concentration
         b. Requires transporters
      2. Endocytosis—movement of bulk amounts of material into the cell in vesicles
         a. Phagocytosis—engulfing of large particles
         b. Pinocytosis—intake of fluid droplets
      3. Exocytosis—movement of bulk amounts of materials out of the cell in vesicles
   C. How osmosis affects cells
      1. Isotonic solution—same concentration as cell fluids; cell remains the same

2. Hypotonic solution—lower concentration than cell fluids; cell swells and may undergo hemolysis (bursting)
3. Hypertonic solution—higher concentration than cell fluids; cell undergoes crenation (shrinking)

VII. CELL AGING

A. Mutations (changes) occur in genes
B. Slowing of cellular activity
C. Apoptosis—programmed cell death

VIII. CELLS AND CANCER

A. Cancer
  1. Uncontrolled growth of cells
  2. Spread (metastasize) to other tissues
B. Cancer risk factors
  1. Heredity
  2. Chemicals—carcinogens
  3. Ionizing radiation
  4. Physical irritation
  5. Diet
  6. Viruses

Questions for Study and Review

BUILDING UNDERSTANDING

Fill in the blanks

1. The part of the cell that regulates what can enter or leave is the _____.
2. Distinct segments of DNA that code for specific proteins are called _____.
3. The cytosol and organelles make up the _____.
4. If Solution A has more solute and less water than Solution B, then Solution A is _____ to Solution B.
5. Mechanisms that require energy to move substances across the plasma membrane are called _____ transport mechanisms.

Matching > Match each numbered item with the most closely related lettered item.

___ **6.** DNA duplication takes place
___ **7.** DNA is tightly wound into chromosomes
___ **8.** Chromosomes line up along the cell's equator
___ **9.** Chromosomes separate and move toward opposite ends of the cell
___ **10.** Cell membrane pinches off, dividing the cell into two new daughter cells

a. metaphase
b. anaphase
c. telophase
d. interphase
e. prophase

Multiple Choice

___ **11.** The main component of the plasma membrane is
  a. phospholipid
  b. cholesterol
  c. carbohydrate
  d. protein

___ **12.** ATP is synthesized in the
  a. nucleus
  b. Golgi apparatus
  c. endoplasmic reticulum
  d. mitochondria

___ **13.** Transcription of the DNA strand TGAAC would produce an mRNA strand with the sequence
  a. CAGGU
  b. ACTTG

  c. CAGGT
  d. ACUUG

___ **14.** Somatic cells divide by the process called
  a. mitosis
  b. meiosis
  c. crenation
  d. hemolysis

___ **15.** Movement of solute from a region of high concentration to one of lower concentration is called
  a. exocytosis
  b. diffusion
  c. endocytosis
  d. osmosis

UNDERSTANDING CONCEPTS

16. List the components of the plasma membrane and state a function for each.

17. Compare and contrast the following cellular components:
    a. microvilli and cilia
    b. nucleus and nucleolus
    c. rough ER and smooth ER
    d. lysosome and peroxisome
    e. DNA and RNA
    f. chromosome and gene

18. Describe the role of each of the following in protein synthesis: DNA, nucleotide, RNA, ribosomes, rough ER, and Golgi apparatus.

19. List and define six methods by which materials cross the plasma membrane. Which of these requires cellular energy?

20. Why is the plasma membrane described as selectively permeable?

21. What will happen to a red blood cell placed in a 5.0% salt solution? In distilled water?

22. Discuss the link between genetic mutation and cancer. List six risk factors associated with cancer.

CONCEPTUAL THINKING

23. Cigarette smoke paralyzes the cilia of cells lining the respiratory tract. Explain the effects of this on respiratory system function.

24. In the Disease in Context case story, Jim's cardiac muscle cells adapted to his unhealthy lifestyle by synthesizing more contractile proteins. Beginning with events in the nucleus, describe the process of manufacturing a contractile protein.

25. In Jim's case, we saw that changes at the cellular level can ultimately affect the entire organism. Explain why this is so.

26. Kidney failure causes a buildup of waste and water in the blood. A procedure called hemodialysis removes these substances from the blood. During this procedure, the patient's blood passes by a semipermeable membrane within the dialysis machine. Waste and water from the blood diffuse across the membrane into dialysis fluid on the other side. Based on this information, compare the osmotic concentration of the blood with that of the dialysis fluid.

Tissues are groups of cells similar in structure, arranged in a characteristic pattern, and specialized for the performance of specific tasks. The study of tissues is known as **histology** (his-TOL-o-je). This study shows that the form, arrangement, and composition of cells in different tissues account for their properties.

The tissues in our bodies might be compared with the different materials used to construct a building. Think for a moment of the great variety of building materials used according to need—wood, stone, steel, plaster, insulation, and others. Each of these has different properties, but together they contribute to the building as a whole. The same may be said of tissues. To read about the origin of the different tissues, see Box 4-1, Stem Cells: So Much Potential.

Tissue Classification

The four main tissue groups are the following:

- **Epithelial** (ep-ih-THE-le-al) **tissue** covers surfaces, lines cavities, and forms glands.
- **Connective tissue** supports and forms the framework of all parts of the body.
- **Muscle tissue** contracts and produces movement.
- **Nervous tissue** conducts nerve impulses.

This chapter concentrates mainly on epithelial and connective tissues; muscle and nervous tissues receive more attention in later chapters.

Epithelial Tissue

Epithelial tissue, or **epithelium** (ep-ih-THE-le-um), forms a protective covering for the body. It is the main tissue of the skin's outer layer. It also forms membranes, ducts, and the lining of body cavities and hollow organs, such as the organs of the digestive, respiratory, and urinary tracts.

Structure of Epithelial Tissue

Epithelial cells are tightly packed to better protect underlying tissue or form barriers between systems. The cells vary in shape and arrangement according to their function. Epithelial tissue is classified on the basis of these characteristics. In shape, the cells may be described as follows:

- **Squamous** (SKWA-mus)—flat and irregular
- **Cuboidal**—square
- **Columnar**—long and narrow

The cells may be arranged in a single layer, in which case it is described as **simple** (Fig. 4-1). Simple epithelium functions as a thin barrier through which materials can pass fairly easily. For example, simple epithelium allows for absorption of materials from the lining of the digestive tract into the blood and allows for passage of oxygen from the blood to body tissues. Areas subject to wear-and-tear that require protection are covered with epithelial cells in multiple layers, an arrangement described as **stratified** (Fig. 4-2). If the cells are staggered so that they appear to be in multiple layers but really are not, they are termed

---

Box 4-1 — Hot Topics

Stem Cells: So Much Potential

At least 200 different types of cells are found in the human body, each with its own unique structure and function. All originate from unspecialized precursors called **stem cells**, which exhibit two important characteristics: they can divide repeatedly and have the potential to become specialized cells.

Stem cells come in two types. **Embryonic stem cells**, found in early embryos, are the source of all body cells and potentially can differentiate into any cell type. **Adult stem cells**, found in babies and children as well as adults, are stem cells that remain in the body after birth and can differentiate into only a few cell types. They assist with tissue growth and repair. For example, in red bone marrow, these cells differentiate into blood cells, whereas in the skin, they differentiate into new skin cells after a cut or scrape.

The potential healthcare applications of stem cell research are numerous. In the near future, stem cell transplants

may be used to repair damaged tissues in treating illnesses such as diabetes, cancer, heart disease, Parkinson disease, and spinal cord injury. This research may also help explain how cells develop and why some cells develop abnormally, causing birth defects and cancer. Scientists may also use stem cells to test drugs before trying them on animals and humans.

But stem cell research is controversial. Some argue that it is unethical to use embryonic stem cells because they are obtained from aborted fetuses or fertilized eggs left over from in vitro fertilization. Others argue that these cells would be discarded anyway and have the potential to improve lives. A possible solution is the use of adult stem cells. However, adult stem cells are less abundant and lack embryonic stem cells' potential to differentiate, so more research is needed to make this a viable option.

pseudostratified. Terms for both shape and arrangement are used to describe epithelial tissue. Thus, a single layer of flat, irregular cells would be described as *simple squamous epithelium*, whereas tissue with many layers of these same cells would be described as *stratified squamous epithelium*.

Some organs, such as the urinary bladder, must vary a great deal in size as they work. These organs are lined with **transitional epithelium**, which is capable of great expansion but returns to its original form once tension is relaxed—as when, in this case, the urinary bladder is emptied.

Special Functions of Epithelial Tissue

Some epithelial tissues produce secretions, including **mucus** (MU-kus) (a clear, sticky fluid), digestive juices, sweat, and other substances. The air that we breathe passes over epithelium that lines the respiratory passageways. Mucus-secreting **goblet cells**, named for their shape, are scattered among the pseudostratified epithelial cells (Fig. 4-3A). The epithelial cells also have tiny hairlike projections called **cilia** (SIL-e-ah). Together, the mucus and the cilia help trap bits of dust and other foreign particles that could otherwise reach and damage the lungs. The digestive tract is lined with simple columnar epithelium that also contains goblet cells. They secrete mucus that protects the lining of the digestive organs (Fig. 4-3B).

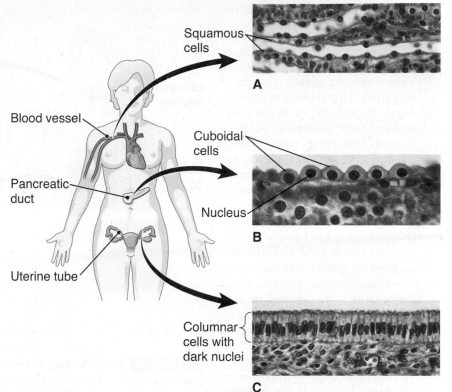

Figure 4-1 **Simple epithelial tissues. (A)** Simple squamous has flat, irregular cells with flat nuclei. **(B)** Cuboidal cells are square in shape with round nuclei. **(C)** Columnar cells are long and narrow with ovoid nuclei. (Reprinted with permission from Cormack DH. *Essential Histology*, 2nd ed. Philadelphia: Lippincott Williams & Wilkins, 2001.) [**ZOOMING IN ➤** In how many layers are these epithelial cells?]

PASSport to Success Visit **thePoint** or see the Student Resource CD in the back of this book for a summary chart on epithelial tissue.

Epithelium repairs itself quickly after it is injured. In areas of the body subject to normal wear-and-tear, such as the skin, the inside of the mouth, and the lining of the intestinal tract, epithelial cells reproduce frequently, replacing damaged tissue. Certain areas of the epithelium that form the outer layer of the skin are capable of modifying themselves for greater strength whenever they are subjected to unusual wear-and-tear; the growth of calluses is a good example of this response.

Glands

The active cells of many glands are epithelial cells. A gland is an organ specialized to produce a substance that is sent out to other parts of the body. The gland manufactures these secretions from materials removed from the blood. Glands

Figure 4-2 **Stratified squamous epithelium.** Cells are arranged in multiple layers. (Reprinted with permission from Cormack DH. *Essential Histology*, 2nd ed. Philadelphia: Lippincott Williams & Wilkins, 2001.)

are divided into two categories based on how they release their secretions:

- **Exocrine** (EK-so-krin) **glands** have ducts or tubes to carry secretions away from the gland. The ducts may carry the secretions to another organ, to a cavity, or to the body surface. These substances act in a limited area near their source. Examples of exocrine glands include the glands in the gastrointestinal tract that secrete digestive juices, the sebaceous (oil) glands of the skin, and the lacrimal glands that produce tears. These and other exocrine glands are discussed in the chapters on specific systems.

  In structure, an exocrine gland may consist of a single cell, such as the goblet cells that secrete mucus into the digestive and respiratory tracts. Most, however, are composed of multiple cells in various arrangements (Fig. 4-4). They may be tubular, in a simple straight form, or in a branched formation, as are found in the digestive tract. They may also be coiled, as are the sweat glands of the skin. They may be saclike, as are the sebaceous (oil) glands of the skin, or compound formations of tubes and sacs, as are the salivary glands in the mouth.

- **Endocrine** (EN-do-krin) **glands** secrete not through ducts, but directly into surrounding tissue fluid. Most often the secretions are then absorbed into the bloodstream, which carries them throughout the body. These secretions, called **hormones**, have effects on specific tissues known as the *target tissues*. Endocrine glands have an extensive network of blood vessels. These so-called *ductless glands* include the pituitary, thyroid, adrenal glands, and others described in greater detail in Chapter 12.

CHECKPOINT **4-1** ➤ Epithelium is classified according to cell shape. What are the three basic shapes?

CHECKPOINT **4-2** ➤ Glands are classified according to whether they secrete through ducts or secrete directly into surrounding fluid and the bloodstream. What are these two categories of glands?

Connective Tissue

The supporting fabric everywhere in the body is connective tissue. This is so extensive and widely distributed that

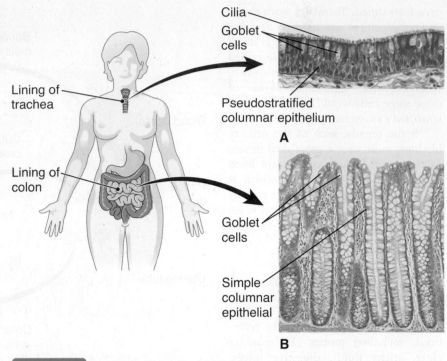

Figure 4-3 **Special features of epithelial tissues. (A)** The lining of the trachea showing cilia and goblet cells that secrete mucus. **(B)** The lining of the intestine showing goblet cells. (Reprinted with permission from Cormack DH. *Essential Histology*, 2nd ed. Philadelphia: Lippincott Williams & Wilkins, 2001.)

if we were able to dissolve all the tissues except connective tissue, we would still be able to recognize the entire body's contours. Connective tissue has large amounts of nonliving material between the cells. This intercellular background material or **matrix** (MA-trix) contains varying amounts of water, fibers, and hard minerals.

Histologists, specialists in the study of tissues, have numerous ways of classifying connective tissues based on their structure or function. Here we describe the different types according to their distribution and function, while listing them in order of increasing hardness.

- Circulating connective tissue has a fluid consistency; its cells are suspended in a liquid environment. The two types are blood, which circulates in blood vessels (Fig. 4-5), and lymph, a fluid derived from blood that circulates in lymphatic vessels. Chapters 13 and 16 have more information on circulating connective tissue.

- Generalized connective tissue is widely distributed. It supports and protects structures. Some is loosely held together in a semi-liquid matrix. Some is denser and contains many fibers. Cells called **fibroblasts** produce the various fibers in all connective tissue. (The word ending –*blast* refers to a young and active cell). Examples of structures composed of this denser connective tissue are tendons, ligaments, and the capsules (coverings) around some organs.

- Structural connective tissue is mainly associated with the skeleton. Examples are cartilage, which has a very

4

Tissue surface

Duct

Secretory portion

A Simple tubular

B Branched tubular

C Coiled tubular

D Simple saclike (alveolar)

E Compound

Figure 4-4 **Some structural types of exocrine glands. (A)** Simple tubular, as found in the intestine. **(B)** Branched tubular, as found in the stomach. **(C)** Coiled tubular, such as the sweat glands of the skin. **(D)** Simple saclike (alveolar), such as the oil glands of the skin. **(E)** Compound, with tubes and sacs, such as the salivary glands.

firm consistency, and bone tissue, which is hardened by minerals in the matrix.

The generalized and structural connective tissues are described in greater detail below.

PASSport to Success   Visit *thePoint* or see the Student Resource CD in the back of this book for a summary chart of the connective tissue types.

CHECKPOINT **4-3** ➤ Connective tissues vary according to the composition of the material that is between the cells. What is the general name for this intercellular material?

Generalized Connective Tissue

This tissue is found throughout the body and is less specific in function than other types. There are two forms: loose and dense.

Loose connective tissue, as the name implies, has a soft or semi-liquid consistency. The types are:

- **Areolar** (ah-RE-o-lar) **tissue** is named from a word that means "space" because of its open composition (see Fig. 4-5B). It contains cells and fibers in a soft, jellylike matrix. This tissue is found in membranes, around vessels and organs, between muscles, and under the skin. It is the most common type of connective tissue.

- **Adipose** (AD-ih-pose) **tissue** contains cells (adipocytes) that are able to store large amounts of fat (see Fig. 4-5C). The fat in this tissue is a reserve energy supply for the body. Adipose tissue is also a heat insulator, as in the underlying layers of the skin, and is protective padding for organs and joints.

Dense connective tissue is more firm and is characterized by the many fibers that give it strength and flexibility. The main type of fiber in this and other connective tissue is **collagen** (KOL-ah-jen), a flexible white protein. (See Box 4-2, Collagen: The Body's Scaffolding.) The different types vary in the main fibers they contain and how they are arranged:

- **Irregular dense connective tissue** has mostly collagenous fibers in random arrangement. This tissue makes up the fibrous membranes that cover various organs, as described later in this chapter. Particularly strong forms make up the tough capsules around certain organs, such as the kidney, the liver, and some glands.

- **Regular dense connective tissue** also has mostly collagenous fibers, but they are in a regular, parallel alignment like the strands of a cable. This tissue can pull in one direction. Examples are the cordlike **tendons**, which connect muscles to bones, and the **ligaments**, which connect bones to other bones (Fig. 4-6A).

- **Elastic connective tissue** has many elastic fibers that allow it to stretch and then return to its original length. This tissue appears in the vocal cords, the respiratory passageways, and the walls of blood vessels.

Structural Connective Tissue

The structural connective tissues are mainly associated with the skeleton and are stronger and more solid than all the other groups.

CARTILAGE Because of its strength and flexibility, cartilage is a structural material and provides reinforcement. It is also a shock absorber and a bearing surface that reduces friction between moving parts, as at joints. The cells that produce cartilage are **chondrocytes** (KON-dro-sites), a name derived from the word root *chondro*, meaning "cartilage" and the root *cyto*, meaning "cell." There are three forms of cartilage:

- **Hyaline** (HI-ah-lin) **cartilage** is the tough translucent material, popularly called gristle, that covers the ends of the long bones (see Fig. 4-6B). Hyaline cartilage also makes up the tip of the nose and reinforces the larynx ("voicebox") and the trachea ("windpipe").

- **Fibrocartilage** (fi-bro-KAR-tih-laj) is firm and rigid, and is found between vertebrae (segments) of the spine, at the anterior joint between the pubic bones of the hip, and in the knee joint.

- **Elastic cartilage** can spring back into shape after it is bent. An easy place to observe the properties of elastic cartilage is in the outer portion of the ear. It is also located in the larynx.

Figure 4-5 **Circulating and generalized (loose) connective tissue. (A)** Blood smear showing various blood cells in a liquid matrix. **(B)** Areolar connective tissue, a mixture of cells and fibers in a jellylike matrix. **(C)** Adipose tissue shown here surrounding darkstaining glandular tissue. The slide shows areas where fat is stored and nuclei at the edge of the cells. (A, reprinted with permission from McClatchey KD. *Clinical Laboratory Medicine*, 2nd ed. Baltimore: Lippincott Williams & Wilkins, 2001; B, reprinted with permission from Cormack DH. *Essential Histology*, 2nd ed. Philadelphia: Lippincott Williams & Wilkins, 2001; C, Reprinted with permission from Mills SE. *Histology for Pathologists*, 3rd ed. Philadelphia: Lippincott Williams & Wilkins, 2006.) **[ZOOMING IN ➤** Which of these tissues has the most fibers? Which of these tissues is modified for storage? **]**

CHECKPOINT **4-4** ➤ Connective tissue is characterized by the presence of fibers. The main fibers in connective tissue are made of what protein?

BONE The tissue that composes bones, called **osseous** (OS-e-us) **tissue**, is much like cartilage in its cellular structure (see Fig. 4-6C). In fact, the skeleton of the fetus in the early stages of development is made almost entirely

Box 4-2   A Closer Look

Collagen: The Body's Scaffolding

The most abundant protein in the body, making up about 25% of total protein, is collagen. Its name, derived from a Greek word meaning "glue," reveals its role as the main structural protein in connective tissue.

Fibroblasts secrete collagen molecules into the surrounding matrix, where the molecules are then assembled into fibers. These fibers give the matrix its strength and its flexibility. Collagen fibers' high tensile strength makes them stronger than steel fibers of the same size, and their flexibility confers resilience on the tissues that contain them. For example, collagen in skin, bone, tendons, and ligaments resists pulling forces, whereas collagen found in joint cartilage and between vertebrae resists compression. Based on amino acid structure, there are at least 19 types of collagen, each of which imparts a different property to the connective tissue containing it.

The arrangement of collagen fibers in the matrix reveals much about the tissue's function. In the skin and membranes covering muscles and organs, collagen fibers are arranged irregularly, with fibers running in all directions. The result is a tissue that can resist stretching forces in many different directions. In tendons and ligaments, collagen fibers have a parallel arrangement, forming strong ropelike cords that can resist longitudinal pulling forces. In bone tissue, collagen fibers' meshlike arrangement promotes deposition of calcium salts into the tissue, which gives bone strength while also providing flexibility.

Collagen's varied properties are also evident in the preparation of a gelatin dessert. Gelatin is a collagen extract made by boiling animal bones and other connective tissue. It is a viscous liquid in hot water but forms a semisolid gel on cooling.

---

of cartilage. This tissue gradually becomes impregnated with salts of calcium and phosphorus that make bone characteristically solid and hard. The cells that form bone are called **osteoblasts** (OS-te-o-blasts), a name that combines the root for bone (*osteo*) with a root (*blast*) that means an immature cell. As these cells mature, they are referred to as **osteocytes** (OS-te-o-sites). Within the osseous tissue are nerves and blood vessels. A specialized type of tissue, the bone marrow, is enclosed within bones. The red bone marrow contained in certain regions produces blood cells. Chapter 7 has more information on bones.

CHECKPOINT **4-5** ➤ Connective tissue is the supportive and protective material found throughout the body. What are some examples of circulating, generalized, and structural connective tissue?

Muscle Tissue

Muscle tissue is designed to produce movement by contraction of its cells, which are called **muscle fibers** because most of them are long and threadlike. If a piece of well-cooked meat is pulled apart, small groups of these muscle fibers may be seen. Muscle tissue is usually classified as follows:

■ **Skeletal muscle,** which works with tendons and bones to move the body (Fig. 4-7A). This type of tissue is described as **voluntary muscle** because it can be made to

contract by conscious thought. The cells in skeletal muscle are very large and are remarkable in having multiple nuclei and a pattern of dark and light banding described as **striations**. This type of muscle is also called striated muscle. Chapter 8 has more details on skeletal muscles.

■ **Cardiac muscle,** which forms the bulk of the heart wall and is known also as **myocardium** (mi-o-KAR-de-um) (see Fig. 4-7B). This is the muscle that produces the regular contractions known as *heartbeats*. Cardiac muscle is described as **involuntary muscle** because it typically contracts independently of thought. Most of the time we are not aware of its actions at all. Cardiac muscle has branching cells and specialized membranes between the cells that appear as dark lines under the microscope. Their technical name is *intercalated* (in-TER-cal-a-ted) *disks*. The heart and cardiac muscle are discussed in Chapter 14.

■ **Smooth muscle** is also involuntary muscle (see Fig. 4-7C). It forms the walls of the hollow organs in the ventral body cavities, including the stomach, intestines, gallbladder, and urinary bladder. Together these organs are known as viscera (VIS-eh-rah), so smooth muscle is sometimes referred to as *visceral muscle*. Smooth muscle is also found in the walls of many tubular structures, such as the blood vessels and the tubes that carry urine from the kidneys. A smooth muscle is attached to the base of each body hair. Contraction of these muscles causes the condition of the skin that we call *gooseflesh*. Smooth muscle cells are of a typical size and taper at each end. They are not striated and have only one nu-

Figure 4-6

Generalized (dense) and structural connective tissue. (A) Fibrous connective tissue. In tendons and ligaments, collagenous fibers are arranged in the same direction. **(B)** In cartilage, the cells (chondrocytes) are enclosed in a firm matrix. **(C)** Bone is the hardest connective tissue. The cells (osteocytes) are within the hard matrix. (A and B, reprinted with permission from Mills SE. *Histology for Pathologists*, 3rd ed. Philadelphia: Lippincott Williams & Wilkins, 2006; C, reprinted with permission from Gartner LP, Hiatt JL. *Color Atlas of Histology*, 4th ed. Baltimore: Lippincott Williams & Wilkins, 2005.)

cleus per cell. Structures containing smooth muscle are discussed in the chapters on the various body systems.

Muscle tissue, like nervous tissue, repairs itself only with difficulty or not at all once an injury has been sustained. When injured, muscle tissue is frequently replaced with connective tissue.

CHECKPOINT 4-6 ➤ What are the three types of muscle tissue?

Nervous Tissue

The human body is made up of countless structures, each of which contributes to the action of the whole organism. This aggregation of structures might be compared to a large corporation. For all the workers in the corporation to coordinate their efforts, there must be some central control, such as the president or CEO. In the body, this central agent is the **brain** (Fig. 4-8A). Each body struc-

ture is in direct communication with the brain by means of its own set of "wires," called **nerves** (see Fig. 4-8B). Nerves from even the most remote parts of the body come together and feed into a great trunk cable called the **spinal cord,** which in turn leads into the central switchboard of the brain. Here, messages come in and orders go out 24 hours a day. Some nerves, the cranial nerves, connect directly with the brain and do not communicate with the spinal cord. This entire control system, including the brain, is made of nervous tissue.

The Neuron

The basic unit of nervous tissue is the **neuron** (NU-ron), or nerve cell (Fig. 4-8C). A neuron consists of a nerve cell body plus small branches from the cell called *fibers*. One type of fiber, the **dendrite** (DEN-drite), is generally short and forms tree-like branches. This type of fiber carries messages in the form of nerve impulses to the nerve cell body. A single fiber, the **axon** (AK-son), carries impulses away from the nerve cell body. Neurons may be quite long; their fibers can extend for several feet. A **nerve** is a bundle of such nerve cell fibers held together with connective tissue (see Fig. 4-8B).

Just as wires are insulated to keep them from being short-circuited, some axons are insulated and protected by a coating of material called **myelin** (MI-eh-lin). Groups of myelinated fibers form "white matter," named for the color of the myelin, which is much like fat in appearance and consistency.

Not all neurons have myelin, however; some axons are unmyelinated, as are all dendrites and all cell bodies. These areas appear gray in color. Because the outer layer of the brain has large collections of cell bodies and unmyelinated fibers, the brain is popularly termed *gray matter,* even though its interior is composed of white matter (see Fig. 4-8A).

Neuroglia

Nervous tissue is supported and protected by specialized cells known as **neuroglia** (nu-ROG-le-ah) or *glial* (GLI-al) *cells,* which are named from the Greek word *glia* meaning "glue." Some of these cells protect the brain from harmful substances; others get rid of foreign organisms and cellular debris; still others form the myelin sheath around axons. They do not, however, transmit nerve impulses.

Membranes

Membranes are thin sheets of tissue. Their properties vary: some are fragile, others tough; some are transparent, others opaque (i.e., they cannot be seen through). Membranes may cover a surface, may be a dividing partition, may line a hollow organ or body cavity, or may anchor an organ. They may contain cells that secrete lubricants to ease the movement of organs, such as the heart and lung, and the movement of joints. Epithelial membranes and connective tissue membranes are described below.

Epithelial Membranes

An **epithelial membrane** is so named because its outer surface is made of epithelium. Underneath, however, there is a layer of connective tissue that strengthens the membrane, and in some cases, there is a thin layer of smooth muscle under that. Epithelial membranes are made of closely packed active cells that manufacture lubricants and protect the deeper tissues from invasion by microorganisms. Epithelial membranes are of several types:

- **Serous** (SE-rus) **membranes** line the walls of body cavities and are folded back onto the surface of internal organs, forming their outermost layer.

- **Mucous** (MU-kus) **membranes** line tubes and other spaces that open to the outside of the body.

- The **cutaneous** (ku-TA-ne-us) **membrane**, commonly known as the **skin**, has an outer layer of epithelium. This membrane is complex and is discussed in detail in Chapter 6.

SEROUS MEMBRANES Serous membranes line the closed ventral body cavities and do not connect with the outside of the body. They secrete a thin, watery lubricant, known as serous fluid, that allows organs to move with a minimum of friction. The thin epithelium of serous membranes is a smooth, glistening kind of tissue called **mesothelium** (mes-o-THE-le-um). The membrane itself may be referred to as the **serosa** (se-RO-sah).

There are three serous membranes:

- The **pleurae** (PLU-re), or **pleuras** (PLU-rahs), line the thoracic cavity and cover each lung.

Figure 4-7 **Muscle tissue. (A)** Skeletal muscle cells have bands (striations) and multiple nuclei. **(B)** Cardiac muscle makes up the wall of the heart. **(C)** Smooth muscle is found in soft body organs and in vessels. (A and C, reprinted with permission from Cormack DH. *Essential Histology*, 2nd ed. Philadelphia: Lippincott Williams & Wilkins, 2001; B, reprinted with permission from Gartner LP, Hiatt JL. *Color Atlas of Histology*, 4th ed. Baltimore: Lippincott Williams & Wilkins, 2005.)

A more detailed discussion of nervous tissue and the nervous system can be found in Chapters 9 and 10.

CHECKPOINT **4-7** ➤ What is the basic cellular unit of the nervous system and what is its function?

CHECKPOINT **4-8** ➤ What are the nonconducting support cells of the nervous system called?

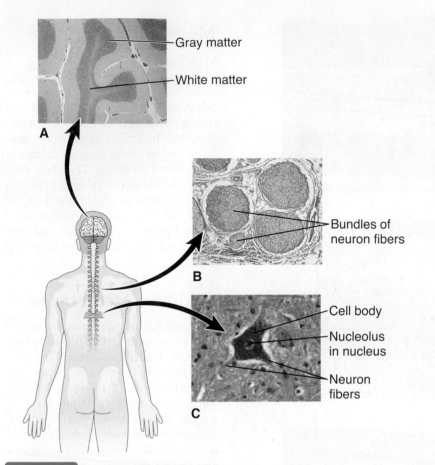

A

- Gray matter
- White matter

B

- Bundles of neuron fibers

C

- Cell body
- Nucleolus in nucleus
- Neuron fibers

Figure 4-8 **Nervous tissue. (A)** Brain tissue. **(B)** Cross-section of a nerve. **(C)** A neuron, or nerve cell. (Reprinted with permission from Cormack DH. *Essential Histology*, 2nd ed. Philadelphia: Lippincott Williams & Wilkins, 2001.)

- The **serous pericardium** (per-ih-KAR-de-um) forms part of a sac that encloses the heart, which is located in the chest between the lungs.

- The **peritoneum** (per-ih-to-NE-um) is the largest serous membrane. It lines the walls of the abdominal cavity, covers the abdominal organs, and forms supporting and protective structures within the abdomen (see Fig. 19-3 in Chapter 19).

Serous membranes are arranged so that one portion forms the lining of a closed cavity, while another part folds back to cover the surface of the organ contained in that cavity. The relationship between an organ and the serous membrane around it can be visualized by imagining your fist punching into a large, soft balloon (Fig. 4-9). Your fist is the organ and the serous membrane around it is in two layers, one against your fist and one folded back to form an outer layer. Although in two layers, each serous membrane is continuous.

The portion of the serous membrane attached to the wall of a cavity or sac is known as the **parietal** (pah-RI-eh-tal) **layer**; the word *parietal* refers to a wall. In the example above, the parietal layer is represented by the outermost layer of the balloon. Parietal pleura lines the thoracic (chest) cavity, and parietal pericardium lines the fibrous

sac (the fibrous pericardium) that encloses the heart (see Fig. 4-9).

Because internal organs are called *viscera*, the portion of the serous membrane attached to an organ is the **visceral layer**. Visceral pericardium is on the surface of the heart, and each lung surface is covered by visceral pleura. Portions of the peritoneum that cover organs in the abdomen are named according to the particular organ involved. The visceral layer in our balloon example is in direct contact with your fist.

A serous membrane's visceral and parietal layers normally are in direct contact with a minimal amount of lubricant between them. The area between the two layers forms a **potential space**. That is, it is *possible* for a space to exist there, although normally one does not. Only if substances accumulate between the layers, as when inflammation causes the production of excessive amounts of fluid, is there an actual space.

MUCOUS MEMBRANES Mucous membranes are so named because they produce a thick and sticky substance called **mucus** (MU-kus). (Note that the adjective *mucous* contains an "o," whereas the noun *mucus* does not.) These membranes form extensive continuous linings in the digestive, respiratory, urinary, and reproductive systems, all of which are connected with the outside of the body. These membranes vary somewhat in both structure and function. The cells that line the nasal cavities and the respiratory passageways are supplied with tiny, hairlike extensions called *cilia*, described in Chapter 3. The microscopic cilia move in waves that force secretions outward. In this way, foreign particles, such as bacteria, dust, and other impurities trapped in the sticky mucus, are prevented from entering the lungs and causing harm. Ciliated epithelium is also found in certain tubes of both the male and the female reproductive systems.

The mucous membranes that line the digestive tract have special functions. For example, the stomach's mucous membrane protects the deeper tissues from the action of powerful digestive juices. If for some reason a portion of this membrane is injured, these juices begin to digest a part of the stomach itself—as happens in cases of peptic ulcers. Mucous membranes located farther along in the digestive system are designed to absorb nutrients, which the blood then transports to all cells.

The noun **mucosa** (mu-KO-sah) refers to the mucous membrane of an organ.

the ends of bones, thus permitting free movement of the joints. Synovial membranes also line small cushioning sacs near the joints called **bursae** (BUR-se).

■ The **meninges** (men-IN-jeze) are several membranous layers covering the brain and the spinal cord.

Fascia (FASH-e-ah) refers to fibrous bands or sheets that support organs and hold them in place. Fascia is found in two regions:

■ **Superficial fascia** is the continuous sheet of tissue that underlies the skin and contains adipose (fat) tissue that insulates the body and protects the skin. This tissue is also called *subcutaneous fascia* because it is located beneath the skin.

■ **Deep fascia** covers, separates, and protects skeletal muscles.

Finally, there are membranes whose names all start with the prefix *peri-* because they are around organs:

■ The **fibrous pericardium** (per-e-KAR-de-um) forms the cavity that encloses the heart, the pericardial cavity. This fibrous sac and the serous pericardial membranes described above are often described together as the pericardium (see Fig. 4-9B).

■ The **periosteum** (per-e-OS-te-um) is the membrane around a bone.

■ The **perichondrium** (per-e-KON-dre-um) is the membrane around cartilage.

Membranes and Disease

We are all familiar with a number of diseases that directly affect membranes. These range from the common cold, which is an inflammation of the nasal mucosa, to the sometimes fatal condition known as **peritonitis**, an infection of the peritoneum, which can follow rupture of the appendix and other mishaps in the abdominal region.

Although membranes usually help to prevent the spread of infection from one area of the body to another, they may sometimes act as pathways along which disease may travel. In general, epithelial membranes appear to have more resistance to infections than do layers made of connective tissue. Lowered resistance, however, may allow the transmission of infection along any membrane. For exam-

Figure 4-9 **Organization of serous membranes. (A)** An organ fits into a serous membrane like a fist punching into a soft balloon. **(B)** The outer layer of a serous membrane is the parietal layer. The inner layer is the visceral layer. The fibrous pericardium reinforces the parietal pericardium.

CHECKPOINT **4-9** ► Epithelial membranes have an outer layer of epithelium. What are the three types of epithelial membranes?

Connective Tissue Membranes

The following list is an overview of membranes that consist of connective tissue with no epithelium. These membranes are described in greater detail in later chapters.

■ **Synovial** (sin-O-ve-al) **membranes** are thin connective tissue membranes that line the joint cavities. They secrete a lubricating fluid that reduces friction between ple, throat infections may travel along mucous membranes into other parts of the upper respiratory tract and even into the sinuses and the ears. In females, an infection may travel up the tubes and spaces of the reproductive system into the peritoneal cavity (see Fig. 23-14 in Chapter 23).

The connective tissue (or collagen) diseases, such as **systemic lupus erythematosus** (LU-pus er-ih-them-ah-TO-sus) (SLE) and **rheumatoid** (RU-mah-toyd) **arthritis**, may affect many parts of the body because collagen is the major intercellular protein in solid connective tissue. In SLE, serous membranes, such as the pleura, pericardium, and peritoneum, are often involved. In rheumatoid arthritis, the synovial membrane becomes inflamed and swollen, and the cartilage in the joints is gradually replaced with fibrous connective tissue.

Benign and Malignant Tumors

For a variety of reasons, the normal pattern of cell and tissue development may be broken by an uncontrolled growth of cells having no purpose in the body. Any abnormal growth of cells is called a **tumor**, or **neoplasm**. If the tumor is confined to a local area and does not spread, it is a **benign** (be-NINE) tumor. If the tumor spreads to neighboring

tissues or to distant parts of the body, it is a **malignant** (mah-LIG-nant) tumor. The general term for any type of malignant tumor is **cancer**. The process of tumor cell spread is called **metastasis** (meh-TAS-tah-sis).

Tumors are found in all kinds of tissue, but they occur most frequently in those tissues that repair themselves most quickly, specifically epithelium and connective tissue, in that order.

Benign Tumors

Benign tumors, theoretically at least, are not dangerous in themselves; they do not spread. Their cells stick together, and often they are encapsulated, that is, surrounded by a containing membrane. The cells in a benign tumor are very similar in appearance to the normal cells from which they are derived (Fig. 4-10A,B). Benign tumors grow as a single mass within a tissue, lending them neatly to complete surgical removal. Medically, they are described as growing *in situ* (SI-tu), meaning that they are confined to their place of origin and do not invade other tissues or spread to other sites. Of course, some benign tumors can be quite harmful; they may grow within an organ, increase in size, and cause considerable mechanical damage. A benign brain tumor, for example, can kill a person just as a malignant one can because

Figure 4-10 **Benign and malignant tumors. (A)** Normal cartilage. **(B)** A benign chondroma closely resembles normal cartilage. **(C)** Chondrosarcoma of bone. The tumor is composed of malignant chondrocytes, which have bizarre shapes and abnormal nuclei. (A and B, Reprinted with permission from Rubin E, Farber JL. *Pathology*, 3rd ed. Philadelphia: Lippincott Williams & Wilkins, 1999; C, Reprinted from Bullough PG, Vigorita VJ. *Atlas of Orthopaedic Pathology*. New York: Gower Medical Publishing, 1984. With permission from Elsevier.)

it grows in an enclosed area and compresses vital brain tissue. Some examples of benign tumors are given below (note that most of the names end in *-oma*, which means "tumor").

- **Papilloma** (pap-ih-LO-mah)—a tumor that grows in epithelium as a projecting mass. One example is a wart.

- **Adenoma** (ad-eh-NO-mah)—an epithelial tumor that grows in and about the glands (*adeno-* means "gland").

- **Lipoma** (lip-O-mah)—a connective tissue tumor originating in fatty (adipose) tissue.

- **Osteoma** (os-te-O-mah)—a connective tissue tumor that originates in the bones.

- **Myoma** (mi-O-mah)—a tumor of muscle tissue. Rare in voluntary muscle, it is common in some types of involuntary muscle, particularly in the uterus (womb). When found in the uterus, however, it is ordinarily called a *fibroid*.

- **Angioma** (an-je-O-mah)—a tumor that usually is composed of small blood or lymphatic vessels; an example is a birthmark.

- **Nevus** (NE-vus)—a small skin tumor that can appear in a variety of tissues. Some nevi are better known as moles; some are angiomas. Ordinarily, these tumors are harmless, but they can become malignant.

- **Chondroma** (kon-DRO-mah)—a tumor of cartilage cells that may remain within the cartilage or develop on the surface, as in the joints (see Fig. 4-10B).

Malignant Tumors

Malignant tumors, unlike benign tumors, can cause death no matter where they occur. Malignant cells are very different in appearance from their parent cells and are unable to function normally (see Fig. 4-10C). Malignant tumors, moreover, grow much more rapidly than benign tumors. The word *cancer* means "crab," and this is descriptive: a cancer sends out clawlike extensions into neighboring tissue. Cancer cells also spread by either the blood or the lymph (another circulating fluid), and when they arrive at other sites, they form new (secondary) growths, or **metastases** (meh-TAS-tah-seze).

Malignant tumors are classified into two main categories according to whether they originate in epithelial or connective tissue:

- **Carcinoma** (kar-sih-NO-mah). This type of cancer originates in epithelium and is by far the most common form of cancer. Usual sites of carcinoma are the skin, mouth, lung, breast, stomach, colon, prostate, and uterus. Carcinomas are usually spread by the lymphatic system (see Chapter 16).

- **Sarcoma** (sar-KO-mah). These are cancers of connective tissue and therefore may be found anywhere in the body. Their cells are usually spread by the blood, and they often form metastases in the lungs. The cells of a chondrosarcoma, a tumor that arises from cartilage cells, is shown in Figure 4-10C.

Cancers of the nervous system, lymphatic system, and blood are classified differently according to the cells in which they originate as well as other clinical features. A **neuroma** (nu-RO-mah) is a tumor that arises from a nerve. Because nervous tissue does not multiply throughout life, however, it is rarely involved in cancer. Usually, a nervous system tumor originates in the support (neuroglial) tissue of the brain or spinal cord and is called a **glioma** (gli-O-mah). A malignant neoplasm of lymphatic tissue is called a **lymphoma** (lim-FO-mah), and cancer of white blood cells is **leukemia** (lu-KE-me-ah).

CHECKPOINT 4-10 ➤ What is the difference between a benign and a malignant tumor?

Symptoms of Cancer

Everyone should be familiar with certain signs that may indicate early cancer and should report these signs for further investigation by their healthcare provider. Early symptoms may include unusual bleeding or discharge, persistent indigestion, chronic hoarseness or cough, changes in the color or size of moles, a sore that does not heal in a reasonable time, the presence of an unusual lump, and the presence of white patches inside the mouth or white spots on the tongue. Late symptoms of cancer include weight loss and pain. Many cancers are now diagnosed by routine screening tests that are part of the standard physical examination.

Diagnosis of Cancer

Improved methods of cancer detection lead to earlier and more successful treatment. These methods include the following:

- **Microscopic study** of tissue or cells removed from the body. **Biopsy** (BI-op-se) is the removal of living tissue for the purpose of microscopic examination. Specimens can be obtained by needle withdrawal (aspiration) of fluid; by a small punch, as of the skin; by an endoscope (lighted tube) introduced into a body cavity; or by surgical removal (excision). In some cases, fluids can be examined for signs of cancerous cells, as these cells often slough off into surrounding fluids. The most common example of this type of cytologic study is the Pap (Papanicolaou) test for cancer of the uterine cervix. Pleural or peritoneal fluids also may be studied for signs of cancerous cells.

- **Radiography** is the use of x-rays to obtain images of internal structures. A common application of this method is mammography, x-ray study of the breast. Radiologists can examine other structures such as the lungs, nervous system, and digestive system by this method, although they often need a contrast medium to show changes in soft tissues.

- **Ultrasound** (ultrasonography) is the use of reflected high-frequency sound waves to differentiate various kinds of tissue.

- **Computed tomography** (CT) is the use of x-rays to produce a cross-sectional picture of body parts, such as the brain (see Fig. 10-12A in Chapter 10).

- **Magnetic resonance imaging** (MRI) is the use of magnetic fields and radio waves to show changes in soft tissues.

- **Positron emission tomography** (PET) shows activity within an organ by computerized interpretation of the radiation emitted following administration of a radioactive substance, such as glucose. This method has been used to diagnose lung and brain tumors.

 PASSport to Success Visit *thePoint* or see the Student Resource CD in the back of this book for information on careers in histotechnology—the laboratory study of tissues.

NEW METHODS OF DIAGNOSIS Tests for tumor markers are newer approaches to cancer diagnosis. Tumor markers are substances, such as hormones, enzymes, or other proteins, produced in greater than normal quantity by cancerous cells. Laboratories can detect these markers in cells or in body fluids, such as blood. The most widely used of these screenings is for PSA (prostate-specific antigen), a protein produced in large quantity by prostatic tumors. Some others are CA 125 in ovarian cancer, AFP (alpha-fetoprotein) in liver cancer, CEA (carcinoembryonic antigen) in digestive system and breast cancers, and CD antigens (proteins) in blood and lymphatic cancers. Although tumor markers are often produced in amounts too small to be detected early in the disease process, physicians can still use them to monitor treatment.

In some instances, cancer has been linked to changes in a person's genetic makeup. In these cases, a certain type of cancer would "run in families," and people could be genetically tested for a predisposition to that form of the disease. The clearest correlation between genetics and cancer has been established in a small percentage of breast cancers.

STAGING Oncologists (cancer specialists) use diagnostic studies for a process called staging, which is a procedure for establishing the extent of tumor spread, both at the original site and in other locations (metastases). **Staging** is important for selecting and evaluating therapy and for predicting the disease's outcome. The method commonly used for staging is the TNM system. These letters stand for primary tumor (T), regional lymph nodes (N), and distant metastases (M). Based on TNM results, a stage ranging in Roman numerals from I to IV in severity is assigned. Cancers of the blood, lymphatic system, and nervous system are evaluated by different methods.

Treatment of Cancer

Some standard cancer treatments are described first, followed by some newer approaches. Note that various treatment methods may be combined. For example, chemotherapy alone or with radiation therapy may precede surgery, or surgery may be performed before other treatment is given.

SURGERY Benign tumors usually can be removed completely by surgery. Malignant tumors cannot be treated so easily. If cancerous tissue is removed surgically, there is always the possibility that a few hidden cells will be left behind to resume tumor growth. If the cells have metastasized (spread) to distant locations, the predicted outcome is usually much less favorable.

The **laser** (LA-zer) is a device that produces a highly concentrated and intense beam of light. It is used to destroy tumors or as a cutting device for removing a tumorous growth. The laser's important advantages are its ability to coagulate blood and prevent bleeding and its capacity to direct a narrow beam of light accurately and attack harmful cells while avoiding normal cells.

Other methods for destroying cancerous tissue include electrosurgery, which uses high-frequency current; cryosurgery, which uses extreme cold generated by liquid nitrogen; and chemosurgery, which employs chemicals.

RADIATION Sometimes, surgery is preceded or followed by radiation. Radiation therapy is administered by x-ray machines or by the placement of small amounts of radioactive material within the involved organ. These materials can be in the form of needles, beads, seeds, or other devices. Some radioactive chemicals can be injected or taken orally. Radiation destroys the more rapidly dividing cancer cells while causing less damage to the more slowly dividing normal cells. A goal in radiation therapy is accurate focus of the radiation beam to reduce damage to normal body structures.

CHEMOTHERAPY Chemotherapy is a general term for treatment with drugs, but often the term is understood to mean the treatment of cancer with **antineoplastic** (an-ti-ne-o-PLAS-tik) **agents**. These agents are drugs that act selectively on actively growing cells, and they are most effective when used in combination. Certain types of leukemia, various cancers of the lymphatic system, and other forms of cancer often are treated effectively by this means. Researchers continue to develop new drugs and more effective drug combinations. Although antineoplastic agents are more toxic to tumor cells than to normal cells, they do also damage normal cells and must be administered under careful control by health professionals who understand the complications they may cause. Patients who receive these drugs, because of their weakened state, are subject to the development of opportunistic infections; that is, infections that develop in a person who has been weakened by disease.

NEWER APPROACHES TO CANCER TREATMENT The immune system constantly works to protect the body against abnormal and unwanted cells, a category that includes tumor cells. **Immunotherapy** involves the use of substances that stimulate the immune system as a whole or vaccines prepared specifically against a tumor to control growth. In certain types of breast cancer, antibodies have been used to block receptor sites for a factor that stimulates tumor growth.

Some cancers, such as those of the breast, testis, and prostate, are stimulated to grow more rapidly by hormones. Counteracting hormones or other chemicals that block receptors for the stimulants can be used to restrict tumor growth in these tissues.

For a tumor to establish itself, new blood vessels must develop and supply the rapidly growing cells with nutrients and oxygen. Some attempts have been made to block tumor growth by preventing this process of angiogenesis (growth of blood vessels).

CHECKPOINT 4-11 ➤ What are the three standard approaches to the treatment of cancer?

Tissues and Aging

With aging, tissues lose elasticity and collagen becomes less flexible. These changes affect the skin most noticeably, but internal changes occur as well. The blood vessels, for example, have a reduced capacity to expand. Less blood supply and lower metabolism slow the healing process. Tendons and ligaments stretch, causing a stooped posture and joint instability. Bones may lose calcium salts, becoming brittle and prone to fracture. With age,

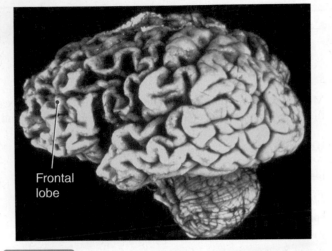

Frontal lobe

Figure 4-11 Atrophy of the brain. Brain tissue has thinned and larger spaces appear between sections of tissue, especially in the frontal lobe. (Reprinted with permission from Okazaki H, Scheithauer BW. *Atlas of Neuropathology.* New York: Gower Medical Publishing, 1988. By permission of the author.)

muscles and other tissues waste from loss of cells, a process termed *atrophy* (AT-ro-fe) (Fig. 4-11). Changes that apply to specific organs and systems are described in later chapters.

Disease in Context revisited

➤ Ben's Cystic Fibrosis

Ben's parents were shocked when the doctor diagnosed their 2-year-old with cystic fibrosis. Their immediate concern was, of course, for their son. The doctor reassured them that with proper treatment their son could lead a relatively normal life and that in the future, new therapies might even offer a cure. He asserted that they were not to blame for Ben's condition. Cystic fibrosis is an inherited disease—Ben's parents each carried a defective gene in their DNA and both had, by chance, passed copies to Ben. As a result, Ben was unable to synthesize a channel protein found in the plasma membranes of exocrine gland cells. Normally, this channel regulates the movement of chloride into the cell. Because the channels did not work in Ben's epithelial cells, chloride was trapped outside the cells. The negatively charged chloride ions attract positively charged sodium ions normally found in extracellular fluid. These two ions form the salt, sodium chloride, which is lost in high amounts in the sweat of individuals with cystic fibrosis.

Although the exact reason is still unclear, abnormal chloride channel function causes epithelial glands in many organs to produce thick, sticky mucus. In the lungs, this mucus causes difficulty breathing, inflammation, and bacterial infection. The thick mucus also decreases the ability of the large and small intestines to absorb nutrients, resulting in low weight gain, poor growth, and vitamin deficiencies. This problem is compounded by damage to the pancreas, preventing production of essential digestive enzymes.

During this case, we saw that a defective membrane channel in Ben's epithelial cells had wide-spread effects on his whole body. In later chapters, as you learn about the body's organs, remember that their structure and function are closely related to the condition of their constituent tissues. Cystic fibrosis is an inherited disease. The case study in Chapter 25, Heredity and Hereditary Diseases, will follow Alison as she learns more about Ben's condition.

Word Anatomy

Medical terms are built from standardized word parts (prefixes, roots, and suffixes). Learning the meanings of these parts can help you remember words and interpret unfamiliar terms.

WORD PART	MEANING	EXAMPLE
hist/o	tissue	*Histology* is the study of tissues.
Epithelial Tissue		
epi-	on, upon	*Epithelial* tissue covers body surfaces.
pseud/o-	false	*Pseudostratified* epithelium appears to be in multiple layers but is not.
Connective Tissue		
-blast	immature cell, early stage of cell	A *fibroblast* is a cell that produces fibers.
chondr/o	cartilage	A *chondrocyte* is a cartilage cell.
oss, osse/o	bone, bone tissue	*Osseous* tissue is bone tissue.
oste/o	bone, bone tissue	An *osteocyte* is a mature bone cell.
Muscle Tissue		
my/o	muscle	The *myocardium* is the heart muscle.
cardi/o	heart	See preceding example.
Nervous Tissue		
neur/o	nerve, nervous system	A *neuron* is a nerve cell.
Membranes		
pleur/o	side, rib	The *pleurae* are membranes that line the chest cavity.
peri-	around	The *peritoneum* wraps around the abdominal organs.
-itis	inflammation	*Peritonitis* is inflammation of the peritoneum.
arthr/o	joint	*Arthritis* is inflammation of a joint.
Benign and Malignant Tumors		
neo-	new	A *neoplasm* is an abnormal growth of new cells, a tumor.
mal-	bad, disordered, diseased, abnormal	A *malignant* tumor spreads to other parts of the body.
-oma	tumor, swelling	A *lipoma* is a tumor that originates in adipose (fatty) tissue.
onc/o	tumor	An *oncologist* is a specialist in cancer treatment.
papill/o	nipple	A *papilloma* is a projecting (nipple-like) tumor, such as a wart.
aden/o	gland	An *adenoma* is a tumor of a gland.
angi/o	vessel	An *angioma* is a tumor composed of small vessels.
leuk/o-	white, colorless	*Leukemia* is a cancer of white blood cells.
graph/o	writing, record	*Mammography* is x-ray imaging (radiography) of the breast (mamm/o).
ultra-	beyond	*Ultrasound* is high-frequency sound waves.
ant/i-	against	An *antineoplastic* agent is a drug active against cancer.

Summary

I.   **TISSUE CLASSIFICATION**—epithelial tissue, connective tissue, muscle tissue, nervous tissue

II. **EPITHELIAL TISSUE**—covers surfaces; lines cavities, organs, and ducts
   A. Cells—squamous, cuboidal, columnar
   B. Arrangement—simple or stratified
   C. Special functions
      1. Produces secretions, e.g., mucus, digestive juices, sweat
      2. Filters impurities using cilia
   D. Glands—active cells are epithelial cells
      1. Exocrine
         a. Secrete through ducts
         b. Examples: digestive glands, tear glands, sweat and oil glands of skin
      2. Endocrine
         a. Secrete into body fluids and bloodstream
         b. Produce hormones

III. **CONNECTIVE TISSUE**—supports, binds, forms framework of body
   A. Circulating—fluid matrix; travels in vessels
      1. Blood
      2. Lymph
   B. Generalized—widely distributed; not specialized
      1. Loose—cells and fibers in semiliquid matrix
         a. Areolar—in membranes, around vessels and organs, under skin
         b. Adipose—stores fat; insulation, padding, energy reserve
      2. Dense—has many fibers (e.g. collagenous, elastic) made by fibroblasts
         a. Irregular—fibers not organized; in membranes, capsules
         b. Regular—fibers in parallel alignment; in tendons, ligaments
         c. Elastic—fibers can stretch and return to shape; in vocal cords, respiratory passageways, blood vessel walls
   C. Structural—mainly associated with skeleton
      1. Cartilage
         a. Strong and flexible
         b. Cushions and absorbs shock
         c. Produced by chondrocytes
         d. Types
            (1) Hyaline—covers ends of bones, makes up tip of nose, reinforces larynx and trachea
            (2) Fibrocartilage—in certain joints
            (3) Elastic—in outer ear, larynx
      2. Bone
         a. Matrix contains mineral salts

         b. Cells
            (1) Osteoblasts—produce bone
            (2) Osteocytes—mature bone cells

IV. **MUSCLE TISSUE**—contracts to produce movement
   A. Types
      1. Skeletal muscle—voluntary; moves skeleton
      2. Cardiac muscle—involuntary; forms main part of the heart
      3. Smooth muscle—involuntary; forms visceral organs

V.   **NERVOUS TISSUE**
   A. Neuron—nerve cell
      1. Cell body—contains nucleus
      2. Dendrite—fiber carrying impulses toward cell body
      3. Axon—fiber carrying impulses away from cell body
         a. Myelin—fatty material that insulates some axons
            (1) Myelinated fibers—make up white matter
            (2) Unmyelinated cells and fibers—make up gray matter
   B. Neuroglia—support and protect nervous tissue

VI. **MEMBRANES**—thin sheets of tissue
   A. Epithelial membranes—outer layer epithelium
      1. Serous membrane—secretes watery fluid
         a. Parietal layer—lines body cavity
         b. Visceral layer—covers internal organs
         c. Examples—pleurae, pericardium, peritoneum
      2. Mucous membrane
         a. Secretes mucus
         b. Lines tube or space that opens to the outside (e.g., respiratory, digestive, reproductive tracts)
      3. Cutaneous membrane—skin
   B. Connective tissue membranes
      1. Synovial membrane—lines joint cavity
      2. Meninges—around brain and spinal cord
      3. Fascia—under skin and around muscles
      4. Pericardium—around heart; periosteum—around bone; perichondrium—around cartilage
   C. Membranes and disease—may confine infection, but may be route for spread

VII. **BENIGN AND MALIGNANT TUMORS**—tumor (neoplasm) results from uncontrolled growth of cells
   A. Benign tumor—localized
   B. Malignant tumor—invades tissue and metastasizes (spreads) to other locations
      1. Carcinoma—originates in epithelium
      2. Sarcoma—cancer of connective tissue

3. Others—cancers of nervous system, lymphatic system, blood
C. Symptoms of cancer—bleeding, persistent indigestion, hoarseness or cough, change in mole, lump, nonhealing sore, pain, weight loss
D. Diagnosis of cancer
  1. Microscopic study (biopsy to obtain specimen), ultrasound, CT, MRI, PET
    a. Also blood tests for markers, genetic tests

2. Staging—classification based on size of tumor and extent of invasion
E. Treatment of cancer
  1. Surgical removal
  2. Radiation
  3. Chemotherapy—drugs
  4. Others—immunotherapy, hormones, inhibitors of blood vessel formation
VIII. TISSUES AND AGING

Questions for Study and Review

BUILDING UNDERSTANDING

Fill in the blanks

1. A group of similar cells arranged in a characteristic pattern is called a(n) _____.

2. Glands that secrete their products directly into the blood are called _____ glands.

3. Tissue that supports and forms the framework of the body is called _____ tissue.

4. A tumor that is confined to a local area and does not spread is a(n) _____ tumor.

5. The removal of living tissue for the purpose of microscopic examination is called _____.

Matching > Match each numbered item with the most closely related lettered item.

___ 6. Membrane around the heart

___ 7. Membrane around each lung

___ 8. Membrane around bone

___ 9. Membrane around cartilage

___ 10. Membrane around abdominal organs

a. perichondrium
b. pericardium
c. peritoneum
d. periosteum
e. pleura

Multiple Choice

___ 11. Epithelium composed of a single layer of long and narrow cells is called
  a. simple cuboidal epithelium
  b. simple columnar epithelium
  c. stratified cuboidal epithelium
  d. stratified columnar epithelium

___ 12. Tendons and ligaments are examples of
  a. areolar connective tissue
  b. loose connective tissue
  c. regular, dense connective tissue
  d. cartilage

___ 13. A tissue composed of long striated cells with multiple nuclei is
  a. smooth muscle tissue
  b. cardiac muscle tissue
  c. skeletal muscle tissue
  d. nervous tissue

___ 14. A bundle of nerve cell fibers held together with connective tissue is called a(n)
  a. dendrite
  b. axon
  c. nerve
  d. myelin

___ 15. All of the following are types of epithelial membranes except
  a. cutaneous membrane
  b. mucous membrane
  c. serous membrane
  d. synovial membrane

UNDERSTANDING CONCEPTS

16. Explain how epithelium is classified and discuss at least three functions of this tissue type.

17. Compare the structure and function of exocrine and endocrine glands and give two examples of each type.

18. Describe the functions of connective tissue. Name two kinds of fibers found in connective tissue and discuss how their presence affects tissue function.

19. Compare and contrast the three different types of muscle tissue.

20. Compare serous and mucous membranes.

21. Describe the difference between a benign tumor and a malignant tumor.

22. Define the term *cancer* and name some of its early symptoms. How is cancer diagnosed? How is it treated?

CONCEPTUAL THINKING

23. Prolonged exposure to cigarette smoke causes damage to ciliated epithelium that lines portions of the respiratory tract. Discuss the implications of this damage.

24. The middle ear is connected to the throat by a tube called the eustachian (auditory) tube. All are lined by a continuous mucous membrane. Using this information, describe why a throat infection (pharyngitis) may lead to an ear infection (otitis media).

25. In cystic fibrosis, the production of abnormally thick sticky mucus results in lung and digestive disorders. What are some of the normal functions of mucus in the body?

26. In Ben's case, an abnormal epithelial channel protein had widespread effects. Another hereditary disease, osteogenesis imperfecta, is characterized by abnormal collagen fiber synthesis. Which tissue type would be most affected by this disorder? List some possible symptoms of this disease.

Disease and the First Line of Defense

II

The first chapter in this unit discusses deviation from the normal, which is the basis for disease. After a general discussion of different types of diseases, the chapter concentrates on infectious diseases and the organisms that cause them, including bacteria, viruses, fungi, protozoa, and worms. Other forms of disease are discussed in chapters on the individual body systems. The skin is the first defense against infections, organisms, and other sources of injury. The properties and functions of the skin are discussed in the second chapter of this unit.

CHAPTER 5

Disease and Disease-Producing Organisms

Learning Outcomes

After careful study of this chapter, you should be able to:

1. Define *disease* and list seven categories of disease
2. List seven predisposing causes of disease
3. Define terminology used in describing and treating disease
4. Define *complementary and alternative medicine*; cite several alternative or complementary fields of practice
5. Explain methods by which microorganisms can be transmitted from one host to another
6. List four types of organisms studied in microbiology and give the characteristics of each
7. List some diseases caused by each type of microorganism
8. Define *normal flora* and explain the value of the normal flora
9. Describe the three types of bacteria according to shape
10. List several diseases in humans caused by worms
11. Give some reasons for the emergence and spread of microorganisms today
12. Describe several public health measures taken to prevent the spread of disease
13. Differentiate *sterilization*, *disinfection*, and *antisepsis*
14. Describe techniques included as part of body substance precautions
15. List some antimicrobial agents and describe how they work
16. Describe several methods used to identify microorganisms in the laboratory
17. Show how word parts are used to build words related to disease (see Word Anatomy at the end of the chapter)

Selected Key Terms

The following terms and other boldface terms in the chapter are defined in the Glossary

acute
antisepsis
asepsis
chronic
diagnosis
disease
disinfection
epidemic
etiology
helminth
microorganism
nosocomial infection
opportunistic infection
pathogen
pathophysiology
prion
prognosis
sign
spore
sterilization
symptom
syndrome
systemic
therapy
toxin
vector

Disease
in Context

> ## Maria's Case: When Pathogens Attack

The man sharing the elevator with Maria Sanchez looked terrible—watery eyes, runny nose, and a sickly, run-down appearance. As the elevator opened and the man stepped toward the doors, he let out a loud sneeze. "Pardon me," he said, as the elevator closed behind him. *If I was that sick, I'd stay in bed*, Maria thought. Maria didn't know it yet, but soon she would be.

The passenger left something behind when he exited the elevator. Microscopic droplets of mucus and water from his sneeze floated in the air. Inside each droplet were thousands of microorganisms, called viruses, capable of making Maria very sick. She inhaled several of these germ-laden droplets into her respiratory system as she waited for the elevator to reach her floor. Maria exited the elevator unaware that her body had been invaded.

Maria's warm, moist respiratory tract was a perfect environment for this microorganism. When a virus landed on the epithelial tissue lining her throat, protein spikes protruding from its surface fit snugly into receptors on an epithelial cell, stimulating endocytosis of the virus. Having successfully "picked the lock" on the cell's plasma membrane, the virus was inside the cell and ready to begin the second phase of its attack!

Shortly after entering the cell, the virus released its RNA, which was then transported into the cell's nucleus. Unable to recognize the viral RNA as foreign, the nucleus transcribed it into viral messenger RNA. Returning to the cytoplasm, this new RNA was translated into viral proteins at the ribosomes. Some of these proteins were combined with viral RNA to make new viruses. Others took over the machinery of the host cell to make more viral components.

Since entering the epithelial cell about 24 hours ago, the virus had successfully hijacked cellular RNA and protein synthesis. The cell had been turned into a virus-making factory! With the cell nearly exhausted, the new viruses that filled its cytoplasm exited to infect new hosts. Although finally free of the pathogen, the cell had no more resources left and died.

Maria Sanchez' body has been invaded by the influenza virus. In this chapter, we'll learn more about viruses as well as other disease-producing organisms. Later in the case, we'll see how Maria's body is coping with its unwanted visitors.

Box 5-1 A Closer Look

The CDC: Making People Safer and Healthier

The Centers for Disease Control and Prevention (CDC) in Atlanta, Georgia, is responsible for protecting and improving the health of the American public—at home and abroad. Established in 1946, the CDC has become a world leader in the fight against infectious disease, with an expanded role that now includes control and prevention of chronic diseases such as cancer, heart disease, and stroke. The CDC also works to protect the public from environmental hazards such as waterborne illnesses, weather emergencies, biologic and chemical terrorism, and dangers in the home and workplace. In addition, the CDC provides education to guide informed health and lifestyle decisions.

The CDC's stated goal is "healthy people in a healthy world—through prevention." During the 1940s, the newly created CDC joined state and local health officials in the fight against malaria. In the 1950s, it participated in the fight against polio, which has virtually been eliminated in the

United States and elsewhere. In the 1960s, the CDC joined the World Health Organization in efforts to eradicate smallpox worldwide, and in the 1970s, it identified the pathogen responsible for Legionnaires disease. In the 1980s, the CDC reported the first cases of AIDS and began intensive research on the disease, which continues today. During the 1990s, CDC researchers rapidly identified the strain of hantavirus that caused a serious and often fatal pulmonary disease in people in the southwestern U.S. and investigated an outbreak of deadly Ebola virus in Zaire. Currently, the CDC is working with laboratories throughout the U.S. to identify and control the organisms that cause West Nile disease and influenza.

The CDC employs about 8,500 people in state, federal, and foreign locations. They work in more than 170 occupations, including health information, laboratory science, and microbiology.

Frequently, the physician uses laboratory tests to help establish the diagnosis. Common methods used for diagnosis include imaging studies, blood tests, and study of tissues removed in biopsy. A **prognosis** (prog-NO-sis) is a prediction of the probable outcome of a disease based on the patient's condition and the physician's knowledge about the disease (*prognosis* is from the Greek word *gnosis* meaning "knowledge").

Nurses and other healthcare professionals play an extremely valuable role in the diagnostic process by observing closely for signs, collecting and organizing information from the patient about his or her symptoms, and then reporting this information to the physician. Once a patient's disorder is known, the physician prescribes a course of treatment, known as **therapy**. Treatment may include drugs, surgery, radiation, counseling, physical or occupational therapy, and many other measures, alone or in combinations. Specific measures in a course of treatment include those carried out by the nurse and other healthcare providers under the physician's orders.

Complementary and Alternative Medicine

The term *complementary and alternative medicine* (CAM) refers to methods of disease prevention or treatment that can be used along with or instead of traditional modern medical practices. Many of these nontraditional approaches have a long history in ancient philosophies and practices. Some examples of complementary and alternative practices are:

- **Naturopathy** (na-chur-OP-a-the), a philosophy of helping people to heal themselves by developing healthy lifestyles
- **Chiropractic** (ki-ro-PRAK-tik), a field that stresses manipulation to correct misalignment for treatment of musculoskeletal disorders
- **Acupuncture** (AK-u-punk-chur), an ancient Chinese method of inserting thin needles into the body at specific points to relieve pain or promote healing
- **Biofeedback** (bi-o-FEED-bak), which teaches people to control involuntary responses, such as heart rate and blood pressure, by means of electronic devices that monitor changes and feed information back to a person

Exercise, massage, yoga, meditation, nutritional counseling, and other health-promoting practices are also included under this heading.

The U.S. National Institutes of Health (NIH) has established the National Center for Complementary and Alternative Medicine (NCCAM) to study the value of these therapies.

HERBAL REMEDIES The use of plant-derived remedies has increased in industrialized countries in recent years. Many plant products are used as conventional drugs, but typically they are measured, purified, and often modified instead of being used in their natural state. Questions of purity, safety, dosage, and effectiveness have arisen in the use of herbal remedies as, to date, they have not been tested as rigorously as conventional drugs. The U.S. government does not test or regulate herbal remedies, and there are no requirements to report their adverse effects. There are, however, restrictions on the health claims that can be made by the manufacturers, and the U.S. Food and Drug Administration (FDA) can withdraw products from the market that cause unreasonable risk of harm at the recommended doses. The U.S. Office of Dietary Supplements (ODS) supports and coordinates research on herbal preparations.

Prevention of Disease

In recent years, physicians, nurses, and other healthcare workers have taken on increasing responsibilities in disease prevention. Throughout most of medical history, the physician's aim has been to cure patients of existing diseases. The modern concept of prevention, however, seeks to stop disease before it actually happens—to keep people well through the promotion of health. Areas of improvement include cessation of smoking, improved diet, weight control, and adequate exercise. A vast number of organizations exist for the purpose of promoting health, ranging from the World Health Organization (WHO) on an international level to local private, governmental, and community health programs. In the U.S., the Centers for Disease Control and Prevention (CDC) plays an important role in the study of disease (see Box 5-1). A rapidly growing responsibility of all people in health occupations is educating patients on the maintenance of total health, both physical and mental.

CHECKPOINT 5-5 ➤ A physician uses signs and symptoms to identify an illness. What is this identification called?

Infectious Disease

A predominant cause of disease in humans is the invasion of the body by disease-producing **microorganisms** (mi-kro-OR-gan-izms). The word *organism* means "anything having life"; *micro* means "very small." Thus, a microorganism is a tiny living thing, too small to be seen by the naked eye. Other terms for microorganism are *microbe* and, more popularly, *germ*. A microbe, or any other organism, that lives on or within a living **host** and at the host's expense is called a **parasite**.

Although most microorganisms are harmless to humans, and many are beneficial, a few types cause illness; that is, they are **pathogenic** (path-o-JEN-ic). Any disease-causing organism is a **pathogen** (PATH-o-jen). If the body is invaded by pathogens, with adverse effects, the condition is called an **infection**. If the infection is restricted to a relatively small area of the body, it is local; a generalized, or **systemic** (sis-TEM-ik), infection is one that affects the whole body. Systemic infections are usually spread by the blood.

An infection that takes hold because the host has been compromised (weakened) by disease is described as an **opportunistic infection**. For example, people with depressed immune systems, such as those with AIDS, become infected with organisms that are ordinarily harmless.

MODES OF TRANSMISSION A **communicable** disease is one that can be transmitted from one person to another; it is contagious or "catching." Organisms may be transmitted from an infected host to a new host by direct or indirect contact. For example, infected human hosts may transfer their microorganisms directly to other individuals by touching, shaking hands, kissing, or having sexual intercourse. Microorganisms may be transferred indirectly through touched objects, such as bedding, toys, food, and dishes.

The atmosphere is a carrier of microorganisms. Although microbes cannot fly, the dust in the air is alive with them. In close quarters, germ-laden droplets discharged by sneezing, coughing, and even normal conversation contaminate the atmosphere. Insects and other pests may deposit infectious material on food, skin, or clothing. Pathogens are also spread by such pests as rats, mice, fleas, lice, flies, and mosquitoes. Pets may be an indirect source of some infections.

An insect bite may introduce infectious organisms into the body. An insect or other animal that transmits a disease-causing organism from one host to another is termed a **vector** (VEK-tor). Crowded conditions and poor sanitation increase the spread of disease organisms by all of these mechanisms. (See Box 5-2, The Cold Facts about the Common Cold.)

PORTALS OF ENTRY AND EXIT There are several avenues through which microorganisms may enter the body: the skin, respiratory tract, and digestive system, as well as the urinary and reproductive systems. These portals of entry may also serve as exit routes, leading to the spread of infection. For example, discharges from the respiratory and intestinal tracts may spread infection through air, by contamination of hands, and by contamination of food and water supplies.

Control of infectious disease involves breaking the "chain of infection" by which microorganisms spread through a population. Microbial control is discussed later in this chapter.

> **PASSport to Success**
> Visit *thePoint* or see the Student Resource CD in the back of this book for a chart and illustrations pertaining to disease transmission.

CHECKPOINT 5-6 ➤ What is the relationship between a parasite and a host?

CHECKPOINT 5-7 ➤ What term describes any disease-causing organism?

Box 5-2   Health Maintenance

The Cold Facts about the Common Cold

Every year, an estimated one billion Americans suffer from the symptoms of the common cold—runny nose, sneezing, coughing, and headache. Although most cases are mild and usually last about a week, colds are the leading cause of doctor visits and missed days at work and school.

Colds are caused by a viral infection of the mucous membranes of the upper respiratory tract. More than 200 different viruses are known to cause cold symptoms. While most colds occur in winter, scientists think that cold weather does not increase the risk of "catching" a cold; the incidence is probably higher in winter because people spend more time indoors, increasing the chances that the virus will spread from person to person.

Colds spread primarily from contact with a contaminated surface. When an infected person coughs or sneezes, small droplets of water filled with viral particles are propelled through the air. One unshielded sneeze may spread hundreds of thousands of viral particles several feet. Depending upon temperature and humidity, these particles may live as long as 3 to 6 hours, and others who touch the contaminated surface may pick up the particles on their hands.

To help prevent the transmission of cold viruses:

- Avoid close contact with someone who is sneezing or coughing.
- Wash hands frequently to remove any viral particles you may have picked up.
- Avoid touching or rubbing your eyes, nose, or mouth with contaminated hands.
- Clean contaminated surfaces with disinfectant.

There are currently no medically proven cures for the common cold and treatments only ease the symptoms. Because viruses cause the common cold, antibiotics are of no benefit. Getting plenty of rest and drinking lots of fluids are the best ways to speed recovery.

CHECKPOINT **5-8** ➤ What are some portals of entry and exit for microorganisms?

Microbiology—The Study of Microorganisms

Microorganisms are simple, usually single-cell, forms of life. The group includes bacteria, viruses, fungi, protozoa, and algae. The study of these microscopic organisms is **microbiology** (mi-kro-bi-OL-o-je). The organisms included in the study of microbiology along with their scientific specialties are listed here and summarized in Table 5-1:

- **Bacteria** (bak-te-re-ah) are primitive, single-cell organisms that grow in a wide variety of environments. The study of bacteria, both beneficial and disease producing, is **bacteriology** (bak-te-re-OL-o-je). The group includes rickettsiae and chlamydiae, which are extremely small bacteria that multiply within living cells.

- **Viruses** (VI-rus-es) are extremely small infectious agents that can multiply only within living cells. **Virology** (vi-ROL-o-je) is the study of viruses.

- **Fungi** (FUN-ji) are a group that included yeasts and molds. **Mycology** (mi-KOL-o-je) is the study of fungi (the root *myco-* refers to a fungus).

- **Protozoa** (pro-to-ZO-ah) are single-cell animals. Their study is **protozoology** (pro-to-zo-OL-o-je). Although the term *parasitology* (par-ah-si-TOL-o-je) is the study of parasites in general, in practice, it usually refers to the study of protozoa and worms (helminths).

- **Algae** (AL-je) are very simple multicellular or single-cell aquatic plants. Their study is **algology** (al-GOL-o-je). These organisms rarely cause diseases and will not be described any further in this chapter.

Despite the fact that this discussion centers on pathogens, most microorganisms are harmless to humans and are actually essential to the continuation of all life on earth. Algae, single-cell plants, produce a large proportion of the oxygen we breathe, and they are food for aquatic animals. Through the actions of microorganisms, dead animals and plants are decomposed and transformed into substances that enrich the soil. Sewage is rendered harmless by microorganisms. Several bacterial groups transform atmospheric nitrogen into a form that plants can use, a process called *nitrogen fixation*. Farmers take advantage of this capacity by allowing a field to lie fallow (untilled) so that microorganisms can replenish the nitrogen in its soil. Certain bacteria and fungi produce the antibiotics that make our lives safer. Others produce the fermented products that make our lives more enjoyable, such as beer, wine, cheeses, and yogurt.

Normal Flora

We have a population of microorganisms that normally grows on and within our bodies. We live in balance with these organisms, which make up the **normal flora**. These

| Table 5-1 | Organisms Studied in Microbiology |

Type of Organism	Name of Study	Characteristics of Organisms	Representative Examples
Bacteria	Bacteriology	Simple, single-cell organisms. Grow in many environments. Lack a true nucleus and most organelles.	Bacteria
Viruses	Virology	Composed of nucleic acid (DNA or RNA) and protein. Can reproduce only within living cells—obligate intracellular parasites.	Viruses
Fungi	Mycology	Very simple, non-green, plantlike organisms. Single-cell forms are yeasts; filamentous forms are molds.	Fungi
Protozoa	Protozoology	Single-cell, animal-like organisms.	Protozoa
Algae	Algology	Simple aquatic plants. Not parasitic.	Algae

populations are beneficial because they crowd out and prevent the growth of other harmful varieties of organisms. Some microorganisms that are normally harmless may become pathogenic if the normal flora are destroyed, as by the administration of antibiotics that act on a wide range of microoganisms.

CHECKPOINT 5-9 ➤ What are the categories of organisms studied in microbiology?

CHECKPOINT 5-10 ➤ What term refers to the microorganisms that normally live in or on the body?

Bacteria

Bacteria are single-cell organisms that are among the most primitive forms of life on earth. They are unique in that their genetic material is not enclosed in a membrane, that is, they do not have a true nucleus. They also lack most of the organelles found in plant and animal cells. They can be seen only with a microscope; from 10 to 1,000 bacteria (depending on the species) would, if lined up, span a pinhead. Staining of the cells with dyes helps make their structures more visible and reveals information about their properties.

Bacteria are found everywhere: in soil, in hot springs, in polar ice, and on and within plants and animals. Their requirements for water, nutrients, oxygen, temperature, and other factors vary widely according to species. Some are capable of carrying out photosynthesis, as do green plants; others must take in organic nutrients, as do animals. Some, described as **anaerobic** (an-air-O-bik), can grow in the absence of oxygen; others, called **aerobic** (air-O-bik), require oxygen. Other groups of bacteria are described as **facultative anaerobes**. These cells will use oxygen if it is present but are able to grow without oxygen

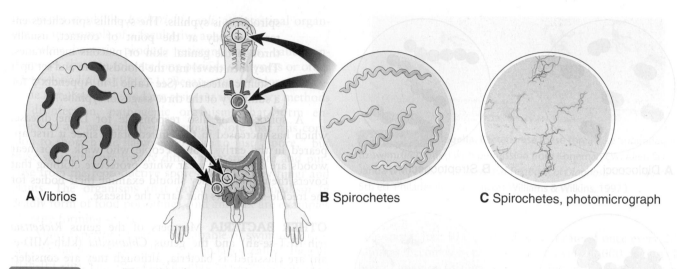

A Vibrios   **B** Spirochetes   **C** Spirochetes, photomicrograph

Figure 5-5 **Curved rods. (A)** Vibrios, comma-shaped organisms. A vibrio causes Asiatic cholera. **(B)** Spirochetes, spiral-shaped organisms that move with a twisting motion. A spirochete causes syphilis. **(C)** Spirochetes as seen under a microscope. (C, Reprinted with permission from Koneman EW, Alien SD, Janda WM, et al. *Color Atlas and Textbook of Diagnostic Microbiology*, 5th ed. Philadelphia: Lippincott Williams & Wilkins, 1997.) **[ZOOMING IN ➤** What feature indicates that the cells in A are capable of movement? **]**

size to large molecules, but unlike other molecules, they contain genetic material and are able to reproduce. Viruses are so tiny that they are invisible with a light microscope; they can be seen only with an electron microscope. Because of their small size and the difficulties associated with growing them in the laboratory, viruses were not studied with much success until the middle of the 20th century.

Viruses have some of the fundamental properties of living matter, but they are not cellular, and they have no enzyme system. They consist of a nucleic acid core, either DNA or RNA, surrounded by a coat of protein (Fig. 5-7). Like the rickettsiae and the chlamydiae, they can grow

only within living cells—they are obligate intracellular parasites. Unlike these other organisms, however, viruses are not susceptible to antibacterial agents (antibiotics) and must be treated with antiviral drugs.

Viruses are classified according to the type of nucleic acid they contain—DNA or RNA—and whether that nucleic acid is single stranded (ss) or double stranded (ds). They are further grouped according to the diseases they cause, of which there are a considerable number—measles, poliomyelitis, hepatitis, chickenpox, and the common cold, to name just a few. **AIDS** is a very serious viral disease discussed in Chapter 17. The virus that causes AIDS and other representative viruses are listed in Table 2 in Appendix 5.

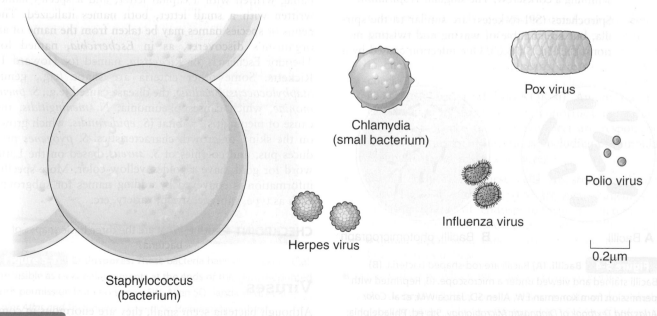

Pox virus

Chlamydia (small bacterium)

Polio virus

Influenza virus

Herpes virus

0.2μm

Staphylococcus (bacterium)

Figure 5-6 **Virus size comparison.** A chlamydia and a staphylococcus are shown for reference.

Figure 5-7 **Virus structure.** Note the regular arrangement of units in the protein coat. Magnified ×234,000. (Reprinted with permission from Koneman EW, Alien SD, Janda WM, et al. *Color Atlas and Textbook of Diagnostic Microbiology*, 5th ed. Philadelphia: Lippincott Williams & Wilkins, 1997.)

Viruses are named according to where they were isolated (Hanta, Ebola, West Nile), the symptoms they cause (yellow fever virus, which causes jaundice; hepatitis virus, which causes inflammation of the liver), the host (chickenpox, human immunodeficiency virus, swine influenza), or the vector that caries them (Colorado tick fever).

INFECTIOUS AGENTS SMALLER THAN VIRUSES
Viruses were considered the smallest known infectious agents until the discovery of two even smaller and simpler agents of disease. **Prions** (PRI-ons) are infectious particles composed solely of protein (the name comes from **proteinaceous infectious agent**). Researchers have linked prions to several fatal diseases in humans and animals. They are very slow-growing and hard to destroy, producing spongy degeneration of brain tissue, described as *spongiform encephalopathy* (en-sef-ah-LOP-a-the). Some examples of diseases caused by prions are Creutzfeldt-Jacob disease (CJD) in humans; bovine spongiform encephalopathy (BSE), the so-called "mad cow disease," in cows, a variant of which affects humans; and scrapie in sheep. Some diseases caused by prions are described in Table 3 of Appendix 5.

Viroids (VI-royds), in contrast, are composed of RNA alone with no protein coat. They are also intracellular par-

asites, but so far, they have been linked only to diseases in plants.

CHECKPOINT **5-13** ➤ How do viruses differ from bacteria?

Fungi

The true **fungi** (FUN-ji) are a large group of simple plant-like organisms. Only a few types are pathogenic. Although fungi are much larger and more complicated than bacteria, they are a simple life form. They differ from the higher plants in that they lack the green pigment chlorophyll, which enables most plants to use the energy of sunlight to manufacture food. Like bacteria, fungi grow best in dark, damp places. Single-cell fungi are generally referred to as **yeasts**; the fuzzy, filamentous forms are called **molds** (Fig. 5-8). Molds reproduce in several ways, including by simple cell division and by production of multiple reproductive spores. Yeasts reproduce by simple cell division and can also form buds that pinch off as new cells. Familiar examples of fungi are mushrooms, puffballs, bread molds, and the yeasts used in baking and brewing.

FUNGAL DISEASES Diseases caused by fungi are called **mycotic** (mi-KOT-ik) infections (*myco-* means "fungus"). Examples of these are athlete's foot and ringworm. Common types of ringworm are *Tinea capitis* (TIN-e-ah KAP-ih-tis), which involves the scalp, and *Tinea corporis* (kor-PO-ris), which can grow on almost any nonhairy body surface.

One yeast-like fungus that may infect a weakened host is *Candida*. This is a normal inhabitant of the mouth and digestive tract that may produce skin lesions, an oral infection called *thrush*, digestive upset, or inflammation of the vaginal tract (vaginitis) as an opportunistic infection in a weakened host.

Although fungi cause few systemic diseases, some diseases they cause are very dangerous and may be difficult to cure. Pneumonia can result from the inhalation of fungal spores contained in dust particles. An atypical fungus,

Figure 5-8 **Fungi. (A)** Yeasts. Some of these single-cell fungi are budding to form new cells **(B)** Molds, filamentous forms of fungi. (A, Reprinted with permission from LWW's Organism Central [CD-ROM for Windows]. Philadelphia: Lippincott Williams & Wilkins, 2001; B, Reprinted with permission from Koneman EW, Alien SD, Janda WM, et al. *Color Atlas and Textbook of Diagnostic Microbiology*, 5th ed. Philadelphia: Lippincott Williams & Wilkins, 1997.)

Pneumocystis jiroveci (formerly called *P. carinii*) causes a previously rare pneumonia known as PCP (*Pneumocystis pneumonia*) in people with AIDS and others with weakened immune systems. Table 4 in Appendix 5 lists typical fungal diseases.

Protozoa

With the **protozoa** (pro-to ZO-ah), we come to the only group of microbes that can be described as animal-like. Although protozoa are also single-cell organisms, they are much larger than bacteria (Fig. 5-9).

Protozoa are found all over the world in the soil and in almost any body of water from moist grass to mud puddles to the sea. There are four main divisions of protozoa:

- **Amebas** (ah-ME-bas). An ameba (also spelled *amoeba*) is an irregular mass of cytoplasm that propels itself by extending part of its cell (a pseudopod, or "false foot") and then flowing into the extension. Amebic dysentery is caused by a pathogen of this group (see Fig. 5-9A,B).
- **Ciliates** (SIL-e-ates). This type of protozoon is covered with tiny hairs called cilia that produce a wave action to propel the organism.
- **Flagellates** (FLAJ-eh-lates). Long, whiplike filaments called flagella propel these organisms. One of this group, a **trypanosome** (tri-PAN-o-some), causes African sleeping sickness, which is spread by the tsetse fly (see Fig. 5-9C,D). *Giardia* is a flagellated protozoon that contaminates water supplies throughout the world. It infects the intestinal tract, causing diarrhea. The disease, giardiasis, is the most common waterborne disease in the United States.
- **Sporozoa** (spor-o-ZO-ah) are also known as **apicomplexans** (ap-i-kom-PLEK-sans). Unlike other protozoa, sporozoa cannot propel themselves. They are obligate parasites, unable to grow outside a host. Members of the genus *Plasmodium* (plaz-MO-de-um) cause malaria (see Fig. 5-9E,F). These protozoa, carried by a mosquito vector, cause much serious illness in the tropics, resulting in over 1 million deaths each year. The sporozoon *Cryptosporidium* is an opportunistic pathogen that causes severe and prolonged diarrhea in people suffering from AIDS and others with an inadequate immune system.

Table 5 in Appendix 5 presents a list of typical pathogenic protozoa with the diseases they cause.

CHECKPOINT **5-14** ➤ What group of microorganisms is most animal-like?

Parasitic Worms

Many species of worms, also referred to as **helminths**, are parasites with human hosts. The study of worms, particularly parasitic worms, is called **helminthology** (hel-min-THOL-o-je). Whereas invasion by any form of organism is usually called an *infection*, the presence of parasitic worms in the body also can be termed an *infestation* (Fig. 5-10). Although worms themselves can be seen with the naked eye, one needs a microscope to see their eggs or larval forms.

Roundworms

Many human parasitic worms are classified as roundworms, and the large worm **ascaris** (AS-kah-ris) is one of the most common (see Fig. 5-10A). This worm is prevalent in many parts of Asia, where it is found mostly in larval form. In the United States, it is found most frequently among children (ages 4 to 12 years) in rural areas with warm climates.

> **PASSport to Success** Visit *thePoint* or see the Student Resource CD in the back of this book to see photographs of roundworms.

Ascaris is a long, white-yellow worm pointed at both ends. It may infest the lungs or the intestines, producing intestinal obstruction if present in large numbers. The eggs produced by the adult worms are deposited with feces (excreta) in the soil. These eggs are very resistant; they can live in soil during either freezing or hot, dry weather and cannot be destroyed even by strong antiseptics. New worms develop within the eggs and later reach the digestive system of a host by means of contaminated food. Ascaris infestation may be diagnosed by a routine stool examination.

Another fairly common infestation, particularly in children, is the seat worm, or **pinworm** (*Enterobius vermicularis*), which is also hard to control and eliminate. The worms average 12 mm (somewhat less than 1/2 inch) in length and live in the large intestine. The adult female moves outside the vicinity of the anus to lay its thousands of eggs. A child's fingers often transfer these eggs from the itching anal area to the mouth. In the digestive system of the host, the eggs develop to form new adult worms, and thus a new infestation is begun. A child also may infect others by this means. In addition, pinworm eggs that are expelled from the body constitute a hazard because they may live in the external environment for several months. Patience and every precaution, with careful attention to medical instructions, are necessary to get rid of the worms. It is essential to wash the hands, keep the fingernails clean, and avoid finger sucking.

Hookworms are parasites that live in the small intestine. They are dangerous because they suck blood from the host, causing such a severe anemia (blood deficiency) that the victim becomes sluggish, both physically and mentally. Most victims become susceptible to various chronic infections because of extremely reduced resistance following continuous blood loss.

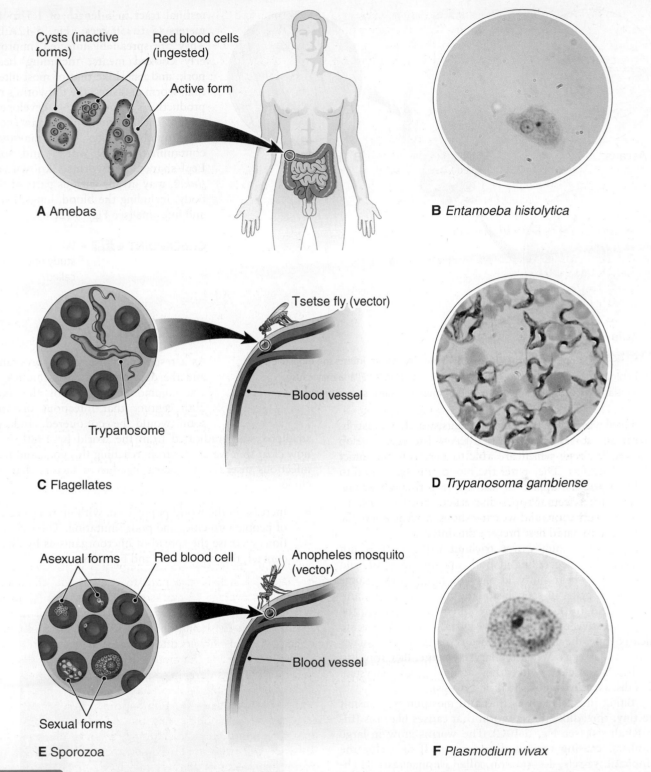

Figure 5-9 **Some parasitic protozoa.** **(A)** Amebas. **(B)** *Entamoeba histolytica*, cause of amebic dysentery, seen under the microscope. **(C)** Flagellates. Trypanosomes cause African sleeping sickness. **(D)** Trypansomes in a blood sample seen under the microscope. **(E)** Sporozoa. *Plasmodium vivax* causes malaria. **(F)** An enlarged red blood cell with a single parasite seen under the microscope. (B, D, F, Reprinted with permission from Koneman EW, Alien SD, Janda WM, et al. *Color Atlas and Textbook of Diagnostic Microbiology*, 5th ed. Philadelphia: Lippincott Williams & Wilkins, 1997.) **[ZOOMING IN ➤** Why are the parasites in E described as intracellular? What is the role of the vectors shown in C and E? **]**

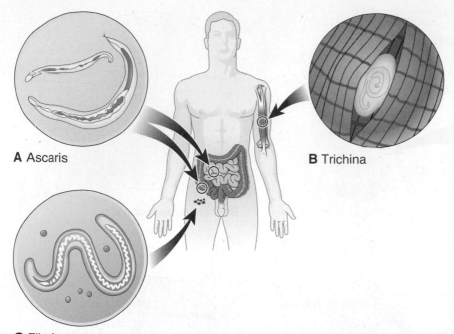

A Ascaris

B Trichina

C Filaria

Figure 5-10 **Common parasitic roundworms. (A)** Ascaris infests the digestive tract. **(B)** Trichina is transmitted in meat and encysts in muscles. **(C)** Filaria may cause elephantiasis. [**ZOOMING IN ➤** What kind of muscle tissue is shown in B?]

Hookworms lay thousands of eggs, which are distributed in the soil by contaminated feces. The eggs develop into small larvae, which are able to penetrate the intact skin of bare feet. They enter the blood and are carried to the lungs and the upper respiratory tract, finally reaching the digestive system. Proper disposal of body wastes, attention to sanitation, and wearing shoes in areas where the soil is contaminated best prevent this infestation.

The small roundworm **trichina** (trik-I-nah) is not transmitted by feces, but in pork and the meat of wild game, such as bear and wild pig. The tiny worms become enclosed in cysts, or sacs, inside the muscles of these animals (Fig. 5-10B). If the undercooked meat is eaten, the host's digestive juices dissolve the cysts, and the worms are released into the intestine. In a day or two, the females mate and lay eggs. When the larvae emerge, they travel to the host's muscles, where they again become encysted. This disease is **trichinosis** (trik-ih-NO-sis).

Biting insects, such as flies and mosquitoes, transmit the tiny, threadlike filaria worm that causes **filariasis** (fil-ah-RI-ah-sis) (see Fig. 5-10C). The worms grow in large numbers, causing various disturbances. If they clog the lymphatic vessels, a condition called **elephantiasis** (el-eh-fan-TI-ah-sis) results, in which the lower extremities, the scrotum, the breasts and other areas may become tremendously enlarged (Fig. 5-11). Filariasis is most common in tropical and subtropical lands, such as southern Asia and many of the South Pacific islands.

Flatworms

Some flatworms resemble long ribbons, whereas others have the shape of a leaf. Tapeworms may grow in the in-

testinal tract to a length of 1.5 to 15 meters (5 to 50 feet) (Fig. 5-12A,B). They are spread by infected, improperly cooked meats, including beef, pork, and fish. Like that of most intestinal worm parasites, the flatworm's reproductive system is highly developed, so that each worm produces an enormous number of eggs, which may then contaminate food, water, and soil. Leaf-shaped flatworms, known as *flukes*, may invade various parts of the body, including the blood, lungs, liver, and intestine (see Fig. 5-12C).

CHECKPOINT 5-15 ➤ What is the study of worms called?

Microbial Control

As a result of immunization programs and the development of antibiotics, it was commonly believed by the mid-20th century that infectious diseases soon would be conquered. Indeed, smallpox was eradicated from the world by 1980. It is now clear that we are far from reaching this goal, and that infectious diseases are increasing due to factors that include:

- Increase in the world population, with more crowding of people into cities and poor sanitation. These conditions increase the spread of microorganisms by direct contact, through the air, and by pests.

Figure 5-11 **Filariasis.** The photo shows massive enlargement (elephantiasis) of the scrotum and left leg. (Reprinted with permission from Rubin E, Farber JL. Pathology, 3rd ed. Philadelphia: Lippincott Williams & Wilkins, 1999.)

Figure 5-12 **Flatworms. (A)** Tapeworms can measure more than 30 feet in length. The arrow shows the headlike attachment point. **(B)** Segments of a tapeworm. **(C)** A fluke. (Reprinted with permission from Koneman EW, Alien SD, Janda WM, et al. *Color Atlas and Textbook of Diagnostic Microbiology*, 5th ed. Philadelphia: Lippincott Williams & Wilkins, 1997.)

■ Disruption of animal habitats, with more contact between humans and animals, allowing the spread of animal pathogens to human hosts. Some organisms that have made this shift include HIV, the cause of AIDS, which originated in chimpanzees; West Nile virus from birds; severe acute respiratory syndrome (SARS), which probably came from a small wild mammal used for food; and various strains of influenza.

■ Increased travel, especially air travel, which can spread an infectious organism throughout the globe in a day. SARS spread rapidly from China to other countries in the spring of 2003.

■ Medical advances that keep people alive longer, but in a debilitated state, subject to opportunistic infections.

■ Changes in food handling that allow foods to be stored, processed, and shipped long distances on a large scale, sometimes with inadequate oversight.

Because of their huge variety and adaptability, there is scarcely a place on earth that is naturally free of microorganisms. One exception is the interior of normal body tissue. However, body surfaces and passageways leading to the outside, such as the mouth, throat, nasal cavities, and large intestine, harbor an abundance of both harmless and potentially pathogenic microbes. If a person's natural defenses are sound, he or she may harbor many microbes

safely. If that person's resistance becomes lowered, however, an infection can result. Although many vaccines are available to protect against disease, inhabitants in poor areas may not have access to them. Lack of immunization in combination with lowered resistance due to poor nutrition and disease create a susceptible host.

Microbes and Public Health

All societies establish and enforce measures designed to protect the health of their populations. Most of these practices are concerned with preventing the spread of infectious organisms. A few examples of fundamental public health considerations are listed below:

■ **Sewage and garbage disposal.** In times past, when people disposed of the household "slops" by simply throwing them out the window, great epidemics were inevitable. Modern practice is to divert sewage into a processing plant in which harmless microbes are put to work destroying the pathogens. The resulting noninfectious "sludge" makes excellent fertilizer.

■ **Water purification.** Drinking water that has become polluted with untreated sewage may be contaminated with such dangerous pathogens as typhoid bacilli, polio and hepatitis viruses, and dysentery amebas. A filtering process usually purifies the municipal water supply, and a close and constant watch is kept on its microbial population. Industrial and chemical wastes, such as asbestos fibers, acids and detergents from homes and from industry, and pesticides used in agriculture, complicate the problem of obtaining pure drinking water.

- **Prevention of food contamination.** Various national, state, and local laws seek to prevent disease outbreaks through contaminated food. Certain animal diseases (e.g., tuberculosis and tularemia) can be passed to humans through food, and food is also a natural breeding place for many dangerous pathogens. Some of the organisms that cause food poisoning are the botulism bacillus (*Clostridium botulinum*) that grows in improperly canned foods, so-called *staph* (*Staphylococcus aureus*), and species of *Salmonella* transmitted in eggs, poultry, and dairy products. In recent years, a variety of the normally harmless intestinal bacillus *Escherichia coli* (*E. coli* 0157:H7) has caused outbreaks of food poisoning from undercooked meat and from produce. For further information, see Table 1 in Appendix 5. Most cities have sanitary regulations requiring, among other things, compulsory periodic inspection of food-handling establishments.

- **Milk pasteurization.** Milk is rendered free of pathogens by pasteurization, a process in which the milk is heated to 63°C (145°F) for 30 minutes and then cooled rapidly before being packaged. Sometimes, slightly higher temperatures are used for a much shorter time with satisfactory results. The entire pasteurization process, including the cooling and packing, is accomplished in a closed system, without any exposure to air. Pasteurized milk still contains microbes, but no harmful ones. Pasteurization is also used to preserve other beverages and dairy products.

Aseptic Methods

In the practice of medicine, surgery, nursing, and other health fields, specialized procedures are followed to reduce or eliminate the growth of pathogenic organisms. The term *sepsis* refers to the presence of pathogenic organisms (or their toxins) in the blood or tissues; **asepsis** (a-SEP-sis) is its opposite—a condition in which no pathogens are present. Procedures that are designed to kill, remove, or prevent the growth of microbes are called *aseptic methods*.

There are several terms designating aseptic practices. These are often confused with one another. Some of the more commonly used terms and their definitions are as follows (Fig. 5-13):

- **Sterilization.** To sterilize an object means to kill *every* living microorganism on it. In operating rooms and delivery rooms especially, staff members keep sterile as much of the environment as possible, including the clothing worn by personnel and the instruments used. The most common sterilization method is by means of steam under pressure in an **autoclave**. Dry heat is also used. Ethylene oxide, a gas, is used to sterilize supplies and equipment that are not able to withstand high temperatures. Most pathogens can be killed by exposure to boiling water for 4 minutes. However, the time and temperature required to ensure the destruction of all spore-forming organisms in sterilization are much greater than those required to kill most pathogens.

- **Disinfection.** Disinfection refers to any measure that kills all pathogens (except spores) but does not necessarily kill all harmless microbes. Most **disinfectants** (disinfecting agents) are chemicals that can be applied directly to nonliving surfaces. Examples are chlorine compounds, such as household bleach, phenol compounds, and mercury compounds. Commercial disinfectant products contain more than one chemical

Figure 5-13 **Aseptic methods.**

agent in order to kill a variety of organisms. Two other terms for bacteria-killing agents, synonymous with disinfectant, are **bactericide** and **germicide**, agents that kill bacteria and germs.

■ **Antisepsis.** This term refers to any process in which pathogens are not necessarily killed but are prevented from multiplying, a state called **bacteriostasis** (bak-te-re-o-STA-sis) (*stasis* means "steady state"). **Antiseptics** are less powerful than disinfectants and are safe to use on living tissues. Examples are alcohol, organic iodine solutions, and hydrogen peroxide.

Infection Control Techniques

In the 1980s, concern about the spread of blood-borne infections, such as hepatitis B and HIV, led to the development of isolation and barrier techniques for the handling of blood and other body fluids that might contain blood. These *universal precautions* have now been extended to include all potentially infective body substances and are entitled *body substance precautions* or *body substance isolation.* According to guidelines established by the CDC (Centers for Disease Control and Prevention), healthcare personnel must use barriers for any contact with moist body substances, mucous membranes, or nonintact skin, whether or not blood is visible and regardless of the patient's diagnosis. Gloves must be worn for each patient contact and changed if necessary during care. Protective coverings such as a mask, eye protection, face shield, or fluid-repellent gown should be worn during procedures that may generate sprays of blood or body fluids. Soiled linen, trash, and other waste must be treated as if contaminated and disposed of properly. Needles and other sharp instruments must be handled safely and disposed of in puncture-proof containers. To avoid the risk of needlestick injuries, **needles are not recapped.** In circumstances when it is necessary to recap, the needle should be slipped into the cap with one hand or by using a recapping device.

Additional isolation precautions are instituted for infections that are spread by airborne routes, such as tuberculosis, measles (rubeola), and SARS; for those spread by droplets or direct contact; and for infections involving antibiotic-resistant organisms. These measures may include keeping a patient in a private room and limiting visitor contact, filtering circulating air, and having health personnel wear protective clothing.

HANDWASHING Handwashing is the single most important measure for preventing the spread of infection in all settings. Thorough washing promptly after patient contact and after contact with any body secretions is of utmost importance in infection control. Standard precautions include handwashing after glove removal due to the rapid multiplication of normal flora inside the gloves. Gloves are not considered a substitute for handwashing because they may have small defects, they may be torn, or hands may become contaminated when the gloves are removed.

OSHA The Occupational Safety and Health Administration (OSHA) is a U.S. government agency that establishes minimum health and safety standards for workers. The agency has issued regulations for protection against infectious materials based on the CDC guidelines and has enforced these regulations. Employers at healthcare facilities must provide workers with the equipment and supplies needed to prevent their exposure to infectious materials.

CHECKPOINT 5-16 ➤ Aseptic practices are intended to eliminate pathogens. What are the three levels of asepsis?

CHECKPOINT 5-17 ➤ What is the single most important measure for preventing the spread of infection?

Antimicrobial Agents

Antimicrobial (antiinfective) agents are drugs that act to kill or inhibit infectious microorganisms. These include antibacterial, antiviral, antifungal, and antiparasitic substances, which interfere with vital metabolic processes that the infecting agents need to survive and reproduce. A drug that acts on intestinal worms is an anthelmintic (ant-hel-MIN-tik) agent or vermifuge (VER-mih-fuj). The term *antibiotic*, in its most general sense, refers to any substance that acts against a living organism, but the term has come to be used only for drugs that act against bacteria.

ANTIBIOTICS (ANTIBACTERIAL AGENTS) An **antibiotic** is a substance produced by living cells that has the power to kill or arrest the growth of bacteria. Most antibiotics are derived from fungi (molds) and soil bacteria. Penicillin, the first widely used antibiotic, is made from a common blue mold, *Penicillium.* Often, the drugs derived from penicillin can be recognized by the ending *-cillin* in the name. Other fungi that produce a large number of antibiotics are members of the group *Cephalosporium.* The soil bacteria *Streptomyces* produce some frequently used antibiotics. These drug names often end in *-mycetin.*

The development of antibiotics has been of incalculable benefit to humanity. Since the time that penicillin saved many lives on the battlefields of World War II in the 1940s, antibiotics have been considered miracle drugs. Enthusiasm for their use, however, has given rise to some undesirable effects.

One danger of antibiotic use is the development of opportunistic infections. As noted, there is a normal flora of microorganisms in the body that competes with pathogens. Antibiotics, especially those that kill a wide variety of bacteria (broad-spectrum antibiotics), eliminate these competitors and allow pathogens to thrive. For example, antibiotics often destroy the normal flora of the vaginal tract and allow a troublesome yeast infection to develop.

The widespread use of antibiotics has resulted in the natural selection of pathogens that are resistant to these medications. Under some circumstances, bacteria can even transfer genes for resistance directly from one cell to another. Some strains of common organisms, such as streptococci, staphylococci, pneumococci, *E. coli*, and tuberculosis are now resistant to most antibiotics (see Appendix 5 for diseases caused by these microorganisms).

The prevalence of antibiotic-resistant pathogens is a serious problem in hospitals today. These organisms cause infections that do not respond to drugs. In the United States, about 5% of acute care hospital patients contract one or more such infections. Patients who are elderly or severely debilitated are most susceptible to these **nosocomial** (nos-o-KO-me-al) (hospital-acquired) infections (the word *nosocomial* comes from a Greek word for hospital). Some strains currently causing nosocomial infections are methicillin-resistant *Staphylococcus aureus* (MRSA) and vancomycin-resistant enterococci (VRE).

When taking antibiotics, it is important to complete the entire course of treatment to guarantee the destruction of all pathogens. If not, the more resistant cells will be able to survive treatment and grow out in great numbers, leading to the development of strains that do not respond to that antibiotic. Also, patients should not press physicians to prescribe antibiotics when they will do no good, as for the treatment of viral infections such as colds and flu.

Pharmaceutical companies may be able to find new antibiotics. Also, using these drugs in combinations may help to eliminate all the bacteria causing an infection. We may be able to reverse the trend toward resistance by using these drugs with more care. Large quantities of antibiotics are now used in agriculture to control disease among farm animals and increase productivity. Some people now shop for meats that are free of antibiotics. There is some evidence that susceptibility to a given drug will reappear when a bacterial population is no longer exposed to it.

CHECKPOINT **5-18** ➤ What is an antibiotic?

ANTIVIRAL AGENTS There are not many effective antiviral drugs, and each one has a limited range of action. These agents function to:

- block removal of the protein coat of the virus after it enters a cell, as in treatment of influenza A virus.

- block production of viral nucleic acid, as does the drug AZT (zidovudine). The reverse transcriptase inhibitors used to treat HIV infections block the enzyme needed for viral RNA to function in the host cell.

- block enzymes that are needed to assemble and release new virus particles, as does the drug indinavir, a so-called *protease inhibitor*, used to treat HIV infection.

Note that viruses mutate rapidly to become resistant to these drugs, and none can eliminate latent (temporarily inactive) infections. In treating AIDS, the drugs are commonly used in combinations.

Laboratory Identification of Pathogens

The nurse, physician, or laboratory worker often obtains specimens from patients to identify bacteria and other organisms. Specimens most frequently studied are blood, spinal fluid, feces, urine, and sputum, along with swabbings from other areas. Swabs are used to collect specimens from the nose, throat, eyes, and cervix as well as from ulcers or other infected areas. The healthcare worker must label each specimen completely and accurately with the patient's name, appropriate identification, source of the specimen, physician's name, the date, and time. He or she must then deliver it to the laboratory promptly.

Bacterial Isolations and Tests

In the lab, bacterial cells are grown out in cultures using substances called **media**, such as nutrient broth or agar, that the bacteria can use as food. Individual organisms are then isolated, that is, separated from other cells in the specimen, usually by streaking the cultures over the surface of a solid medium. The isolated cells then multiply to form separate colonies (clones) on the surface of the medium (Fig. 5-14). The laboratory technicians then perform a variety of tests to identify the organism or organisms obtained from the specimen. At this time, the organism is usually tested for sensitivity to various antibiotics that might be used to treat the infection. This whole procedure is described as a culture and sensitivity (C & S).

> ☼ **PASSport to Success** Visit *thePoint* or see the Student Resource CD in the back of this book for more information on careers in medical technology.

Figure 5-14 **Isolated colonies of bacteria growing on a solid medium.** Each colony contains all the offspring of a single cell. (Reprinted with permission from Koneman EW, Alien SD, Janda WM, et al. *Color Atlas and Textbook of Diagnostic Microbiology*, 5th ed. Philadelphia: Lippincott Williams & Wilkins, 1997.)

Figure 5-15 **Gram's stained bacteria. (A)** Gram-positive diplococci. **(B)** Gram-negative bacilli among white blood cells in a urine sediment. (Reprinted with permission from Koneman EW, Alien SD, Janda WM, et al. *Color Atlas and Textbook of Diagnostic Microbiology*, 5th ed. Philadelphia: Lippincott Williams & Wilkins, 1997.)

5

Staining Techniques

One of the most frequently used methods for beginning the process of identification involves examining the cells under the microscope. To make the cells visible under the microscope, they must first be stained with colored dyes (stains), which are applied to a thin smear of the culture on a glass slide. The most commonly used staining procedure is known as the **Gram's stain** (Fig. 5-15). A bluish purple dye (such as crystal violet) is applied, and then a weak iodine solution is added. This causes a colorfast combination within certain organisms, so that washing with alcohol does not remove the dye. These bacteria are said to be *Gram positive* and appear bluish purple under the microscope (Fig. 5-15A). Examples are the pathogenic staphylococci and streptococci; the cocci that cause certain types of pneumonia; and the bacilli that produce diphtheria, tetanus, and anthrax. Other organisms are said to be *Gram negative* because the coloring can be removed from them with a solvent. These are then stained for visibility, usually with a red dye (see Fig. 5-15B). Examples of gram-negative organisms are the diplococci that cause gonorrhea and epidemic meningitis and the bacilli that produce typhoid fever, pneumonia, and one type of dysentery. The colon bacillus (*E. coli*) normally found in the intestine is also Gram negative, as is the cholera vibrio. Can you tell which of the organisms in Figure 5-3 are Gram positive and which are Gram negative?

Another stain used to identify organisms is the **acid-fast stain**. After being stained with a reddish dye (carbolfuchsin), the smear is treated with acid. Most bacteria quickly lose their stain upon application of the acid, but the organisms that cause tuberculosis and other acid-fast cells retain the red stain. The negative cells are then stained with a different dye, usually a blue one.

A few organisms, such as the spirochetes of syphilis and the rickettsiae, do not stain with any of the commonly used dyes. Special techniques must be used to identify these organisms.

Other Methods of Identification

In addition to the various staining procedures, laboratory techniques for identifying bacteria include:

- observing the cultures' growth characteristics in liquid and solid medium.
- studying the cells' oxygen requirements.
- observing the ability of the bacteria to utilize (ferment) various carbohydrates (sugars).
- analyzing reactions to various test chemicals.
- studying the bacteria by serologic (immunologic) tests based on the antigen–antibody reaction (see Chapter 17).

Laboratories now use modern techniques of genetic analysis to identify organisms based on their nucleic acids. They use the polymerase chain reaction (PCR) to make multiple copies of an organism's unique DNA or RNA sequences. These sequences are then identified by so-called "genetic fingerprinting" methods. Genetic tests are faster and cheaper than standard culturing procedures and can be used directly on a patient specimen. Scientists have used PCR to identify the infectious agent for diseases such as AIDS, hepatitis, and Lyme disease, and for identifying the pathogens that cause emerging diseases such as West Nile disease and severe acute respiratory syndrome (SARS). Epidemiologists use PCR to identify the source and monitor the spread of infections in a population, because it can identify individuals infected with the same strain of an organism.

CHECKPOINT 5-19 ➤ One way of identifying microorganisms is to examine them under a microscope. Before examination, the cells are colored so they can be seen. What are the dyes used to color the cells called?

Disease in Context revisited

▸ Maria Succumbs to the Influenza Virus

Maria Sanchez looked terrible—watery eyes, runny nose, and a sickly, run-down appearance. Just yesterday, she felt fine. But today, she was so fa-tigued that she could hardly get out of bed. She had a fever, chills, and a cough that left her throat aching. Maria was certainly feeling the effects of the in-fluenza virus that had invaded the epithelial lining of her respiratory tract about 3 days ago.

Many of Maria's local symptoms were due to the virus. Her watery eyes and runny nose were the result of extracellular fluid leaking from holes in the mucous membrane lining her respiratory tract—holes left from the death and shedding of millions of epithelial cells! Without these ciliated cells, Maria wasn't able to move the extra fluid up and out of her respiratory tract, so she periodically coughed in an effort to do so. Maria's systemic symptoms were due, in large part, to her body's counter-attack against the virus. Since viruses work most efficiently at near-normal body temperature, her fever actually slowed viral replication. Her fa-tigue helped beat the virus too. By staying in bed, her body was able to conserve energy that her immune system could use to fight the virus. In a few days, that system would beat the virus and she would make a complete recovery.

During this case, we saw that the influenza virus that invaded Maria's body is designed to hijack her epithelial cells and force them to make new viruses. Maria's body is also well-designed to combat the virus. In Chapter 17, Body Defenses, Immunity, and Vaccines, we'll revisit Maria again and learn how immu-nization can help protect Maria from influenza in the future.

Word Anatomy

Medical terms are built from standardized word parts (prefixes, roots, and suffixes). Learning the meanings of these parts can help you remember words and interpret unfamiliar terms.

WORD PART	MEANING	EXAMPLE
Categories of Disease		
psych/o	mind	The medical field of *psychiatry* specializes in treatment of mental disorders.
pre-	before	A *predisposing* cause enters into production of disease.
Study of Disease		
idio-	self, separate, distinct	An *idiopathic* disease has no known cause; it is "self-originating."
iatro	physician, medicine	An *iatrogenic* disease results from the adverse effects of treatment.
pan-	all	A *pandemic* disease is prevalent throughout an entire country, continent, or the world.
syn-	together	A *syndrome* is a group of symptoms and signs that together characterize a disease.
chir/o	hand	*Chiropractic* treatment involves use of the hands for manipulation to correct misalignment of the body.
Infectious Disease		
myc/o	fungus	*Mycology* is the study of fungi.
aer/o	air, gas	An *aerobic* organism requires air (oxygen) to grow.
an-	absent, deficient, lack of	An *anaerobic* organism does not require air (oxygen) to grow.
tox/o	poison	Bacteria can harm the body by producing *toxins*.
diplo-	double	*Diplococci* are round bacteria arranged in pairs.
strepto-	chain	*Streptococci* are round bacteria arranged in chains.
staphylo-	grapelike cluster	*Staphylococci* are bacteria in clusters.
py/o	pus	The species name *pyogenes* indicates that an organism produces pus.
Microbial Control		
septic	poison, rot, decay	*Aseptic* methods are used to kill or prevent the growth of microorganisms.
–cide	kill or destroy	A *bactericide* is an agent that kills bacteria.

5

Summary

I. **CATEGORIES OF DISEASE**—infection, degenerative disease, nutritional disorders, metabolic disorders, immune disorders, neoplasms, psychiatric disorders
   A. Predisposing causes of disease—age, gender, heredity, living conditions and habits, emotional disturbance, physical and chemical damage, preexisting illness
II. **THE STUDY OF DISEASE**—pathophysiology
   A. Disease terminology
      1. Etiology—study of origin or causation
      2. Terms related to severity and duration
         a. Acute—severe, of short duration
         b. Chronic—less severe, of long duration
         c. Subacute—intermediate, between acute and chronic
      3. Idiopathic—of unknown cause
      4. Iatrogenic—results from adverse effects of treatment
      5. Epidemiology—study of diseases in populations
         a. Statistics
            (1) Incidence—number of new cases in a population during specific time
            (2) Prevalence—number of cases in a population at a given time
            (3) Mortality rate—percentage of the population that dies from disease within a given period
         b. Categories
            (1) Epidemic—widespread in a given region
            (2) Endemic—found at lesser level but continuously in a population
            (3) Pandemic—prevalent throughout an entire country or the world
III. **TREATMENT AND PREVENTION OF DISEASE**
   A. Diagnosis—determination of the nature of the illness
      1. Symptom—change in body function felt by the patient
      2. Sign—change in body function observable by others
      3. Syndrome—group of signs and symptoms that characterize a disease
   B. Prognosis—prediction of probable outcome of disease
   C. Therapy—course of treatment
   D. Complementary and alternative medicine (CAM)—methods of disease prevention or treatment used along with or instead of traditional modern medical practices—e.g. naturopathy, chiropractic, acupuncture, biofeedback
      1. Herbal remedies—plant products

E. Prevention of disease—removal of potential causes of disease
IV. **INFECTIOUS DISEASE**
   A. Parasite—organism that lives on or within a host at host's expense
   B. Pathogen—disease-causing organism
   C. Infection—invasion by pathogens with adverse effects
      1. Local—small area
      2. Systemic—generalized; usually spread by blood
   D. Opportunistic infection—takes hold in a weakened host
   E. Communicable infection—can be spread from person to person; is contagious
   F. Modes of transmission
      1. Direct contact
      2. Indirect—touched objects, air, pests
         a. Vector—animal that transfers organisms from host to host
      3. Portals of entry and exit—skin, respiratory, digestive, urinary, and reproductive systems
V. **MICROBIOLOGY—THE STUDY OF MICROORGANISMS**
   A. Normal flora—population of microorganisms normally growing on and within the body
   B. Bacteria
      1. Some features
         a. Oxygen requirements—aerobic, anaerobic, facultative anaerobes
         b. Endospores—resistant forms
         c. Flagella—used for swimming
         d. Pili—short, threadlike; used for attachment
      2. Shape and arrangement
         a. Cocci—round
            (1) Diplococci—pairs
            (2) Streptococci—chains
            (3) Staphylococci—clusters
         b. Bacilli—straight rods; some produce endospores
         c. Curved rods
            (1) Vibrios—comma shaped
            (2) Spirilla—corkscrew or wavy
            (3) Spirochetes—flexible spirals
      3. Other bacteria—obligate intracellular parasites
         a. Rickettsiae
         b. Chlamydiae
   C. Viruses
      1. Contain only nucleic acid and protein
      2. Obligate intracellular parasites
      3. Infectious agents smaller than viruses
         a. Prions—contain only protein; cause slow-growing brain diseases

b.   Viroids—contain only RNA
D.   Fungi—simple, plantlike organisms
   1.   Yeasts—single cell
   2.   Molds—filamentous
E.   Protozoa—single-cell, animal-like organisms
   1.   Amebas—dysentery
   2.   Ciliates
   3.   Flagellates—African sleeping sickness, giardiasis
   4.   Sporozoa (apicomplexans)—malaria, *Cryptosporidium* infection

VI. PARASITIC WORMS (HELMINTHS)
A.   Roundworms
   1.   Ascaris
   2.   Pinworms
   3.   Hookworms
   4.   Trichina—transmitted in undercooked meat
   5.   Filaria—causes filariasis (elephantiasis)
B.   Flatworms
   1.   Tapeworms
   2.   Flukes

VII. MICROBIAL CONTROL
A.   Emergence and spread of microorganisms—factors related to population growth, technology
B.   Microbes and public health
   1.   Sewage and garbage disposal
   2.   Water purification
   3.   Prevention of food contamination
   4.   Milk pasteurization
C.   Aseptic methods
   1.   Sterilization—killing of all organisms
   2.   Disinfection—destruction of all pathogens (except endospores); bactericidal
   3.   Antisepsis—pathogens killed or prevented from multiplying (bacteriostasis); safe for living tissue

D.   Infection control techniques
   1.   Body substance precautions (body substance isolation)
     a.   Assume all body fluids potentially infective
     b.   Barriers—gloves, masks, eye protection, gowns
     c.   Handwashing stressed
     d.   OSHA—Occupational Safety and Health Administration
E.   Antimicrobial agents—interfere with essential metabolism
   1.   Antibiotics—antibacterial agents
     a.   Disadvantages—opportunistic infections, bacterial resistance, nosocomial (hospital-acquired) infections
   2.   Antivirals—block removal of protein coat, production of nucleic acid, assembly and release of new virus

VIII. LABORATORY IDENTIFICATION OF PATHOGENS
A.   Collection of specimens; accurate labeling and prompt delivery to lab
B.   Bacterial isolations and tests
C.   Staining techniques (e.g., Gram's, acid-fast)
D.   Other methods of identification
   1.   Growth characteristics
   2.   Oxygen requirements
   3.   Fermentation
   4.   Reactions to test chemicals
   5.   Serologic (immunologic) tests
   6.   Genetic analysis
     a.   PCR (polymerase chain reaction) duplicates unique nucleic acids
     b.   Segments identified for a genetic "fingerprint"

Questions for Study and Review

BUILDING UNDERSTANDING

Fill in the blanks

1. An inadequate diet may result in _____ disorders such as scurvy or rickets.

2. The study of the cause of any disease or the theory of its origin is _____.

3. A(n) _____ infection attacks an individual already weakened by disease.

4. Mycotic infections are caused by _____.

5. Certain molds and soil bacteria produce bacteria-killing substances called _____.

Matching > Match each numbered item with the most closely related lettered item.

___ **6.** Organisms that cause pneumonia, diphtheria, and syphilis

___ **7.** Organisms that cause AIDS, hepatitis, and the common cold

___ **8.** Organisms that cause athlete's foot, ringworm, and thrush

___ **9.** Organisms that cause amebic dysentery, giardiasis, and malaria

___ **10.** Organisms that cause pinworm, trichinosis, and filariasis

a. protozoa

b. helminths

c. viruses

d. fungi

e. bacteria

Multiple Choice

___ **11.** The incidence of early heart disease is higher in men than women. A predisposing cause of this disease appears to be

    a. age

    b. gender

    c. heredity

    d. living conditions and habits

___ **12.** A syndrome is defined as a

    a. disease accompanied by a characteristic group of signs and symptoms

    b. widespread disease

    c. disease that is neither acute nor chronic

    d. communicable disease

___ **13.** Structures that allow some bacteria to move along solid surfaces are called

    a. endospores

    b. flagella

    c. pili

    d. vibrios

___ **14.** Which of the following protozoa are obligate parasites?

    a. amebas

    b. flagellates

    c. sporozoa

    d. ciliates

___ **15.** An antibiotic should be prescribed only for a

    a. fungal infection

    b. viral infection

    c. parasitic infection

    d. bacterial infection

UNDERSTANDING CONCEPTS

16. Explain the difference between the terms in each of the following pairs:

    a. acute and chronic

    b. epidemic and endemic

    c. symptom and sign

    d. host and parasite

    e. pathogen and vector

17. List five portals that pathogens may use to enter or exit the body.

18. Classify bacteria into three groups based on oxygen requirements and three groups based on shape.

19. How do rickettsiae and chlamydiae differ from other bacteria in size and living habits? Name some diseases caused by rickettsiae and chlamydiae.

20. What is the difference between a virus and a prion?

21. Explain how an infectious disease can emerge and spread across the country and the world. Name some public health measures that can prevent disease outbreaks.

22. Why are standard precautions followed? What measures are included in the use of standard precautions?

CONCEPTUAL THINKING

23. While you are on a work-exchange program in the tropics, a cholera epidemic sweeps through the area where you are staying. Of the 1,000 people living in the area, 100 people contract cholera and 10 die of it in 1 month. What is the percentage incidence and mortality rate of cholera during that time? What precautions could you take to lessen your risk of contracting this bacterial disease?

24. Mr. Baker is in the hospital with severe burns to more than half of his body. His chart calls for close adherence to aseptic methods. Describe three procedures used in healthcare facilities to ensure asepsis. What kind of infection is Mr. Baker at increased risk of contracting during his long recovery in the hospital?

25. While working in the lab, you are given the job of identifying bacteria cultured from a patient's sputum sample. You smear a sample of the bacteria onto a glass slide and Gram's stain it. Microscopic examination reveals bluish purple cells arranged in chains. What do you think the bacteria could be? What disease could the patient have? What kind of drug therapy may be prescribed?

26. In Maria's case, what was the virus' portal of entry? To prevent Maria from spreading the virus to other people, what infection control technique would you suggest?

5

CHAPTER 6

The Skin in Health and Disease

Learning Outcomes

After careful study of this chapter, you should be able to:

1. Name and describe the layers of the skin
2. Describe the subcutaneous tissue
3. Give the location and function of the accessory structures of the skin
4. List the main functions of the skin
5. Summarize the information to be gained by observation of the skin
6. List the main disorders of the skin
7. Show how word parts are used to build words related to the skin (see Word Anatomy at the end of the chapter)

Selected Key Terms

The following terms and other boldface terms in the chapter are defined in the Glossary

alopecia
arrector pili
cicatrix
dermatitis
dermis
epidermis
erythema
exfoliation
integument
keloid
keratin
lesion
melanin
scar
sebaceous
sebum
stratum
subcutaneous
sudoriferous

PASSport to Success

Visit *thePoint* or see the Student Resource CD in the back of this book for definitions and pronunciations of key terms as well as a pretest for this chapter.

Disease in Context

▶ Paul's Case: Sun-Damaged Skin

"Wait a minute," Paul said to his reflection in the mirror as he trimmed his goatee after shaving. He had noticed a small nodule to the side of his left nostril. The lump was mostly pink with a pearly-white border, and painless to the touch. *I haven't seen that before. Probably just a pimple, or maybe a small cyst,* Paul thought, although he couldn't help thinking back to the many hours he had spent as a kid sailing competitively at the seashore. *I know sun exposure isn't great for your skin, even dangerous, and I wasn't real careful about wearing sunscreen. Even if I did, it would have washed off anyway while I was sailing,* he rationalized. Paul finished his trimming and decided the lump was probably nothing.

Despite his attempts to forget about the lump, Paul was concerned. Over the next several days he showed the small, rounded mass to several people to get their opinions. No one had an answer when he asked, "What do you think this is?" When several weeks produced no change, except maybe a little depression in the center of the mass, worry led him to make an appointment with a dermatologist.

"Well Paul, I'm not sure. It could be nothing, but we better look a little closer," said Dr. Nielsen. "It could be benign, but we have to be sure that it's not a small skin cancer. This is a very common site for such a lesion. Basal cell and squamous cell carcinomas arise from the underlying epithelial cells of the skin, especially in sun-exposed areas. UV rays from the sun can damage DNA, causing the cells to divide more rapidly than normal, resulting in an abnormal growth. Basal cell and squamous cell carcinomas are the most common forms of cancer but are usually completely treatable. We'll remove this and send it to the pathology lab to see what's going on." Paul left Dr. Nielsen's office with a small bandage over the site of excision, some ointment to apply, and instructions to call the office in 3 days.

Paul's dermatologist suspects that Paul may have skin cancer—a disease affecting the integumentary system. In this chapter, we'll learn that skin is just one part of the system. Later in the chapter, we'll revisit Paul and learn the final diagnosis of that lump on his nose.

The skin is the one system that can be inspected in its entirety without requiring surgery or special equipment. The skin not only gives clues to its own health but also reflects the health of other body systems. Although the skin may be viewed simply as a membrane enveloping the body, it is far more complex than the other epithelial membranes described in Chapter 4.

The skin is associated with accessory structures, also known as appendages, which include glands, hair, and nails. Together with blood vessels, nerves, and sensory organs, the skin and its associated structures form the **integumentary** (in-teg-u-MEN-tar-e) **system**. This name is from the word integument (in-TEG-u-ment), which means "covering." The term cutaneous (ku-TA-ne-us) also refers to the skin. The functions of this system are discussed later in the chapter after a description of its structure.

> PASSport to Success
> Visit **thePoint** or see the Student Resource CD in the back of this book for a summary chart of skin structures.

Structure of the Skin

The skin consists of two layers (Fig. 6-1):

- The **epidermis** (ep-ih-DER-mis), the outermost portion, which itself is subdivided into thin layers called **strata** (STRA-tah) (sing. stratum). The epidermis is composed entirely of epithelial cells and contains no blood vessels.

- The **dermis,** or true skin, has a framework of connective tissue and contains many blood vessels, nerve endings, and glands.

Figure 6-2 is a photograph of the skin as seen through a microscope showing the layers and some accessory structures.

Epidermis

The epidermis is the surface portion of the skin, the outermost cells of which are constantly lost through wear and tear. Because there are no blood vessels in the epidermis,

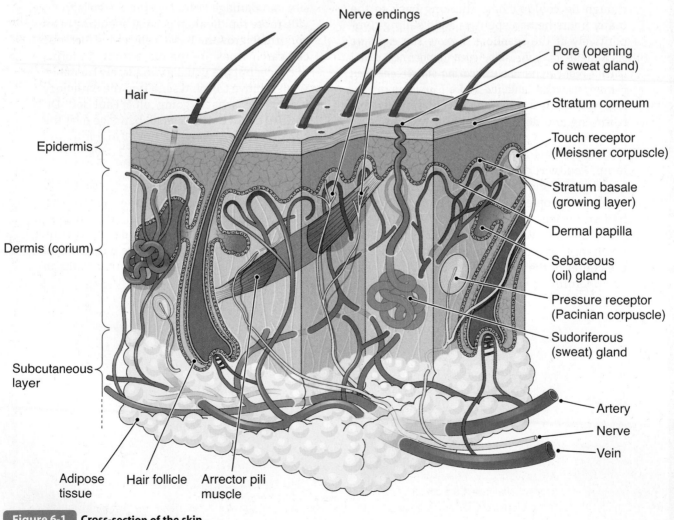

Figure 6-1 **Cross-section of the skin.**

Figure 6-2 **Microscopic view of thin skin.** Tissue layers and some accessory structures are labeled. (Reprinted with permission from Cormack DH. *Essential Histology*, 2nd ed. Philadelphia: Lippincott Williams & Wilkins, 2001.)

the cells must be nourished by capillaries in the underlying dermis. New epidermal cells are produced in the deepest layer, which is closest to the dermis. The cells in this layer, the **stratum basale** (bas-A-le), or **stratum germinativum** (jer-min-a-TI-vum), are constantly dividing and producing daughter cells, which are then pushed upward toward the skin's surface. As the epidermal cells die from the gradual loss of nourishment, they undergo changes. Mainly, their cytoplasm is replaced by large amounts of a protein called **keratin** (KER-ah-tin), which thickens and protects the skin (Fig. 6-3).

By the time epidermal cells approach the surface, they have become flat, filled with keratin, and horny, forming the uppermost layer of the epidermis, the **stratum corneum**

Figure 6-3 **Upper portion of the skin.** Layers of keratin in the stratum corneum are visible at the surface. Below are layers of stratified squamous epithelium making up the remainder of the epidermis. (Reprinted with permission from Cormack DH. *Essential Histology*, 2nd ed. Philadelphia: Lippincott Williams & Wilkins, 2001.)

(KOR-ne-um). The stratum corneum is a protective layer and is more prominent in thick skin than in thin skin. Cells at the surface are constantly being lost and replaced from below, especially in areas of the skin that are subject to wear and tear, as on the scalp, face, soles of the feet, and palms of the hands. Although this process of **exfoliation** (eks-fo-le-A-shun) occurs naturally at all times, many cosmetics companies sell products to promote exfoliation, presumably to "enliven" and "refresh" the skin.

Between the stratum basale and the stratum corneum there are additional layers of stratified epithelium that vary in number and quantity depending on the skin's thickness.

Cells in the deepest layer of the epidermis produce **melanin** (MEL-ah-nin), a dark pigment that colors the skin and protects it from the harmful rays of sunlight. The cells that produce this pigment are the **melanocytes** (MEL-ah-no-sites). Irregular patches of melanin are called freckles.

Dermis

The **dermis,** the so-called "true skin," has a framework of elastic connective tissue and is well supplied with blood vessels and nerves. Because of its elasticity, the skin can stretch, even dramatically as in pregnancy, with little damage. Most of the skin's accessory structures, including the sweat glands, the oil glands, and the hair, are located in the dermis and may extend into the subcutaneous layer under the skin.

The thickness of the dermis also varies in different areas. Some places, such as the soles of the feet and the palms of the hands, are covered with very thick layers of skin, whereas others, such as the eyelids, are covered with very thin and delicate layers. (See Box 6-1, Thick and Thin Skin: Getting a Grip on Their Differences.)

Portions of the dermis extend upward into the epidermis, allowing blood vessels to get closer to the surface cells (see Figs. 6-1 and 6-2). These extensions, or **dermal papillae,** can be seen on the surface of thick skin, such as at the tips of the fingers and toes. Here they form a distinct pattern of ridges that help to prevent slipping, such as when grasping an object. The unchanging patterns of the ridges are determined by heredity. Because they are unique to each person, fingerprints and footprints can be used for identification.

CHECKPOINT 6-1 ➤ The skin and all its associated structures comprise a body system. What is the name of this system?

CHECKPOINT 6-2 ➤ The skin itself is composed of two layers. Moving from the superficial to the deeper layer, what are the names of these two layers?

Subcutaneous Layer

The dermis rests on the **subcutaneous** (sub-ku-TA-ne-us) **layer,** sometimes referred to as the hypodermis or the su-

Thick and Thin Skin: Getting a Grip on Their Differences

The skin is the largest organ in the body, weighing about 4 kg. Though it appears uniform in structure and function, its thickness in fact varies, from less than 1 mm covering the eyelids to more than 5 mm on the upper back. Many of the functional differences between skin regions reflect the thickness of the epidermis and not the skin's overall thickness. Based on epidermal thickness, skin can be categorized as **thick** (about 1 mm deep) or **thin** (about 0.1 mm deep).

Areas of the body exposed to significant wear-and-tear (the palms, fingertips, and bottoms of the feet and toes) are covered with thick skin. It is composed of a thick stratum corneum and an extra layer not found in thin skin, the stratum lucidum, both of which make thick skin resistant to abrasion. Thick skin is also characterized by epidermal ridges (e.g., fingerprints) and numerous sweat glands, but lacks hair and

sebaceous (oil) glands. These adaptations make the thick skin covering the hands and feet effective for grasping or gripping. Thick skin's dermis also contains many sensory receptors, giving the hands and feet a superior sense of touch.

Thin skin covers body areas not exposed to much wear-and-tear. It has a very thin stratum corneum and lacks a distinct stratum lucidum. Though thin skin lacks epidermal ridges and has fewer sensory receptors than thick skin, it has several specializations that thick skin does not. Thin skin is covered with hair, which may help prevent heat loss from the body. In fact, hair is most densely distributed in skin that covers regions of great heat loss—the head, axillae (armpits), and groin. Thin skin also contains numerous sebaceous glands, making it supple and free of cracks that might let infectious organisms enter.

---

perficial fascia (see Fig. 6-1). This layer connects the skin to the surface muscles. It consists of loose connective tissue and large amounts of adipose (fat) tissue. The fat serves as insulation and as a reserve energy supply. Continuous bundles of elastic fibers connect the subcutaneous tissue with the dermis, so there is no clear boundary between the two.

The blood vessels that supply the skin with nutrients and oxygen and help to regulate body temperature run through the subcutaneous layer. This tissue is also rich in nerves and nerve endings, including those that supply nerve impulses to and from the dermis and epidermis. The thickness of the subcutaneous layer varies in different parts of the body; it is thinnest on the eyelids and thickest on the abdomen.

CHECKPOINT 6-3 ➤ What is the composition of the subcutaneous layer?

Accessory Structures of the Skin

The integumentary system includes some structures associated with the skin—glands, hair, and nails—that not only protect the skin itself but have some more generalized functions as well.

 PASSport to Success   Visit **thePoint** or see the Student Resource CD in the back of this book for a summary of the skin's accessory structures.

Sebaceous (Oil) Glands

The **sebaceous** (se-BA-shus) **glands** are saclike in structure, and their oily secretion, **sebum** (SE-bum), lubricates the skin and hair and prevents drying. The ducts of the sebaceous glands open into the hair follicles (Fig. 6-4A).

Babies are born with a covering produced by these glands that resembles cream cheese; this secretion is called the **vernix caseosa** (VER-niks ka-se-O-sah), which literally means "cheesy varnish." Modified sebaceous glands, **meibomian** (mi-BO-me-an) **glands**, are associated with the eyelashes and produce a secretion that lubricates the eyes.

Blackheads consist of a mixture of dried sebum and keratin that may collect at the openings of the sebaceous glands. If these glands become infected, pimples result. If a sebaceous gland becomes blocked, a sac of accumulated sebum may form and gradually increase in size. Such a sac is referred to as a **sebaceous cyst**. Usually, it is not difficult to remove such tumorlike cysts by surgery.

Sudoriferous (Sweat) Glands

The **sudoriferous** (su-do-RIF-er-us) **glands**, or sweat glands, are coiled, tubelike structures located in the dermis and the subcutaneous tissue (see Fig. 6-4B). Most of the sudoriferous glands function to cool the body. They release sweat, or perspiration, that draws heat from the skin as the moisture evaporates at the surface. These **eccrine** (EK-rin) type sweat glands are distributed throughout the skin. Each gland has a secretory portion and an excretory tube that extends directly to the surface and opens at a pore (see also Fig. 6-1). Because sweat contains small

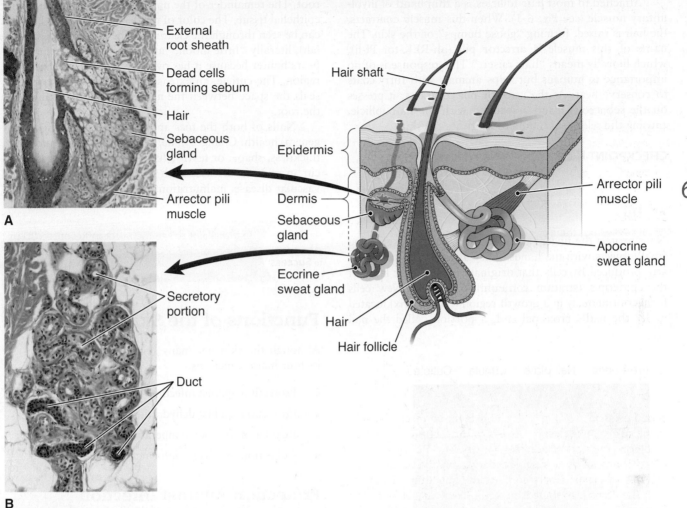

External root sheath

Dead cells forming sebum

Hair

Sebaceous gland

Arrector pili muscle

A

Secretory portion

Duct

B

Hair shaft

Epidermis

Dermis

Sebaceous gland

Eccrine sweat gland

Hair

Hair follicle

Arrector pili muscle

Apocrine sweat gland

6

Figure 6-4 **Portion of skin showing associated glands and hair. (A)** A sebaceous (oil) gland and its associated hair follicle. **(B)** An eccrine (temperature-regulating) sweat gland. (A and B, Reprinted with permission from Cormack DH. *Essential Histology*, 2nd ed. Philadelphia: Lippincott Williams & Wilkins, 2001.) **[ZOOMING IN ➤** How do the sebaceous glands and apocrine sweat glands secrete to the outside? What kind of epithelium makes up the sweat glands? **]**

amounts of dissolved salts and other wastes in addition to water, these glands also serve a minor excretory function.

Present in smaller number, the **apocrine** (AP-o-krin) sweat glands are located mainly in the armpits (axillae) and groin area. These glands become active at puberty and release their secretions through the hair follicles in response to emotional stress and sexual stimulation. The apocrine glands release some cellular material in their secretions. Body odor develops from the action of bacteria in breaking down these organic cellular materials.

Several types of glands associated with the skin are modified sweat glands. These are the **ceruminous** (seh-RU-min-us) **glands** in the ear canal that produce ear wax, or **cerumen**; the **ciliary** (SIL-e-er-e) **glands** at the edges of the eyelids; and the **mammary glands**.

CHECKPOINT 6-4 ➤ Some skin glands produce an oily secretion called sebum. What is the name of these glands?

CHECKPOINT 6-5 ➤ What is the scientific name for the sweat glands?

Hair

Almost all of the body is covered with hair, which in most areas is soft and fine. Hairless regions are the palms of the hands, soles of the feet, lips, nipples, and parts of the external genital areas. Hair is composed mainly of keratin and is not living. Each hair develops, however, from living cells located in a bulb at the base of the **hair follicle**, a sheath of epithelial and connective tissue that encloses the hair (see Fig. 6-4). Melanocytes in this growth region add pigment to the developing hair. Different shades of melanin produce the various hair colors we see in the population. The part of the hair that projects above the skin is the **shaft**; the portion below the skin is the **root** of the hair.

Attached to most hair follicles is a thin band of involuntary muscle (see Fig. 6-1). When this muscle contracts, the hair is raised, forming "goose bumps" on the skin. The name of this muscle is **arrector pili** (ah-REK-tor PI-li), which literally means "hair raiser." This response is of no importance to humans but helps animals with furry coats to conserve heat. As the arrector pili contracts, it presses on the sebaceous gland associated with the hair follicle, causing the release of sebum to lubricate the skin.

CHECKPOINT 6-6 ➤ Each hair develops within a sheath. What is this sheath called?

Nails

Nails protect the fingers and toes and also help in grasping small objects with the hands. They are made of hard keratin produced by cells that originate in the outer layer of the epidermis (stratum corneum) (Fig. 6-5). New cells form continuously in a growth region (nail matrix) located under the nail's proximal end, a portion called the **nail**

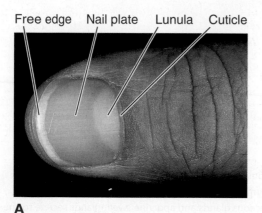

A

Free edge   Nail plate   Lunula   Cuticle

B

Nail bed   Lunula
Nail plate
Cuticle   Nail root
Distal bone of finger   Growth region (nail matrix)

Figure 6-5 **Nail structure. (A)** Photograph of a nail, superior view. **(B)** Midsagittal section of a fingertip. (A, Reprinted with permission from Bickley LS. *Bates' Guide to Physical Examination and History Taking*, 8th ed. Philadelphia: Lippincott Williams & Wilkins, 2003.)

root. The remainder of the **nail plate** rests on a **nail bed** of epithelial tissue. The color of the dermis below the nail bed can be seen through the clear nail. The pale **lunula** (LU-nu-lah), literally "little moon," at the nail's proximal end appears lighter because it lies over the nail's thicker growing region. The **cuticle**, an extension of the stratum corneum, seals the space between the nail plate and the skin above the root.

Nails of both the toes and the fingers are affected by general health. Changes in nails, including abnormal color, thickness, shape, or texture (e.g., grooves or splitting), occur in chronic diseases such as heart disease, peripheral vascular disease, malnutrition, and anemia.

PASSport to Success — Visit **thePoint** or see the Student Resource CD in the back of this book to view some of these conditions.

Functions of the Skin

Although the skin has many functions, the following are its four major functions:

- Protection against infection
- Protection against dehydration (drying)
- Regulation of body temperature
- Collection of sensory information

Protection Against Infection

Intact skin forms a primary barrier against invasion of pathogens. The cells of the stratum corneum form a tight interlocking pattern that resists penetration. The surface cells are constantly shed, thus mechanically removing pathogens. Rupture of this barrier, as in cases of wounds or burns, invites infection of deep tissues. The skin also protects against bacterial toxins (poisons) and some harmful chemicals in the environment.

Protection Against Dehydration

Both keratin in the epidermis and the oily sebum released to the skin's surface from the sebaceous glands help to waterproof the skin and prevent water loss by evaporation.

Regulation of Body Temperature

Both the loss of excess heat and protection from cold are important functions of the skin. Indeed, most of the skin's blood flow is concerned with temperature regulation. In cold conditions, vessels in the skin constrict (become narrower) to reduce blood flow to the surface and diminish heat loss. The skin may become visibly pale under these conditions. Special vessels that directly connect arteries and veins in the skin of the ears, nose, and other exposed locations provide the volume of blood flow needed to prevent freezing.

To cool the body, the skin forms a large surface for radiating body heat to the surrounding air. When the blood vessels dilate (widen), more blood is brought to the surface so that heat can be dissipated.

The other mechanism for cooling the body involves the sweat glands, as noted above. The evaporation of perspiration draws heat from the skin. A person feels uncomfortable on a hot and humid day because water does not evaporate as readily from the skin into the surrounding air. A dehumidifier makes one more comfortable even when the temperature remains high.

As is the case with so many body functions, temperature regulation is complex and involves other areas, including certain centers in the brain.

Collection of Sensory Information

Because of its many nerve endings and other special receptors, the skin may be regarded as one of the body's chief sensory organs. Free nerve endings detect pain and moderate changes in temperature. Other types of sensory receptors in the skin respond to light touch and deep pressure. Figure 6-1 shows some free nerve endings, a touch receptor (Meissner corpuscle), and a deep pressure receptor (Pacinian corpuscle) in a section of skin.

Many of the reflexes that make it possible for humans to adjust themselves to the environment begin as sensory impulses from the skin. As elsewhere in the body, the skin works with the brain and the spinal cord to accomplish these important functions.

Other Activities of the Skin

Substances can be absorbed through the skin in limited amounts. Some drugs—for example, estrogens, other steroids, anesthetics, and medications to control motion sickness—can be absorbed from patches placed on the skin. (See Box 6-2, Medication Patches: No Bitter Pill to Swallow.) Most medicated ointments used on the skin, however, are for the treatment of local conditions only. Even medication injected into the subcutaneous tissues is absorbed very slowly.

There is also a minimal amount of excretion through the skin. Water and electrolytes (salts) are excreted in sweat (perspiration). Some nitrogen-containing wastes are eliminated through the skin, but even in disease, the amount of waste products excreted by the skin is small.

Vitamin D needed for the development and maintenance of bone tissue is manufactured in the skin under the effects of ultraviolet radiation in sunlight.

Note that the human skin does not "breathe." The pores of the epidermis serve only as outlets for perspiration from the sweat glands and sebum (oil) from the sebaceous glands. They are not used for exchange of gases.

CHECKPOINT 6-7 ➤ What two mechanisms are used to regulate temperature through the skin?

Box 6-2   ☤   Clinical Perspectives

Medication Patches: No Bitter Pill to Swallow

For most people, pills are a convenient way to take medication, but for others, they have drawbacks. Pills must be taken at regular intervals to ensure consistent dosing, and they must be digested and absorbed into the bloodstream before they can begin to work. For those who have difficulty swallowing or digesting pills, **transdermal (TD) patches** offer an effective alternative to oral medications.

TD patches deliver a consistent dose of medication that diffuses at a constant rate through the skin into the bloodstream. There is no daily schedule to follow, nothing to swallow, and no stomach upset. TD patches can also deliver medication to unconscious patients, who would otherwise require intravenous drug delivery. TD patches are used in hormone replacement therapy, to treat heart disease, to manage pain, and to suppress motion sickness. Nicotine patches are also used as part of programs to quit smoking.

TD patches must be used carefully. Drug diffusion through the skin takes time, so it is important to know how long the patch must be in place before it is effective. It is also important to know how long the medication's effects take to disappear after the patch is removed. Because the body continues to absorb what has already diffused into the skin, removing the patch does not entirely remove the medicine. Also, increased heat may elevate drug absorption to dangerous levels.

A recent advance in TD drug delivery is **iontophoresis**. Based on the principle that like charges repel each other, this method uses a mild electrical current to move ionic drugs through the skin. A small electrical device attached to the patch uses positive current to "push" positively charged drug molecules through the skin, and a negative current to push negatively charged ones. Even though very low levels of electricity are used, people with pacemakers should not use iontophoretic patches. Another disadvantage is that they can move only ionic drugs through the skin.

Observation of the Skin

What can the skin tell you? What do its color, texture, and other attributes indicate? Is there any damage? Much can be learned by an astute observer. In fact, the first indication of a serious systemic disease (such as syphilis) may be a skin disorder.

Color

The color of the skin depends on a number of factors, including the following:

■ Amount of pigment in the epidermis

■ Quantity of blood circulating in the surface blood vessels

■ Composition of the circulating blood, including:

> Quantity of oxygen

> Concentration of hemoglobin

> Presence of bile, silver compounds, or other chemicals

PIGMENT The skin's main pigment, as we have noted, is called **melanin**. This pigment is also found in the hair, the middle coat of the eyeball, the iris of the eye, and certain tumors. Melanin is common to all races, but darker people have a much larger quantity in their tissues. The melanin in the skin helps to protect against the sun's damaging ultraviolet radiation. Thus, skin that is exposed to the sun shows a normal increase in this pigment, a response we call tanning.

Sometimes, there are abnormal increases in the quantity of melanin, which may occur either in localized areas or over the entire body surface. For example, diffuse spots of pigmentation may be characteristic of some endocrine disorders. In **albinism** (AL-bih-nizm), a hereditary disorder that affects melanin production, there is lack of pigment in the skin, hair, and eyes.

Another pigment that imparts color to the skin is carotene, a pigment obtained from carrots and other orange and yellow vegetables. Carotene is stored in fatty tissue and skin. Also visible is hemoglobin, the pigment that gives blood its color, which can be seen through the vessels in the dermis.

DISCOLORATION Pallor (PAL-or) is paleness of the skin, often caused by reduced blood flow or by reduction in hemoglobin, as occurs in cases of anemia. Pallor is most easily noted in the lips, nail beds, and mucous membranes. **Flushing** is redness of the skin, often related to fever. Signs of flushing are most noticeable in the face and neck.

When there is not enough oxygen in circulating blood, the skin may take on a bluish discoloration termed **cyanosis** (si-ah-NO-sis) (Fig. 6-6A). This is a symptom of heart failure and of breathing problems, such as asthma or respiratory obstruction.

A yellowish discoloration of the skin may be caused by excessive amounts of bile pigments, mainly bilirubin (BIL-ih-ru-bin), in the blood (Fig. 6-6B). (Bile is a substance produced by the liver that aids in fat digestion; see Chapter 19.) This condition, called **jaundice** (JAWN-dis) (from the French word for "yellow"), may be a symptom of certain disorders, including:

■ A tumor pressing on the common bile duct or a stone within the duct, either of which would obstruct bile flow into the small intestine

■ Inflammation of the liver (hepatitis), commonly caused by a virus

■ Certain blood diseases in which red blood cells are rapidly destroyed (hemolyzed)

■ Immaturity of the liver. Neonatal (newborn) jaundice occurs when the liver is not yet capable of processing bilirubin (bile pigment). Most such cases correct themselves without treatment in about a week, but this form of jaundice may be treated by exposure to special fluorescent light that helps the body to eliminate bilirubin.

Another possible cause of a yellowish skin discoloration is the excessive intake of carrots and other deeply colored vegetables. This condition is known as **carotenemia** (kar-o-te-NE-me-ah).

A   B

Figure 6-6 **Discoloration of the skin.** **(A)** Cyanosis is a bluish discoloration caused by lack of oxygen. It is seen here in the toes as compared to normal fingertips. **(B)** Jaundice is a yellowish discoloration caused by bile pigments in the blood. (Reprinted with permission from Bickley LS. *Bates' Guide to Physical Examination and History Taking*, 8th ed. Philadelphia: Lippincott Williams & Wilkins, 2003.) [**ZOOMING IN ➤** What color is associated with cyanosis? What color is associated with jaundice?]

Certain types of chronic poisoning may cause gray or brown discoloration of the skin. A peculiar bronze cast is present in Addison disease (malfunction of the adrenal gland). Many other disorders cause skin discoloration, but their discussion is beyond the scope of this chapter.

CHECKPOINT 6-8 ➤ What are some pigments that impart color to the skin?

Lesions

A **lesion** (LE-zhun) is any wound or local damage to tissue. In examining the skin for lesions, it is important to make note of their type, arrangement, and location. Lesions may be flat or raised or may extend below the skin's surface.

SURFACE LESIONS A surface lesion is often called a **rash** or, if raised, an **eruption** (e-RUP-shun). Skin rashes may be localized, as in diaper rash, or generalized, as in measles and other systemic infections. Often, these lesions are accompanied by **erythema** (er-eh-THE-mah), or redness of the skin. The following are some terms used to describe surface skin lesions:

- **Macule** (MAK-ule)—a spot that is neither raised nor depressed. Macules are typical of measles and descriptive of freckles (Fig. 6-7A).
- **Papule** (PAP-ule)—a firm, raised area, as in some stages of chickenpox and in the second stage of syphilis (see Fig. 6-7B). A pimple is a papule. A large firm papule is called a **nodule** (NOD-ule).
- **Vesicle** (VES-ih-kl)—a blister or small fluid-filled sac as seen in chickenpox or shingles eruptions (see Fig. 6-7C). Another term for a vesicle is a **bulla** (BUL-ah).
- **Pustule** (PUS-tule)—a vesicle filled with pus. Pustules may develop if vesicles become infected (see Fig. 6-7D).

DEEPER LESIONS A deeper skin lesion may develop from a surface lesion or may be caused by **trauma** (TRAW-mah), that is, a wound or injury. Because such breaks may be followed by infection, wounds should be cared for to prevent the entrance of pathogens and toxins into deeper tissues and body fluids. Deeper injuries to the skin include the following:

- **Excoriation** (eks-ko-re-A-shun)—a scratch into the skin
- **Laceration** (las-er-A-shun)—a rough, jagged wound made by tearing of the skin
- **Ulcer** (UL-ser)—a sore associated with disintegration and death of tissue (Fig. 6-8A)
- **Fissure** (FISH-ure)—a crack in the skin. Athlete's foot, for example, can produce fissures. Tongue fissures may be normal variations in the tongue's surface (see Fig. 6-8B), but may also appear on the lips or tongue as a result of injury or disease.

CHECKPOINT 6-9 ➤ What is a lesion?

A Macule

B Papule

C Vesicle

D Pustule

Figure 6-7 **Surface lesions. (A)** Macules on the dorsal surface of the hand, wrist, and forearm. **(B)** Papules on the knee. **(C)** Vesicles on the chin. **(D)** Pustules on the palm. (Photographs reprinted with permission from Bickley LS. *Bates' Guide to Physical Examination and History Taking*, 8th ed. Philadelphia: Lippincott Williams & Wilkins, 2003. Line drawings reprinted with permission from Cohen BJ. *Medical Terminology*, 5th ed. Philadelphia: Lippincott Williams & Wilkins, 2008.)

6

A Ulcer

B Fissures

Figure 6-8 **Deeper lesions. (A)** Tongue ulcer. **(B)** Tongue fissures. (Photographs reprinted with permission from Langlais RP, Miller CS. *Color Atlas of Common Oral Diseases*, 3rd ed. Philadelphia: Lippincott Williams & Wilkins, 2002. Line drawings reprinted with permission from Cohen BJ. *Medical Terminology*, 5th ed. Philadelphia: Lippincott Williams & Wilkins, 2008.)

Burns

Most burns are caused by contact with hot objects, explosions, or scalding with hot liquids. They may also be caused by electrical injuries, contact with harmful chemicals, or abrasion. Burns are assessed by the depth of damage and the percentage of body surface area (BSA) involved. Depth of tissue destruction is categorized as follows:

■ **Superficial partial-thickness**—involves the epidermis and perhaps a portion of the dermis. The tissue is reddened and may blister, as in cases of sunburn.

■ **Deep partial-thickness**—involves the epidermis and portions of the dermis. The tissue is blistered and broken, with a weeping surface. Causes include scalding and exposure to flame.

■ **Full-thickness**—involves the full skin and sometimes subcutaneous tissue and underlying tissues as well. The tissue is broken, dry and pale, or charred. These injuries may require skin grafting and may result in loss of digits or limbs.

The above classification replaces an older system of ranking burns as first-, second-, and third-degree according to the depth of tissue damage.

The amount of body surface area involved in a burn may be estimated by using the **rule of nines**, in which surface areas are assigned percentages in multiples of nine (Fig. 6-9). The more accurate Lund and Browder method divides the body into small areas and estimates the proportion of BSA that each contributes.

Infection is a common complication of burns, because the skin, a major defense against invasion of microorganisms, is damaged. Respiratory complications may be caused by inhalation of smoke and toxic chemicals, and circulatory problems may result from loss of fluids and electrolytes. Treatment of burns includes respiratory care, administration of fluids, wound care, and pain control. Patients must be monitored for circulatory complications, infections, and signs of posttraumatic stress.

SUNBURN Sunlight can cause chemical and biologic changes in the skin. On exposure, the skin first becomes reddened (erythematous) and then may become swollen and blistered. Sunlight can cause severe burns that result in serious illness.

Excessive exposure to the ultraviolet (UV) radiation in sunlight causes genetic mutations in skin cells that interfere with repair mechanisms and may lead to cancer. It also causes premature skin aging involving wrinkling, discoloration ("age spots" or "liver spots") and a "leathery" texture. Note that radiation exposure in tanning booths is no safer than sun tanning.

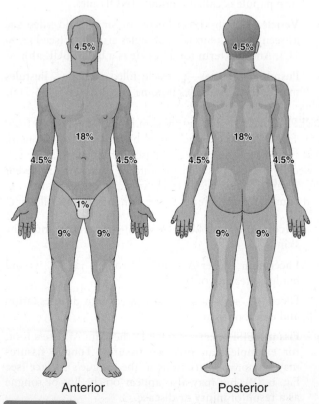

Anterior　　　　Posterior

Figure 6-9 **The rule of nines.** This method is used to estimate percentages of body surface area (BSA) in treatment of burns.

Disease in Context revisited

► Squamous Cell Carcinoma

Paul was edgy during the 3 days before he called back at the dermatologist's office. *What if I have skin cancer? Even if it's treatable, I may have a scar—and right smack in the center of my face!* Finally, he made the call, and learned from Dr. Nielsen that he did indeed have a small squamous cell carcinoma.

"I recommend that you consult Dr. Morris, a local surgeon who specializes in a procedure that guarantees the removal of all abnormal cells," the dermatologist advised. "Mohs surgery is done in stages, with the surgeon first removing just the visible lesion and then checking microscopically to be sure that the margins of the excised tissue are free of cancerous cells. If not, additional tissue is removed by degrees until the margins are clean."

Fortunately, Dr. Morris had to repeat the procedure only once after the first pathology examination to be sure of success. Paul left reassured after several hours. Dr. Morris was confident that Paul was safe from the cancer and that scarring would be minimal. "Let's make an appointment for a follow-up visit when I'll remove the stitches and you can see for yourself," he said.

That evening Paul described his day to his wife and told of his additional instructions. "I need to see my regular dermatologist every 6 months now, as I may be prone to these types of carcinomas." Paul can't undo earlier damage, but he can prevent further insult to his skin by wearing sunscreen outdoors and reapplying it often. The doctor also advised him to cover up in the sun and avoid times of high sun intensity. "Come to think of it," Paul said to his wife, "that's good advice for you too!"

In this case, we saw the carcinogenic effect of sun damage on the integumentary system. (To review the topics of neoplasms and malignancy, refer back to Chapters 3 and 4.) Unfortunately for Paul, the effects of years of sun damage are not limited to his skin. In Chapter 11, *The Sensory System*, we'll learn how sun exposure can affect other systems as well.

Tissue Repair

True tissue regeneration after injury can occur only in areas that have actively dividing cells or cells that can be triggered to divide by injury. Specifically, these tissues are the epithelial and connective tissues. Even among the connective tissues, repair occurs more slowly in tissues that are not very active metabolically, in cartilage for example. Muscle tissue and nervous tissue, which stop dividing early in life, generally do not restore themselves, although some types can carry out minimal regeneration. When muscle and nervous tissues are injured, they are generally replaced by connective tissue.

Repair of a skin wound or lesion begins after blood has clotted and a scab has formed at the surface to protect underlying tissue. From damaged capillaries, new vessels branch and grow into the injured tissue. Fibroblasts (fiber-producing cells) manufacture collagen to close the gap made by the wound. A large wound requires extensive growth of new connective tissue, which develops from within the wound. This new tissue forms a **scar**, also called a **cicatrix** (SIK-ah-triks).

After the upper layer of epithelium has regenerated, the scab is released. The underlying scar tissue may then continue to show at the surface as a white line. Scar tissue is strong but is not as flexible as normal tissue and does not function like the tissue it replaces. Suturing (sewing) the edges of a clean wound together, as is done in the case of operative wounds, decreases the amount of connective tissue needed for repair and thus reduces the size of the resulting scar.

Excess collagen production in the formation of a scar may result in the development of **keloids** (KE-loyds), tumorlike masses or sharply raised areas on the skin surface. These are not dangerous but may be removed for the sake of appearance.

Wound healing is affected by:

- Nutrition—A complete and balanced diet will provide the nutrients needed for cell regeneration. All required vitamins and minerals are important, but especially vitamins A and C, which are needed for collagen.

- Blood supply—The blood brings oxygen and nutrients to the tissues and also carries away waste materials and toxins (poisons) that might form during the healing process. White blood cells attack invading bacteria at the site of the injury. Poor circulation, as occurs in cases of diabetes, for example, will delay wound healing.

- Infection—Contamination prolongs inflammation and interferes with the formation of materials needed for wound repair.

■ Age—Healing is generally slower among the elderly due to a slower rate of cell replacement. The elderly also may have a lowered immune response to infection.

CHECKPOINT 6-10 ➤ What two categories of tissues repair themselves most easily?

PASSport to Success — Visit *thePoint* or see the Student Resource CD in the back of this book to view an animation on wound healing.

Effects of Aging on the Integumentary System

As people age, wrinkles, or crow's feet, develop around the eyes and mouth owing to the loss of fat and collagen in the underlying tissues. The dermis becomes thinner, and the skin may become transparent and lose its elasticity, an effect sometimes called "parchment skin." Pigment formation decreases with age. However, there may be localized areas of extra pigmentation in the skin with the formation of brown spots ("liver spots"), especially on areas exposed to the sun (e.g., the back of the hands). Circulation to the dermis decreases, so white skin looks paler.

The hair does not replace itself as rapidly as before and thus becomes thinner on the scalp and elsewhere on the body. Decreased melanin production leads to gray or white hair. Hair texture changes as the hair shaft becomes less dense, and hair, like the skin, becomes drier as sebum production decreases.

The sweat glands decrease in number, so there is less output of perspiration and lowered ability to withstand heat. The elderly are also more sensitive to cold because of less fat in the skin and poor circulation. The fingernails may flake, become brittle, or develop ridges, and toenails may become discolored or abnormally thickened.

Care of the Skin

The most important factors in caring for the skin are those that ensure good general health. Proper nutrition and adequate circulation are vital to skin maintenance. Regular cleansing removes dirt and dead skin debris and sustains the slightly acid environment that inhibits bacterial growth. Careful hand washing with soap and water, with attention to the under-nail areas, is a simple measure that reduces the spread of disease.

The skin needs protection from continued exposure to sunlight to prevent premature aging and cancerous changes. Appropriate applications of sunscreens before and during time spent in the sun, especially after swimming, can prevent skin damage. Limiting sun exposure during midday and covering up with protective clothing are also important.

Skin Disorders

Skin disorders range from simple superficial nuisances, such as acne and rashes, to more deep-seated problems that may lead to systemic disease.

Dermatitis

Dermatosis (der-mah-TO-sis) is a general term referring to any skin disease. Inflammation of the skin is called **dermatitis** (der-mah-TI-tis). It may be caused by many kinds of irritants, such as the oil of poison oak or poison ivy plants, detergents, and strong acids, alkalis, or other chemicals. Prompt removal of the irritant is the most effective method of prevention and treatment. A thorough cleansing as soon as possible after contact with plant oils may prevent the development of itching eruptions.

ATOPIC DERMATITIS Atopic dermatitis (ah-TOP-ik der-mah-TI-tis) or **eczema** (EK-ze-mah) is characterized by intense itching and skin inflammation (Fig. 6-10). The affected areas show redness (erythema), blisters (vesicles), pimplelike lesions (papules), and scaling and crusting of the skin surface. Scratching (excoriation) of the skin can lead to a secondary bacterial infection. Atopic dermatitis commonly first occurs in early childhood, with the recurrence of acute episodes throughout life. The skin may be excessively sensitive to many soaps, detergents, rough fabrics, or perspiration. The person with atopic dermatitis may also be subject to allergic disorders, such as hay fever, asthma, and food allergies.

Figure 6-10 **Atopic dermatitis (eczema).** Scratches (excoriation) are visible in the photo. (Reprinted with permission from Bickley LS. *Bates' Guide to Physical Examination and History Taking*, 8th ed. Philadelphia: Lippincott Williams & Wilkins, 2003.)

Figure 6-11 **Psoriasis.** Silvery surface scales are visible. (Reprinted with permission from Bickley LS. *Bates' Guide to Physical Examination and History Taking*, 8th ed. Philadelphia: Lippincott Williams & Wilkins, 2003.)

Psoriasis

Psoriasis (so-RI-ah-sis) is a chronic overgrowth of the epidermis leading to large, sharply outlined, red (erythematous), flat areas (plaques) covered with silvery scales (Fig. 6-11). The cause of this chronic, recurrent skin disease is unknown, but there is sometimes a hereditary pattern, and an immune disorder may be involved. Psoriasis is treated with topical corticosteroids and exposure to ultraviolet (UV) light.

CHECKPOINT 6-11 ➤ What is the difference between dermatosis and dermatitis?

Cancer

Skin cancer is the most common form of cancer in the United States. Exposure to sunlight predisposes to development of skin cancer, which, in the United States, is most common among people who have fair skin and who live in the Southwest, where exposure to the sun is consistent and may be intense.

Basal cell and squamous cell carcinomas arise in the epidermis and generally appear on the face, neck, and hands (Fig. 6-12A,B). Early detection and treatment in these cases usually results in cure, although squamous cell carcinoma is the more likely to metastasize.

Melanoma (mel-ah-NO-mah) is a malignant tumor of melanocytes (melanin-forming cells). This type of cancer originates in a **nevus** (NE-vus), a mole or birthmark, anywhere in the body (see Fig. 6-12C). Unlike a normal mole, which has an evenly round shape and well-defined border, a melanoma may show irregularity in shape. Other signs of melanoma are a change in color or uneven color and increase in size of a mole. A predisposing factor for melanoma is severe, blistering sunburn, although these cancers can appear in areas not sun-exposed, such as the soles of the feet, between fingers and toes, and in mucous membranes.

CHECKPOINT 6-12 ➤ What is the name for a cancer of the skin's pigment-producing cells?

Acne and Other Skin Infections

Acne (AK-ne) is a disease of the sebaceous (oil) glands connected with the hair follicles. The common type, called **acne vulgaris** (vul-GA-ris), is found most often in people between the ages of 14 and 25 years. The infection takes the form of pimples, which generally surround blackheads. Acne is usually most severe at adolescence, when certain endocrine glands that control sebaceous secretions are particularly active.

IMPETIGO Impetigo (im-peh-TI-go) is an acute contagious disease of staphylococcal or streptococcal origin that may be serious enough to cause death in newborn infants. It takes the form of blisterlike lesions that become filled with pus and contain millions of virulent bacteria. It is found most frequently among poor and undernourished children. Affected people may reinfect themselves or infect others.

VIRAL INFECTIONS One virus that involves the skin is **herpes** (HER-peze) **simplex virus**, which causes the forma-

Figure 6-12   **Skin cancer. (A)** Basal cell carcinoma. **(B)** Squamous cell carcinoma. **(C)** Malignant melanoma. (A, Reprinted with permission from Goodheart HP. *Goodheart's Photoguide of Common Skin Disorders; Diagnosis and Management*, 2nd ed. Philadelphia: Lippincott Williams & Wilkins, 2003; B, Reprinted with permission from Bickley LS. *Bates' Guide to Physical Examination and History Taking*, 8th ed. Philadelphia: Lippincott Williams & Wilkins, 2003; C, Reprinted with permission from Rubin E, Farber JL. *Pathology*, 3rd ed. Philadelphia: Lippincott Williams & Wilkins, 1999.)

tion of watery vesicles (cold sores, fever blisters) on the skin and mucous membranes. Type I herpes causes lesions around the nose and mouth; type II is responsible for genital infections (see Table 2 in Appendix 5).

Shingles (herpes zoster) is seen in adults and is caused by the same virus that causes chickenpox (varicella). Infection follows nerve pathways, producing small lesions on the skin. Vesicular lesions may be noted along the course of a nerve. Pain, increased sensitivity, and itching are common symptoms that usually last longer than a year. Prompt treatment with antiviral drugs decreases the disease's severity.

A **wart**, or **verruca** (veh-RU-kah), is a small tumor caused by a virus of the human papillomavirus (HPV) group. Warts may appear anywhere on the body, including the genital region and the soles of the feet (plantar wart). They can be removed by chemical treatment or surgery. Usually benign, warts have been associated with cancer, especially in the case of genital warts and cancer of the cervix (neck of the uterus).

FUNGAL INFECTIONS Fungi are non-green, plantlike microorganisms that may cause surface infections of the skin. These superficial mycotic (fungal) infections, commonly known as tinea or ringworm, may appear on the face, body, scalp, hands, or feet (Fig. 6-13). When on the foot, the condition is usually called **athlete's foot**, as fungal growth is promoted by the dampness of perspiration. Fungal nail infections commonly result from wearing false nails or acrylic nails, as fungal growth is promoted by the moisture that accumulates under the artificial nails.

Fungal infections are difficult to treat. Topical antifungal agents may be effective, but often the patient must take an oral antifungal drug.

CHECKPOINT 6-13 ➤ What are some viruses that affect the skin?

Figure 6-13 **Tinea (ringworm) of the body.** (Reprinted with permission from Hall JC. *Sauer's Manual of Skin Diseases*, 8th ed. Philadelphia: Lippincott Williams & Wilkins, 1999.)

CHECKPOINT 6-14 ➤ What causes tinea or ringworm infections?

Alopecia (Baldness)

Alopecia (al-o-PE-she-ah), or baldness, may be caused by a number of factors. The most common type, known as male pattern baldness, is an expression of heredity and aging; it is influenced by male sex hormones. Topical applications of the drug minoxidil (used as an oral medication to control blood pressure) have produced hair growth in this type of baldness. Alopecia also may result from a systemic disease, such as uncontrolled diabetes, thyroid disease, or malnutrition. In such cases, control of the disease results in regrowth of hair. An expanding list of drugs has been linked with baldness, including the chemotherapeutic drugs used in treating neoplasms.

Allergy and Other Immune Disorders

Allergy, also known as hypersensitivity, is an unfavorable immune response to a substance that is normally harmless to most people (see Chapter 17). Foods, drugs, cosmetics, and a variety of industrial substances can provoke allergic responses in some people. Often the skin is involved in such responses, showing inflammation, rashes, vesicles, or other forms of eruptions, usually accompanied by severe **pruritus** (pru-RI-tus), or itching.

Urticaria (ur-tih-KA-re-ah), or hives, is an allergic reaction characterized by the temporary appearance of elevated red patches known as *wheals*.

AUTOIMMUNE DISORDERS An autoimmune disease results from an immune reaction to one's own tissues. The following diseases that involve the skin are believed to be caused, at least in part, by autoimmune reactions.

Pemphigus (PEM-fi-gus) is characterized by the formation of blisters, or bullae (BUL-e) in the skin and mucous membranes caused by a separation of epidermal cells from underlying tissue layers. Rupture of these lesions leaves deeper areas of the skin unprotected from infection and fluid loss, much as in cases of burns. Pemphigus is fatal unless treated by methods to suppress the immune system.

Lupus erythematosus (LU-pus er-ih-the-mah-TO-sus) (LE) is a chronic, inflammatory, autoimmune disease of connective tissue. The more widespread form of the disease, systemic lupus erythematosus (SLE), involves the skin and other organs. The discoid form (DLE) involves only the skin. It is seen as rough, raised, violet-tinted papules, usually limited to the face and scalp. There may also be a butterfly-shaped rash across the nose and cheeks, described as a malar (cheekbone) rash. The skin lesions of lupus are worsened by exposure to sunlight's ultraviolet radiation. SLE is more prevalent in women than in men and has a higher incidence among Asians and African Americans than in other populations.

Scleroderma is a disease of unknown cause that involves overproduction of collagen with thickening and tightening of the skin. Sweat glands and hair follicles are also involved. A very early sign of scleroderma is numbness, pain, and tingling on exposure to cold caused by constriction of blood vessels in the fingers and toes. Skin symptoms first appear on the forearms and around the mouth. Internal organs become involved in a diffuse form of scleroderma called progressive systemic sclerosis (PSS).

Pressure Ulcers

Pressure ulcers are skin lesions that appear where the body rests on skin that covers bony projections, such as the spine, heel, elbow, or hip. The pressure interrupts circulation leading to ulceration and death of tissue. Poor general health, malnutrition, age, obesity, and infection contribute to the development of pressure ulcers.

Lesions first appear as redness of the skin. If ignored, they may penetrate the skin and underlying muscle, extending even to bone and requiring months to heal.

Pads or mattresses to relieve pressure, regular cleansing and drying of the skin, frequent change in position, and good nutrition help to prevent pressure ulcers. Prevention of pressure ulcer by these methods is far easier than treatment of an established ulcer.

Other terms for pressure ulcers are *decubitus ulcer* and *bedsore*. Both of these terms refer to lying down, although pressure ulcers may appear in anyone with limited movement, not only those who are confined to bed.

CHECKPOINT 6-15 ➤ What are several autoimmune disorders that involve the skin?

PASSport to Success Visit **thePoint** or see the Student Resource CD in the back of this book for an illustration of systemic lupus erythematosus. Observation and care of the skin are important in nursing as well as other healthcare professions. These resources also have information on nursing careers.

Word Anatomy

Medical terms are built from standardized word parts (prefixes, roots, and suffixes). Learning the meanings of these parts can help you remember words and interpret unfamiliar terms.

WORD PART	MEANING	EXAMPLE
Structure of the Skin		
derm/o	skin	The *epidermis* is the outermost layer of the skin.
corne/o	horny	The stratum *corneum* is the outermost thickened, horny layer of the skin.
melan/o	dark, black	A *melanocyte* is a cell that produces the dark pigment melanin.
sub-	under, below	The *subcutaneous* layer is under the skin.
Accessory Structures of the Skin		
ap/o-	separation from, derivation from	The *apocrine* sweat glands release some cellular material in their secretions.
pil/o	hair	The *arrector pili* muscle raises the hair to produce "goose bumps."
Observation of the Skin		
alb/i	white	*Albinism* is a condition associated with a lack of pigment, so the skin appears white.
-ism	state of	See preceding example.
cyan/o	blue	*Cyanosis* is a bluish discoloration of the skin caused by lack of oxygen.
-sis	condition, process	See preceding example.
bili	bile	*Bilirubin* is a pigment found in bile.

WORD PART	MEANING	EXAMPLE
Observation of the Skin		
-emia	condition of blood	In *carotenemia*, vegetable pigments, as from carrots, appear in the blood and give color to the skin.
eryth	red	*Erythema* is redness of the skin.
Skin Disorders		
dermat/o	skin	*Dermatosis* is any skin disease.
scler/o	hard	*Scleroderma* is associated with a hardening of the skin.

Summary

I. **STRUCTURE OF THE SKIN**
  A. Epidermis—surface layer of the skin
    1. Stratum basale (stratum germinativum)
      a. Produces new cells
      b. Melanocytes produce melanin—dark pigment
    2. Stratum corneum
      a. Surface layer of dead cells
      b. Contain keratin
  B. Dermis (true skin)
    1. Deeper layer of the skin
    2. Has blood vessels and accessory structures
  C. Subcutaneous layer
    1. Under the skin
    2. Made of connective tissue and adipose (fat) tissue

II. **ACCESSORY STRUCTURES OF THE SKIN**
  A. Sebaceous (oil) glands
    1. Release sebum—lubricates skin and hair
  B. Sudoriferous (sweat) glands
    1. Eccrine type
      a. Control body temperature
      b. Widely distributed
      c. Vent directly to surface
    2. Apocrine type
      a. Respond to stress
      b. In armpit and groin
      c. Excrete through hair follicle
  C. Hair
    1. Develop in hair follicle (sheath)
    2. Active cells at base of follicle
  D. Nails
    1. Grow from nail matrix at proximal end

III. **FUNCTIONS OF THE SKIN**
  A. Protection against infection—barrier
  B. Protection against dehydration—keratin and sebum waterproof skin
  C. Regulation of body temperature—blood supply and sweat glands
  D. Collection of sensory information—receptors in skin
  E. Other activities of the skin—absorption, excretion, manufacture of vitamin D

IV. **OBSERVATION OF THE SKIN**
  A. Color
    1. Pigment—mainly melanin, also carotene, hemoglobin
    2. Discoloration—pallor, flushing, cyanosis, jaundice, poisoning
  B. Lesions—wound or local damage
    1. Surface lesions (rash, eruption)
      a. Macule (spot), papule (firm, raised), vesicle (blister), pustule (pus-filled)
    2. Deeper lesions
      b. excoriation (scratch), laceration (tear), ulcer (sore), fissure (crack)
  C. Burns
    1. Evaluated by depth of damage and amount of body surface area (BSA) involved
    2. Sunburn—risk factor in skin cancer and causes premature skin aging

V. **TISSUE REPAIR**
    1. Requires actively dividing cells
    2. Easiest in epithelial and connective tissue
    3. Fibrous material forms scar (cicatrix)
    4. Influenced by nutrition, blood supply, infection, age

VI. **EFFECTS OF AGING ON THE INTEGUMENTARY SYSTEM**

VII. **CARE OF THE SKIN**
  A. Good nutrition
  B. Cleansing
  C. Sun protection

VIII. **SKIN DISORDERS**
  A. Dermatitis—inflammation
    1. Atopic dermatitis (eczema)
  B. Psoriasis
  C. Cancer
    1. Basal cell carcinoma
    2. Squamous cell carcinoma
    3. Melanoma—cancer of melanocytes
  D. Acne and other skin infections
    1. Acne—disease of sebaceous glands related to increased endocrine secretions

2. Impetigo—infectious disease of infants and children
3. Viral infections—herpes viruses, shingles, human papilloma virus
4. Fungal (mycotic) infections—tinea (ringworm)

E. Alopecia—baldness

F. Allergy and other immune disorders
   1. Allergy—hypersensitivity
      a. Urticaria (hives)
   2. Autoimmune disorders—pemphigus, lupus erythematosus, scleroderma
G. Pressure ulcers (decubitus ulcer, bedsore)
   1. Caused by pressure on skin over bone

Questions for Study and Review   6

BUILDING UNDERSTANDING

Fill in the blanks

1. Cells of the stratum corneum contain large amounts of a protein called _____.
2. Sweat glands located in the axillae and groin are called _____ sweat glands.
3. The name of the muscle that raises the hair is _____.
4. A dark-colored pigment that protects the skin from ultraviolet light is called _____.
5. A medical term that means "scar" is _____.

Matching > Match each numbered item with the most closely related lettered item.

___ **6.** Skin sensitivity characterized by intense itching and inflammation
___ **7.** A viral infection that follows nerve pathways, producing small lesions on the overlying skin
___ **8.** Severe itching of the skin
___ **9.** Allergic reaction characterized by the appearance of wheals
___ **10.** Chronic skin disease characterized by red flat areas covered with silvery scales

a. urticaria
b. pruritis
c. shingles
d. psoriasis
e. eczema

Multiple Choice

___ **11.** The epidermis is _____ to the dermis.
   a. superficial
   b. deep
   c. lateral
   d. medial

___ **12.** Acne is an infection of a
   a. sudoriferous gland
   b. sebaceous gland
   c. ceruminous gland
   d. meibomian gland

___ **13.** The medical term for baldness is
   a. alopecia
   b. pemphigus
   c. verruca
   d. dermatitis

___ **14.** Accumulation of bile pigments in the blood causes
   a. pallor
   b. cyanosis
   c. jaundice
   d. carotenemia

___ **15.** Basal cell and squamous cell carcinomas are cancers of
   a. epidermal cells
   b. dermal cells
   c. melanocytes
   d. subcutaneous fat

UNDERSTANDING CONCEPTS

16. Compare and contrast the epidermis, dermis, and hypodermis. How are the outermost cells of the epidermis replaced?

17. What are the four most important functions of the skin?

18. Describe the location and function of the two types of skin glands.

19. Describe the events associated with skin wound healing.

20. What changes may occur in the skin with age?

21. What is the difference between the terms *dermatosis* and *dermatitis*? List examples of irritants that can cause dermatitis.

22. Discuss some ways to prevent and control athlete's foot.

23. What is a decubitus ulcer? List the two best measures for preventing decubitus ulcer.

CONCEPTUAL THINKING

24. Skin is the largest organ in your body. Explain why it is an organ.

25. Remember Mr. Baker from the last chapter? He sustained full-thickness burns to his legs while lighting a fire with gasoline. After Mr. Baker is informed that he will require skin grafting, he asks you why his own skin won't heal by itself. How would you answer his question? Using the rule of nines, estimate Mr. Baker's percentage of body surface area burned.

26. In Paul's case, sun damage caused skin cancer. Which layer of skin was damaged? Why is this layer most likely to become cancerous?

Movement and Support

This unit deals with the skeletal and muscular systems, which work together to execute movement and to support and protect vital organs. It covers the additional functions of the skeletal system in housing the blood-forming tissue and storing some minerals. The chapter on muscles describes the characteristics of all types of muscles and then concentrates on the muscles that are attached to the skeleton and how they function. The main skeletal muscles are named and located and their actions are described.

The Skeleton: Bones and Joints

Learning Outcomes

After careful study of this chapter, you should be able to:

1. List the functions of bones
2. Describe the structure of a long bone
3. Differentiate between compact bone and spongy bone with respect to structure and location
4. Differentiate between red and yellow marrow with respect to function and location
5. Name the three different types of cells in bone and describe the functions of each
6. Explain how a long bone grows
7. Name and describe various markings found on bones
8. List the bones in the axial skeleton
9. Explain the purpose of the infant fontanels
10. Describe the normal curves of the spine and explain their purpose
11. List the bones in the appendicular skeleton
12. Compare the structure of the female pelvis and the male pelvis
13. Describe five types of bone disorders
14. Name and describe eight types of fractures
15. Describe how the skeleton changes with age
16. Describe the three types of joints
17. Describe the structure of a synovial joint and give six examples of synovial joints
18. Demonstrate six types of movement that occur at synovial joints
19. Describe four types of arthritis
20. List some causes of backache
21. Describe methods used to correct diseased joints
22. Show how word parts are used to build words related to the skeleton (see Word Anatomy at the end of the chapter)

Selected Key Terms

The following terms and other boldface terms in the chapter are defined in the Glossary

amphiarthrosis
arthritis
arthroscope
arthroplasty
bursa
circumduction
diaphysis
diarthrosis
endosteum
epiphysis
fontanel
joint
osteoblast
osteoclast
osteocyte
osteon
osteopenia
osteoporosis
periosteum
resorption
skeleton
synarthrosis
synovial

PASSport to Success

Visit *thePoint* or see the Student Resource CD in the back of this book for definitions and pronunciations of key terms as well as a pretest for this chapter.

Disease in Context

➤ Reggie's Case: A Footballer's Fractured Femur

"Donnelly throws deep for a touchdown. Wilson makes a beautiful catch! Ooh, a nasty hit from number 34." The crowd roared their approval for the wide receiver. On the ground, Reggie Wilson knew that something was wrong with his hip. In fact, he thought he had actually heard the bone break! It didn't take long for the coaches and medical staff to realize that Reggie needed help. And it didn't take long for the ambulance to get him to the trauma center closest to the stadium.

At the hospital, the emergency team examined Reggie. His injured leg appeared shorter than the other and was adducted and laterally rotated—all signs of a hip fracture. An x-ray confirmed the team's suspicions: Reggie had sustained an intertrochanteric fracture of his right femur. He would need surgery, but luckily for Reggie, the fracture line extended from the greater trochanter to the lesser trochanter and didn't involve the femoral neck. This meant that the blood supply to the femoral head was not in danger, so the surgery would be more straightforward.

In the operating room, the surgical team applied traction to Reggie's right leg, pulling on it to reposition the broken ends of his proximal femur back into anatomic position (verified with another x-ray). Then, the orthopedic surgeon made an incision beginning at the tip of the greater trochanter and continuing distally along the lateral thigh through the skin, subcutaneous fat, and vastus lateralis muscle. After exposing the proximal femur, the surgeon drilled a hole and installed a titanium screw through the greater trochanter, neck, and into the femoral head. He then positioned a titanium plate over the screw and fastened it to the femoral shaft with four more screws. Confident that the broken ends of the femur were firmly held together, the surgeon closed the wound with sutures and skin staples. Reggie was then wheeled into the recovery room.

The surgical team successfully realigned the fractured ends of Reggie's femur. Now Reggie's body will begin the healing process. In this chapter we'll learn more about bones and joints. Later in the chapter we'll see how Reggie's skeletal system is repairing itself.

The skeleton is the strong framework on which the body is constructed. Much like the frame of a building, the skeleton must be strong enough to support and protect all the body structures. Bone tissue is the most dense form of the connective tissues described in Chapter 4. Bones work with muscles to produce movement at the joints. The bones and joints, together with supporting connective tissue, form the skeletal system. See Appendix 7: Dissection Atlas for pictures of a complete human skeleton, both anterior and posterior views. You can refer to these pictures as you study this chapter.

Bones

Bones have a number of functions, several of which are not evident in looking at the skeleton:

- To serve as a firm framework for the entire body
- To protect such delicate structures as the brain and the spinal cord
- To work as levers with attached muscles to produce movement
- To store calcium salts, which may be resorbed into the blood if calcium is needed
- To produce blood cells (in the red marrow)

Bone Structure

The complete bony framework of the body, known as the **skeleton** (Fig. 7-1), consists of 206 bones. It is divided into a central portion, the axial skeleton, and the extremities, which make up the appendicular skeleton. The individual bones in these two divisions will be described in detail later in this chapter. The bones of the skeleton can be of several different shapes. They may be flat (ribs, cranium), short (carpals of wrist, tarsals of ankle), or irregular (vertebrae, facial bones). The most familiar shape, however, is the **long bone**, the type of bone that makes up almost all of the skeleton of the arms and legs. The long narrow shaft of this type of bone is called the **diaphysis** (di-AF-ih-sis). At the center of the diaphysis is a **medullary** (MED-u-lar-e) **cavity**, which contains bone marrow. The long bone also has two irregular ends, a proximal and a distal **epiphysis** (eh-PIF-ih-sis) (Fig. 7-2).

BONE TISSUE Bones are not lifeless. Even though the spaces between the cells of bone tissue are permeated with stony deposits of calcium salts, the bone cells themselves are very much alive. Bones are organs, with their own system of blood vessels, lymphatic vessels, and nerves.

There are two types of bone tissue, also known as **osseous** (OS-e-us) **tissue.** One type is **compact bone,** which is hard and dense (Fig. 7-3). This tissue makes up the main shaft of a long bone and the outer layer of other bones. The cells in this type of bone are located in rings of bone

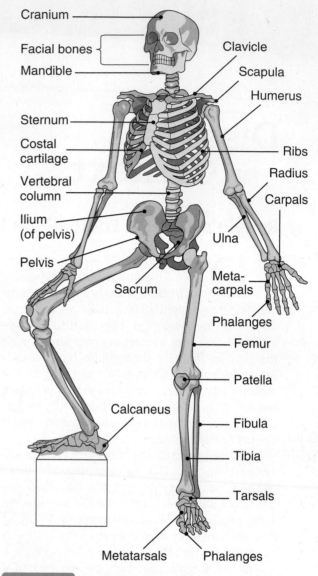

Figure 7-1 **The skeleton.** The axial skeleton is shown in yellow; the appendicular, in blue.

tissue around a central **haversian** (ha-VER-shan) **canal** containing nerves and blood vessels. The bone cells live in spaces (lacunae) between the rings and extend out into many small radiating channels so that they can be in contact with nearby cells. Each ringlike unit with its central canal makes up a **haversian system,** also known as an **osteon** (OS-te-on) (see Fig. 7-3B). Forming a channel across the bone, from one side of the shaft to the other, are many **perforating** (Volkmann) **canals,** which also house blood vessels and nerves.

The second type of bone tissue, called **spongy bone,** or **cancellous bone,** has more spaces than compact bone. It is made of a meshwork of small, bony plates filled with red marrow. Spongy bone is found at the epiphyses (ends) of the long bones and at the center of other bones. Figure 7-4 shows a photograph of both compact and spongy tissue in a bone section.

Cartilage

Epiphyseal line (growth line)

Proximal epiphysis

Spongy (cancellous) bone (containing red marrow)

Endosteum

Compact bone

Medullary (marrow) cavity

Artery and vein

Diaphysis

Yellow marrow

Periosteum

Distal epiphysis

Figure 7-2 **The structure of a long bone.**

CHECKPOINT **7-1** ➤ A long bone has a long, narrow shaft and two irregular ends. What are the scientific names for the shaft and the ends of a long bone?

CHECKPOINT **7-2** ➤ What are the two types of osseous (bone) tissue and where is each type found?

BONE MARROW Bones contain two kinds of marrow. **Red marrow** is found at the ends of the long bones and at the center of other bones (see Fig. 7-2). Red bone marrow manufactures blood cells. **Yellow marrow** is found chiefly in the central cavities of the long bones. Yellow marrow is composed largely of fat.

BONE MEMBRANES Bones are covered on the outside (except at the joint region) by a membrane called the **periosteum** (per-e-OS-te-um) (see Fig. 7-2). This membrane's inner layer contains cells (osteoblasts) that are essential in bone formation, not only during growth but also in the repair of injuries. Blood vessels and lymphatic vessels in the periosteum play an important role in the nourishment of bone tissue. Nerve fibers in the periosteum make their

presence known when one suffers a fracture, or when one receives a blow, such as on the shinbone. A thinner membrane, the **endosteum** (en-DOS-te-um), lines the bone's marrow cavity; it too contains cells that aid in the growth and repair of bone tissue.

Bone Growth and Repair

During early development, the embryonic skeleton is at first composed almost entirely of cartilage. (Portions of the skull develop from fibrous connective tissue.) The conversion of cartilage to bone, a process known as **ossification**, begins during the second and third months of embryonic life. At this time, bone-building cells, called **osteoblasts** (OS-te-o-blasts), become active. First, they begin to manufacture the **matrix**, which is the material located between the cells. This intercellular substance contains large quantities of **collagen**, a fibrous protein that gives the tissue strength and resilience. Then, with the help of enzymes, calcium compounds are deposited within the matrix.

Once this intercellular material has hardened, the cells remain enclosed within the lacunae (small spaces) in the matrix. These cells, now known as **osteocytes** (OS-te-o-sites), are still living and continue to maintain the existing bone matrix, but they do not produce new bone tissue. When bone has to be remodeled or repaired later in life, new osteoblasts develop from stem cells in the endosteum and periosteum.

One other cell type found in bone develops from a type of white blood cell (monocyte). These large, multinucleated **osteoclasts** (OS-te-o-klasts) are responsible for the process of **resorption**, which is the breakdown of bone tissue. Resorption is necessary for bone remodeling and repair, as occurs during growth and after injury. Bone tissue is also resorbed when its stored minerals are needed by the body.

Both the formation and resorption of bone tissue are regulated by hormones. Vitamin D promotes calcium absorption from the intestine. Other hormones involved in these processes are produced by glands in the neck. Calcitonin from the thyroid gland promotes the uptake of calcium by bone tissue. Parathyroid hormone (PTH) from the parathyroid glands at the posterior of the thyroid causes bone resorption and release of calcium into the blood. These hormones are discussed more fully in Chapter 12.

CHECKPOINT **7-3** ➤ What are the three types of cells found in bone and what is the role of each?

FORMATION OF A LONG BONE In a long bone, the transformation of cartilage into bone begins at the center of the shaft during fetal development. Around the time of birth, secondary bone-forming centers, or **epiphyseal** (ep-ih-FIZ-e-al) **plates**, develop across the ends of the bones (see Figs. 7-2 and 7-4). The long bones continue to grow in length at these centers by calcification of new cartilage

7

Figure 7-3 **Compact bone tissue. (A)** This section shows osteocytes (bone cells) within osteons (haversian systems). It also shows the canals that penetrate the tissue. **(B)** Microscopic view of compact bone in cross section (×300) showing a complete osteon. In living tissue, osteocytes (bone cells) reside in spaces (lacunae) and extend out into channels that radiate from these spaces. (B, Reprinted with permission from Gartner LP, Hiatt JL. *Color Atlas of Histology*, 4th ed. Baltimore: Lippincott Williams & Wilkins, 2005.)

through childhood and into the late teens. Finally, by the late teens or early 20s, the bones stop growing in length. Each epiphyseal plate hardens and can be seen in x-ray films as a thin line, the epiphyseal line, across the end of the bone. Physicians can judge a bone's future growth by the appearance of these lines on x-ray films.

As a bone grows in length, the shaft is remodeled so that it grows wider as the central marrow cavity increases in size. Thus, alterations in a bone's shape result from the addition of bone tissue to some surfaces and its resorption from others.

The processes of bone resorption and bone formation continue throughout life, more actively in some places than in others, as bones are subjected to wear-and-tear or injuries. The bones of small children are relatively pliable because they contain a larger proportion of cartilage and are undergoing active bone formation. In elderly people, there is a slowing of bone tissue renewal. As a result, the bones are weaker and more fragile. Elderly people also have a de-

creased ability to form the protein framework on which calcium salts are deposited. Fractures in elderly people heal more slowly because of these decreases in bone metabolism.

PASSport to Success — Visit **the*Point*** or see the Student Resource CD in the back of this book to view the animation *Bone Growth*, showing the growth process in a long bone.

CHECKPOINT **7-4** ➤ As the embryonic skeleton is converted from cartilage to bone, the intercellular matrix becomes hardened. What compounds are deposited in the matrix to harden it?

CHECKPOINT **7-5** ➤ After birth, long bones continue to grow in length at secondary centers. What are these centers called?

Figure 7-4 **Bone tissue, longitudinal section.** The epiphysis (end) of this long bone has an outer layer of compact bone. The remainder of the tissue is spongy (cancellous) bone, shown by the arrows. Transverse growth lines are also visible. (Reprinted with permission from Rubin R, Strayer DS. *Rubin's Pathology: Clinicopathologic Foundations of Medicine,* 5th ed. Baltimore: Lippincott Williams & Wilkins, 2007.)

Bone Markings

In addition to their general shape, bones have other distinguishing features, or **bone markings**. These markings include raised areas and depressions, which help to form joints or serve as points for muscle attachments, and various holes, which allow the passage of nerves and blood vessels. Some of these identifying features are described next.

PROJECTIONS
- **Head**—a rounded, knoblike end separated from the rest of the bone by a slender region, the neck.
- **Process**—a large projection of a bone, such as the superior part of the ulna in the forearm that creates the elbow.
- **Condyle** (KON-dile)—a rounded projection; a small projection above a condyle is an epicondyle.
- **Crest**—a distinct border or ridge, often rough, such as over the top of the hip bone.
- **Spine**—a sharp projection from the surface of a bone, such as the spine of the scapula (shoulder blade).

DEPRESSIONS OR HOLES
- **Foramen** (fo-RA-men)—a hole that allows a vessel or a nerve to pass through or between bones. The plural is foramina (fo-RAM-ih-nah).

- **Sinus** (SI-nus)—an air space found in some skull bones.
- **Fossa** (FOS-sah)—a depression on a bone surface. The plural is fossae (FOS-se).
- **Meatus** (me-A-tus)—a short channel or passageway, such as the channel in the temporal bone of the skull that leads to the inner ear.

Examples of these and other markings can be seen on the bones illustrated in this chapter. To find out how these markings can be used in healthcare, see Box 7-1, Landmarking: Seeing with Your Fingers.

CHECKPOINT 7-6 ➤ Bones have a number of projections, depressions, and holes. What are some functions of these markings?

PASSport to Success — Visit *thePoint* or see the Student Resource CD in the back of this book to view bone markings on an illustration of a whole skeleton.

Bones of the Axial Skeleton

The skeleton may be divided into two main groups of bones (see Fig. 7-1):

- The **axial** (AK-se-al) **skeleton** consists of 80 bones and includes the bony framework of the head and the trunk.
- The **appendicular** (ap-en-DIK-u-lar) **skeleton** consists of 126 bones and forms the framework for the extremities (limbs) and for the shoulders and hips.

We describe the axial skeleton first and then proceed to the appendicular skeleton. Table 7-1 provides an outline of all the bones included in this discussion.

Framework of the Skull

The bony framework of the head, called the **skull,** is subdivided into two parts: the cranium and the facial portion. Refer to Figures 7-5 through 7-8, which show different views of the skull, as you study the following descriptions. Color-coding of the bones will aid in identification as the skull is seen from different positions.

CRANIUM This rounded chamber that encloses the brain is composed of eight distinct cranial bones.

- The **frontal bone** forms the forehead, the anterior of the skull's roof, and the roof of the eye orbit (socket). The **frontal sinuses** (air spaces) communicate with the nasal cavities (see Figs. 7-7 and 7-8). These sinuses and others near the nose are described as **paranasal sinuses.**

Box 7-1   🩺   **Clinical Perspectives**

Landmarking: Seeing with Your Fingers

Most body structures lie beneath the skin, hidden from direct view except in dissection. A technique called **landmarking** allows healthcare providers to locate hidden structures simply and easily. Bony prominences, or landmarks, can be palpated (felt) beneath the skin to serve as reference points for locating other internal structures. Landmarking is used during physical examinations and surgeries, when giving injections, and for many other clinical procedures. The lower tip of the sternum, the xiphoid process, is a reference point in the administration of cardiopulmonary resuscitation (CPR).

Practice landmarking by feeling for some of the other bony prominences. You can feel the joint between the mandible and the temporal bone of the skull (the temporomandibular joint, or TMJ) anterior to the ear canal as you move your lower jaw up and down. Feel for the notch in the sternum (breast bone) between the clavicles (collar bones).

Approximately 4 cm below this notch you will feel a bump called the sternal angle. This prominence is an important landmark because its location marks where the trachea splits to deliver air to both lungs. Move your fingers lateral to the sternal angle to palpate the second ribs, important landmarks for locating the heart and lungs. Feel for the most lateral bony prominence of the shoulder, the acromion process of the scapula (shoulder blade). Two to three fingerbreadths down from this point is the correct injection site into the deltoid muscle of the shoulder. Place your hands on your hips and palpate the iliac crest of the hip bone. Move your hands forward until you reach the anterior end of the crest, the anterior superior iliac spine (ASIS). Feel for the part of the bony pelvis that you sit on. This is the ischial tuberosity. It and the ASIS are important landmarks for locating safe injection sites in the gluteal region.

- The two **parietal** (pah-RI-eh-tal) bones form most of the top and the side walls of the cranium.

- The two **temporal bones** form part of the sides and some of the base of the skull. Each one contains **mastoid sinuses** as well as the ear canal, the eardrum, and the ear's entire middle and internal portions. The **mastoid process** of the temporal bone projects downward immediately behind the external part of the ear. It contains the mastoid air cells and is a place for muscle attachment.

- The **ethmoid** (ETH-moyd) **bone** is a light, fragile bone located between the eyes (see Fig. 7-7). It forms a part of the eye orbit's medial wall, a small portion of the cranial floor, and most of the nasal cavity roof. It contains several air spaces, comprising some of the paranasal sinuses. A thin, platelike, downward extension of this bone (the perpendicular plate) forms much of the nasal septum, a midline partition in the nose (see Fig. 7-5A).

- The **sphenoid** (SFE-noyd) **bone,** when seen from a superior view, resembles a bat with its wings extended. It lies at the base of the skull anterior to the temporal bones and forms part of the eye socket. The sphenoid contains a saddlelike depression, the **sella turcica** (SEL-ah TUR-sih-ka), that holds and protects the pituitary gland (see Fig. 7-7).

- The **occipital** (ok-SIP-ih-tal) **bone** forms the skull's posterior and a part of its base. The **foramen magnum,** located at the base of the occipital bone, is a large opening through which the spinal cord communicates with the brain (see Figs. 7-6 and 7-7).

Uniting the skull bones is a type of flat, immovable joint known as a **suture** (SU-chur) (see Fig. 7-5). Some of the most prominent cranial sutures are these:

- The coronal (ko-RO-nal) suture joins the frontal bone with the two parietal bones along the coronal plane.

- The squamous (SKWA-mus) suture joins the temporal bone to the parietal bone on the cranium's lateral surface (named because it is in a flat portion of the skull).

- The lambdoid (LAM-doyd) suture joins the occipital bone with the parietal bones in the posterior cranium (named because it resembles the Greek letter lambda).

- The sagittal (SAJ-ih-tal) suture joins the two parietal bones along the superior midline of the cranium, along the sagittal plane (see Fig. 7-5C).

FACIAL BONES The facial portion of the skull is composed of 14 bones (see Fig. 7-5):

- The **mandible** (MAN-dih-bl), or lower jaw bone, is the skull's only movable bone.

- The two **maxillae** (mak-SIL-e) fuse in the midline to form the upper jaw bone, including the anterior part of the hard palate (roof of the mouth). Each maxilla contains a large air space, called the **maxillary sinus,** that communicates with the nasal cavity.

- The two **zygomatic** (zi-go-MAT-ik) **bones,** one on each side, form the prominences of the cheeks.

- Two slender **nasal bones** lie side by side, forming the bridge of the nose.

Table 7-1	Bones of the Skeleton	
Region	**Bones**	**Description**
Axial Skeleton		
Skull		
Cranium	Cranial bones (8)	Chamber enclosing the brain; houses the ear and forms part of the eye socket
Facial portion	Facial bones (14)	Form the face and chambers for sensory organs
Hyoid		U-shaped bone under lower jaw; used for muscle attachments
Ossicles	Ear bones (3)	Transmit sound waves in inner ear
Trunk		
Vertebral column	Vertebrae (26)	Enclose the spinal cord
Thorax	Sternum	Anterior bone of the thorax
	Ribs (12 pair)	Enclose the organs of the thorax
Appendicular Skeleton		
Upper division		
Shoulder girdle	Clavicle	Anterior; between sternum and scapula
	Scapula	Posterior; anchors muscles that move arm
Upper extremity	Humerus	Proximal arm bone
	Ulna	Medial bone of forearm
	Radius	Lateral bone of forearm
	Carpals (8)	Wrist bones
	Metacarpals (5)	Bones of palm
	Phalanges (14)	Bones of fingers
Lower division		
Pelvis	Os coxae (2)	Join sacrum and coccyx of vertebral column to form the bony pelvis
Lower extremity	Femur	Thigh bone
	Patella	Kneecap
	Tibia	Medial bone of leg
	Fibula	Lateral bone of leg
	Tarsal bones (7)	Ankle bones
	Metatarsals (5)	Bones of instep
	Phalanges (14)	Bones of toes

7

- The two **lacrimal** (LAK-rih-mal) **bones,** each about the size of a fingernail, form the anterior medial wall of each orbital cavity.

- The **vomer** (VO-mer), shaped like the blade of a plow, forms the inferior part of the nasal septum (see Fig. 7-5A).

- The paired **palatine** (PAL-ah-tine) **bones** form the posterior part of the hard palate (see Figs. 7-6 and 7-8).

- The two **inferior nasal conchae** (KON-ke) extend horizontally along the lateral wall (side) of the nasal cavities. The paired superior and middle conchae are part of the ethmoid bone (see Figs. 7-5A and 7-8).

In addition to the cranial and facial bones, there are three tiny bones, or **ossicles** (OS-sik-ls), in each middle ear (see Chapter 11) and, just below the mandible (lower jaw), a single horseshoe, or U-shaped, bone called the **hyoid** (HI-oyd) **bone,** to which the tongue and other muscles are attached (see Fig. 7-5B).

Openings in the base of the skull provide spaces for the entrance and exit of many blood vessels, nerves, and other structures. Bone projections and depressions (fossae) provide for muscle attachment. Some portions protect delicate structures, for example, the eye orbit and the part of the temporal bone that encloses the inner ear. The sinuses provide lightness and serve as resonating chambers for the voice (which is why your voice sounds better to you as you are speaking than it sounds when you hear it played back as a recording).

INFANT SKULL The infant's skull has areas in which the bone formation is incomplete, leaving so-called soft spots, properly called **fontanels** (fon-tah-NELS) (Fig. 7-9). These flexible regions allow the skull to compress and change shape during the birth process. They also allow for rapid

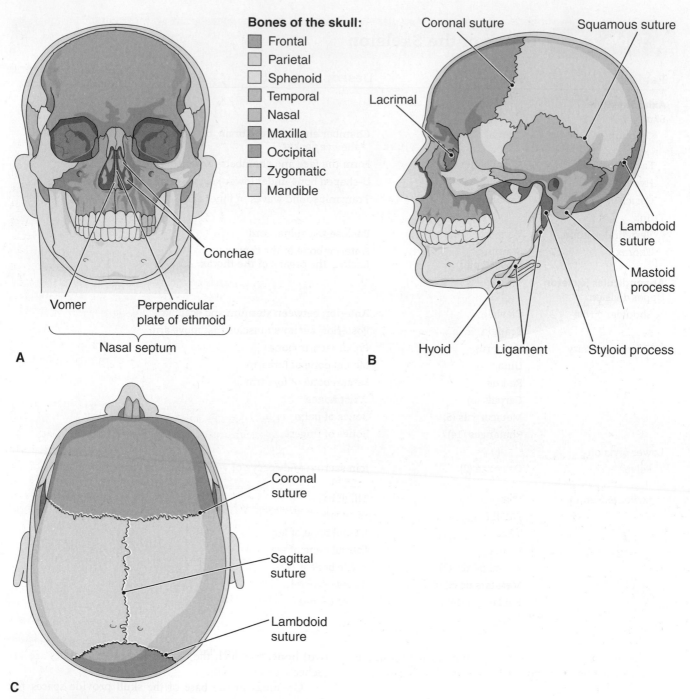

Bones of the skull:
- Frontal
- Parietal
- Sphenoid
- Temporal
- Nasal
- Maxilla
- Occipital
- Zygomatic
- Mandible

Conchae

Vomer   Perpendicular plate of ethmoid

Nasal septum

A

Coronal suture   Squamous suture

Lacrimal

Lambdoid suture

Mastoid process

Hyoid   Ligament   Styloid process

B

Coronal suture

Sagittal suture

Lambdoid suture

C

Figure 7-5 **The skull. (A)** Anterior view. **(B)** Left lateral view. **(C)** Superior view. **[ZOOMING IN ➤** What type of joint is between the bones of the skull? **]**

brain growth during infancy. Although there are a number of fontanels, the largest and most recognizable is near the front of the skull at the junction of the two parietal bones and the frontal bone. This anterior fontanel usually does not close until the child is about 18 months old.

PASSport to Success Visit **thePoint** or see the Student Resource CD in the back of this book for supplementary pictures of the anterior and posterior head and neck.

Framework of the Trunk

The bones of the trunk include the spine, or **vertebral** (VER-teh-bral), **column**, and the bones of the chest, or **thorax** (THO-raks).

VERTEBRAL COLUMN This bony sheath for the spinal cord is made of a series of irregularly shaped bones. These number 33 or 34 in the child, but because of fusions that occur later in the lower part of the spine, there usually are

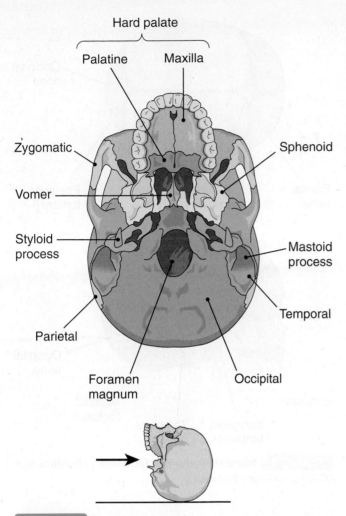

Figure 7-6 **The skull, inferior view.** The mandible (lower jaw) has been removed. **[ZOOMING IN ➤** What two bones make up each side of the hard palate? **]**

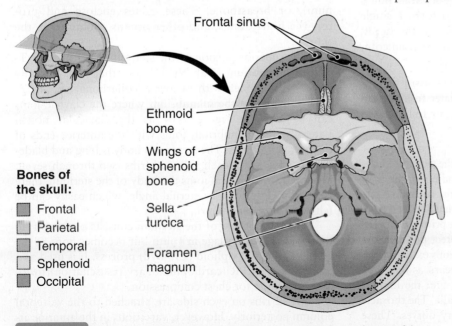

Bones of the skull:

- ■ Frontal
- ■ Parietal
- ■ Temporal
- □ Sphenoid
- ■ Occipital

Figure 7-7 **Floor of cranium, superior view.** The internal surfaces of some of the cranial bones are visible. **[ZOOMING IN ➤** What is a foramen? **]**

just 26 separate bones in the adult spinal column. Figures 7-10 and 7-11 show the vertebral column from lateral and anterior views.

The **vertebrae** (VER-teh-bre) have a drum-shaped **body** (centrum) located anteriorly (toward the front) that serves as the weight-bearing part; disks of cartilage between the vertebral bodies absorb shock and provide flexibility (see Fig. 7-11). In the center of each vertebra is a large hole, or foramen. When all the vertebrae are linked in series by strong connective tissue bands (ligaments), these spaces form the spinal canal, a bony cylinder that protects the spinal cord. Projecting posteriorly (toward the back) from the bony arch that encircles the spinal cord is the **spinous process**, which usually can be felt just under the skin of the back. Projecting laterally is a **transverse process** on each side. These processes are attachment points for muscles. When viewed from a lateral aspect, one can see that the vertebral column has a series of **intervertebral foramina**, formed between the vertebrae as they join together, through which spinal nerves emerge from the spinal cord (see Fig. 7-10).

The bones of the vertebral column are named and numbered from superior to inferior and according to location. There are five groups:

- The **cervical** (SER-vih-kal) **vertebrae,** seven in number (C1 to C7), are located in the neck (see Fig. 7-11). The first vertebra, called the **atlas,** supports the head (Fig. 7-12). (This vertebra is named for the mythologic character who was able to support the world in his hands.) When one nods the head, the skull rocks on the atlas at the occipital bone. The second cervical vertebra, the **axis** (see Fig. 7-12), serves as a pivot when the head is turned from side to side. It has an upright toothlike part, the **dens,** that projects into the atlas as a pivot point. The absence of a body in these vertebrae allows for the extra movement. Only the cervical vertebrae have a hole in the transverse process on each side (see Fig. 7-11). These **transverse foramina** accommodate blood vessels and nerves that supply the neck and head.

- The **thoracic vertebrae,** 12 in number (T1 to T12), are located in the chest. They are larger and stronger than the cervical vertebrae and each has a longer spinous process that points downward (see Fig. 7-11). The posterior ends of the 12 pairs of ribs are attached to these vertebrae.

- The **lumbar vertebrae,** five in number (L1 to L5), are located in the small of the back. They are larger and heavier than the vertebrae superior to them and can support more weight (see Fig. 7-11). All of their processes are shorter and thicker.

7

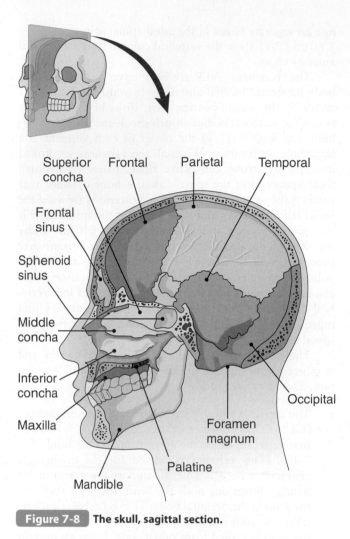

Figure 7-8 The skull, sagittal section.

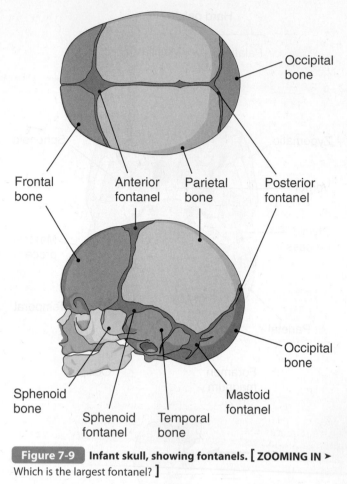

Figure 7-9 Infant skull, showing fontanels. [ZOOMING IN ➤ Which is the largest fontanel?]

- The **sacral** (SA-kral) **vertebrae** are five separate bones in the child. They eventually fuse to form a single bone, called the **sacrum** (SA-krum), in the adult. Wedged between the two hip bones, the sacrum completes the posterior part of the bony pelvis.

- The **coccygeal** (kok-SIJ-e-al) **vertebrae** consist of four or five tiny bones in the child. These later fuse to form a single bone, the **coccyx** (KOK-siks), or tail bone, in the adult.

Curves of the Spine When viewed from the side, the vertebral column shows four curves, corresponding to the four vertebral groups (see Fig. 7-10). In the fetus, the entire column is concave forward (curves away from a viewer facing the fetus), as seen in Figure 7-13. This is the primary curve.

When an infant begins to assume an erect posture, secondary curves develop. These curves are convex (curve toward the viewer). The cervical curve appears as the baby holds its head up at about 3 months of age; the lumbar curve appears when the child begins to walk. The thoracic and sacral curves remain the two primary curves. These curves of the vertebral column provide some of the resilience and spring so essential in balance and movement.

THORAX The bones of the thorax form a cone-shaped cage (Fig. 7-14). Twelve pairs of **ribs** form the bars of this cage, completed anteriorly by the **sternum** (STER-num), or breastbone. These bones enclose and protect the heart, lungs, and other organs contained in the thorax.

The superior portion of the sternum is the broadly T-shaped **manubrium** (mah-NU-bre-um) that joins laterally on the right and left with a clavicle (collarbone) (see Fig. 7-1). The point on the manubrium where the clavicle joins can be seen on Figure 7-14 as the clavicular notch. Laterally, the manubrium joins with the anterior ends of the first pair of ribs. The sternum's **body** is long and blade-like. It joins along each side with ribs two through seven. Where the manubrium joins the body of the sternum, there is a slight elevation, the **sternal angle**, which easily can be felt as a surface landmark.

The inferior end of the sternum consists of a small tip that is made of cartilage in youth but becomes bone in the adult. This is the **xiphoid** (ZIF-oyd) **process**. It is used as a landmark for CPR (cardiopulmonary resuscitation) to locate the region for chest compression.

All 12 ribs on each side are attached to the vertebral column posteriorly. However, variations in the anterior attachment of these slender, curved bones have led to the following classification:

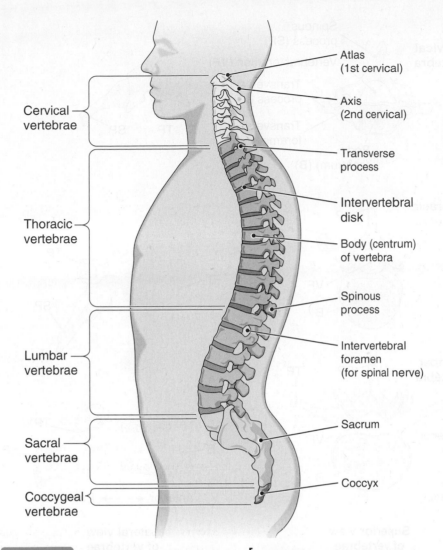

Figure 7-10   **Vertebral column, left lateral view.** [**ZOOMING IN ➤** From an anterior view, which group(s) of vertebrae form a convex curve? Which group(s) form a concave curve?]

Labels (top to bottom):

Cervical vertebrae

Thoracic vertebrae

Lumbar vertebrae

Sacral vertebrae

Coccygeal vertebrae

Atlas (1st cervical)

Axis (2nd cervical)

Transverse process

Intervertebral disk

Body (centrum) of vertebra

Spinous process

Intervertebral foramen (for spinal nerve)

Sacrum

Coccyx

CHECKPOINT 7-8 ➤ What are the five regions of the vertebral column?

Bones of the Appendicular Skeleton

The appendicular skeleton may be considered in two divisions: upper and lower. The upper division on each side includes the shoulder, the arm (between the shoulder and the elbow), the forearm (between the elbow and the wrist), the wrist, the hand, and the fingers. The lower division includes the hip (part of the pelvic girdle), the thigh (between the hip and the knee), the leg (between the knee and the ankle), the ankle, the foot, and the toes.

The Upper Division of the Appendicular Skeleton

The bones of the upper division may be divided into two groups, the shoulder girdle and the upper extremity.

THE SHOULDER GIRDLE The shoulder girdle consists of two bones (Fig. 7-15):

- True ribs, the first seven pairs, are those that attach directly to the sternum by means of individual extensions called **costal** (KOS-tal) **cartilages**.

- False ribs are the remaining five pairs. Of these, the 8th, 9th, and 10th pairs attach to the cartilage of the rib above. The last two pairs have no anterior attachment at all and are known as **floating ribs**.

The spaces between the ribs, called **intercostal spaces**, contain muscles, blood vessels, and nerves.

PASSport to Success Visit *thePoint* or see the Student Resource CD in the back of this book for additional pictures of the skeleton of the torso.

CHECKPOINT 7-7 ➤ The axial skeleton consists of the bones of the skull and the trunk. What bones make up the skeleton of the trunk?

- The **clavicle** (KLAV-ih-kl), or collarbone, is a slender bone with two shallow curves. It joins the sternum anteriorly and the scapula laterally and helps to support the shoulder. Because it often receives the full force of falls on outstretched arms or of blows to the shoulder, it is the most frequently broken bone.

- The **scapula** (SKAP-u-lah), or shoulder blade, is shown from anterior and posterior views in Figure 7-15. The **spine** of the scapula is the posterior raised ridge that can be felt behind the shoulder in the upper portion of the back. Muscles that move the arm attach to **fossae** (depressions), known as the **supraspinous fossa** and the **infraspinous fossa**, superior and inferior to the scapular spine. The **acromion** (ah-KRO-me-on) is the process that joins the clavicle. This can be felt as the highest point of the shoulder. Below the acromion there is a shallow socket, the **glenoid cavity**, that forms a ball-and-socket joint with the arm bone (humerus). Medial to the glenoid cavity is the **coracoid** (KOR-ah-koyd) **process**, to which muscles attach.

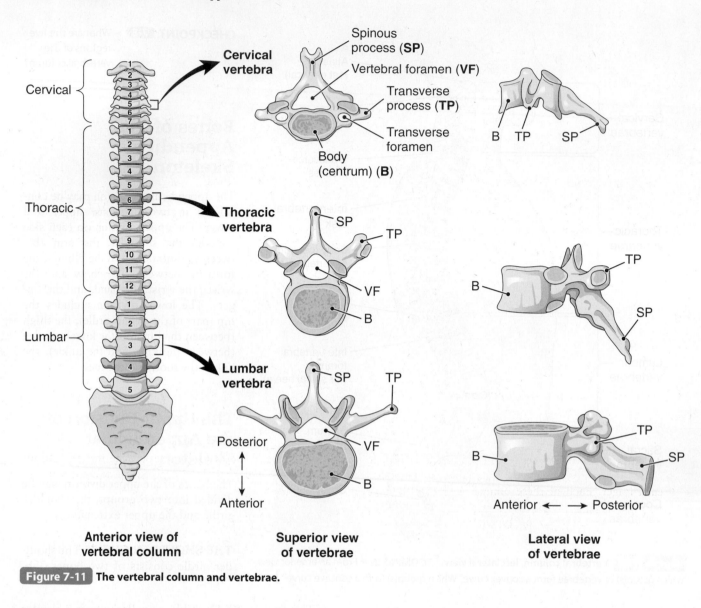

Figure 7-11 The vertebral column and vertebrae.

THE UPPER EXTREMITY The upper extremity is also referred to as the upper limb, or simply the arm, although technically, the arm is only the region between the shoulder and the elbow. The region between the elbow and wrist is the forearm. The upper extremity consists of the following bones:

■ The proximal bone is the **humerus** (HU-mer-us), or arm bone (Fig. 7-16). The head of the humerus forms a joint with the glenoid cavity of the scapula. The distal end has a projection on each side, the medial and lateral **epicondyles** (ep-ih-KON-diles), to which tendons attach, and a pulley-shaped midportion, the **trochlea** (TROK-le-ah), that forms a joint with the ulna of the forearm.

■ The forearm bones are the **ulna** (UL-nah) and the **radius** (RA-de-us). In the anatomic position, the ulna lies on the medial side of the forearm in line with the little finger, and the radius lies laterally, above the thumb (Fig. 7-17). When the forearm is supine, with the palm

up or forward, the two bones are parallel; when the forearm is prone, with the palm down or back, the distal end of the radius rotates around the ulna so that the shafts of the two bones are crossed (Fig. 7-18). In this position, a distal projection (styloid process) of the ulna shows at the outside of the wrist.

■ The proximal end of the ulna has the large **olecranon** (o-LEK-rah-non) that forms the point of the elbow (see Fig. 7-17). The trochlea of the distal humerus fits into the ulna's deep **trochlear notch**, allowing a hinge action at the elbow joint. This ulnar depression, because of its deep half-moon shape, is also known as the semilunar notch (Fig. 7-19).

■ The wrist contains eight small **carpal** (KAR-pal) **bones** arranged in two rows of four each. The names of these eight different bones are given in Figure 7-20.

■ Five **metacarpal bones** are the framework for the palm of each hand. Their rounded distal ends form the knuckles.

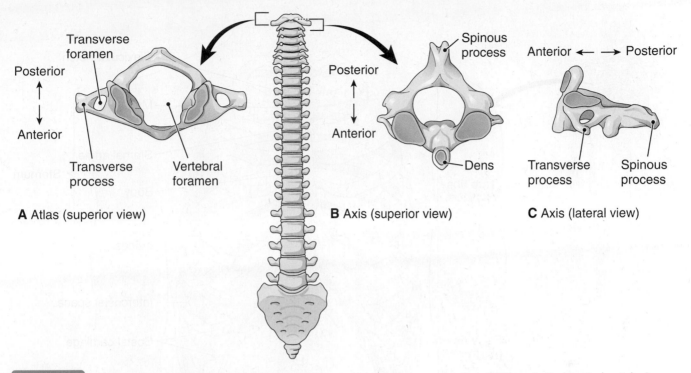

Figure 7-12 **The first two cervical vertebrae. (A)** The atlas (1st cervical vertebra), superior view. **(B)** The axis (2nd cervical vertebra), superior view. **(C)** The axis, lateral view.

- There are 14 **phalanges** (fah-LAN-jeze), or finger bones, in each hand, two for the thumb and three for each finger. Each of these bones is called a **phalanx** (FA-lanx). They are identified as the first, or proximal, which is attached to a metacarpal; the second, or

middle; and the third, or distal. Note that the thumb has only two phalanges, a proximal and a distal (see Fig. 7-20).

> **PASSport to Success** Visit *thePoint* or see the Student Resource CD in the back of this book for additional pictures of the upper extremity skeleton.

The Lower Division of the Appendicular Skeleton

The bones of the lower division also fall into two groups, the pelvis and the lower extremity.

THE PELVIC BONES The hip bone, or **os coxae**, begins its development as three separate bones that later fuse (Fig. 7-21). These individual bones are:

- The **ilium** (IL-e-um) forms the upper, flared portion. The **iliac** (IL-e-ak) **crest** is the curved rim along the ilium's superior border. It can be felt just below the waist. At either end of the crest are two bony projections. The most prominent of these is the **anterior superior iliac spine**, which is often used as a surface landmark in diagnosis and treatment.

- The **ischium** (IS-ke-um) is the lowest and strongest part. The **ischial** (IS-ke-al) **spine** at the posterior of the pelvic outlet is used as a reference point during childbirth to indicate the progress of the presenting

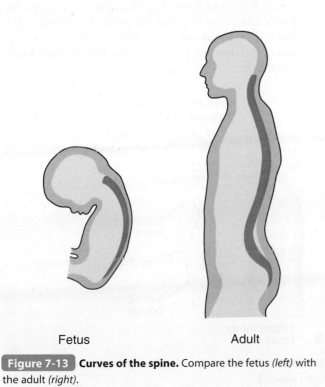

Fetus   Adult

Figure 7-13 **Curves of the spine.** Compare the fetus *(left)* with the adult *(right)*.

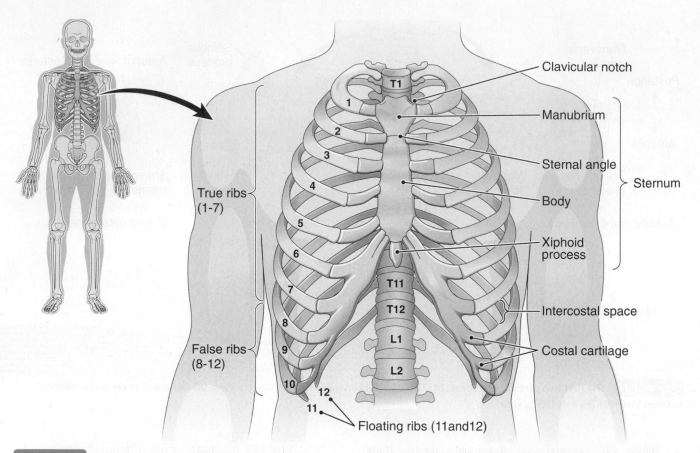

Figure 7-14 **Bones of the thorax, anterior view.** The first 7 pairs of ribs are the true ribs; pairs 8 through 12 are the false ribs, of which the last 2 pairs are also called floating ribs. [**ZOOMING IN ➤** To what bones do the costal cartilages attach?]

part (usually the baby's head) down the birth canal. Just inferior to this spine is the large **ischial tuberosity**, which helps support the trunk's weight when a person sits down. One is sometimes aware of this ischial projection when sitting on a hard surface for a while.

■ The **pubis** (PU-bis) forms the anterior part of the os coxae. The joint formed by the union of the two hip bones anteriorly is called the **pubic symphysis** (SIM-fih-sis). This joint becomes more flexible late in pregnancy to allow for passage of the baby's head during childbirth.

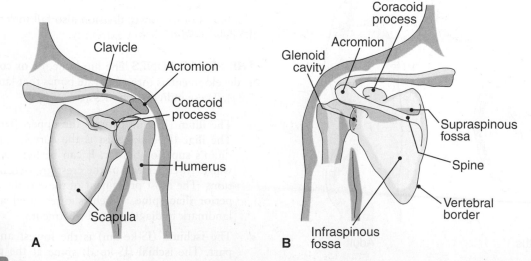

Figure 7-15 **The shoulder girdle and scapula. (A)** Bones of the shoulder girdle, left anterior view. **(B)** Left scapula, posterior view. [**ZOOMING IN ➤** What does the prefix *supra* mean? What does the prefix *infra* mean?]

The largest foramina in the entire body are found near the anterior of each hip bone on either side of the pubic symphysis. Each opening is partially covered by a membrane and is called an **obturator** (OB-tu-ra-tor) **foramen** (see Fig. 7-21).

The two ossa coxae join in forming the pelvis, a strong bony girdle completed posteriorly by the sacrum and coccyx of the spine. The pelvis supports the trunk and the organs in the lower abdomen, or pelvic cavity, including the urinary bladder, the internal reproductive organs, and parts of the intestine.

The female pelvis is adapted for pregnancy and childbirth (Fig. 7-22). Some ways in which the female pelvis differs from that of the male are:

- It is lighter in weight.
- The ilia are wider and more flared.
- The pubic arch, the anterior angle between the pubic bones, is wider.
- The pelvic opening is wider and more rounded.
- The lower diameter, the pelvic outlet, is larger.
- The sacrum and coccyx are shorter and less curved.

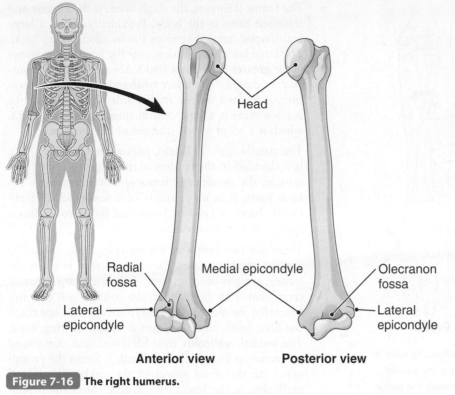

Head

Radial fossa

Medial epicondyle

Olecranon fossa

Lateral epicondyle

Lateral epicondyle

Anterior view   **Posterior view**

Figure 7-16 **The right humerus.**

Portions of all three pelvic bones contribute to the formation of the **acetabulum** (as-eh-TAB-u-lum), the deep socket that holds the head of the femur (thigh bone) to form the hip joint.

7

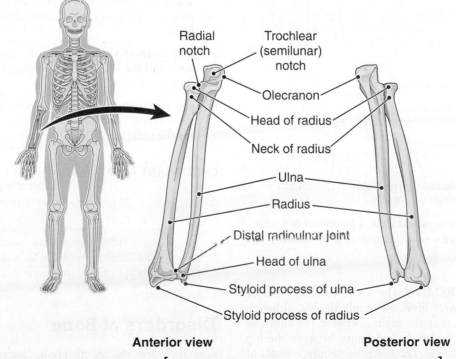

Radial notch

Trochlear (semilunar) notch

Olecranon

Head of radius

Neck of radius

Ulna

Radius

Distal radioulnar joint

Head of ulna

Styloid process of ulna

Styloid process of radius

Anterior view   **Posterior view**

Figure 7-17 **Radius and ulna of the right forearm.** [**ZOOMING IN ➤** What is the lateral bone of the forearm?]

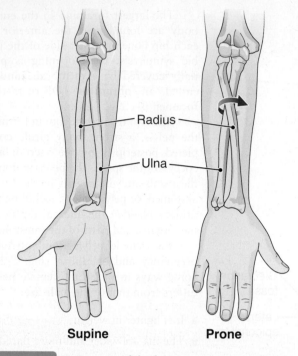

Radius

Ulna

Supine   **Prone**

Figure 7-18 **Movements of the forearm.** When the palm is supine (facing up or forward), the radius and ulna are parallel. When the palm is prone (facing down or to the rear), the radius crosses over the ulna.

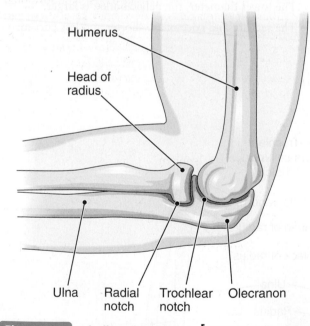

Humerus

Head of radius

Ulna   Radial notch   Trochlear notch   Olecranon

Figure 7-19 **Left elbow, lateral view.** [**ZOOMING IN ➤** What part of what bone forms the bony prominence of the elbow?]

THE LOWER EXTREMITY The lower extremity is also referred to as the lower limb, or simply the leg, although technically the leg is only the region between the knee and the ankle. The portion of the extremity between the hip and the knee is the thigh. The lower extremity consists of the following bones:

- The **femur** (FE-mer), the thigh bone, is the longest and strongest bone in the body. Proximally, it has a large ball-shaped head that joins the os coxae (Fig. 7-23). The large lateral projection near the head of the femur is the **greater trochanter** (tro-KAN-ter), used as a surface landmark. The **lesser trochanter**, a smaller elevation, is located on the medial side. On the posterior surface there is a long central ridge, the **linea aspera**, which is a point for attachment of hip muscles.

- The **patella** (pah-TEL-lah), or kneecap (see Fig. 7-1), is embedded in the tendon of the large anterior thigh muscle, the quadriceps femoris, where it crosses the knee joint. It is an example of a **sesamoid** (SES-ah-moyd) **bone**, a type of bone that develops within a tendon or a joint capsule.

- There are two bones in the leg (Fig. 7-24). Medially (on the great toe side), the **tibia**, or shin bone, is the longer, weight-bearing bone. It has a sharp anterior crest that can be felt at the surface of the leg. Laterally, the slender **fibula** (FIB-u-lah) does not reach the knee joint; thus, it is not a weight-bearing bone. The **medial malleolus** (mal-LE-o-lus) is a downward projection at the tibia's distal end; it forms the prominence on the inner aspect of the ankle. The **lateral malleolus**, at the fibula's distal end, forms the prominence on the outer aspect of the ankle. Most people think of these projections as their "ankle bones," whereas, in truth, they are features of the tibia and fibula.

- The structure of the foot is similar to that of the hand. However, the foot supports the body's weight, so it is stronger and less mobile than the hand. There are seven **tarsal bones** associated with the ankle and foot. These are named and illustrated in Figure 7-25. The largest of these is the **calcaneus** (kal-KA-ne-us), or heel bone.

- Five **metatarsal bones** form the framework of the instep, and the heads of these bones form the ball of the foot (see Fig. 7-25).

- The **phalanges** of the toes are counterparts of those in the fingers. There are three of these in each toe except for the great toe, which has only two.

CHECKPOINT **7-9** ➤ What division of the skeleton consists of the bones of the shoulder girdle, hip, and extremities?

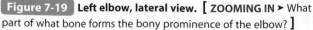

PASSport to Success   Visit **thePoint** or see the Student Resource CD in the back of this book for additional pictures of the skeleton of the pelvis and lower extremity.

Disorders of Bone

Bone disorders include metabolic diseases, in which there is a lack of normal bone formation or excess loss of bone

Figure 7-20 **Bones of the right hand, anterior view.**

Metabolic Disorders

Osteoporosis (os-te-o-po-RO-sis) is a disorder of bone formation in which there is a lack of normal calcium salt deposits and a decrease in bone protein. There is an increased breakdown of bone tissue without an increase in the deposit of new bone by osteoblasts (Fig. 7-26). The bones thus become fragile and break easily, most often involving the spine, pelvis, and long bones.

Although everyone loses bone tissue with age, this loss is most apparent in postmenopausal women, presumably because of decline in estrogen. The early stages of bone loss involve a reduction in bone density to below average levels, a condition known as **osteopenia** (os-te-o-PE-ne-ah). Several treatments for osteopenia are available, but medical experts are not in agreement about when treatment should be given and what that treatment should be. Hormone replacement therapy (HRT) is now in question because long-term studies have cast doubt on the safety and effectiveness of the most commonly used form of the drugs. Nonhormonal medications are available to reduce bone resorption and even promote the development of new bone tissue. With regard to nondrug measures, an increase in calcium intake throughout life delays the onset and decreases the severity of this disorder. Weight-bearing exercises, such as weight lifting and brisk walking, are also important to stimulate

tissue; tumors; infections; and structural problems, such as malformation or fractures. Many bone disorders can be diagnosed by x-ray studies.

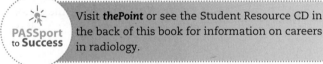

Visit **thePoint** or see the Student Resource CD in the back of this book for information on careers in radiology.

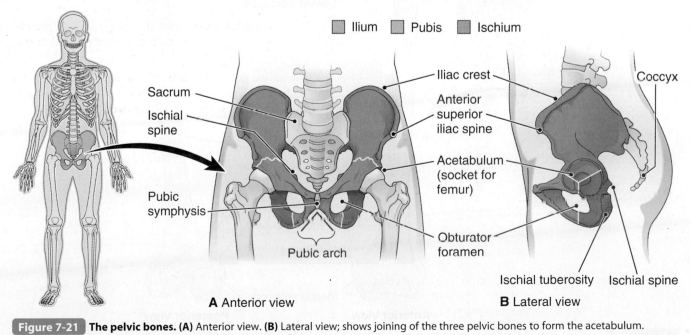

Figure 7-21 **The pelvic bones. (A)** Anterior view. **(B)** Lateral view; shows joining of the three pelvic bones to form the acetabulum.
[ZOOMING IN ➤ What bone is nicknamed the "sit bone"? **]**

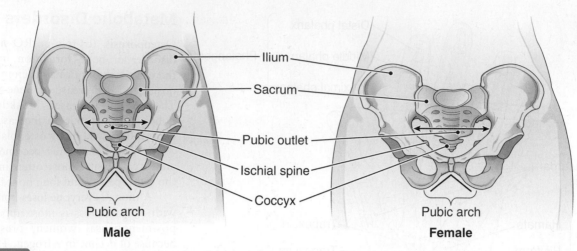

Figure 7-22 **Comparison of male and female pelvis, anterior view.** Note the broader angle of the pubic arch and the wider pelvic outlet in the female. Also, the ilia are wider and more flared; the sacrum and coccyx are shorter and less curved.

growth of bone tissue. (See Box 7-2, Three Steps Toward a Strong and Healthy Skeleton.)

Changes in bone can be followed with radiographic bone mineral density (BMD) tests to determine possible loss of bone mass. However, there is no clear correlation between bone density alone and fracture risk among post-menopausal women.

Other conditions that can lead to osteoporosis include nutritional deficiencies; disuse, as in paralysis or immobilization in a cast; and excess steroids from the adrenal gland.

Abnormal calcium metabolism may cause various bone disorders. In one of these, called Paget disease, or **osteitis deformans** (os-te-I-tis de-FOR-mans), the bones un-

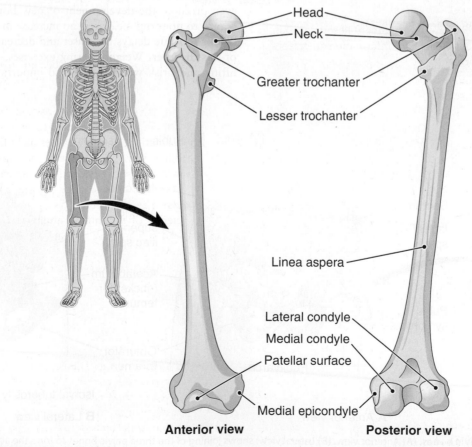

Figure 7-23 **The right femur (thigh bone).**

Lateral condyle
Head of fibula
Proximal tibiofibular joint

Articular surface
Medial condyle
Head of fibula

Anterior crest

Tibia

Fibula

Distal tibiofibular joint

Medial malleolus

Articular surface
Lateral malleolus

Anterior view **Posterior view**

Figure 7-24 **Tibia and fibula of the right leg.** [**ZOOMING IN** ➤ What is the medial bone of the leg?]

7

dergo periods of calcium loss followed by periods of excessive deposition of calcium salts. As a result, the bones become deformed. Cause and cure are not known at the present time. The bones also can become decalcified owing to the effect of a tumor of the parathyroid gland (see Chapter 12).

In **osteomalacia** (os-te-o-mah-LA-she-ah) bone tissue softens due to lack of calcium salt formation. Possible causes include vitamin D deficiency, renal disorders, liver disease, and certain intestinal disorders. When osteomalacia occurs in children, the disease is known as **rickets**. The disorder is usually caused by a deficiency of vitamin D and was common among children in past centuries who had poor diets and inadequate exposure to sunlight. Rickets affects the bones and their growth plates, causing the skeleton to remain soft and become distorted.

Tumors

Tumors, or neoplasms, that develop in bone tissue may be benign, as is the case with certain cysts, or they may be malignant, as are **osteosarcomas** and **chondrosarcomas**. Osteosarcoma most commonly occurs in a young person in a bone's growing region, especially around the knee. Chondrosarcoma arises in cartilage and

Fibula
Tibia

Lateral malleous
Medial malleolus

Tarsal bones
Cuboid
Cuneiforms

Talus
Calcaneus
Navicular
Tarsal bones

Metatarsal bones

Phalanges

Figure 7-25 **Bones of the right foot.** [**ZOOMING IN** ➤ Which tarsal bone is the heel bone?]

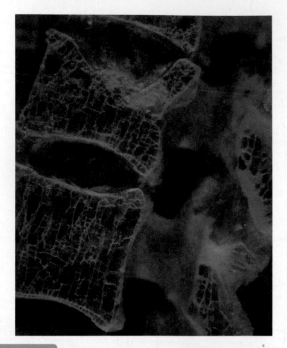

Figure 7-26 **Osteoporosis.** A section of the vertebral column showing loss of bone tissue and a compression fracture of a vertebral body (top). (Reprinted with permission from Rubin E, Farber JL. *Pathology*, 3rd ed. Philadelphia: Lippincott Williams & Wilkins, 1999.)

usually appears in midlife. In older people, tumors at other sites often metastasize (spread) to bones, most commonly to the spine.

Infection

Osteomyelitis (os-te-o-mi-eh-LI-tis) is an inflammation of bone caused by **pyogenic** (pi-o-JEN-ik) (pus-producing) bacteria. These organisms may reach the bone through the bloodstream or by way of an injury in which the skin has been broken. The infection may remain localized, or it may spread through the bone to involve the marrow and the periosteum.

Before the advent of antibiotics, bone infections were resistant to treatment, and the prognosis for people with such infections was poor. Now, there are fewer cases because many blood-borne infections are prevented or treated early and do not progress to affect the bones. If those bone infections that do appear are treated promptly, the chance of a cure is usually excellent.

Tuberculosis may spread to bones, especially the long bones of the extremities and the wrist and ankle bones. Tuberculosis of the spine is **Pott disease**. Infected vertebrae are weakened and may collapse, causing pain, deformity, and pressure on the spinal cord. Antibiotics can control the disease if the strains involved are not resistant to the drugs and the host is not weakened by other diseases.

Structural Disorders

Abnormalities of the spinal curves are known as **curvatures of the spine** (Fig. 7-27) and include:

■ **Kyphosis** (ki-FO-sis), an exaggeration of the thoracic curve, commonly referred to as "hunchback"

Box 7-2 **Health Maintenance**

Three Steps Toward a Strong and Healthy Skeleton

The skeleton is the body's framework. It supports and protects internal organs, helps to produce movement, and manufactures blood cells. Bone also stores nearly all of the body's calcium, releasing it into the blood when needed for processes such as nerve transmission, muscle contraction, and blood clotting. Proper nutrition, exercise, and a healthy lifestyle can help the skeleton perform all these essential roles.

A well-balanced diet supplies the nutrients and energy needed for strong, healthy bones. Calcium and phosphorus confer strength and rigidity. Protein supplies the amino acids needed to make collagen, which gives bone tissue flexibility, and vitamin C helps stimulate collagen synthesis. Foods rich in both calcium and phosphorus include dairy products, fish, beans, and leafy green vegetables. Meat is an excellent source of protein, whereas citrus fruits are rich in vitamin C. Vitamin D helps the digestive system absorb calcium into the

bloodstream, making it available for bone. Foods rich in vitamin D include fish, liver, and eggs.

When body fluids become too acidic, bone releases calcium and phosphate and is weakened. Both magnesium and potassium help regulate the pH of body fluids, with magnesium also helping bone absorb calcium. Foods rich in magnesium and potassium include beans, potatoes, and leafy green vegetables. Bananas and dairy products are high in potassium.

Like muscle, bone becomes weakened with disuse. Consistent exercise promotes a stronger, denser skeleton by stimulating bone to absorb more calcium and phosphate from the blood, reducing the risk of osteoporosis. A healthy lifestyle also includes avoiding smoking and excessive alcohol consumption, both of which decrease bone calcium and inhibit bone growth. High levels of caffeine in the diet may also rob the skeleton of calcium.

Kyphosis   Lordosis   Scoliosis

Figure 7-27 **Abnormalities of the spinal curves.**

- **Lordosis** (lor-DO-sis), an excessive lumbar curve, commonly known as "swayback"
- **Scoliosis** (sko-le-O-sis), a lateral curvature of the vertebral column

Scoliosis is the most common of these disorders. In extreme cases, it may cause compression of internal organs. Scoliosis occurs in the rapid growth period of the teens, more often in girls than in boys. Early discovery and treatment produce good results.

PASSport to **Success** · Visit **thePoint** or see the Student Resource CD in the back of this book for pictures of scoliosis and other spinal curvatures.

Cleft palate is a congenital deformity in which there is an opening in the roof of the mouth owing to faulty union of the maxillary bones. An infant born with this defect has difficulty nursing because the mouth communicates with the nasal cavity above, and the baby therefore sucks in air rather than milk. Surgery is usually performed to correct the condition.

Flatfoot is a common disorder in which the tendons and ligaments that support the foot's long arch are weakened and the curve of the arch flattens (see Fig. 7-25). This arch normally helps to absorb shock and distribute body weight and aids in walking. Flatfoot may be brought on by excess weight or poor posture and may also result from a hereditary failure of arch formation. It may cause difficulty or pain in walking. An arch support may be helpful in treating flatfoot.

Fractures

A **fracture** is a break in a bone, usually caused by trauma (Fig. 7-28). Almost any bone can be fractured with sufficient force. Such injuries may be classified as follows:

- **Closed fracture**—a simple bone fracture with no open wound
- **Open fracture**—a broken bone protrudes through the skin or an external wound leads to a broken bone
- **Greenstick fracture**—one side of the bone is broken and the other is bent. These are most common in children.
- **Impacted fracture**—the broken ends of the bone are jammed into each other
- **Comminuted** (KOM-ih-nu-ted) **fracture**—there is more than one fracture line and the bone is splintered or crushed
- **Spiral fracture**—the bone has been twisted apart. These are relatively common in skiing accidents.
- **Transverse fracture**—the fracture goes straight across the bone

7

Closed   Open   Greenstick   Impacted   Comminuted   Spiral   Transverse   Oblique

Figure 7-28 **Types of fractures.**

■ **Oblique fracture**—the break occurs at an angle across the bone

The most important step in first aid care of fractures is to prevent movement of the affected parts. Protection by simple splinting after careful evaluation of the situation, leaving as much as possible "as is," and a call for expert help are usually the safest measures. People who have back injuries may be spared serious spinal cord damage if they are carefully and correctly moved on a firm board or door. If trained paramedics or rescue personnel can reach the scene, untrained people should follow a "hands off" rule. If there is no external bleeding, covering the victim with blankets may help combat shock. First aid should always be immediately directed toward the control of hemorrhage.

Skeletal Changes in the Aging

The aging process includes significant changes in all connective tissues, including bone. There is a loss of calcium salts and a decrease in the amount of protein formed in bone tissue. The reduction of collagen in bone and in tendons, ligaments, and skin contributes to the stiffness so often experienced by older people. Muscle tissue is also lost throughout adult life. Thus, there is a tendency to decrease the exercise that is so important to the maintenance of bone tissue.

Changes in the vertebral column with age lead to a loss in height. Approximately 1.2 cm (about 0.5 inches)

are lost each 20 years beginning at 40 years of age, owing primarily to a thinning of the intervertebral disks (between the bodies of the vertebrae). Even the vertebral bodies themselves may lose height in later years. The costal (rib) cartilages become calcified and less flexible, and the chest may decrease in diameter by 2 to 3 cm (about 1 inch), mostly in the lower part.

The Joints

An **articulation**, or **joint**, is an area of junction or union between two or more bones. Joints are classified into three main types on the basis of the material between the adjoining bones. They may also be classified according to the degree of movement permitted (Table 7-2):

■ **Fibrous joint.** The bones in this type of joint are held together by fibrous connective tissue. An example is a **suture** (SU-chur) between bones of the skull. This type of joint is immovable and is termed a **synarthrosis** (sin-ar-THRO-sis).

■ **Cartilaginous joint.** The bones in this type of joint are connected by cartilage. Examples are the joint between the pubic bones of the pelvis—the pubic symphysis—and the joints between the bodies of the vertebrae. This type of joint is slightly movable and is termed an **amphiarthrosis** (am-fe-ar-THRO-sis).

Table 7-2	**Joints**		
Type	**Movement**	**Material Between the Bones**	**Examples**
Fibrous	Immovable (synarthrosis)	No joint cavity; fibrous connective tissue between bones	Sutures between skull bones
Cartilaginous	Slightly movable (amphiarthrosis)	No joint cavity; cartilage between bones	Pubic symphysis; joints between vertebral bodies
Synovial	Freely movable (diarthrosis)	Joint cavity containing synovial fluid	Gliding, hinge, pivot, condyloid, saddle, ball-and-socket joints

■ **Synovial** (sin-O-ve-al) **joint.** The bones in this type of joint have a potential space between them called the **joint cavity,** which contains a small amount of thick, colorless fluid. This lubricant, **synovial fluid,** resembles uncooked egg white (*ov* is the root, meaning "egg") and is secreted by the membrane that lines the joint cavity. The synovial joint is freely movable and is termed a **diarthrosis** (di-ar-THRO-sis). Most joints are synovial joints; they are described in more detail next.

CHECKPOINT 7-10 ➤ What are the three types of joints classified according to the type of material between the adjoining bones?

More About Synovial Joints

The bones in freely movable joints are held together by **ligaments,** bands of fibrous connective tissue. Additional ligaments reinforce and help stabilize the joints at various points (Fig. 7-29A). Also, for strength and protection, there is a **joint capsule** of connective tissue that encloses each joint and is continuous with the periosteum of the bones (see Fig. 7-29B). The bone surfaces in freely movable joints are protected by a smooth layer of hyaline cartilage called the **articular** (ar-TIK-u-lar) **cartilage** (see Fig. 7-29B). Some complex joints may have cartilage between the bones that acts as a cushion, such as the crescent-shaped medial meniscus (meh-NIS-kus) and lateral meniscus in the knee joint (Fig. 7-30). Fat may also appear as padding around a joint.

Near some joints are small sacs called **bursae** (BER-se), which are filled with synovial fluid (see Fig. 7-30). These lie in areas subject to stress and help ease movement over and around the joints. Inflammation of a bursa, as a result of injury or irritation, is called **bursitis.**

TYPES OF SYNOVIAL JOINTS
Synovial joints are classified according to the types of movement they allow, as described and illustrated in Table 7-3. Listed in order of increasing range of motion, they are:

■ Gliding joint
■ Hinge joint
■ Pivot joint

■ Condyloid joint
■ Saddle joint
■ Ball-and-socket joint

MOVEMENT AT SYNOVIAL JOINTS The chief function of the freely movable joints is to allow for changes of position and so provide for motion. These movements are named to describe changes in the positions of body parts (Fig. 7-31). For example, there are four kinds of angular movement, or movement that changes the angle between bones, as listed on the following page:

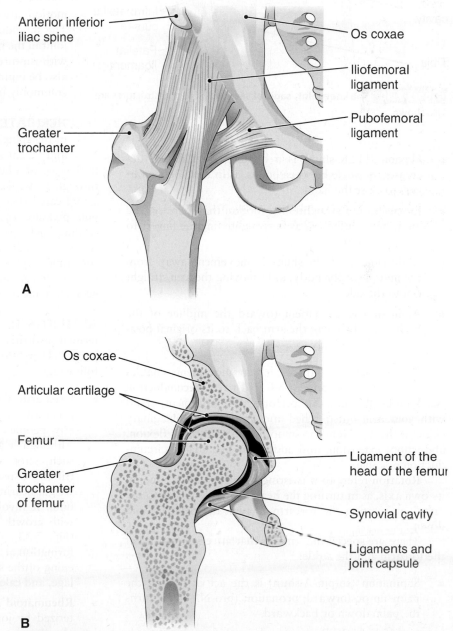

Figure 7-29 Structure of a synovial joint. (A) Anterior view of the hip joint showing ligaments that reinforce and stabilize the joint. **(B)** Frontal section through right hip joint showing protective structures.

Figure 7-30 **The knee joint, sagittal section.** Protective structures are also shown.

- **Flexion** (FLEK-shun) is a bending motion that decreases the angle between bones, as in bending the fingers to close the hand.

- **Extension** is a straightening motion that increases the angle between bones, as in straightening the fingers to open the hand.

- **Abduction** (ab-DUK-shun) is movement away from the midline of the body, as in moving the arm straight out to the side.

- **Adduction** is movement toward the midline of the body, as in bringing the arm back to its original position beside the body.

A combination of these angular movements enables one to execute a movement referred to as **circumduction** (ser-kum-DUK-shun). To perform this movement, stand with your arm outstretched and draw a large imaginary circle in the air. Note the smooth combination of flexion, abduction, extension, and adduction that makes circumduction possible.

Rotation refers to a twisting or turning of a bone on its own axis, as in turning the head from side to side to say "no," or rotating the forearm to turn the palm up and down.

There are special movements that are characteristic of the forearm and the ankle:

- **Supination** (su-pin-A-shun) is the act of turning the palm up or forward; **pronation** (pro-NA-shun) turns the palm down or backward.

- **Inversion** (in-VER-zhun) is the act of turning the sole inward, so that it faces the opposite foot; **eversion** (e-VER-zhun) turns the sole outward, away from the body.

- In **dorsiflexion** (dor-sih-FLEK-shun), the foot is bent upward at the ankle, narrowing the angle between the leg and the top of the foot; in **plantar flexion**, the toes point downward, as in toe dancing, flexing the arch of the foot.

CHECKPOINT **7-11** ➤ What is the most freely movable type of joint?

Disorders of Joints

Joints are subject to certain mechanical disorders. A **dislocation** is a derangement of the joint parts. Ball-and-socket joints, which have the widest range of motion, also have the greatest tendency to dislocate. The shoulder joint is the most frequently dislocated joint in the body. A **sprain** is the wrenching of a joint with rupture or tearing of the ligaments. There may also be injuries to the cartilage within the joint, most commonly in the knee joint.

HERNIATED DISK The disks between the vertebrae of the spine consist of an outer ring of fibrocartilage and a central mass known as the nucleus pulposus. In the case of a **herniated disk**, this central mass protrudes through a weakened outer cartilaginous ring into the spinal canal (Fig. 7-32). The herniated or "slipped" disk puts pressure on the spinal cord or spinal nerves, often causing back spasms or pain along the sciatic nerve that travels through the leg, a pain known as sciatica. It is sometimes necessary to remove the disk and fuse the vertebrae involved. Newer techniques make it possible for surgeons to remove only a specific portion of the disk.

ARTHRITIS The most common type of joint disorder is termed **arthritis**, which means "inflammation of the joints." There are different kinds of arthritis, including the following:

- **Osteoarthritis** (os-te-o-arth-RI-tis), also known as degenerative joint disease (DJD), usually occurs in elderly people as a result of normal wear and tear. Although it appears to be a natural result of aging, such factors as obesity and repeated trauma can contribute. Osteoarthritis occurs mostly in joints used in weight bearing, such as the hips, knees, and spinal column. It involves degeneration of the joint cartilage, with growth of new bone at the edges of the joints (Fig. 7-33). Degenerative changes include bone spur formation at the edges of the articular surfaces, thickening of the synovial membrane, atrophy of the cartilage, and calcification of the ligaments.

- **Rheumatoid arthritis** is a crippling condition characterized by joint swelling in the hands, the feet, and elsewhere as a result of inflammation and overgrowth of the synovial membranes and other joint tissues. The articular cartilage is gradually destroyed, and the joint cavity develops adhesions—that is, the surfaces tend

Table 7-3	Synovial Joints	
Type of Joint	**Type of Movement**	**Examples**
Gliding joint	Bone surfaces slide over one another	Joints in the wrist and ankles (Figs. 7-20 and 7-25)
Hinge joint	Allows movement in one direction, changing the angle of the bones at the joint	Elbow joint; joints between phalanges of fingers and toes (Figs. 7-19, 7-20, and 7-25)
Pivot joint	Allows rotation around the length of the bone	Joint between the first and second cervical vertebrae; joint at proximal ends of the radius and ulna (Figs. 7-10 and 7-19)
Condyloid joint	Allows movement in two directions	Joint between the metacarpal and the first phalanx of the finger (knuckle) (Fig. 7-20); joint between the occipital bone of the skull and the first cervical vertebra (atlas) (Fig. 7-10)
Saddle joint	Like a condyloid joint, but with deeper articulating surfaces	Joint between the wrist and the metacarpal bone of the thumb (Fig. 7-20)
Ball-and-socket joint	Allows movement in many directions around a central point. Gives the greatest freedom of movement	Shoulder joint and hip joint (Figs. 7-15 and 7-29)

to stick together—so that the joints stiffen and ultimately become useless. The exact cause of rheumatoid arthritis is uncertain. However, the disease shares many characteristics of autoimmune disorders, in which antibodies are produced that attack the body's own tissues. The role of inherited susceptibility is clear. Treatment includes rest, appropriate exercise, and medications to reduce pain and swelling. Removal of specific antibodies from the blood and administration of drugs to suppress abnormal antibody production have been successful.

■ **Septic (infectious) arthritis** arises when bacteria spread to involve joint tissue, usually by way of the bloodstream. Bacteria introduced during invasive medical procedures, illegal drug injections, or by other means can settle in joints. A variety of organisms are commonly involved, including *Streptococcus*, *Staphylococcus*, and *Neisseria* species. The joints and the bones themselves are subject to attack by the tuberculosis organism, and the result may be gradual bone destruction near the joint.

Flexion/extension

Pronation/supination

Abduction/adduction

Circumduction

Dorsiflexion/plantar flexion

Rotation

Inversion/eversion

Figure 7-31 **Movements at synovial joints.**

Spinous process

Spinal nerve root

Spinal nerves

Nucleus pulposus

Herniated disk compresses nerve root

Fibrocartilage

Erosion of cartilage and bone

Joint space narrows

Bone spur

Figure 7-32 **Herniated disk.** The central portion (nucleus pulposus) of an intervertebral disk protrudes through the outer rim of cartilage to put pressure on a spinal nerve. (Reprinted with permission from Cohen BJ. *Medical Terminology*, 5th ed. Philadelphia: Lippincott Williams & Wilkins, 2008.)

Figure 7-33 **Joint changes in osteoarthritis (DJD).** The left side shows early changes with breakdown of cartilage and narrowing of the joint space. The right side shows progression of the disease with loss of cartilage and formation of bone spurs.

Figure 7-34 **Arthroscopic examination of the knee.**
Endoscope is inserted between projections at the end of the femur to view the posterior of the knee. (Reprinted with permission from Cohen BJ. *Medical Terminology*, 5th ed. Philadelphia: Lippincott Williams & Wilkins, 2008.)

- **Gout** is a kind of arthritis caused by a metabolic disturbance. One product of metabolism is uric acid, which normally is excreted in the urine. If there happens to be an overproduction of uric acid, or for some reason not enough is excreted, the accumulated uric acid forms crystals that are deposited as masses around the joints and in other areas. As a result, the joints become inflamed and extremely painful. Any joint can be involved, but the one most commonly affected is the big toe. Most gout sufferers are men past middle life.

BACKACHE Backache is another common complaint. Some of its causes are listed below:

- Diseases of the vertebrae, such as infections or tumors, and in older people, osteoarthritis or bone atrophy (wasting away) following long illnesses and lack of exercise.

- Disorders of the intervertebral disks, especially those in the lower lumbar region. Pain may be very severe, with muscle spasms and the extension of symptoms along the course of the sciatic nerve in the leg.

- Abnormalities of the lower vertebrae or of the ligaments and other supporting structures.

- Disorders involving abdominopelvic organs or those in the space behind the peritoneum (such as the kidney). Variations in the position of the uterus are seldom a cause.

- Strains on the lumbosacral joint (where the lumbar region joins the sacrum) or strains on the sacroiliac joint (where the sacrum joins the ilium of the pelvis).

Backache can be prevented by attention to proper movement and good posture. It is most important that the back itself not be used for lifting. A weight to be lifted should be brought close to the body and then the legs should do the actual lifting. An adequate exercise program and control of body weight are also important.

CHECKPOINT 7-12 ➤ What is the most common type of joint disorder?

Joint Repair

Physicians can examine injured joints from outside and even repair them surgically with a lighted instrument known as an **arthroscope** (AR-thro-skope), a type of endoscope (Fig. 7-34). Using arthroscopic techniques, orthopedic surgeons (specialists in the treatment of musculoskeletal disorders) can repair or replace ligaments and remove or reshape cartilage with minimal invasion. Abnormal amounts of fluid that accumulate in a joint cavity as a result of injury can be drained by a tapping procedure called **arthrocentesis** (ar-thro-sen-TE-sis).

If joint degeneration is severe, and conservative therapies, such as medication, physical therapy, and weight loss have failed, a joint replacement or **arthroplasty** (AR-thro-plas-te) may be required. Millions of such surgeries have been performed successfully to restore function in cases of injury, arthritis, and other chronic degenerative bone diseases. Hips and knees are the joints most commonly replaced, but surgeons can also replace shoulder, elbow, wrist, hand, ankle, and foot joints.

The strong, non-toxic, and corrosion-resistant prosthetic (artificial) joints are made of plastic, ceramic, or metal alloys, and are bonded in place with screws or glue. Some are designed to promote bone growth into them to aid in attachment. Computer-controlled machines now produce individualized joints. Until recently, arthroplasty was rarely performed on young people because prosthetic joints had a lifespan of only about 10 years. Current methods have increased this range to 20 years or more, so arthroplasties will require fewer replacements.

7

Disease in Context revisited

▶ Reggie's Fracture Begins to Heal Itself

"So, Doc, what's the chance my leg's going to heal up enough to play football again?" asked Reggie. "Well," replied the doctor, "It's going to take some time before you're catching footballs again, but once your hip heals, it will be better than new."

The surgeon knew that even before the surgery to realign its broken ends, Reggie's femur had already begun to heal itself. Immediately after the injury occurred on the football field, a blood clot formed around the fracture. A day or two later, chemical messengers within the clot would stimulate blood vessels from the periosteum and endosteum to invade the clot, bringing connective tissue cells with them. Over the next several weeks, fibroblasts and chondroblasts in the clot would secrete collagen and cartilage, converting it into a soft callus. Meanwhile, macrophages would remove the remains of the

blood clot and osteoclasts would digest dead bone tissue. Soon after, osteoblasts in the callus would convert it into spongy bone called a hard callus. Months after the injury, osteoclasts and osteoblasts would work together to remodel the outer layers of the hard callus into compact bone, resulting in a repair even stronger than the original bone tissue in Reggie's femur.

During this case, we saw how fractured bones are repaired using screws and plates. We also saw that the body has its own "orthopedic surgeons"—cells like osteoblasts and osteoclasts, which can engineer a bone repair that is even stronger than the original. Although Reggie's skeletal system is beginning to repair itself, he is not out of danger yet. In Chapter 15, a blood clot puts Reggie's life in jeopardy.

Word Anatomy

Medical terms are built from standardized word parts (prefixes, roots, and suffixes). Learning the meanings of these parts can help you remember words and interpret unfamiliar terms.

WORD PART	MEANING	EXAMPLE
Bones		
dia-	through, between	The *diaphysis*, or shaft, of a long bone is between the two ends, or epiphyses.
oss, osse/o	bone, bone tissue	*Osseous* tissue is another name for bone tissue.
oste/o	bone, bone tissue	The *periosteum* is the fibrous membrane around a bone.
-clast	break	An *osteoclast* breaks down bone in the process of resorption.
Bones of the Axial Skeleton		
para-	near	The *paranasal* sinuses are near the nose.
pariet/o	wall	The *parietal* bones form the side walls of the skull.
cost/o	rib	*Intercostal* spaces are located between the ribs.
Bones of the Appendicular Skeleton		
supra-	above, superior	The *supraspinous* fossa is a depression superior to the spine of the scapula.
infra-	below, inferior	The *infraspinous* fossa is a depression inferior to the spine of the scapula.
meta-	near, beyond	The *metacarpal* bones of the palm are near and distal to the carpal bones of the wrist.

WORD PART	MEANING	EXAMPLE
Disorders of Bone		
-penia	lack of	In *osteopenia*, there is a lack of bone density.
-malacia	softening	*Osteomalacia* is a softening of bone tissue.
The Joints		
arthr/o	joint, articulation	A *synarthrosis* is an immovable joint, such as a suture.
amphi-	on both sides, around, double	An *amphiarthrosis* is a slightly movable joint.
ab-	away from	*Abduction* is movement away from the midline of the body.
ad-	toward, added to	*Adduction* is movement toward the midline of the body.
circum-	around	*Circumduction* is movement around a joint in a circle.

Summary

I. **BONES**
   A. Main functions
      1. Serve as body framework
      2. Protect organs
      3. Serve as levers for movement
      4. Store calcium salts
      5. Form blood cells
   B. Bone structure
      1. Long bone
         a. Diaphysis—shaft
         b. Epiphysis—end
      2. Bone tissue
         a. Compact—in shaft of long bones; outside of other bones
         b. Spongy (cancellous)—in end of long bones; center of other bones
      3. Bone marrow
         a. Red—in spongy bone
         b. Yellow—in central cavity of long bones
      4. Bone membranes—contain bone-forming cells
         a. Periosteum—covers bone
         b. Endosteum—lines marrow cavity
   C. Bone growth and repair
      1. Bone cells
         a. Osteoblasts—bone-forming cells
         b. Osteocytes—mature bone cells that maintain bone
         c. Osteoclasts—cells that break down (resorb) bone; derived from monocytes, types of white blood cells
      2. Formation of a long bone—begins in center of shaft and continues at epiphyseal plate
   D. Bone markings
      1. Projections—head, process, condyle, crest, spine
      2. Depressions and holes—foramen, sinus, fossa, meatus

II. **BONES OF THE AXIAL SKELETON**
   A. Framework of the skull
      1. Cranium—frontal, parietal, temporal, ethmoid, sphenoid, occipital
      2. Facial bones—mandible, maxilla, zygomatic, nasal, lacrimal, vomer, palatine, inferior nasal conchae
      3. Other—ossicles (of ear), hyoid
      4. Infant skull—fontanels (soft spots)
   B. Framework of the trunk
      1. Vertebral column—divisions: cervical, thoracic, lumbar, sacral, coccygeal
         a. Curves
            (1) Thoracic and sacral—concave, primary
            (2) Cervical and lumbar—convex, secondary
      2. Thorax
         a. Sternum—manubrium, body, xiphoid process
         b. Ribs
            (1) True—first seven pairs
            (2) False—remaining five pairs, including two floating ribs

III. **BONES OF THE APPENDICULAR SKELETON**
   A. Upper division
      1. Shoulder girdle—clavicle, scapula
      2. Upper extremity—humerus, ulna, radius, carpals, metacarpals, phalanges
   B. Lower division
      1. Pelvic bones—os coxae (hip bone): ilium, ischium, pubis
         a. Female pelvis lighter, wider, more rounded than male
      2. Lower extremity—femur, patella, tibia, fibula, tarsals, metatarsals, phalanges

IV. **DISORDERS OF BONE**
   A. Metabolic—osteoporosis, osteopenia, osteitis deformans, osteomalacia, rickets

B. Tumors

C. Infection—osteomyelitis, tuberculosis (in spine is called Pott disease)

D. Structural disorders—curvature of the spine, cleft palate, flat foot

E. Fractures—closed, open, greenstick, impacted, comminuted, spiral, transverse, oblique

F. Changes in aging—loss of calcium salts, decreased collagen production, thinning of intervertebral disks, loss of flexibility

V. **THE JOINTS (ARTICULATIONS)**

A. Kinds of joints

1. Fibrous—immovable (synarthrosis)

2. Cartilaginous—slightly movable (amphiarthrosis)

3. Synovial—freely movable (diarthrosis)

B. More about synovial joints

1. Structure of synovial joints

a. Joint cavity—contains synovial fluid

b. Ligaments—hold joint together

c. Joint capsule—strengthens and protects joint

d. Articular cartilage—covers ends of bones

e. Bursae—fluid-filled sacs near joints; cushion and protect joints and surrounding tissue

2. Types of synovial joints—gliding, hinge, pivot, condyloid, saddle, ball-and-socket

3. Movement at synovial joints

a. Angular—flexion, extension, abduction, adduction

b. Circular—circumduction, rotation

c. Special at forearm—supination, pronation

d. Special at ankle—inversion, eversion, dorsiflexion, plantar flexion

C. Disorders of Joints

1. Dislocations and sprains

2. Herniated disk—central portion of intervertebral disk projects through outer cartilage

3. Arthritis—osteoarthritis, rheumatoid arthritis, infectious arthritis, gout

4. Backache

D. Joint repair

1. Arthroscope—endoscope used to examine and repair joints

2. Arthroplasty—joint replacement

Questions for Study and Review

BUILDING UNDERSTANDING

Fill in the blanks

1. The shaft of a long bone is called the _____.

2. The structural unit of compact bone is the _____.

3. Red bone marrow manufactures _____.

4. Bones are covered by a connective tissue membrane called _____.

5. Bone matrix is produced by _____.

Matching > Match each numbered item with the most closely related lettered item.

___ 6. A rounded bony projection

___ 7. A sharp bony prominence

___ 8. A hole through bone

___ 9. A bony depression

___ 10. An air-filled bony cavity

a. condyle

b. foramen

c. fossa

d. sinus

e. spine

Multiple Choice

___ 11. On which of the following bones would the mastoid process be found?

a. occipital bone

b. femur

c. temporal bone

d. humerus

___ 12. An abnormal exaggeration of the thoracic curve is called

a. kyphosis

b. lordosis

c. osteitis deformans

d. Pott disease

___ **13.** A splintered or crushed bone with multiple fractures is classified as having a(n) _____ fracture.

    a. open
    b. impacted
    c. comminuted
    d. greenstick

___ **14.** A joint that is freely moveable is called a(n) _____ joint.

    a. arthrotic
    b. amphiarthrotic
    c. diarthrotic
    d. synarthrotic

___ **15.** Which of the following synovial joints describes the hip?

    a. gliding
    b. hinge
    c. pivot
    d. ball-and-socket

UNDERSTANDING CONCEPTS

16. List five functions of bone and describe how a long bone's structure enables it to carry out each of these functions.

17. Explain the differences between the terms in each of the following pairs:

    a. osteoblast and osteocyte
    b. periosteum and endosteum
    c. compact bone and spongy bone
    d. epiphysis and diaphysis
    e. axial skeleton and appendicular skeleton

18. Discuss the process of long bone formation during fetal development and childhood. What role does resorption play in bone formation?

19. Name the bones of the:

    a. cranium and face
    b. thoracic cavity, vertebral column, and pelvis
    c. upper and lower limbs

20. Compare and contrast osteoporosis, osteomalacia, and osteomyelitis.

21. Name three effects of aging on the skeletal system.

22. What are the similarities and differences between osteoarthritis, rheumatoid arthritis, and gout?

23. Differentiate between the terms in each of the following pairs:

    a. flexion and extension
    b. abduction and adduction
    c. supination and pronation
    d. inversion and eversion
    e. circumduction and rotation
    f. dorsiflexion and plantar flexion

7

CONCEPTUAL THINKING

24. The vertebral bodies are much larger in the lower back than the neck. What is the functional significance of this structural difference?

25. Nine-year-old Alek is admitted to the emergency room with a closed fracture of the right femur. Radiography reveals that the fracture crosses the distal epiphyseal plate. What concerns should Alek's healthcare team have about the location of his injury?

26. In the case story, Reggie presented with three typical signs of hip fracture—shortening, adduction, and lateral rotation of the affected limb. What causes these signs? (HINT—the skeleton is part of the musculoskeletal system.)

27. In Reggie's case, he fractured the proximal end of his right femur, an integral component of his hip. Name the joint disorders that Reggie is more at risk of in (a) the short term, and (b) the long term.

CHAPTER 8

The Muscular System

Learning Outcomes

After careful study of this chapter, you should be able to:

1. Compare the three types of muscle tissue
2. Describe three functions of skeletal muscle
3. Briefly describe how skeletal muscles contract
4. List the substances needed in muscle contraction and describe the function of each
5. Define the term *oxygen debt*
6. Describe three compounds stored in muscle that are needed to generate energy in highly active muscle cells
7. Cite the effects of exercise on muscles
8. Compare isotonic and isometric contractions
9. Explain how muscles work in pairs to produce movement
10. Compare the workings of muscles and bones to lever systems
11. Explain how muscles are named
12. Name some of the major muscles in each muscle group and describe the main function of each
13. Describe how muscles change with age
14. List the major muscular disorders
15. Show how word parts are used to build words related to the muscular system (see Word Anatomy at the end of the chapter)

Selected Key Terms

The following terms and other boldface terms in the chapter are defined in the Glossary

acetylcholine
actin
antagonist
bursitis
fascicle
glycogen
insertion
lactic acid
motor unit
myalgia
myoglobin
myosin
neuromuscular junction
neurotransmitter
origin
oxygen debt
prime mover
spasm
synapse
synergist
tendon
tonus

PASSport to Success

Visit *thePoint* or see the Student Resource CD in the back of this book for definitions and pronunciations of key terms as well as a pretest for this chapter.

Disease in Context

➤ Sue's Case: A Muscle Mystery

Dr. Mathews glanced at his patient's chart as he stepped into the consulting room to see her. Sue Pritchard was 26 years old, white, and, according to her medical history, relatively healthy. "Hi Sue. It's been a while since your last visit. What can I do for you today?" asked the doctor.

"I'm probably making a mountain out of a molehill," Sue replied. "But, I've been having some odd symptoms that got me worried. For the last couple of weeks I've noticed that my right hand is getting weak. Just the other day, I had barely enough strength to hold my coffee cup! On top of that, I've had trouble walking. I haven't fallen down or anything, but I feel like I'm off balance."

Based on Sue's description of her symptoms, Dr. Mathews initially suspected a problem with her muscular system. He checked her hand strength and verified that her right hand was weaker than her left—unusual since she was right-handed. He compared both of Sue's arms and observed slight atrophy of the flexor muscles in her right forearm. He tested several of her reflexes and noted that the responses in her biceps brachii and quadriceps femoris muscles were exaggerated in her right limbs. He had Sue do a few simple coordination tests like touching her nose and standing on one foot. As in the previous tests, Sue seemed to have more difficulty with right-sided tasks than left. "Have you had any pain or tingling in your arms or legs lately?" the doctor asked.

"Yes!" answered Sue. "In fact, last night I had a cramp in my right leg that was so painful I had to get out of bed and walk it off. And, my fingertips have been tingling on and off for the last few days too."

Dr. Mathews quickly recognized that Sue's problem was not just limited to her muscular system. It also appeared that her nervous system was involved.

Dr. Mathews' knowledge of the structure and function of the muscular system helps him to diagnose medical conditions. In this chapter you will learn about muscle tissue and the connection it has with nervous tissue. Later in the chapter, we'll find out more about Sue's condition.

Types of Muscle

There are three kinds of muscle tissue: smooth, cardiac, and skeletal muscle, as introduced in Chapter 4. After a brief description of all three types (Table 8-1), this chapter concentrates on skeletal muscle, which has been studied the most.

Smooth Muscle

Smooth muscle makes up the walls of the hollow body organs as well as those of the blood vessels and respiratory passageways. It moves involuntarily and produces the wave-like motions of peristalsis that move substances through a system. Smooth muscle can also regulate the diameter of an opening, such as the central opening of blood vessels, or produce contractions of hollow organs, such as the uterus. Smooth muscle fibers (cells) are tapered at each end and have a single, central nucleus. The cells appear smooth under the microscope because they do not contain the visible bands, or **striations**, that are seen in the other types of muscle cells. Smooth muscle may contract in response to a nerve impulse, hormonal stimulation, stretching, and other stimuli. The muscle contracts and relaxes slowly and can remain contracted for a long time.

Cardiac Muscle

Cardiac muscle, also involuntary, makes up the heart's wall and creates the pulsing action of that organ. The cells of cardiac muscle are striated, like those of skeletal muscle. They differ in having one nucleus per cell and branching interconnections. The membranes between the cells are specialized to allow electrical impulses to travel rapidly through them, so that contractions can be better coordinated. These membranes appear as dark lines between the cells (see Table 8-1) and are called intercalated (in-TER-kah-la-ted) disks, because they are "inserted between" the cells. The electrical impulses that produce cardiac muscle contractions are generated within the muscle itself but can be modified by nervous stimuli and hormones.

Skeletal Muscle

When viewed under the microscope, skeletal muscle cells appear heavily striated. The arrangement of protein threads within the cell that produces these striations is described later. The cells are very long and cylindrical and have multiple nuclei per cell. During development, the nuclei of these cells divide repeatedly by mitosis without division of the cell contents, resulting in a large, multinucleated cell. Such cells can contract as a large unit when stimulated. The nervous system stimulates skeletal muscle to contract, and the tissue usually contracts and relaxes rapidly. Because it is under conscious control, skeletal muscle is described as voluntary.

Skeletal muscle is so named because most of these muscles are attached to bones and produce movement at the joints. There are a few exceptions. The muscles of the abdominal wall, for example, are partly attached to other muscles, and the muscles of facial expression are attached to the skin. Skeletal muscles constitute the largest amount of the body's muscle tissue, making up about 40% of the total body weight. This muscular system is composed of more than 600 individual skeletal muscles. Although each one is a distinct structure, muscles usually act in groups to execute body movements.

Table 8-1	Comparison of the Different Types of Muscle		
	Smooth	**Cardiac**	**Skeletal**
Location	Wall of hollow organs, vessels, respiratory passageways	Wall of heart	Attached to bones
Cell characteristics	Tapered at each end, branching networks, nonstriated	Branching networks; special membranes (intercalated disks) between cells; single nucleus; lightly striated	Long and cylindrical; multinucleated; heavily striated
Control	Involuntary	Involuntary	Voluntary
Action	Produces peristalsis; contracts and relaxes slowly; may sustain contraction	Pumps blood out of heart; self-excitatory but influenced by nervous system and hormones	Produces movement at joints; stimulated by nervous system; contracts and relaxes rapidly

CHECKPOINT **8-1** ➤ What are the three types of muscle?

The Muscular System

The three primary functions of skeletal muscles are:

- Movement of the skeleton. Muscles are attached to bones and contract to change the position of the bones at a joint.

- Maintenance of posture. A steady partial contraction of muscle, known as **muscle tone**, keeps the body in position. Some of the muscles involved in maintaining posture are the large muscles of the thighs, back, neck, and shoulders as well as the abdominal muscles.

- Generation of heat. Muscles generate most of the heat needed to keep the body at 37°C (98.6°F). Heat is a natural by-product of muscle cell metabolism. When we are cold, muscles can boost their heat output by the rapid small contractions we know of as shivering.

CHECKPOINT **8-2** ➤ What are the three main functions of skeletal muscle?

Structure of a Muscle

In forming whole muscles, individual muscle fibers are arranged in bundles, or **fascicles** (FAS-ih-kls), held to-gether by fibrous connective tissue (Fig. 8-1, Table 8-2). The deepest layer of this connective tissue, the **endomysium** (en-do-MIS-e-um) surrounds the individual fibers in the fascicles. Around each fascicle is a connective tissue layer known as the **perimysium** (per-ih-MIS-e-um). The entire muscle is then encased in a tough connective tissue sheath, the **epimysium** (ep-ih-MIS-e-um), which forms the innermost layer of the **deep fascia**, the tough, fibrous sheath that encloses a muscle. (Note that all these layers are named with prefixes that describe their position added to the root *my/o*, meaning "muscle.") All of these supporting tissues merge to form the **tendon**, the band of connective tissue that attaches a muscle to a bone (see Fig. 8-1).

Muscle Cells in Action

Nerve impulses coming from the brain and the spinal cord stimulate skeletal muscle fibers (see Chapter 9). Because these impulses are traveling away from the central nervous system (CNS), they are described as **motor** impulses (as contrasted to sensory impulses traveling toward the CNS), and the neurons (nerve cells) that carry these impulses are described as motor neurons. As the neuron contacts the muscle, its axon (fiber) branches to supply from a few to hundreds of individual muscle cells, or in some cases more than 1,000 (Fig. 8-2).

A single neuron and all the muscle fibers it stimulates comprise a **motor unit**. Small motor units are used in fine coordination, as in movements of the eye. Larger motor

Figure 8-1 **Structure of a skeletal muscle. (A)** Structure of a muscle showing the tendon that attaches it to a bone. **(B)** Muscle tissue seen under a microscope. Portions of several fascicles are shown with connective tissue coverings. (B, Reprinted with permission from Gartner LP, Hiatt JL. *Color Atlas of Histology*, 3rd ed. Philadelphia: Lippincott Williams & Wilkins, 2000.) **[ZOOMING IN ➤** What is the innermost layer of connective tissue in a muscle? What layer of connective tissue surrounds a fascicle of muscle fibers? **]**

Table 8-2	Connective Tissue Layers in Skeletal Muscle	
Name of Layer	**Location**	
Endomysium	Around each individual muscle fiber	
Perimysium	Around fascicles (bundles) of muscle fibers	
Epimysium	Around entire muscle; forms the innermost layer of the deep fascia	

units are used for maintaining posture or for broad movements, such as walking or swinging a tennis racquet.

THE NEUROMUSCULAR JUNCTION The point at which a nerve fiber contacts a muscle cell is called the **neuromuscular junction** (NMJ) (Fig. 8-3). It is here that a chemical classified as a **neurotransmitter** is released from the neuron to stimulate the muscle fiber. The specific neurotransmitter released here is **acetylcholine** (as-e-til-KO-lene), abbreviated ACh, which is found elsewhere in the body as well. A great deal is known about the events that occur at this junction, and this information is important in understanding muscle action.

The neuromuscular junction is an example of a **synapse** (SIN-aps), a point of communication between cells. Between the cells there is a tiny space, the **synaptic cleft,** across which the neurotransmitter must travel. Until its release, the neurotransmitter is stored in tiny membranous sacs, called vesicles, in the nerve fiber's endings. Once released, the neurotransmitter crosses the synaptic cleft and attaches to receptors, which are proteins embedded in the muscle cell membrane.

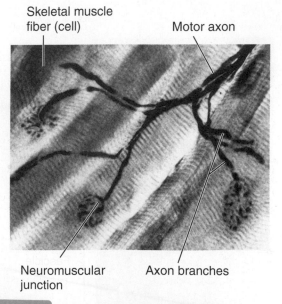

Skeletal muscle fiber (cell)

Motor axon

Neuromuscular junction

Axon branches

Figure 8-2 **Nervous stimulation of skeletal muscle.** A motor axon branches to stimulate multiple muscle fibers (cells). The point of contact between the neuron and the muscle cell is the neuromuscular junction. (Reprinted with permission from Cormack DH. *Essential Histology*, 2nd ed. Philadelphia: Lippincott Williams & Wilkins, 2001.)

The membrane forms multiple folds at this point that increase surface area and hold a maximum number of receptors. The muscle cell's receiving membrane is known as the **motor end plate**.

Muscle fibers, like nerve cells, show the property of **excitability**; that is, they are able to transmit electrical current along the plasma membrane. When the muscle is stimulated at the neuromuscular junction, an electrical impulse is generated that spreads rapidly along the muscle cell membrane. This spreading wave of electrical current is called the **action potential** because it calls the muscle cell into action. Chapter 9 provides more information on synapses and the action potential.

CHECKPOINT 8-3 ➤ Muscles are activated by the nervous system. What is the name of the special synapse where a nerve cell makes contact with a muscle cell?

CHECKPOINT 8-4 ➤ What neurotransmitter is involved in the stimulation of skeletal muscle cells?

PASSport to Success Visit **thePoint** or see the Student Resource CD in the back of this book for the animation *The Neuromuscular Junction and Neurotransmitters.*

CONTRACTION Another important property of muscle tissue is **contractility**. This is a muscle fiber's capacity to undergo shortening and to change its shape, becoming thicker. Studies of muscle chemistry and observation of cells under the powerful electron microscope have given a concept of how muscle cells work.

These studies reveal that each skeletal muscle fiber contains many threads, or filaments, made of two kinds of proteins, called **actin** (AK-tin) and **myosin** (MI-o-sin). Filaments made of actin are thin and light; those made of myosin are thick and dark. The filaments are present in alternating bundles within the muscle cell (Fig. 8-4). It is the alternating bands of light actin and heavy myosin filaments that give skeletal muscle its striated appearance. They also give a view of what occurs when muscles contract.

Note that the actin and myosin filaments overlap where they meet, just as your fingers overlap when you fold your hands together. A contracting subunit of skeletal muscle is called a **sarcomere** (SAR-ko-mere). It consists of a band of myosin filaments and the actin filaments on each side of them (see Fig. 8-4). In movement, the myosin filaments "latch on" to the actin filaments in their overlapping region by means of many paddlelike extensions called myosin heads. In this way, the myosin heads form attachments between the actin and myosin filaments that are described as cross-bridges. Using the energy of ATP for

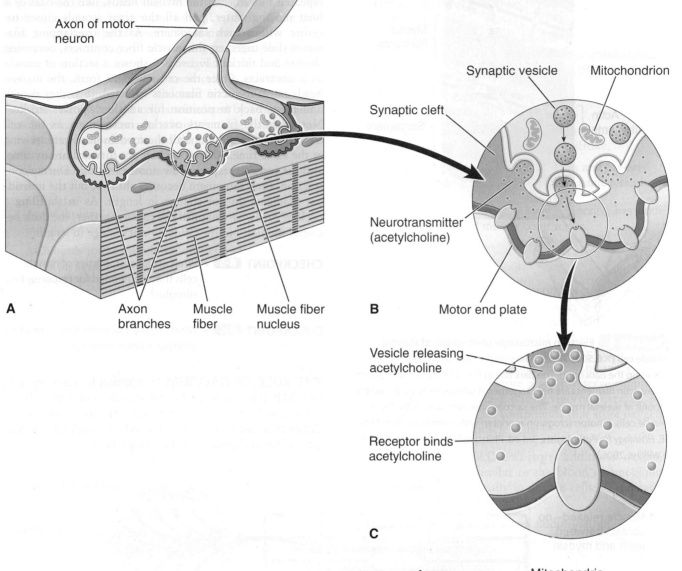

A

Axon of motor neuron

Axon branches

Muscle fiber

Muscle fiber nucleus

B

Synaptic cleft

Synaptic vesicle

Mitochondrion

Neurotransmitter (acetylcholine)

Motor end plate

C

Vesicle releasing acetylcholine

Receptor binds acetylcholine

8

D

Axon

Mitochondria

Vesicles with neurotransmitter

Folds in motor end plate of muscle cell

Figure 8-3 **Neuromuscular junction (NMJ).** **(A)** The branched end of a motor neuron makes contact with the membrane of a muscle fiber (cell). **(B)** Enlarged view of the NMJ showing release of neurotransmitter (acetylcholine) into the synaptic cleft. **(C)** Acetylcholine attaches to receptors in the motor end plate, whose folds increase surface area. **(D)** Electron microscope photograph of the neuromuscular junction. (D, Courtesy of A. Sima.)

Box 8-1   A Closer Look

Muscle Contraction and Energy

When we think of muscle contraction, we might imagine a runner's rippling muscles. But muscle contraction actually occurs at a microscopic level within the sarcomere's working parts: the thick and thin filaments.

Thick filaments are composed of many myosin molecules, each shaped like two golf clubs twisted together with the myosin heads projecting away from the sarcomere's center (see Fig. 8-6). Each myosin head can bind ATP and convert it into ADP and a phosphate molecule, which remain bound. The chemical energy released during this reaction charges the myosin head, enabling it to do work.

Thin filaments' actin molecules are twisted together like two strands of beads. Each "bead" has a myosin-binding site, but the two regulatory proteins, troponin and tropomyosin, cover the binding sites when the muscle is at rest. When calcium shifts these proteins away from the binding sites, the following cycle of events occurs:

1. The charged myosin heads attach to the actin molecules and form cross-bridges between the thick and thin filaments.
2. Using their stored energy, the myosin heads pull the thin filaments to the center of the sarcomere, releasing the ADP and phosphate molecules.
3. New ATP molecules bind to the myosin heads, causing them to detach from actin and breaking the cross-bridges.
4. The myosin heads convert ATP into ADP and phosphate, which recharges them.

After death, muscles enter a stage of rigidity known as rigor mortis. This phenomenon illustrates ATP's crucial role in muscle contraction. Shortly after death, muscle cells begin to degrade. Calcium escapes into the cytoplasm, and the muscle filaments slide together. Metabolism has ceased, however, and there is no ATP to disengage the filaments, so they remain locked in a contracted state. Rigor mortis lasts about 24 hours, gradually fading as enzymes break down the muscle filaments.

---

phosphate stored in the tissues meet the increased demands, but continual exercise depletes these stores.

For a short time, glucose may be used anaerobically, that is, without the benefit of oxygen. This anaerobic process generates ATP rapidly and permits greater magnitude of activity than would otherwise be possible, as, for example, allowing sprinting instead of jogging. However, anaerobic metabolism is inefficient; it does not produce as much ATP as does metabolism in the presence of oxygen. Also, an organic acid called **lactic acid** accumulates in the cells when this alternate metabolic pathway is used. Anaerobic metabolism can continue only until the buildup of lactic acid causes the muscles to fatigue.

Muscles operating anaerobically are in a state of **oxygen debt**. After stopping exercise, a person must continue to take in extra oxygen by continued rapid breathing (panting) until the debt is paid in full. That is, enough oxygen must be taken in to convert the lactic acid to other substances that can be metabolized further. In addition, the glycogen, myoglobin, and creatine phosphate that are stored in the cells must be replenished. The time after strenuous exercise during which extra oxygen is needed is known as the period of recovery oxygen consumption.

CHECKPOINT 8-9 ➤ When muscles work without oxygen, a compound is produced that causes muscle fatigue. What is the name of this compound?

Effects of Exercise

Regular exercise results in a number of changes in muscle tissue. These changes correspond to the three components of exercise: stretching, aerobics, and resistance training. When muscles are stretched, they contract more forcefully, as the internal filaments can interact over a greater length. Stretching also helps with balance and promotes flexibility at the joints. Aerobic exercise, that is, exercise that increases oxygen consumption, such as running, biking, or swimming, leads to improved endurance. Resistance training, such as weight lifting, causes muscle cells to increase in size, a condition known as hypertrophy (hi-PER-tro-fe). One can see this change in the enlarged muscles of bodybuilders. Some of the changes in muscle tissue that lead to improved endurance and strength include:

- Increase in the number of capillaries, which brings more blood to the cells
- Increase in the number of mitochondria to increase production of ATP
- Increase in reserves of myoglobin, glycogen, and creatine phosphate to promote endurance

An exercise program should include all three methods—stretching, aerobic exercise, and resistance training—with periods of warm-up and cool-down before and after working out. This type of varied program is described as cross-training or interval training.

In addition to affecting muscle tissue itself, exercise causes some systemic changes. The **vasodilation** (vas-o-di-LA-shun), or widening of blood vessel diameter, that occurs during exercise allows blood to flow more easily to muscle tissue. With continued work, more blood is pumped back to the heart. The heart's temporarily increased load strengthens the myocardium and improves its circulation. With exercise training, the heart's chambers gradually enlarge to accommodate more blood. A trained athlete's resting heart rate is lower than the average rate because the heart can function more efficiently.

Regular exercise also improves breathing and respiratory efficiency. Circulation in the capillaries surrounding the alveoli (air sacs) is increased, and this brings about enhanced gas exchange. The more efficient distribution and use of oxygen delays the onset of oxygen debt. Even moderate regular exercise has the additional benefits of weight control, strengthening of the bones, decreased blood pressure, and decreased risk of heart attacks. The effects of exercise on the body are studied in the fields of sports medicine and exercise physiology. Box 8-2, Anabolic Steroids: Winning at All Costs?, has information on how steroids affect muscles.

Types of Muscle Contractions

Muscle **tone** refers to a muscle's partially contracted state that is normal even when the muscle is not in use. The maintenance of this tone, or **tonus** (TO-nus), is due to the action of the nervous system in keeping the muscles in a constant state of readiness for action. Muscles that are little used soon become flabby, weak, and lacking in tone.

In addition to the partial contractions that are responsible for muscle tone, there are two other types of contractions on which the body depends:

- In **isotonic** (i-so-TON-ik) **contractions,** the tone or tension within the muscle remains the same but the muscle as a whole shortens, producing movement; that is, work is accomplished. Lifting weights, walking, running, or any other activity in which the muscles become shorter and thicker (forming bulges) are isotonic contractions.

- In **isometric** (i-so-MET-rik) **contractions,** there is no change in muscle length but there is a great increase in muscle tension. Pushing against an immovable force produces an isometric contraction. For example, if you push the palms of your hands hard against each other, there is no movement, but you can feel the increased tension in your arm muscles.

Most body movements involve a combination of both isotonic and isometric contractions. When walking, for example, some muscles contract isotonically to propel the body forward, but at the same time, other muscles are contracting isometrically to keep your body in position.

The Mechanics of Muscle Movement

Most muscles have two or more points of attachment to the skeleton. The muscle is attached to a bone at each end by means of a cordlike extension called a **tendon** (Fig. 8-7). All of the connective tissue within and around the muscle merges to form the tendon, which then attaches directly to the bone's periosteum (see Fig. 8-1). In some instances, a broad sheet called an **aponeurosis** (ap-o-nu-RO-sis) may attach muscles to bones or to other muscles.

In moving the bones, one end of a muscle is attached to a more freely movable part of the skeleton, and the other end is attached to a relatively stable part. The less

8

Box 8-2   Hot Topics

Anabolic Steroids: Winning at All Costs?

Anabolic steroids mimic the effects of the male sex hormone testosterone by promoting metabolism and stimulating growth. These drugs are legally prescribed to promote muscle regeneration and prevent atrophy from disuse after surgery. However, athletes also purchase them illegally, using them to increase muscle size and strength and improve endurance.

When steroids are used illegally to enhance athletic performance, the doses needed are large enough to cause serious side effects. They increase blood cholesterol levels, which may lead to atherosclerosis, heart disease, kidney failure, and

stroke. Steroids damage the liver, making it more susceptible to disease and cancer, and suppress the immune system, increasing the risk of infection and cancer. In men, steroids cause impotence, testicular atrophy, low sperm count, infertility, and the development of female sex characteristics such as breasts (gynecomastia). In women, steroids disrupt ovulation and menstruation and produce male sex characteristics such as breast atrophy, enlargement of the clitoris, increased body hair, and deepening of the voice. In both sexes steroids increase the risk for baldness and, especially in men, cause mood swings, depression, and violence.

Often, more than one feature is used in naming. Refer to Figures 8-9 and 8-10 as you study the locations and functions of the superficial skeletal muscles and try to figure out the basis for each name. Although they are described in the singular, most of the muscles are present on both sides of the body.

Muscles of the Head

The principal muscles of the head are those of facial expression and of mastication (chewing) (Fig. 8-11, Table 8-3).

The muscles of facial expression include ring-shaped ones around the eyes and the lips, called the **orbicularis**

Orbicularis oculi

Masseter

Sternocleidomastoid

Deltoid

Pectoralis major

Serratus anterior

Biceps brachii

Brachioradialis

Flexor carpi

Extensor carpi

Abdominal aponeurosis (tendon)

Adductors of thigh

Peroneus longus

Tibialis anterior

Temporalis

Orbicularis oris

Trapezius

External oblique

Intercostals

Internal oblique

Rectus abdominis

Sartorius

Quadriceps femoris

Gastrocnemius

Soleus

Anterior view

Figure 8-9 **Superficial muscles, anterior view.** Associated structure is labeled in parentheses.

Posterior view

Figure 8-10 **Superficial muscles, posterior view.** Associated structures are labeled in parentheses.

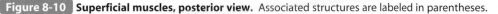

(or-bik-u-LAH-ris) **muscles** because of their shape (think of "orbit"). The muscle surrounding each eye is called the **orbicularis oculi** (OK-u-li), whereas the lip muscle is the **orbicularis oris**. These muscles, of course, all have antagonists. For example, the **levator palpebrae** (PAL-pe-bre) **superioris**, or lifter of the upper eyelid, is the antagonist for the orbicularis oculi.

One of the largest muscles of expression forms the fleshy part of the cheek and is called the **buccinator** (BUK-se-na-tor). Used in whistling or blowing, it is sometimes referred to as the trumpeter's muscle. You can readily think of other muscles of facial expression: for instance, the an-

tagonists of the orbicularis oris can produce a smile, a sneer, or a grimace. There are a number of scalp muscles that lift the eyebrows or draw them together into a frown.

There are four pairs of mastication (chewing) muscles, all of which insert on and move the mandible. The largest are the **temporalis** (TEM-po-ral-is), which is superior to the ear, and the **masseter** (mas-SE-ter) at the angle of the jaw.

The tongue has two muscle groups. The first group, called the **intrinsic muscles**, is located entirely within the tongue. The second group, the **extrinsic muscles**, originates outside the tongue. It is because of these many muscles that the tongue has such remarkable flexibility and can perform

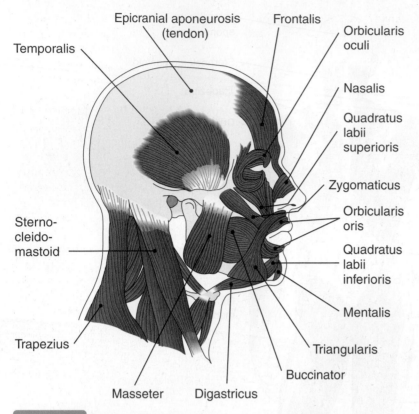

Temporalis
Epicranial aponeurosis (tendon)
Frontalis
Orbicularis oculi
Nasalis
Quadratus labii superioris
Zygomaticus
Orbicularis oris
Quadratus labii inferioris
Mentalis
Triangularis
Buccinator
Digastricus
Masseter
Trapezius
Sterno-cleido-mastoid

Figure 8-11 **Muscles of the head.** Associated structure is labeled in parentheses. [**ZOOMING IN ➤** Which of the muscles in this illustration is named for a bone it is near?]

so many different functions. Consider the intricate tongue motions involved in speaking, chewing, and swallowing. Figure 8-11 shows some additional muscles of the face.

PASSport to Success Visit *thePoint* or see the Student Resource CD in the back of this book for additional pictures of head and neck musculature.

Muscles of the Neck

The neck muscles tend to be ribbonlike and extend vertically or obliquely in several layers and in a complex manner (Fig. 8-11, Table 8-3). The one you will hear of most frequently is the **sternocleidomastoid** (ster-no-kli-do-MAS-toyd), sometimes referred to simply as the sternomastoid. This strong muscle extends superiorly from the sternum across the lateral neck to the mastoid process. When the left and right muscles work together, they bring the head forward on the chest (flexion). Working alone, each muscle tilts and rotates the head so as to orient the face toward the side opposite that muscle. If the head is abnormally fixed in this position, the person is said to have **torticollis** (tor-tih-KOL-is), or wryneck; this condition may be caused by muscle injury or spasm.

A portion of the trapezius muscle (described later) is located at the posterior neck, where it helps hold the head up (extension). Other larger deep muscles are the chief extensors of the head and neck.

Muscles of the Upper Extremities

Muscles of the upper extremities include the muscles that determine the position of the shoulder, the anterior and posterior muscles that move the arm, and the muscles that move the forearm and hand.

MUSCLES THAT MOVE THE SHOULDER AND ARM

The position of the shoulder depends to a large extent on the degree of contraction of the **trapezius** (trah-PE-ze-us), a triangular muscle that covers the posterior neck and ex-

Table 8-3	Muscles of the Head and Neck*	
Name	**Location**	**Function**
Orbicularis oculi	Encircles eyelid	Closes eye
Levator palpebrae superioris (deep muscle; not shown)	Posterior orbit to upper eyelid	Opens eye
Orbicularis oris	Encircles mouth	Closes lips
Buccinator	Fleshy part of cheek	Flattens cheek; helps in eating, whistling, and blowing wind instruments
Temporalis	Above and near ear	Closes jaw
Masseter	At angle of jaw	Closes jaw
Sternocleidomastoid	Along lateral neck, to mastoid process	Flexes head; rotates head toward opposite side from muscle

These and other muscles of the face are shown in Figure 8-11.

tends across the posterior shoulder to insert on the clavicle and scapula (Fig. 8-10, Table 8-4). The trapezius muscles enable one to raise the shoulders and pull them back. The superior portion of each trapezius can also extend the head and turn it from side to side.

The **latissimus** (lah-TIS-ih-mus) **dorsi** is the wide muscle of the back and lateral trunk. It originates from the vertebral spine in the middle and lower back and covers the inferior half of the thoracic region, forming the posterior portion of the axilla (armpit). The fibers of each muscle converge to a tendon that inserts on the humerus. The latissimus dorsi powerfully extends the arm, bringing it down forcibly as, for example, in swimming.

A large **pectoralis** (pek-to-RAL-is) **major** is located on either side of the superior chest (see Fig. 8-9). This muscle arises from the sternum, the upper ribs, and the clavicle and forms the anterior "wall" of the axilla; it inserts on the superior humerus. The pectoralis major flexes and adducts the arm, pulling it across the chest.

The **serratus** (ser-RA-tus) **anterior** is below the axilla, on the lateral chest. It originates on the upper eight or nine ribs on the lateral and anterior thorax and inserts in the scapula on the side toward the vertebrae. The serratus anterior moves the scapula forward when, for example, one is pushing something. It also aids in raising the arm above the horizontal level.

The **deltoid** covers the shoulder joint and is responsible for the roundness of the upper arm just inferior to the shoulder (see Figs. 8-9 and 8-10). This muscle is named for its triangular shape, which resembles the Greek letter delta. The deltoid is often used as an injection site. Arising from the shoulder girdle (clavicle and scapula), the deltoid fibers converge to insert on the lateral surface of the humerus. Contraction of this muscle abducts the arm, raising it laterally to the horizontal position.

The shoulder joint allows for a very wide range of movement. This freedom of movement is possible because the humerus fits into a shallow socket, the scapula's glenoid cavity. This joint requires the support of four deep muscles and their tendons, which compose the **rotator cuff**. The four muscles are the supraspinatus, infraspinatus, teres minor, and subscapularis, known together as SITS, based on the first letters of their names. In certain activities, such as swinging a golf club, playing tennis, or pitching a baseball, the rotator cuff muscles may be injured, even torn, and may require surgery for repair.

PASSport to Success Visit **thePoint** or see the Student Resource CD in the back of this book for additional pictures of muscles that move the shoulder and arm and also the muscles of the rotator cuff.

Table 8-4	Muscles of the Upper Extremities*	
Name	**Location**	**Function**
Trapezius	Posterior neck and upper back, to clavicle and scapula	Raises shoulder and pulls it back; extends head
Latissimus dorsi	Middle and lower back, to humerus	Extends and adducts arm behind back
Pectoralis major	Superior, anterior chest, to humerus	Flexes and adducts arm across chest; pulls shoulder forward and downward
Serratus anterior	Inferior to axilla on lateral chest, to scapula	Moves scapula forward; aids in raising arm, punching, or reaching forward
Deltoid	Covers shoulder joint, to lateral humerus	Abducts arm
Biceps brachii	Anterior arm along humerus, to radius	Flexes forearm at the elbow and supinates hand
Brachialis	Posterior to biceps brachii; inserts at anterior elbow joint	Main flexor of forearm
Brachioradialis	Lateral forearm from distal end of humerus to distal end of radius	Flexes forearm at the elbow
Triceps brachii	Posterior arm, to ulna	Extends forearm to straighten upper extremity
Flexor carpi group	Anterior forearm, to hand	Flexes hand
Extensor carpi group	Posterior forearm, to hand	Extends hand
Flexor digitorum group	Anterior forearm, to fingers	Flexes fingers
Extensor digitorum group	Posterior forearm, to fingers	Extends fingers

*These and other muscles of the upper extremities are shown in Figures 8-9, 8-10, and 8-12.

MUSCLES THAT MOVE THE FOREARM AND HAND

The **biceps brachii** (BRA-ke-i), located at the anterior arm along the humerus, is the muscle you usually display when you want to "flex your muscles" to show your strength (Fig. 8-12A). It inserts on the radius and flexes the forearm. It is a supinator of the hand. The **brachialis** (bra-ke-AL-is) lies deep to the biceps brachii and inserts distally over the anterior elbow joint. It flexes the forearm in all positions, sustains flexion, and steadies the slow extension of the forearm.

Another forearm flexor at the elbow is the **brachioradialis** (bra-ke-o-ra-de-A-lis), a prominent forearm muscle that originates at the distal humerus and inserts on the distal radius.

The **triceps brachii**, located on the posterior arm, inserts on the olecranon of the ulna (Fig. 8-12B). It is used to straighten the arm, as in lowering a weight from an arm curl. It is also important in pushing because it converts the arm and forearm into a sturdy rod.

Most of the muscles that move the hand and fingers originate from the radius and the ulna (see Fig. 8-12).

Some of them insert on the carpal bones of the wrist, whereas others have long tendons that cross the wrist and insert on bones of the hand and the fingers.

The **flexor carpi** and the **extensor carpi muscles** are responsible for many hand movements. Muscles that produce finger movements are the several **flexor digitorum** (dij-e-TO-rum) and the **extensor digitorum muscles**. The names of these muscles may include bones they are near, their action, or their length, for example, longus for long and brevis for short.

Special muscle groups in the fleshy parts of the hand execute the intricate movements that can be performed with the thumb and the fingers. The thumb's freedom of movement has been one of humankind's most useful capacities.

> PASSport to **Success**
> Visit **thePoint** or see the Student Resource CD in the back of this book for additional pictures of the muscles that move the forearm and hand.

Muscles of the Trunk

The trunk muscles include the muscles involved in breathing, the thin muscle layers of the abdomen, and the muscles of the pelvic floor. The following discussion also includes the deep muscles of the back that support and move the vertebral column.

MUSCLES OF RESPIRATION The most important muscle involved in the act of breathing is the **diaphragm**. This dome-shaped muscle forms the partition between the thoracic cavity above and the abdominal cavity below (Fig. 8-13). When the diaphragm contracts, the central dome-shaped portion is pulled downward, thus enlarging the thoracic cavity from top to bottom.

The **intercostal muscles** are attached to and fill the spaces between the ribs. The external and internal intercostals run at angles in opposite directions. Contraction of the intercostal muscles elevates the ribs, thus enlarging the thoracic cavity from side to side and from anterior to posterior. The mechanics of breathing are described in Chapter 18.

CHECKPOINT 8-13 ➤ What muscle is most important in breathing?

Biceps brachii
Brachialis
Brachioradialis
Flexor carpi radialis
Flexor carpi ulnaris
Flexor digitorum superficialis

Triceps brachii
Brachioradialis
Extensor carpi radialis longus
Extensor carpi radialis brevis
Flexor carpi ulnaris
Extensor digitorum
Extensor carpi ulnaris

A Anterior view
B Posterior view

Figure 8-12 **Muscles that move the forearm and hand.**

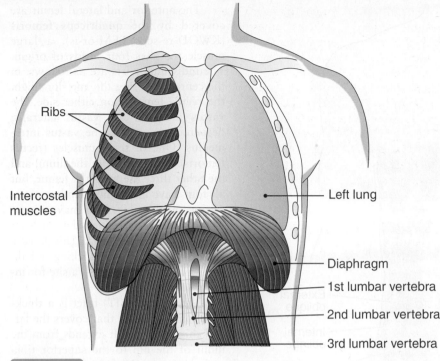

Ribs

Intercostal
muscles

Left lung

Diaphragm
1st lumbar vertebra
2nd lumbar vertebra
3rd lumbar vertebra

Figure 8-13 **Muscles of respiration.** Associated structures are also shown.

DEEP MUSCLES OF THE BACK The deep muscles of the back, which act on the vertebral column itself, are thick vertical masses that lie under the trapezius and latissimus dorsi. The **erector spinae** muscles make up a large group located between the sacrum and the skull. These muscles extend the spine and maintain the vertebral column in an erect posture. The muscles can be strained in lifting heavy objects if the spine is flexed while lifting. One should bend at the hip and knee instead and use the thigh and buttock muscles to help in lifting.

Deeper muscles in the lumbar area extend the vertebral column in that region. These deep back muscles are not shown in the illustrations.

Muscles of the Lower Extremities

8

The muscles in the lower extremities, among the longest and strongest muscles in the body, are specialized for locomotion and balance. They include the muscles that move the thigh and leg and those that control movement of the foot.

MUSCLES THAT MOVE THE THIGH AND LEG The **gluteus maximus** (GLU-te-us MAK-sim-us), which forms much of the buttock's fleshy part, is relatively large in humans because of its support function when a person is standing erect (Fig. 8-10, Table 8-6). This muscle extends the thigh and is important in walking and running. The **gluteus medius**, which is partially covered by the gluteus maximus, abducts the thigh. It is one of the sites used for intramuscular injections.

The **iliopsoas** (il-e-o-SO-as) arises from the ilium and the bodies of the lumbar vertebrae; it crosses the anterior hip joint to insert on the femur (Fig. 8-16A). It is a powerful thigh flexor and helps keep the trunk from falling backward when one is standing erect.

The **adductor muscles** are located on the medial part of the thigh. They arise from the pubis and ischium and insert on the femur. These strong muscles press the thighs together, as in grasping a saddle between the knees when riding a horse. They include the **adductor longus** and **adductor magnus**.

The **sartorius** (sar-TO-re-us) is a long, narrow muscle that begins at the iliac spine, winds downward and medially across the entire thigh, and ends on the tibia's superior medial surface. It is called the tailor's muscle because it is used in crossing the legs in the manner of tailors, who in days gone by sat cross-legged on the floor. The **gracilis** (grah-SIL-is) extends from the pubic bone to the medial tibia. It adducts the thigh at the hip and flexes the leg at the knee.

MUSCLES OF THE ABDOMEN AND PELVIS The abdominal wall has three muscle layers that extend from the back (dorsally) and around the sides (laterally) to the front (ventrally) (Fig. 8-14, Table 8-5). They are the **external oblique** on the exterior, the **internal oblique** in the middle, and the **transversus abdominis**, the innermost. The connective tissue from these muscles extends anteriorly and encloses the vertical **rectus abdominis** of the anterior abdominal wall. The fibers of these muscles, as well as their connective tissue extensions (aponeuroses), run in different directions, resembling the layers in plywood and resulting in a strong abdominal wall. The midline meeting of the aponeuroses forms a whitish area called the **linea alba** (LIN-e-ah AL-ba), which is an important abdominal landmark. It extends from the tip of the sternum to the pubic joint (see Fig. 8-14).

These four pairs of abdominal muscles act together to protect the internal organs and compress the abdominal cavity, as in coughing, emptying the bladder (urination) and bowel (defecation), sneezing, vomiting, and childbirth (labor). The two oblique muscles and the rectus abdominis help bend the trunk forward and sideways.

The pelvic floor, or **perineum** (per-ih-NE-um), has its own form of diaphragm, shaped somewhat like a shallow dish. One of the principal muscles of this pelvic diaphragm is the **levator ani** (le-VA-tor A-ni), which acts on the rectum and thus aids in defecation. The superficial and deep muscles of the female perineum are shown in Figure 8-15 along with some associated structures.

CHECKPOINT **8-14** ➤ What structural feature gives strength to the muscles of the abdominal wall?

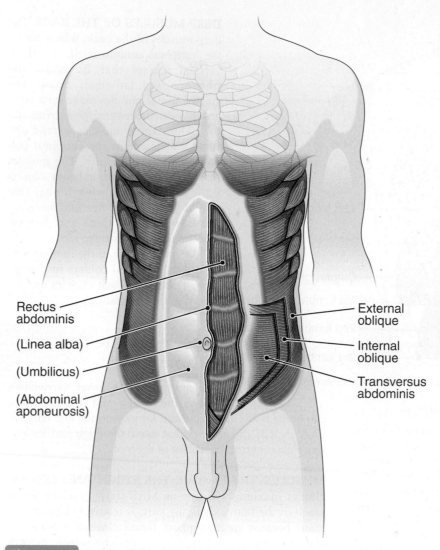

Rectus
abdominis

(Linea alba)

(Umbilicus)

(Abdominal
aponeurosis)

External
oblique

Internal
oblique

Transversus
abdominis

Figure 8-14 **Muscles of the abdominal wall.** Surface tissue is removed on the right side to show deeper muscles. Associated structures are labeled in parentheses.

The anterior and lateral femur are covered by the **quadriceps femoris** (KWOD-re-seps FEM-or-is), a large muscle that has four heads of origin. The individual parts are as follows: in the center, covering the anterior thigh, the **rectus femoris**; on either side, the **vastus medialis** and **vastus lateralis**; deeper in the center, the **vastus intermedius**. One of these muscles (rectus femoris) originates from the ilium, and the other three are from the femur, but all four have a common tendon of insertion on the tibia. You may remember that this is the tendon that encloses the knee cap, or patella. This muscle extends the leg, as in kicking a ball. The vastus lateralis is also a site for intramuscular injections.

The iliotibial (IT) tract is a thickened band of fascia that covers the lateral thigh muscles. It extends from the ilium of the hip to the superior tibia and reinforces the fascia of the thigh (fascia lata) (see Fig. 8-16).

The **hamstring muscles** are located in the posterior part of the thigh (see Fig. 8-16B). Their tendons can be felt behind the knee as they descend to insert on the tibia and fibula. The hamstrings flex the leg on the thigh, as in kneeling. Individually, moving from lateral to medial position, they are the **biceps femoris**, the **semimembranosus**, and the **semitendinosus**. The name of this muscle group refers to the tendons at the posterior of the knee by which these muscles insert on the leg.

Table 8-5	Muscles of the Trunk*	
Name	**Location**	**Function**
Diaphragm	Dome-shaped partition between thoracic and abdominal cavities	Dome descends to enlarge thoracic cavity from top to bottom
Intercostals	Between ribs	Elevate ribs and enlarge thoracic cavity
Muscles of abdominal wall: External oblique Internal oblique Transversus abdominis Rectus abdominis	Anterolateral abdominal wall	Compress abdominal cavity and expel substances from body; flex spinal column
Levator ani	Pelvic floor	Aids defecation
Erector spinae (deep; not shown)	Group of deep vertical muscles between the sacrum and skull	Extends vertebral column to produce erect posture

*These and other muscles of the trunk are shown in Figures 8–13, 8–14, and 8–15.

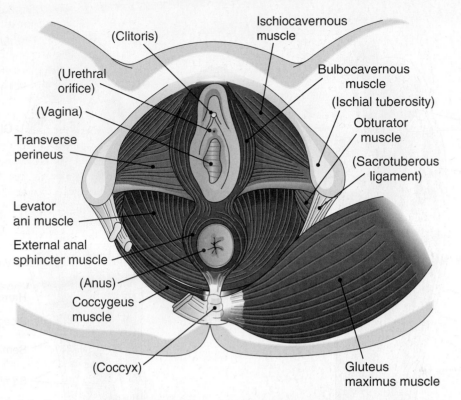

Figure 8-15 **Muscles of the female perineum (pelvic floor).** Associated structures are labeled in parentheses.

Table 8-6 Muscles of the Lower Extremities*

Name	Location	Function
Gluteus maximus	Superficial buttock, to femur	Extends thigh
Gluteus medius	Deep buttock, to femur	Abducts thigh
Iliopsoas	Crosses anterior hip joint, to femur	Flexes thigh
Adductor group (e.g., adductor longus, adductor magnus)	Medial thigh, to femur	Adducts thigh
Sartorius	Winds down thigh, ilium to tibia	Flexes thigh and leg (to sit cross-legged)
Gracilis	Pubic bone to medial surface of tibia	Adducts thigh at hip; flexes leg at knee
Quadriceps femoris: Rectus femoris Vastus medialis Vastus lateralis Vastus intermedius (deep; not shown)	Anterior thigh, to tibia	Extends leg
Hamstring group: Biceps femoris Semimembranosus Semitendinosus	Posterior thigh, to tibia and fibula	Flexes leg
Gastrocnemius	Calf of leg, to calcaneus, inserting by the Achilles tendon	Plantar flexes foot at ankle (as in tiptoeing)
Soleus	Posterior leg deep to gastrocnemius	Plantar flexes foot at ankle
Tibialis anterior	Anterior and lateral shin, to foot	Dorsiflexes foot (as in walking on heels); inverts foot (sole inward)
Peroneus longus	Lateral leg, to foot	Everts foot (sole outward)
Flexor digitorum group	Posterior leg and foot to inferior surface of toe bones	Flexes toes
Extensor digitorum group	Anterior surface of leg bones to superior surface of toe bones	Extends toes

These and other muscles of the lower extremities are shown in Figures 8–16 and 8–17.

Iliopsoas

Sartorius

(Iliotibial tract)

Quadriceps femoris:

Rectus femoris

Vastus lateralis

Vastus medialis

(Vastus intermedius not shown)

(Patella)

Adductor longus

Gracilis

Adductor magnus

A Anterior view

Gluteus medius

Gluteus maximus

Adductor magnus

Gracilis

Sartorius

(Iliotibial tract – cut)

Vastus lateralis

Hamstring group:

Biceps femoris

Semitendinosus

Semimembranosus

B Posterior view

Figure 8-16 **Muscles of the thigh.** Associated structures are labeled in parentheses.

MUSCLES THAT MOVE THE FOOT The **gastrocnemius** (gas-trok-NE-me-us) is the chief muscle of the calf of the leg (its name means "belly of the leg") (Fig. 8-17). It has been called the toe dancer's muscle because it is used in standing on tiptoe. It ends near the heel in a prominent cord called the **Achilles tendon** (see Fig. 8-17B), which attaches to the calcaneus (heel bone). The Achilles tendon is the largest tendon in the body. According to Greek mythology, the region above the heel was the only place that Achilles was vulnerable, and if the Achilles tendon is cut, it is impossible to walk. The soleus (SO-le-us) is a flat muscle deep to the gastrocnemius. It also inserts by means of the Achilles tendon and, like the gastrocnemius, flexes the foot at the ankle.

Another leg muscle that acts on the foot is the **tibialis** (tib-e-A-lis) **anterior**, located on the anterior region of the leg (see Fig. 8-17A). This muscle performs the opposite function of the gastrocnemius. Walking on the heels uses the tibialis anterior to raise the rest of the foot off the ground (dorsiflexion). This muscle is also responsible for inversion of the foot. The muscle for the foot's eversion is the **peroneus** (per-o-NE-us) **longus**, also called the fibularis longus, located on the lateral leg. This muscle's long tendon crosses under the foot, forming a sling that supports the transverse (metatarsal) arch.

The toes, like the fingers, are provided with flexor and extensor muscles. The tendons of the extensor muscles are located in the superior part of the foot and insert on the superior surface of the phalanges (toe bones). The flexor digitorum tendons cross the sole of the foot and insert on the undersurface of the phalanges.

PASSport to **Success** Visit **thePoint** or see the Student Resource CD in the back of this book for additional pictures of the muscles that move the lower extremity.

Effects of Aging on Muscles

Beginning at about 40 years of age, there is a gradual loss of muscle cells with a resulting decrease in the size of each individual muscle. There is also a loss of power, notably in the extensor muscles, such as the large sacrospinalis near the vertebral column. This causes the "bent over" appearance of a hunchback (kyphosis), which in women is often referred to as the *dowager's hump*. Sometimes, there is a tendency to bend (flex) the hips and knees. In addition to causing the previously noted changes in the vertebral column (see Chapter 7), these effects on the extensor muscles

(Patella)

Peroneus longus

Tibialis anterior

Extensor digitorum longus

Gastrocnemius

Soleus

(Tibia)

Gastrocnemius

Soleus

Peroneus longus

(Achilles tendon)

Flexor digitorum longus

(Calcaneus)

A Anterior view

B Posterior view

8

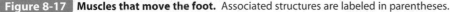

Figure 8-17 **Muscles that move the foot.** Associated structures are labeled in parentheses.

result in a further decrease in the elderly person's height. Activity and exercise throughout life delay and decrease these undesirable effects of aging. Even among the elderly, resistance exercise, such as weight lifting, increases muscle strength and function.

Muscular Disorders

A **spasm** is a sudden and involuntary muscular contraction, which is always painful. A spasm of the visceral muscles is called **colic**, a good example of which is the intestinal muscle spasm often referred to as a *bellyache*. Spasms also occur in the skeletal muscles. If the spasms occur in a series, the condition may be called a **seizure** or **convulsion**.

Cramps are strong, painful muscle contractions, especially of the leg and foot. They are most likely to follow unusually strenuous activity. Cramps that occur during sleep or rest are called *recumbency cramps*.

Strains are common muscle injuries caused by overuse or overstretching. With strains, there is pain, stiffness, and swelling, most commonly in the lower back or neck. The elbow or shoulder may also be affected. Charley horse is soreness and stiffness in a muscle caused by strain, usually referring to strain of the thigh's quadriceps muscle. The

term *Charley horse* comes from the practice of using Charley as a name for old lame horses that were kept around for family use when they were no longer able to do hard work.

Sprains are more severe than strains and involve tearing of the ligaments around a joint, usually as a result of abnormal or excessive joint movement. In severe cases, the ligament can actually tear away from its bone. The ankle is a common site of sprains, as when the ankle is "turned," that is, the foot is turned inward and body weight forces excessive inversion at the joint. The knee is another common site of this type of injury. The pain and swelling accompanying a sprain can be reduced by the immediate application of ice packs, which constrict some of the smaller blood vessels and reduce internal bleeding.

Atrophy (AT-ro-fe) is a wasting or decrease in the size of a muscle when it cannot be used, such as when an extremity must be placed in a cast after a fracture.

Diseases of Muscles

Muscular dystrophy (DIS-tro-fe) is a group of disorders in which there is deterioration of muscles that still have intact nerve function. These disorders all progress at different rates. The most common type, which is found most frequently in male children, causes weakness and paralysis.

Death results from weakness of the cardiac muscle or paralysis of the respiratory muscles. Life expectancy is about 20 years for the most common type of muscular dystrophy, and about 40 years for the other types. Progress toward definitive treatment for some forms of the disease may be possible now that scientists have identified the genetic defects that cause them.

> **PASSport to Success** Visit **thePoint** or see the Student Resource CD in the back of this book for pictures showing the effects of muscular dystrophy.

Myasthenia gravis (mi-as-THE-ne-ah GRA-vis) is characterized by chronic muscular fatigue brought on by the slightest exertion. It affects adults and begins with the muscles of the head. Drooping of the eyelids (ptosis) is a common early sign. This disease is caused by a defect in transmission at the neuromuscular junction.

Myalgia (mi-AL-je-ah) means "muscular pain"; **myositis** (mi-o-SI-tis) is a term that indicates actual inflammation of muscle tissue. **Fibrositis** (fi-bro-SI-tis) means "inflammation of connective tissues" and refers particularly to those tissues associated with muscles and joints. Usually, these disorders appear in combination as **fibromyositis,** which may be acute, with severe pain on motion, or may be chronic. Sometimes, the application of heat, together with massage and rest, relieves the symptoms.

Fibromyalgia syndrome (FMS) is associated with widespread muscle aches, tenderness, and stiffness along with fatigue and sleep disorders. FMS is difficult to diagnose, and there is no known cause, but it may be an autoimmune disease, in which the immune system reacts to one's own tissues. Treatment may include a controlled exercise program and treatment with pain relievers, muscle relaxants, or antidepressants.

Disorders of Associated Structures

Bursitis is inflammation of a bursa, a fluid-filled sac that minimizes friction between tissues and bone. Some bursae communicate with joints; others are closely related to muscles. Sometimes, bursae develop spontaneously in response to prolonged friction. Bursitis can be very painful, with swelling and limitation of motion. Some examples of bursitis are listed below:

- **Olecranon bursitis**—inflammation of the bursa over the point of the elbow (olecranon). Another name for the disorder is student's elbow, as it can be caused by long hours of leaning on the elbows while studying.
- **Ischial bursitis**—common among people who must sit a great deal, such as taxicab drivers and truckers
- **Prepatellar bursitis**—inflammation of the bursa anterior to the patella. This form of bursitis is found in people who must often kneel, hence the name from an earlier time, *housemaid's knee.*
- **Subdeltoid bursitis** and **subacromial bursitis**—appear in the shoulder region and are fairly common forms of bursitis.

> **PASSport to Success** Visit **thePoint** or see the Student Resource CD in the back of this book for information on careers in physical therapy and how physical therapists participate in treatment of muscular disorders.

In some cases a local anesthetic, corticosteroids, or both may be injected to relieve bursitis pain. **Bunions** are enlargements commonly found at the base and medial side of the great toe. Usually, prolonged pressure has caused the development of a bursa, which has then become inflamed. Special shoes may be necessary if surgery is not performed.

Tendinitis (ten-din-I-tis), an inflammation of muscle tendons and their attachments, occurs most often in athletes who overexert themselves. It frequently involves the shoulder, the hamstring muscle tendons at the knee, and the Achilles tendon near the heel. **Tenosynovitis** (ten-o-sin-o-VI-tis), which involves the synovial sheath that encloses tendons, is found most often in women in their 40s after an injury or surgery. It may involve swelling and severe pain with activity.

Shinsplints is experienced as pain and soreness along the tibia ("shin bone") from stress injury of structures in the leg. Some causes of shinsplints are tendinitis at the insertion of the tibialis anterior muscle, sometimes with inflammation of the tibial periosteum, and even stress fracture of the tibia itself. Shinsplints commonly occurs in runners, especially when they run on hard surfaces without adequate shoe support.

Carpal tunnel syndrome involves the tendons of the flexor muscles of the fingers as well as the nerves supplying the hand and fingers. Numbness and weakness of the hand is caused by pressure on the median nerve as it passes through a tunnel formed by the carpal bones of the wrist. Carpal tunnel syndrome is one of the most common repetitive-use disorders. It affects many workers who use their hands and fingers strenuously, such as factory workers, keyboard operators, and musicians.

Disease in Context revisited

➤ Sue's Multiple Sclerosis

Having finished the physical examination of his patient, Dr. Mathews thought carefully about what he had discovered. Sue, a 26-year-old white female, presented with muscle weakness, atrophy, and abnormal reflexes localized to the right side of her body. At first, it seemed likely that Sue was suffering from a muscular system disorder. Muscular dystrophy is characterized by muscle deterioration and weakness, but the doctor knew that the disease is genetic and its effects appear during childhood. Myasthenia gravis, a disorder of the neuromuscular junction, is also characterized by muscle weakness and appears during adulthood. But, it usually begins affecting muscles of the head, not the limbs. Fibromyalgia syndrome affects adults and is associated with widespread muscle aches. This didn't seem to fit either because Sue's disorder was localized to her right side.

It was Sue's report of pain and tingling in her right limbs that provided the last clue Dr. Mathews needed to make his diagnosis. Sue probably had a disorder of the nervous system called multiple sclerosis. The disease is characterized by both muscular and nervous symptoms, which first appear in adults and are sometimes localized to one side of the body. After explaining his findings to Sue, Dr. Mathews ordered an MRI of her brain and spinal cord and referred her to a neurologist for further treatment.

During this case, Dr. Mathews examined Sue's muscular system. He quickly realized that Sue's symptoms suggested that she had a nervous system disorder. The case study in Chapter 9, The Nervous System: The Spinal Cord and Spinal Nerves, will follow Sue as she learns more about multiple sclerosis.

Word Anatomy

Medical terms are built from standardized word parts (prefixes, roots, and suffixes). Learning the meanings of these parts can help you remember words and interpret unfamiliar terms.

WORD PART	MEANING	EXAMPLE
The Muscular System		
my/o	muscle	The *endomysium* is the deepest layer of connective tissue around muscle cells.
sarc/o	flesh	A *sarcomere* is a contracting subunit of skeletal muscle.
troph/o	nutrition, nurture	Muscles undergo *hypertrophy*, an increase in size, under the effects of resistance training.
vas/o	vessel	*Vasodilation* (widening) of the blood vessels in muscle tissue during exercise brings more blood into the tissue.
iso-	same, equal	In an *isotonic* contraction, muscle tone remains the same, but the muscle shortens.
ton/o	tone, tension	See preceding example.
metr/o	measure	In an *isometric* contraction, muscle length remains the same, but muscle tension increases.
The Mechanics of Muscle Movement		
brachi/o	arm	The biceps *brachii* and triceps *brachii* are in the arm.
erg/o	work	*Synergists* are muscles that work together.

WORD PART	MEANING	EXAMPLE
Skeletal Muscle Groups		
quadr/i	four	The *quadriceps* muscle group consists of four muscles.
Muscular Disorders		
a-	absent, lack of	*Atrophy* is a wasting of muscle as a result of disuse (lack of nourishment).
dys-	disordered, difficult	In muscular *dystrophy*, there is deterioration of muscles.
sthen/o	strength	*Myasthenia* gravis is characterized by muscular fatigue (lack of strength).
-algia	pain	*Myalgia* is muscular pain.

Summary

I. **TYPES OF MUSCLE**
  A. Smooth muscle
    1. In walls of hollow organs, vessels, and respiratory passageways
    2. Cells tapered, single nucleus, nonstriated
    3. Involuntary, produces peristalsis, contracts and relaxes slowly
  B. Cardiac muscle
    1. Muscle of heart wall
    2. Cells branch, single nucleus, lightly striated
    3. Involuntary, self-excitatory
  C. Skeletal muscle
    1. Most attached to bones and move skeleton
    2. Cells long, cylindrical; multiple nuclei, heavily striated
    3. Voluntary, contracts and relaxes rapidly

II. **MUSCULAR SYSTEM**
  A. Functions
    1. Movement of skeleton
    2. Maintenance of posture
    3. Generation of heat
  B. Structure of a muscle
    1. Held by connective tissue
      a. Endomysium around individual fibers
      b. Perimysium around fascicles (bundles)
      c. Epimysium around whole muscle
  C. Muscle cells in action
    1. Neuromuscular junction (NMJ)
      a. Point where nerve fiber stimulates muscle cell
      b. Neurotransmitter is acetylcholine (ACh)
        (1) Generates an action potential
      c. Motor end plate—membrane of muscle cell at NMJ
    2. Contraction—sliding together of filaments to shorten muscle
      a. Actin—thin and light
      b. Myosin—thick and dark with projecting heads

3. Role of calcium—uncovers binding sites so cross-bridges can form between actin and myosin
  D. Energy sources
    1. ATP—supplies energy
      a. Myoglobin—stores oxygen
      b. Glycogen—stores glucose
      c. Creatine phosphate—stores energy
    2. Oxygen consumption
      a. Oxygen debt—develops during strenuous exercise
        (1) Anaerobic metabolism
        (2) Yields lactic acid—causes muscle fatigue
      b. Recovery oxygen consumption
        (1) Removes lactic acid
        (2) Replenishes reserved compounds
  E. Effects of exercise
    1. Changes in structure and function of muscle cells
    2. Vasodilation brings blood to tissues
    3. Heart strengthened
    4. Breathing improved
  F. Types of muscle contractions
    1. Tonus—partially contracted state
    2. Isotonic contractions—muscle shortens to produce movement
    3. Isometric contractions—tension increases, but muscle does not shorten

III. **MECHANICS OF MUSCLE MOVEMENT**
  A. Attachments of skeletal muscles
    1. Tendon—cord of connective tissue that attaches muscle to bone
      a. Origin—attached to more fixed part
      b. Insertion—attached to moving part
    2. Aponeurosis—broad band of connective tissue that attaches muscle to bone or other muscle
  B. Muscles work together
    1. Prime mover—performs movement

2. Antagonist—produces opposite movement
3. Synergist—steadies body parts and assists prime mover
C. Levers and body mechanics—muscles function with skeleton as lever systems
   1. Components
      a. Lever—bone
      b. Fulcrum—joint
      c. Force—muscle contraction
   2. Most muscles work as third-class levers (fulcrum-effort-weight)

IV. **SKELETAL MUSCLE GROUPS**
A. Naming of muscles—location, size, shape, direction of fibers, number of heads, action
B. Muscles of the head
C. Muscles of the neck
D. Muscles of the upper extremities
   1. Muscles that move the shoulder and arm
   2. Muscles that move the forearm and hand
E. Muscles of the trunk
   1. Muscles of respiration
   2. Muscles of the abdomen and pelvis

3. Deep muscles of the back
F. Muscles of the lower extremities
   1. Muscles that move the thigh and leg
   2. Muscles that move the foot

V. **EFFECTS OF AGING ON MUSCLES**
A. Decrease in size of muscles
B. Weakening of muscles, especially extensors

VI. **MUSCULAR DISORDERS**
A. Spasms and injuries
   1. Spasm—sudden painful contraction
   2. Strains—overuse injuries
   3. Sprains—tearing of ligament
   4. Atrophy—wasting
B. Diseases of muscles
   1. Muscular dystrophy—group of disorders
   2. Myasthenia gravis
   3. Myalgia, myositis, fibromyositis
   4. Fibromyalgia syndrome (FMS)—generalized disturbance of unknown cause
C. Disorders of associated structures—bursitis, bunions, tendinitis, shinsplints, carpal tunnel syndrome

8

Questions for Study and Review

BUILDING UNDERSTANDING

Fill in the blanks

1. Individual muscle fibers are arranged in bundles called _____.
2. The point at which a nerve fiber contacts a muscle cell is called the _____.
3. A contraction in which there is no change in muscle length but there is a great increase in muscle tension is _____.
4. A term that means "muscular pain" is _____.
5. A disease characterized by chronic muscular fatigue due to defects in neuromuscular transmission is called _____.

Matching > Match each numbered item with the most closely related lettered item.

___ 6. Extends vertebral column to produce erect posture
___ 7. Elevates ribs and enlarges thoracic cavity
___ 8. Flattens cheeks
___ 9. Aids in defecation
___ 10. Closes eye

a. levator ani
b. buccinator
c. orbicularis oris
d. erector spinae
e. intercostal muscles

Multiple Choice

___ 11. From superficial to deep, the correct order of muscle structure is
a. deep fascia, epimysium, perimysium, and endomysium
b. epimysium, perimysium, endomysium, and deep fascia
c. deep fascia, endomysium, perimysium, and epimysium
d. endomysium, perimysium, epimysium, and deep fascia

___ **12.** The function of calcium ions in skeletal muscle contraction is to

    a. bind to receptors on the motor end plate to stimulate muscle contraction

    b. cause a pH change in the cytoplasm to trigger muscle contraction

    c. bind to the myosin binding sites on actin so that myosin will have something to attach to

    d. bind to regulatory proteins so that the myosin binding sites on the actin can be exposed

___ **13.** A broad flat extension that attaches muscle to bone is called a(n)

    a. tendon

    b. fascicle

    c. aponeurosis

    d. motor end plate

___ **14.** Seizures or convulsions are examples of

    a. strains

    b. fibrositis

    c. myositis

    d. spasms

___ **15.** A disease associated with widespread muscle aches, tenderness, and stiffness and with no known cause is

    a. muscular dystrophy

    b. fibromyalgia

    c. myositis

    d. bursitis

UNDERSTANDING CONCEPTS

16. Compare smooth, cardiac, and skeletal muscle with respect to location, structure, and function. Briefly explain how each type of muscle is specialized for its function.

17. Describe three substances stored in skeletal muscle cells that are used to manufacture a constant supply of ATP.

18. Name and describe muscle(s) that

    a. open and close the eye

    b. close the jaw

    c. flex and extend the head

    d. flex and extend the forearm

    e. flex and extend the hand and fingers

    f. flex and extend the leg

    g. flex and extend the foot and toes

19. During a Cesarean section, a transverse incision is made through the abdominal wall. Name the muscles incised and state their functions.

20. What effect does aging have on muscles? What can be done to resist these effects?

21. Define *atrophy* and give one cause.

22. What are muscular dystrophies, and what are some of their effects?

23. Describe bursitis and its several forms.

CONCEPTUAL THINKING

24. Recall that the neurotransmitter acetylcholine initiates skeletal muscle contraction. Normally, acetylcholine is broken down shortly after its release into the synaptic cleft by the enzyme acetylcholinesterase. Many insecticides contain chemicals called organophosphates, which interfere with acetylcholinesterase activity. Based on this information, what could happen to an individual exposed to high concentrations of organophosphates?

25. Margo recently began "working out" and jogs three times a week. After her jog she is breathless and her muscles ache. From your understanding of muscle physiol-

ogy, describe what has happened inside of Margo's skeletal muscle cells. How do Margo's muscles recover from this? If Margo continues to exercise, what changes would you expect to occur in her muscles?

26. Alfred suffered a mild stroke, leaving him partially paralyzed on his left side. Physical therapy was ordered to prevent left-sided atrophy. Prescribe some exercises for Alfred's shoulder and thigh.

27. In Sue's case, her disorder prevents motor impulses from arriving at neuromuscular junctions. With this in mind, explain why one of her symptoms is muscle atrophy.

UNIT IV

Coordination and Control

Two chapters in this unit describe the nervous system and some of its many parts and complex functions. The organs of special sense and other sensory receptors are described in a separate chapter. The last chapter in this unit discusses hormones and the organs that produce them. Working with the nervous system, these hormones play an important role in coordination and control.

CHAPTER 9

The Nervous System: The Spinal Cord and Spinal Nerves

Learning Outcomes

After careful study of this chapter, you should be able to:

1. Describe the organization of the nervous system according to structure and function
2. Describe the structure of a neuron
3. Describe how neuron fibers are built into a nerve
4. Explain the purpose of neuroglia
5. Diagram and describe the steps in an action potential
6. Briefly describe the transmission of a nerve impulse
7. Explain the role of myelin in nerve conduction
8. Briefly describe transmission at a synapse
9. Define *neurotransmitter* and give several examples of neurotransmitters
10. Describe the distribution of gray and white matter in the spinal cord
11. List the components of a reflex arc
12. Define a simple reflex and give several examples of reflexes
13. Describe and name the spinal nerves and three of their main plexuses
14. Compare the location and functions of the sympathetic and parasympathetic nervous systems
15. Explain the role of cellular receptors in the action of neurotransmitters
16. Describe several disorders of the spinal cord and of the spinal nerves
17. Show how word parts are used to build words related to the nervous system (see Word Anatomy at the end of the chapter)

Selected Key Terms

The following terms and other boldface terms in the chapter are defined in the Glossary

acetylcholine
action potential
afferent
autonomic nervous system
axon
dendrite
effector
efferent
epinephrine
ganglion
interneuron
motor
nerve
nerve impulse
neuritis
neuroglia
neurotransmitter
parasympathetic nervous system
plexus
receptor
reflex
sensory
somatic nervous system
sympathetic nervous system
synapse
tract

PASSport to Success

Visit *thePoint* or see the Student Resource CD in the back of this book for definitions and pronunciations of key terms as well as a pretest for this chapter.

Disease in Context

➤ Sue's Second Case: The Importance of Myelin

Dr. Jensen glanced at her patient's chart as she stepped into the consulting room to see her. Sue Pritchard was 26 years old, white, and had been referred to her by Sue's family physician. According to her chart, Sue had presented with motor and sensory deficits, which led her doctor to suspect she had multiple sclerosis (MS). In addition to the referral, her doctor had ordered a magnetic resonance image (MRI) of her brain and spinal cord. "Hi Sue. My name is Dr. Jensen. I'm a neurologist, which means I specialize in the diagnosis and treatment of nervous system disorders like MS. Let's start with a few tests to determine how well your brain and spinal cord communicate with the rest of your body. Then, we'll take a look at your MRI results."

Using a reflex hammer, Dr. Jensen tapped on the tendons of several muscles in Sue's arms and legs to elicit stretch reflexes. She observed abnormal responses—a typical sign of damage to the parts of the spinal cord that control reflexes. The doctor also detected muscle weakness in Sue's limbs—an indication of damage to the descending tracts of white matter in the spinal cord, which carry motor nerve impulses from the brain to skeletal muscle. In addition, the neurologist discovered that Sue's sense of touch was impaired—an indication of damage to the spinal cord's ascending tracts, which carry sensory impulses from receptors in the skin to the brain. Dr. Jensen had discovered that Sue exhibited several of the most common clinical signs of MS.

After the physical examination, Dr. Jensen showed Sue the results of the MRI scan done earlier. "Here's the MRI of your spinal cord. You can see that it is surrounded by bones called vertebrae, which protect it from injury. The nervous tissue making up the spinal cord is organized into two regions—this inner region called gray matter, and this outer one called white matter. If you look closely at the white matter, you can see several damaged areas, which we call lesions. They are causing many of your symptoms because they prevent your spinal cord from transmitting impulses between your brain and the rest of your body. These lesions, or scleroses, are what give multiple sclerosis its name."

The clinical and diagnostic evidence shows that Sue has multiple sclerosis—a disease of neurons in the central nervous system (CNS). In this chapter, we'll learn more about neurons and the spinal cord, one part of the CNS.

Role of the Nervous System

No body system is capable of functioning alone. All are interdependent and work together as one unit to maintain normal conditions, termed *homeostasis*. The nervous system serves as the chief coordinating agency for all systems. Conditions both within and outside the body are constantly changing. The nervous system must detect and respond to these changes (known as *stimuli*) so that the body can adapt itself to new conditions. The nervous system can be compared with a large corporation, in which market researchers (sensory receptors) feed information into middle management (the spinal cord), who then transmit information to the chief executive officer, or CEO (the brain). The CEO organizes and interprets the information and then sends directions out to workers (effectors) who carry out appropriate actions for the good of the company. In this process, memos and e-mails, like the nerves, carry information throughout the system.

Although all parts of the nervous system work in coordination, portions may be grouped together on the basis of either structure or function.

Structural Divisions

The anatomic, or structural, divisions of the nervous system are as follows (Fig. 9-1):

- The **central nervous system** (CNS) includes the brain and spinal cord.
- The **peripheral** (per-IF-er-al) **nervous system** (PNS) is made up of all the nerves outside the CNS. It includes all the **cranial nerves** that carry impulses to and from the brain and all the **spinal nerves** that carry messages to and from the spinal cord.

The CNS and PNS together include all of the nervous tissue in the body.

Functional Divisions

Functionally, the nervous system is divided according to whether control is voluntary or involuntary and according to what type of tissue is stimulated (Table 9-1). Any tissue or organ that carries out a nervous system command is called an **effector**, all of which are muscles or glands.

The **somatic nervous system** is controlled voluntarily (by conscious will), and all its effectors are skeletal muscles (described in Chapter 8). The nervous system's involuntary division is called the **autonomic nervous system** (ANS), making reference to its automatic activity. It is also called the **visceral nervous system** because it controls smooth muscle, cardiac muscle, and glands, which make up most of the soft body organs, the viscera.

The ANS is further subdivided into a **sympathetic nervous system** and a **parasympathetic nervous system** based on organization and how each affects specific organs. The ANS is described later in this chapter.

Although these divisions are helpful for study purposes, the lines that divide the nervous system according to function are not as distinct as those that classify the system structurally. For example, the diaphragm, a skeletal muscle, typically functions in breathing without conscious thought. In addition, we have certain rapid reflex responses involving skeletal muscles—drawing the hand away from a hot stove, for example—that do not involve the brain. In contrast, people can be trained to consciously control involuntary functions, such as blood pressure, heart rate, and breathing rate, by techniques known as *biofeedback*.

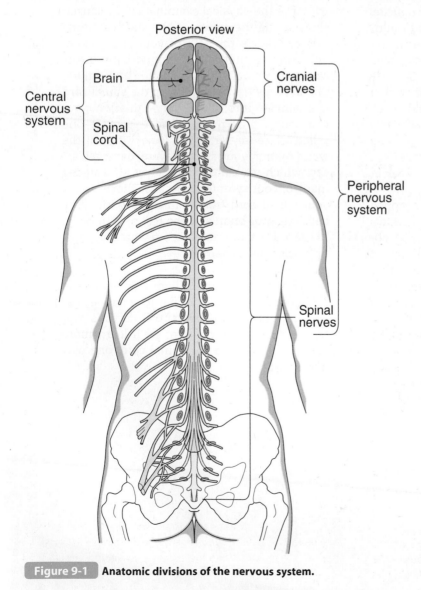

Posterior view

Brain

Central nervous system

Spinal cord

Cranial nerves

Peripheral nervous system

Spinal nerves

Figure 9-1 **Anatomic divisions of the nervous system.**

Table 9-1	Functional Divisions of the Nervous System			
		Characteristics		
Division	**Control**	**Effectors**	**Subdivisions**
Somatic nervous system	Voluntary	Skeletal muscle	None
Autonomic nervous system	Involuntary	Smooth muscle, cardiac muscle, and glands	Sympathetic and parasympathetic systems

CHECKPOINT 9-1 ➤ What are the two divisions of the nervous system based on structure?

CHECKPOINT 9-2 ➤ The nervous system can be divided functionally into two divisions based on type of control and effectors. What division is voluntary and controls skeletal muscle, and what division is involuntary and controls involuntary muscles and glands?

Neurons and Their Functions

The functional cells of the nervous system are highly specialized cells called **neurons** (Fig. 9-2). These cells have a unique structure related to their function.

Structure of a Neuron

The main portion of each neuron, the cell body, contains the nucleus and other organelles typically found in cells. A distinguishing feature of the neurons, however, are the long, threadlike fibers that extend out from the cell body and carry impulses across the cell (Fig. 9-3). There are two kinds of fibers: dendrites and axons.

■ **Dendrites** are neuron fibers that conduct impulses *to* the cell body. Most dendrites have a highly branched, treelike appearance (see Fig. 9-2). In fact, the name comes from a Greek word meaning "tree." Dendrites function as **receptors** in the nervous system. That is, they receive the stimulus that begins a neural pathway. In Chapter 11, we describe how the dendrites of the sensory system may be modified to respond to a specific type of stimulus.

■ **Axons** (AK-sons) are neuron fibers that conduct impulses *away from* the cell body (see Fig. 9-2). These impulses may be delivered to another neuron, to a muscle, or to a gland. An axon is a single fiber, which may be quite long, but it may give off branches and its ending is branched.

THE MYELIN SHEATH Some axons are covered with a fatty material called **myelin** that insulates and protects the fiber (see Fig. 9-2). In the PNS, this covering is produced by

specialized protective cells called **Schwann** (shvahn) **cells** that wrap around the axon like a jelly roll depositing layers of myelin (Fig. 9-4). When the sheath is complete, small

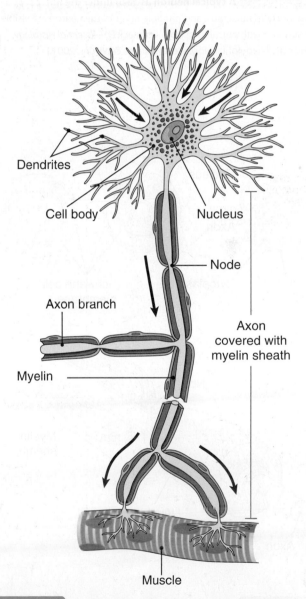

Figure 9-2 **Diagram of a motor neuron.** The break in the axon denotes length. The arrows show the direction of the nerve impulse. [**ZOOMING IN** ➤ Is the neuron shown here a sensory or a motor neuron?]

9

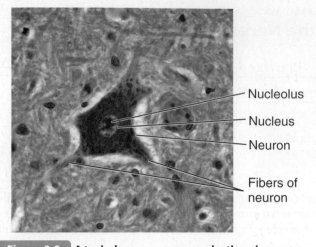

Figure 9-3 **A typical neuron as seen under the microscope.**
The nucleus, nucleolus, and multiple fibers of the neuron are visible.
(Reprinted with permission from Cormack DH. *Essential Histology*,
2nd ed. Philadelphia: Lippincott Williams & Wilkins, 2001.)

A

B

Figure 9-4 **Formation of a myelin sheath. (A)** Schwann cells
wrap around the axon, creating a myelin coating. **(B)** The
outermost layer of the Schwann cell forms the neurilemma. Spaces
between the cells are the nodes (of Ranvier).

spaces remain between the individual cells. These tiny gaps,
called **nodes** (originally, nodes of Ranvier), are important
in speeding nerve impulse conduction.

The Schwann cells' outermost membranes form a thin
coating known as the **neurilemma** (nu-rih-LEM-mah). This
covering is a part of the mechanism by which some peripheral nerves repair themselves when injured. Under some circumstances, damaged nerve cell fibers may regenerate by
growing into the sleeve formed by the neurilemma. Cells of
the brain and the spinal cord are myelinated, not by
Schwann cells, but by other types of protective cells. As a
result, they have no neurilemma. If they are injured, the
damage is permanent. Even in the peripheral nerves, however, repair is a slow and uncertain process.

Myelinated axons, because of myelin's color, are
called **white fibers** and are found in the **white matter** of the
brain and spinal cord as well as most nerves throughout
the body. The fibers and cell bodies of the **gray matter** are
not covered with myelin.

CHECKPOINT **9-3** ➤ The neuron, the functional unit of the
nervous system, has long fibers
extending from the cell body. What is
the name of the fiber that carries
impulses toward the cell body and
what is the name of the fiber that
carries impulses away from the cell
body?

CHECKPOINT **9-4** ➤ Myelin is a substance that covers and
protects some axons. What color
describes myelinated fibers, and what
color describes the nervous system's
unmyelinated tissue?

Types of Neurons

The job of neurons in the PNS is to relay information constantly either to or from the CNS. Neurons that conduct
impulses *to* the spinal cord and brain are described as **sensory neurons**, also called **afferent neurons**. Those cells that
carry impulses *from* the CNS out to muscles and glands
are **motor neurons**, also called **efferent neurons**. Neurons
that relay information within the CNS are **interneurons**,
also called *central* or *association neurons*.

Nerves and Tracts

Everywhere in the nervous system, neuron fibers are collected into bundles of varying size (Fig. 9-5). A fiber bundle located within the PNS is a **nerve**. A similar grouping,
but located within the CNS, is a **tract**. Tracts are located
both in the brain and in the spinal cord, where they conduct impulses to and from the brain.

A nerve or tract can be compared to an electric cable
made up of many wires. The "wires," the nerve cell fibers,
in a nerve or tract are bound together with connective tis-

Figure 9-5 **Cross section of a nerve as seen under the microscope (×132).** Two fascicles (subdivisions) are shown. Perineurium (P) surrounds each fascicle. Epineurium (Ep) is around the entire nerve. Individual axons (Ax) are covered with a myelin sheath (MS), around which is the endoneurium (En) (inset). (Reprinted with permission from Gartner LP, Hiatt JL. *Color Atlas of Histology*, 3rd ed. Philadelphia: Lippincott Williams & Wilkins, 2000.)

sue, just like muscle fibers in a muscle. As in muscles, the individual fibers are organized into subdivisions called *fascicles*. The names of the connective tissue layers are similar to their names in muscles, but the root *neur/o*, meaning "nerve" is substituted for the muscle root *my/o*, as follows:

- Endoneurium is around an individual fiber.
- Perineurium is around a fascicle.
- Epineurium is around the whole nerve.

A nerve may contain all sensory fibers, all motor fibers, or a combination of both types of fibers. A few of the cranial nerves contain only sensory fibers conducting impulses toward the brain. These are described as **sensory (afferent) nerves**. A few of the cranial nerves contain only motor fibers conducting impulses away from the brain and these are classified as **motor (efferent) nerves**. However, most of the cranial nerves and *all* of the spinal nerves contain both sensory *and* motor fibers and are referred to as **mixed nerves**. Note that in a mixed nerve, impulses may be traveling in two directions (toward or away from the CNS), but each individual fiber in the nerve is carrying im-

pulses in one direction only. Think of the nerve as a large highway. Traffic may be going north and south, for example, but each car is going forward in only one direction.

CHECKPOINT **9-5** ➤ Nerves are bundles of neuron fibers in the PNS. These nerves may be carrying impulses either toward or away from the CNS. What name is given to nerves that convey impulses toward the CNS, and what name is given to nerves that transport away from the CNS?

Neuroglia

In addition to conducting tissue, the nervous system contains cells that support and protect the neurons. Collectively, these cells are called **neuroglia** (nu-ROG-le-ah) or **glial** (GLI-al) **cells**, from a Greek word meaning "glue." There are different types of neuroglia, each with specialized functions, some of which are the following:

- Protect and nourish nervous tissue
- Support nervous tissue and bind it to other structures
- Aid in repair of cells
- Act as phagocytes to remove pathogens and impurities
- Regulate the composition of fluids around and between cells

Neuroglia appear throughout the central and peripheral nervous systems. The Schwann cells that produce the myelin sheath in the peripheral nervous system are one type of neuroglia. Another example is shown in Figure 9-6. These cells are astrocytes, named for their star-like appearance. In the brain they attach to capillaries (small blood vessels) to help protect the brain from harmful substances.

Unlike neurons, neuroglia continue to multiply throughout life. Because of their capacity to reproduce, most tumors of the nervous system are tumors of neuroglial tissue and not of nervous tissue itself.

CHECKPOINT **9-6** ➤ The nervous system's nonconducting cells protect, nourish, and support the neurons. What are these cells called?

PASSport to Success — Visit *thePoint* or see the Student Resource CD in the back of this book for a summary of the different neuroglial types.

The Nervous System at Work

The nervous system works by means of electrical impulses sent along neuron fibers and transmitted from cell to cell at highly specialized junctions.

Figure 9-6 **Examples of neuroglia. (A)** Astrocytes in the white matter of the brain. **(B)** Astrocytes attach to capillaries and help to protect the brain from harmful substances. (A, reprinted with permission from Mills SE. *Histology for Pathologists*, 3rd ed. Philadelphia: Lippincott Williams & Wilkins, 2006; B, modified with permission from McConnell TH. *The Nature of Disease: Pathology for the Health Professions*. Baltimore: Lippincott Williams & Wilkins, 2006.)

The Nerve Impulse

The mechanics of nerve impulse conduction are complex but can be compared to the spread of an electric current along a wire. What follows is a brief description of the electrical changes that occur as a resting neuron is stimulated and transmits a nerve impulse.

The plasma membrane of an unstimulated (resting) neuron carries an electrical charge, or **potential**. This resting potential is maintained by ions (charged particles) concentrated on either side of the membrane. At rest, the inside of the membrane is negative as compared with the outside. In this state, the membrane is said to be *polarized*. As in a battery, the separation of charges on either side of the membrane creates a possibility (potential) for generating energy. If there is a way for the charges to move toward each other, electricity (a nerve impulse) will be generated.

A **nerve impulse** starts with a local reversal in the membrane potential caused by changes in the ion concentrations on either side. This sudden electrical change at the membrane is called an **action potential**, as described in Chapter 8 on the muscles. A simple description of the events in an action potential is as follows (Fig. 9-7):

- The resting state. In addition to an electrical difference on the two sides of the plasma membrane at rest, there is also a slight difference in the concentration of ions on either side. At rest, sodium ions (Na^+) are a little more concentrated at the outside of the membrane. At the same time, potassium ions (K^+) are a little more concentrated at the inside of the membrane.

- Depolarization. A stimulus of adequate force, such as electrical, chemical or mechanical energy, causes specific channels in the membrane to open and allow Na^+ ions to flow into the cell. (Remember that substances flow by diffusion from an area where they are in higher concentration to an area where they are in lower concentration.) As these positive ions enter, they raise the charge on the inside of the membrane, a change known as **depolarization** (see Fig. 9-7).

- Repolarization. In the next step of the action potential, K^+ channels open to allow K^+ to leave the cell. As the electrical charge returns to its resting value, the membrane is under-

Figure 9-7 **The action potential.** In depolarization, Na^+ membrane channels open and Na^+ enters the cell. In repolarization, K^+ membrane channels open and K^+ leaves the cell. During the resting stage, the Na^+/K^+ pump returns ion concentrations to their original concentrations so the membrane can be stimulated again.

going **repolarization**. At the same time that the membrane is repolarizing, the cell uses active transport to move Na$^+$ and K$^+$ back to their original concentrations on either side of the membrane. This movement of ions through the plasma membrane against the concentration gradient requires transporters and energy from ATP. As Na$^+$ is transported to the outside of the cell and K$^+$ is transported to the inside of the cell, their concentration gradients are restored so that another action potential can occur. This transport mechanism is described as the **sodium–potassium pump** or Na$^+$–K$^+$ pump.

The action potential occurs rapidly—in less than one thousandth of a second, an is followed by a rapid return to the resting state. However, this local electrical change in the membrane stimulates an action potential at an adjacent point along the membrane (Fig. 9-8). In scientific terms, the channels in the membrane are "voltage dependent," that is, they respond to an electrical stimulus. And so, the action potential spreads along the membrane as a wave of electrical current. The spreading action potential is the nerve impulse, and in fact, the term *action potential* is used to mean the nerve impulse. A stimulus is any force that can start an action potential by opening membrane channels and allowing Na$^+$ to enter the cell.

Figure 9-8 **A nerve impulse.** From a point of stimulation, a wave of depolarization followed by repolarization travels along the membrane of a neuron. This spreading action potential is a nerve impulse.

THE ROLE OF MYELIN IN CONDUCTION As previously noted, some axons are coated with the fatty material myelin. If a fiber is not myelinated, the action potential spreads continuously along the cell's membrane (see Fig. 9-4). When myelin is present on an axon, however, it insulates the fiber against the spread of current. This would appear to slow or stop conduction along these fibers, but in fact, the myelin sheath speeds conduction. The reason is that the action potential must "jump" like a spark from node (space) to node along the sheath (see Fig. 9-3), and this type of conduction, called **saltatory** (SAL-tah-to-re) **conduction**, is actually faster than continuous conduction.

CHECKPOINT **9-7** ➤ An action potential occurs in two stages. In the first stage, the charge on the membrane reverses, and in the second stage, it returns to the resting state. What are the names of these two stages?

CHECKPOINT **9-8** ➤ What ions are involved in generating an action potential?

Visit **thePoint** or see the Student Resource CD in the back of this book for animations *The Synapse and the Nerve Impulse* and *The Myelin Sheath*.

The Synapse

Neurons do not work alone; impulses must be transferred between neurons to convey information within the nervous system. The point of junction for transmitting the nerve impulse is the **synapse** (SIN-aps), a term that comes from a Greek word meaning "to clasp" (Fig. 9-9). At a synapse, transmission of an impulse usually occurs from the axon of one cell, the **presynaptic cell**, to the dendrite of another cell, the **postsynaptic cell**.

As described in Chapter 8, information must be passed from one cell to another at the synapse across a tiny gap between the cells, the **synaptic cleft**. Information usually crosses this gap in the form of a chemical known as a **neurotransmitter**. While the cells at a synapse are at rest, the neurotransmitter is stored in many small vesicles (sacs) within the enlarged axon endings, usually called *end-bulbs* or *terminal knobs*, but known by several other names as well.

When a nerve impulse traveling along a neuron membrane reaches the end of the presynaptic axon, some of those vesicles fuse with the membrane and release their neurotransmitter into the synaptic cleft (an example of exocytosis, as described in Chapter 3). The neurotransmitter then acts as a chemical signal to the postsynaptic cell.

On the postsynaptic receiving membrane, usually that of a dendrite, but sometimes another cell part, there are special sites, or **receptors**, ready to pick up and respond to specific neurotransmitters. Receptors in the postsynaptic cell's membrane influence how or if that cell will respond to a given neurotransmitter.

9

A

B

Axon of presynaptic neuron

Axon

Mitochondria

Vesicles containing neurotransmitter

End bulb of axon

Synaptic cleft

Postsynaptic neuron

Dendrite

Neurotransmitter molecules

Presynaptic membrane

Vesicle

Neurotransmitter

Synaptic cleft

Postsynaptic membrane

Receptor

Figure 9-9 **A synapse. (A)** The end-bulb of the presynaptic (transmitting) axon has vesicles containing neurotransmitter, which is released into the synaptic cleft to the membrane of the postsynaptic (receiving) cell. **(B)** Close-up of a synapse showing receptors for neurotransmitter in the postsynaptic cell membrane.

NEUROTRANSMITTERS Although there are many known neurotransmitters, the main ones are epinephrine (ep-ih-NEF-rin), also called **adrenaline**; a related compound, **norepinephrine** (nor-ep-ih-NEF-rin), or **noradrenaline**; and **acetylcholine** (as-e-til-KO-lene). Acetylcholine (ACh) is the neurotransmitter released at the neuromuscular junction, the synapse between a neuron and a muscle cell. All three of the above neurotransmitters function in the ANS.

It is common to think of neurotransmitters as stimulating the cells they reach; in fact, they have been described as such in this discussion. Note, however, that some of these chemicals inhibit the postsynaptic cell and keep it from reacting, as will be demonstrated later in discussions of the autonomic nervous system.

The connections between neurons can be quite complex. One cell can branch to stimulate many receiving cells, or a single cell may be stimulated by a number of different axons (Fig. 9-10). The cell's response is based on the total effects of all the neurotransmitters it receives at any one time.

After its release into the synaptic cleft, the neurotransmitter may be removed by several methods:

- It may slowly diffuse away from the synapse.
- It may be destroyed rapidly by enzymes in the synaptic cleft.
- It may be taken back into the presynaptic cell to be used again, a process known as *reuptake*.

The method of removal helps determine how long a neurotransmitter will act.

Many drugs that act on the mind, substances known as *psychoactive drugs*, function by affecting neurotransmitter activity in the brain. Prozac, for example, increases the level of the neurotransmitter serotonin by blocking its reuptake into presynaptic cells at synapses. This and other selective serotonin reuptake inhibitors (SSRIs) prolong the neurotransmitter's activity and produce a mood-elevating effect. They are used to treat depression, anxiety, and obsessive-compulsive disorder (OCD). Similar psychoactive drugs prevent the reuptake of the neurotransmitters norepinephrine and dopamine. Another class of antidepressants prevents serotonin's enzymatic breakdown in the synaptic cleft, thus extending its action.

CHECKPOINT **9-9** ➤ Chemicals are needed to carry information across the synaptic cleft at a synapse. As a group, what are all these chemicals called?

ELECTRICAL SYNAPSES Not all synapses are chemically controlled. In smooth muscle, cardiac muscle, and also in the CNS, there is a type of synapse in which electrical energy travels directly from one cell to another. The membranes of the presynaptic and postsynaptic cells are close together and an electrical charge can spread directly between them. These electrical synapses allow more rapid and more coordinated communication. In the heart, for example, it is important that large groups of cells contract together for effective pumping action.

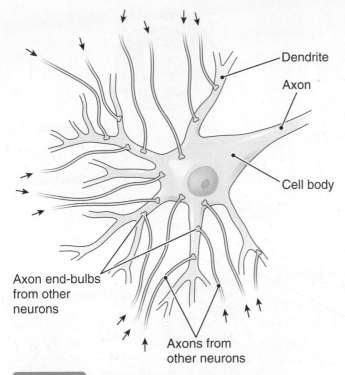

Dendrite

Axon

Cell body

Axon end-bulbs from other neurons

Axons from other neurons

Figure 9-10 **The effects of neurotransmitters on a neuron.** A single neuron is stimulated by axons of many other neurons. The cell responds according to the total of all the excitatory and inhibitory neurotransmitters it receives.

The Spinal Cord

The spinal cord is the link between the peripheral nervous system and the brain. It also helps to coordinate impulses within the CNS. The spinal cord is contained in and protected by the vertebrae, which fit together to form a continuous tube extending from the occipital bone to the coccyx (Fig. 9-11). In the embryo, the spinal cord occupies the entire spinal canal, extending down into the tail portion of the vertebral column. The bony column grows much more rapidly than the nervous tissue of the cord, however, and eventually, the end of the spinal cord no longer reaches the lower part of the spinal canal. This disparity in growth continues to increase, so that in adults, the spinal cord ends in the region just below the area to which the last rib attaches (between the first and second lumbar vertebrae).

Structure of the Spinal Cord

The spinal cord has a small, irregularly shaped internal section of gray matter (unmyelinated tissue) surrounded by a larger area of white matter (myelinated axons) (Fig. 9-12). The internal gray matter is arranged so that a column of gray matter extends up and down dorsally, one on each side; another column is found in the ventral region on each side. These two pairs of columns, called the **dorsal horns** and **ventral horns**, give the gray matter an H-shaped appearance in cross-section. The bridge of gray matter that

connects the right and left horns is the **gray commissure** (KOM-ih-shure). In the center of the gray commissure is a small channel, the **central canal**, that contains cerebrospinal fluid, the liquid that circulates around the brain and spinal cord. A narrow groove, the **posterior median sulcus** (SUL-kus), divides the right and left portions of the posterior white matter. A deeper groove, the **anterior median fissure** (FISH-ure), separates the right and left portions of the anterior white matter.

ASCENDING AND DESCENDING TRACTS The spinal cord is the pathway for sensory and motor impulses traveling to and from the brain. These impulses are carried in the thousands of myelinated axons in the white matter of the spinal cord, which are subdivided into tracts (groups of fibers). Sensory (afferent) impulses entering the spinal cord are transmitted toward the brain in **ascending tracts** of the white matter. Motor (efferent) impulses traveling from the brain are carried in **descending tracts** toward the peripheral nervous system.

CHECKPOINT **9-10** ➤ The spinal cord contains both gray and white matter. How is this tissue arranged in the spinal cord?

CHECKPOINT **9-11** ➤ What is the purpose of the tracts in the white matter of the spinal cord?

9

The Reflex Arc

The nervous system receives, interprets, and acts on both external and internal stimuli. The spinal cord is a relay center for coordinating neural pathways. A complete pathway through the nervous system from stimulus to response is termed a **reflex arc** (Fig. 9-13). This is the nervous system's basic functional pathway. The fundamental parts of a reflex arc are the following (Table 9-2):

1. **Receptor**—the end of a dendrite or some specialized receptor cell, as in a special sense organ, that detects a stimulus

2. **Sensory neuron**, or afferent neuron—a cell that transmits impulses toward the CNS. Sensory impulses enter the dorsal horn of the spinal cord's gray matter.

3. **Central nervous system**—where impulses are coordinated and a response is organized. One or more interneurons may carry impulses to and from the brain, may function within the brain, or may distribute impulses to different regions of the spinal cord. Almost every response involves connecting neurons in the CNS.

4. **Motor neuron**, or efferent neuron—a cell that carries impulses away from the CNS. Motor impulses leave the cord through the ventral horn of the spinal cord's gray matter.

5. **Effector**—a muscle or a gland outside the CNS that carries out a response

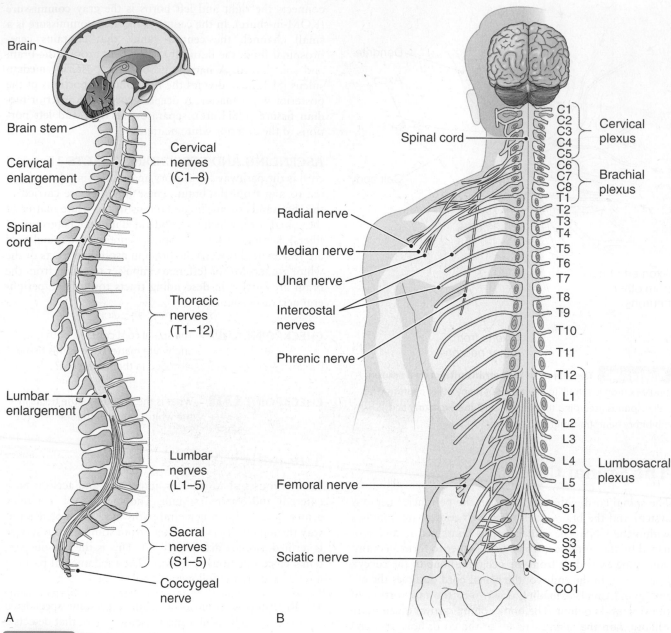

Brain

Brain stem

Cervical enlargement

Spinal cord

Lumbar enlargement

Cervical nerves (C1–8)

Thoracic nerves (T1–12)

Lumbar nerves (L1–5)

Sacral nerves (S1–5)

Coccygeal nerve

A

Spinal cord

Radial nerve

Median nerve

Ulnar nerve

Intercostal nerves

Phrenic nerve

Femoral nerve

Sciatic nerve

C1 C2 C3 C4 C5 — Cervical plexus
C6 C7 C8 T1 — Brachial plexus
T2 T3 T4 T5 T6 T7 T8 T9 T10 T11 T12
L1 L2 L3 L4 L5 — Lumbosacral plexus
S1 S2 S3 S4 S5
CO1

B

Figure 9-11 **Spinal cord and spinal nerves.** Nerve plexuses (networks) are shown. **(A)** Lateral view. **(B)** Posterior view. **[ZOOMING IN ➤** Is the spinal cord the same length as the spinal column? How does the number of cervical vertebrae compare to the number of cervical spinal nerves? **]**

At its simplest, a reflex arc can involve just two neurons, one sensory and one motor, with a synapse in the CNS. Few reflex arcs require only this minimal number of neurons. (The knee-jerk reflex described below is one of the few examples in humans.) Most reflex arcs involve many more, even hundreds, of connecting neurons within the CNS. The many intricate patterns that make the nervous system so responsive and adaptable also make it difficult to study, and investigation of the nervous system is one of the most active areas of research today.

CHECKPOINT 9-12 ➤ What name is given to a pathway through the nervous system from a stimulus to an effector?

Visit *thePoint* or see the Student Resource CD in the back of this book to view the animation *The Reflex Arc.*

REFLEX ACTIVITIES Although reflex pathways may be quite complex, a **simple reflex** is a rapid, uncomplicated, and automatic response involving very few neurons. Reflexes are specific; a given stimulus always produces the same response. When you fling out an arm or leg to catch your balance, withdraw from a painful stimulus, or blink to avoid an object approaching your eyes, you are experiencing reflex behavior. A simple reflex arc that passes

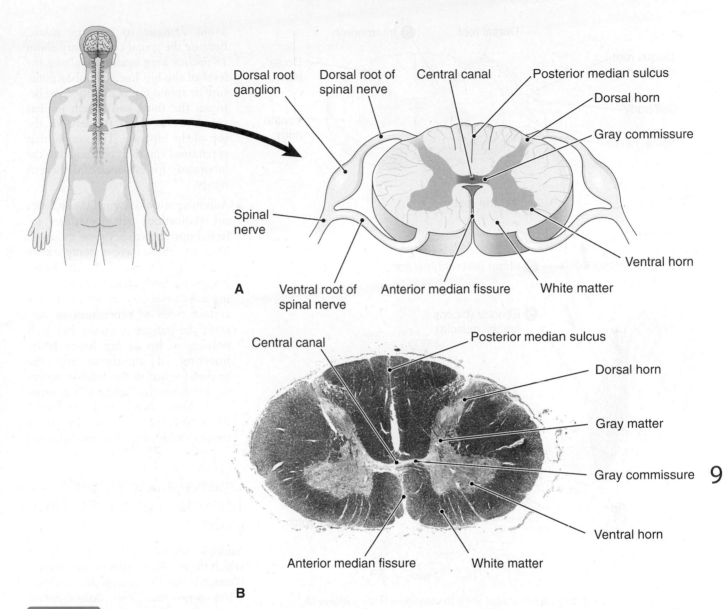

Figure 9-12 **The spinal cord. (A)** Cross section of the spinal cord showing the organization of the gray and white matter. The roots of the spinal nerves are also shown. **(B)** Microscopic view of the spinal cord in cross section (×5). (B, Reprinted with permission from Mills SE. *Histology for Pathologists*, 3rd ed. Philadelphia: Lippincott Williams & Wilkins, 2006.)

through the spinal cord alone and does not involve the brain is termed a **spinal reflex**. Returning to our opening corporation analogy, it's as if middle management makes a decision independently, without involving the CEO.

The **stretch reflex**, in which a muscle is stretched and responds by contracting, is one example of a spinal reflex. If you tap the tendon below the kneecap (the patellar tendon), the muscle of the anterior thigh (quadriceps femoris) contracts, eliciting the knee-jerk reflex (Fig. 9-14). Such stretch reflexes may be evoked by appropriate tapping of most large muscles (such as the triceps brachii in the arm and the gastrocnemius in the calf of the leg). Because reflexes are simple and predictable, they are used in physical examinations to test the condition of the nervous system.

Visit *thePoint* or see the Student Resource CD in the back of this book for an illustration of the following spinal cord procedures.

Medical Procedures Involving the Spinal Cord

■ Lumbar Puncture. It is sometimes necessary to remove a small amount of cerebrospinal fluid (CSF) from the nervous system for testing. CSF is the fluid that circulates in and around the brain and spinal cord. This fluid is taken from the space below the spinal cord to

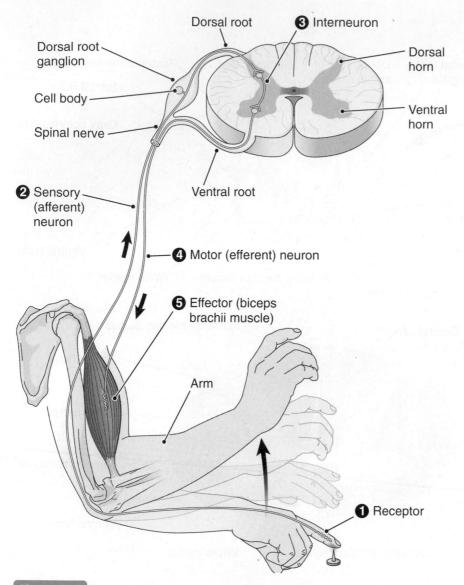

Figure 9-13 **Typical reflex arc.** Numbers show the sequence in the pathway of impulses through the spinal cord (*solid arrows*). Contraction of the biceps brachii results in flexion of the arm at the elbow. **[ZOOMING IN ➤** Is this a somatic or an autonomic reflex arc? What type of neuron is located between the sensory and motor neuron in the CNS? **]**

Table 9-2	Components of a Reflex Arc

Component	Function
Receptor	End of a dendrite or specialized cell that responds to a stimulus
Sensory neuron	Transmits a nerve impulse toward the CNS
Central nervous system	Coordinates sensory impulses and organizes a response. Usually requires interneurons
Motor neuron	Carries impulses away from the CNS toward the effector, a muscle or a gland
Effector	A muscle or gland outside the CNS that carries out a response

avoid damage to nervous tissue. Because the spinal cord is only about 18 inches long and ends above the level of the hip line, a lumbar puncture or spinal tap is usually done between the third and fourth lumbar vertebrae, at about the level of the top of the hipbone. The sample that is removed can then be studied in the laboratory for evidence of disease or injury.

■ Administration of Drugs. Anesthetics or medications are sometimes injected into the space below the cord. The anesthetic agent temporarily blocks all sensation from the lower part of the body. This method of giving anesthesia has an advantage for certain types of procedures or surgery; the patient is awake but feels nothing in his or her lower body. Injection of anesthetic into the epidural space in the lumbar region of the spine (an "epidural") is often used during labor and childbirth. Physicians can also use the spinal route to administer pain medication.

Diseases and Other Disorders of the Spinal Cord

Multiple sclerosis (MS) is a disease in which the myelin sheath around axons is damaged and the neuron fibers themselves degenerate. This demyelination process slows the speed of nerve impulse conduction and disrupts nervous system communication. Both the spinal cord and the brain are affected. Although scientists do not completely understand the cause of MS, there is strong evidence that it involves an attack on the myelin sheath by a person's own immune system, a situation described as *autoimmunity*. Genetic makeup, in combination with environmental factors, may trigger MS. Some research suggests that a prior viral or bacterial infection, even one that occurred many years before, may set off the disease.

MS is the most common chronic CNS disease of young adults in the United States. The disease affects women about twice as often as men, and it is more common in temperate climates and in people of northern

❸ Spinal cord
(CNS)

❷ Sensory
neuron

❶ Receptor

Stimulus

Gray
matter

❹ Motor
neuron

❺ Effector
(quadriceps muscle)

Figure 9-14 **The patellar (knee-jerk) reflex.** Numbers indicate the sequence of a reflex arc. [ZOOMING IN ➤ How many total neurons are involved in this spinal reflex? What neurotransmitter is released at the synapse shown by number 5?]

European ancestry. MS progresses at different rates depending on the individual, and it may be marked by episodes of relapse and remission. At this point, no cure has been found for MS, but drugs that stop the autoimmune response and drugs that relieve MS symptoms are currently under study.

Amyotrophic (ah-mi-o-TROF-ik) **lateral sclerosis** is a nervous system disorder in which motor neurons are destroyed. The progressive destruction causes muscle atrophy and loss of motor control until finally the affected person is unable to swallow or talk.

Poliomyelitis (po-le-o-mi-eh-LI-tis) ("polio") is a viral disease of the nervous system that occurs most commonly in children. Polio is spread by ingestion of water contaminated with feces containing the virus. Infection of the gastrointestinal tract leads to passage of the virus into the blood, from which it spreads to the CNS. Poliovirus tends to multiply in the spinal cord's motor neurons, leading to paralysis, including paralysis of the breathing muscles.

Polio has been virtually eliminated in many countries through the use of vaccines against the disease—first the injected Salk vaccine developed in 1954, followed by the Sabin oral vaccine. A goal of the World Health Organization (WHO) is the total eradication of polio by worldwide vaccination programs, and several philanthropic organizations have joined in this effort.

TUMORS Tumors that affect the spinal cord commonly arise in the support tissue in and around the cord. They are frequently tumors of the nerve sheaths, the meninges, or neuroglia. Symptoms are caused by pressure on the cord

and the roots of the spinal nerves. These include pain, numbness, weakness, and loss of function. Spinal cord tumors are diagnosed by magnetic resonance imaging (MRI) or other imaging techniques, and treatment is by surgery and radiation.

INJURIES Spinal cord injuries may result from wounds, fracture or dislocation of the vertebrae, herniation of intervertebral disks, or tumors. The most common causes of accidental injury to the cord are motor vehicle accidents; falls; sports injuries, especially diving accidents; and job-related injuries. Spinal cord injuries are more common in the young adult age group and many are related to alcohol or drug use.

Cord damage may cause paralysis or loss of sensation in structures supplied by nerves below the level of injury. Different degrees of loss are named using the root *-plegia*, meaning "paralysis," for example:

- Monoplegia (mon-o-PLE-je-ah)- paralysis of one limb
- Diplegia (di-PLE-je-ah)- paralysis of both upper or both lower limbs
- Paraplegia (par-ah-PLE-je-ah)- paralysis of both lower limbs
- Hemiplegia (hem-e-PLE-je-ah)- paralysis of one side of the body
- Tetraplegia (tet-rah-PLE-je-ah) or quadriplegia (kwah-drih-PLE-je-ah)- paralysis of all four limbs

Box 9-1, Spinal Cord Injury: Crossing the Divide, contains information on treatment of these injuries.

The Spinal Nerves

There are 31 pairs of spinal nerves, each pair numbered according to the level of the spinal cord from which it arises (see Fig. 9-11). Note that the nerves that arise near the end of the cord travel in a group within the spinal canal until each exits from its appropriate intervertebral foramen. Each nerve is attached to the spinal cord by two roots: the **dorsal root** and the **ventral root** (see Fig. 9-12). On each dorsal root is a marked swelling of gray matter called the **dorsal root ganglion**, which contains the cell bodies of the sensory neurons. A **ganglion** (GANG-le-on) is any collection of nerve cell bodies located outside the CNS. Fibers from sensory receptors throughout the body lead to the dorsal roots and these dorsal root ganglia

PASSport to Success Visit **thePoint** or see the Student Resource CD in the back of this book for an illustration of the spinal nerves at the end of the spinal cord.

A spinal nerve's ventral root contains motor (efferent) fibers that supply muscles and glands (effectors). The cell bodies of these neurons are located in the cord's ventral gray matter (ventral horns). Because the dorsal (sensory)

9

Box 9-1   Hot Topics

Spinal Cord Injury: Crossing the Divide

Approximately 11,000 new cases of spinal cord injury occur each year in the United States, the majority involving males ages 16 to 30. Because neurons show little, if any, capacity to repair themselves, spinal cord injuries almost always result in a loss of sensory or motor function (or both), and therapy has focused on injury management rather than cure. However, scientists are investigating four improved treatment approaches:

- *Minimizing spinal cord trauma after injury.* Intravenous injection of the steroid methylprednisolone shortly after injury reduces swelling at the site of injury and improves recovery.

- *Using **neurotrophins** to induce repair in damaged nerve tissue.* Certain types of neuroglia produce chemicals called neurotrophins (e.g., nerve growth factor) that have promoted nerve regeneration in experiments.

- *Regulation of inhibitory factors that keep neurons from dividing.* "Turning off" these factors (produced by neuroglia) in the damaged nervous system may promote tissue repair. The factor called Nogo is an example.

- *Nervous tissue transplantation.* Successfully transplanted donor tissue may take over the damaged nervous system's functions.

and ventral (motor) roots combine to form the spinal nerve, all spinal nerves are mixed nerves.

Branches of the Spinal Nerves

Each spinal nerve continues only a short distance away from the spinal cord and then branches into small posterior divisions and larger anterior divisions. The larger anterior branches interlace to form networks called **plexuses** (PLEK-sus-eze), which then distribute branches to the body parts (see Fig. 9-11). The three main plexuses are described as follows:

- The **cervical plexus** supplies motor impulses to the neck muscles and receives sensory impulses from the neck and the back of the head. The phrenic nerve, which activates the diaphragm, arises from this plexus.

- The **brachial** (BRA-ke-al) **plexus** sends numerous branches to the shoulder, arm, forearm, wrist, and hand. The radial nerve emerges from the brachial plexus.

- The **lumbosacral** (lum-bo-SA-kral) **plexus** supplies nerves to the pelvis and legs. The largest branch in this plexus is the **sciatic** (si-AT-ik) **nerve**, which leaves the dorsal part of the pelvis, passes beneath the gluteus maximus muscle, and extends down the posterior thigh. At its beginning, it is nearly 1 inch thick, but it soon branches to the thigh muscles; near the knee, it forms two subdivisions that supply the leg and the foot.

DERMATOMES Sensory neurons from all over the skin, except for the skin of the face and scalp, feed information into the spinal cord through the spinal nerves. The skin surface can be mapped into distinct regions that are supplied by a single spinal nerve. Each of these regions is called a **dermatome** (DER-mah-tome) (Fig. 9-15).

Sensation from a given dermatome is carried over its corresponding spinal nerve. This information can be used to identify the spinal nerve or spinal segment that is involved in an injury, as sensation from its corresponding skin surface will be altered. In some areas, the dermatomes are not absolutely distinct. Some dermatomes may share a nerve supply with neighboring regions. For this reason, it is necessary to numb several adjacent dermatomes to achieve successful anesthesia.

CHECKPOINT 9-13 ➤ How many pairs of spinal nerves are there?

Disorders of the Spinal Nerves

Peripheral neuritis (nu-RI-tis), or peripheral neuropathy, is the degeneration of nerves supplying the distal areas of the extremities. It affects both sensory and motor function, causing symptoms of pain and paralysis. Causes include chronic intoxication (alcohol, lead, drugs), infectious diseases (meningitis), metabolic diseases (diabetes, gout), or nutritional diseases (vitamin deficiency, starvation). Identification and treatment of the underlying disorder is most important. Because peripheral neuritis is a symptom rather than a disease, a complete physical examination may be needed to establish its cause.

Sciatica (si-AT-ih-kah) is a form of peripheral neuritis characterized by severe pain along the sciatic nerve and its branches. The most common causes of this disorder are

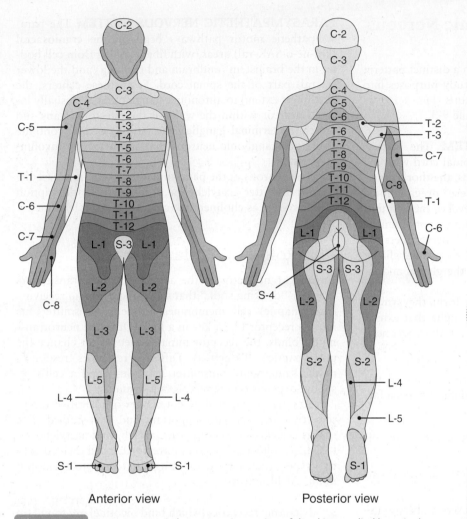

Anterior view   Posterior view

Figure 9-15 **Dermatomes.** A dermatome is a region of the skin supplied by a single spinal nerve. [**ZOOMING IN ➤** Which spinal nerves carry impulses from the skin of the toes? From the anterior hand and fingers?]

rupture of a disk between the lower lumbar vertebrae and arthritis of the lower spinal column.

Herpes zoster, commonly known as *shingles*, is characterized by numerous blisters along the course of certain nerves, most commonly the intercostal nerves, which are branches of the thoracic spinal nerves in the waist area. Shingles is caused by a reactivation of a prior chickenpox virus infection and involves an attack on the sensory cell bodies inside the spinal ganglia. Initial symptoms include fever and pain, followed in 2 to 4 weeks by the appearance of vesicles (fluid-filled skin lesions). The drainage from these vesicles contains highly contagious liquid. The neuralgic pains may persist for years and can be distressing. This infection may also involve the first branch of the fifth cranial nerve and cause pain in the eyeball and surrounding tissues. Early treatment of a recurrent attack with antiviral drugs may reduce the neuralgia.

Guillain-Barré syndrome (ge-YAN bar-RA) is classified as a polyneuropathy (pol-e-nu-ROP-a-the), that is, a disorder involving many nerves. There is progressive muscle weakness caused by loss of myelin, with numbness and paralysis, which may involve the breathing muscles. Sometimes the autonomic nervous system is involved, resulting in problems with involuntary functions. The cause of Guillain-Barré syndrome is not known, but it often follows an infection, usually a viral infection. It may result from an abnormal immune response to one's own nerve tissue. Most people recover completely from the disease with time, but recovery may take months or even years.

> **PASSport to Success**
>
> Occupational therapists often help to care for people with nervous system disorders. Visit *thePoint* or see the Student Resource CD in the back of this book for more information about this career.

The Autonomic Nervous System (ANS)

The autonomic (visceral) nervous system regulates the action of the glands, the smooth muscles of hollow organs and vessels, and the heart muscle. These actions are carried on automatically; whenever a change occurs that calls for a regulatory adjustment, it is made without conscious awareness.

Most ANS studies concentrate on the motor (efferent) portion of the system. All autonomic pathways contain two motor neurons connecting the spinal cord with the effector organ. The two neurons synapse in ganglia that serve as relay stations along the way. The first neuron, the preganglionic neuron, extends from the spinal cord to the ganglion. The second neuron, the postganglionic neuron, travels from the ganglion to the effector. This differs from the voluntary (somatic) nervous system, in which each motor nerve fiber extends all the way from the spinal cord to the skeletal muscle with no intervening synapse. Some of the autonomic fibers are within the spinal nerves; some are within the cranial nerves (see Chapter 10).

CHECKPOINT 9-14 ➤ How many neurons are there in each motor pathway of the ANS?

9

Divisions of the Autonomic Nervous System

The ANS motor neurons are arranged in a distinct pattern, which has led to their separation for study purposes into **sympathetic** and **parasympathetic** divisions (Fig. 9-16), as described below and summarized in Table 9-3.

SYMPATHETIC NERVOUS SYSTEM The sympathetic motor neurons originate in the spinal cord with cell bodies in the thoracic and lumbar regions, the **thoracolumbar** (tho-rah-ko-LUM-bar) area. These preganglionic fibers arise from the spinal cord at the level of the first thoracic spinal nerve down to the level of the second lumbar spinal nerve. From this part of the cord, nerve fibers extend to ganglia where they synapse with postganglionic neurons, the fibers of which extend to the glands and involuntary muscle tissues.

Many of the sympathetic ganglia form the **sympathetic chains**, two cordlike strands of ganglia that extend along either side of the spinal column from the lower neck to the upper abdominal region. (Note that Figure 9-16 shows only one side for each division of the ANS.)

In addition, the nerves that supply the abdominal and pelvic organs synapse in three single **collateral ganglia** farther from the spinal cord. These are the:

- Celiac ganglion, which sends fibers mainly to the digestive organs
- Superior mesenteric ganglion, which sends fibers to the large and small intestines
- Inferior mesenteric ganglion, which sends fibers to the distal large intestine and organs of the urinary and reproductive systems

The postganglionic neurons of the sympathetic system, with few exceptions, act on their effectors by releasing the neurotransmitter epinephrine (adrenaline) and the related compound norepinephrine (noradrenaline). This system is therefore described as **adrenergic**, which means "activated by adrenaline."

PARASYMPATHETIC NERVOUS SYSTEM The parasympathetic motor pathways begin in the **craniosacral** (kra-ne-o-SAK-ral) areas, with fibers arising from cell bodies in the brainstem (midbrain and medulla) and the lower (sacral) part of the spinal cord. From these centers, the first fibers extend to autonomic ganglia that are usually located near or within the walls of the effector organs and are called **terminal ganglia**. The pathways then continue along postganglionic neurons that stimulate the involuntary tissues.

The neurons of the parasympathetic system release the neurotransmitter acetylcholine, leading to the description of this system as **cholinergic** (activated by acetylcholine).

The Role of Cellular Receptors

An important factor in the actions of neurotransmitters are their "docking sites," that is, the receptors on receiving (postsynaptic) cell membranes. A neurotransmitter fits into its receptor like a key in a lock. Once the neurotransmitter binds, the receptor initiates events that change the postsynaptic cell's activity. Different receptors' responses to the same neurotransmitter may vary, and a cell's response depends on the receptors it contains.

Among the many different classes of identified receptors, two are especially important and well-studied. The first is the cholinergic receptors, which bind acetylcholine (ACh). Cholinergic receptors are further subdivided into two types, each named for drugs that bind to them and mimic ACh's effects:

- Nicotinic receptors (which bind nicotine) are found on skeletal muscle cells and stimulate muscle contraction when ACh is present.
- Muscarinic receptors (which bind muscarine, a poison) are found on effector cells of the parasympathetic nervous system. ACh can either stimulate or inhibit muscarinic receptors depending on the effector organ. For example, ACh stimulates digestive organs but inhibits the heart.

Table 9-3	Divisions of the Autonomic Nervous System	
Characteristics	**Divisions**	
	Sympathetic nervous system	**Parasympathetic nervous system**
Origin of fibers	Thoracic and lumbar regions of the spinal cord; thoracolumbar	Brain stem and sacral regions of the spinal cord; craniosacral
Location of ganglia	Sympathetic chains and three single collateral ganglia (celiac, superior mesenteric, inferior mesenteric)	Terminal ganglia in or near the effector organ
Neurotransmitter (see Table 9–4)	Adrenaline and noradrenaline; adrenergic	Acetylcholine; cholinergic
Effects	Response to stress; fight-or-flight response	Reverses fight-or-flight (stress) response; stimulates some activities

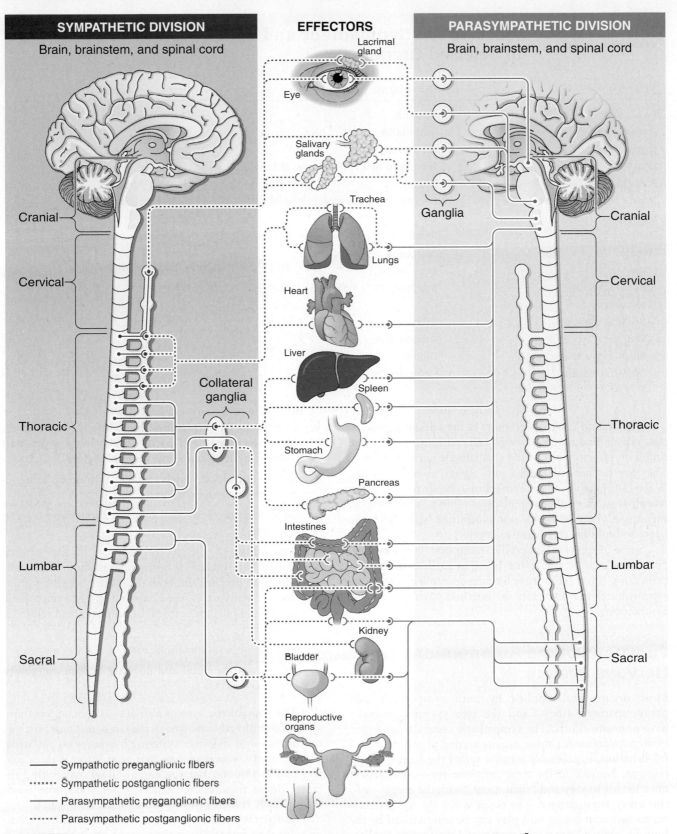

SYMPATHETIC DIVISION
Brain, brainstem, and spinal cord

EFFECTORS

PARASYMPATHETIC DIVISION
Brain, brainstem, and spinal cord

Lacrimal gland

Eye

Salivary glands

Trachea

Ganglia

Lungs

Heart

Collateral ganglia

Liver

Spleen

Stomach

Pancreas

Intestines

Kidney

Bladder

Reproductive organs

Cranial
Cervical
Thoracic
Lumbar
Sacral

Cranial
Cervical
Thoracic
Lumbar
Sacral

—— Sympathetic preganglionic fibers
······ Sympathetic postganglionic fibers
—— Parasympathetic preganglionic fibers
······ Parasympathetic postganglionic fibers

Figure 9-16 **Autonomic nervous system.** The diagram shows only one side of the body for each division. **[ZOOMING IN ➤** Which division of the autonomic nervous system has ganglia closer to the effector organ? **]**

9

Table 9-4	**Effects of the Sympathetic and Parasympathetic Systems on Selected Organs**	
Effector	**Sympathetic system**	**Parasympathetic system**
Pupils of eye	Dilation	Constriction
Sweat glands	Stimulation	None
Digestive glands	Inhibition	Stimulation
Heart	Increased rate and strength of beat	Decreased rate of beat
Bronchi of lungs	Dilation	Constriction
Muscles of digestive system	Decreased contraction (peristalsis)	Increased contraction
Kidneys	Decreased activity	None
Urinary bladder	Relaxation	Contraction and emptying
Liver	Increased release of glucose	None
Penis	Ejaculation	Erection
Adrenal medulla	Stimulation	None
Blood vessels to:		
Skeletal muscles	Dilation	Constriction
Skin	Constriction	None
Respiratory system	Dilation	Constriction
Digestive organs	Constriction	Dilation

The second class of receptors is the adrenergic receptors, which bind norepinephrine and epinephrine. They are found on effector cells of the sympathetic nervous system. They are further subdivided into alpha (α) and beta (β). When norepinephrine (or epinephrine) binds to adrenergic receptors, it can either stimulate or inhibit, depending on the organ. For example, norepinephrine stimulates the heart and inhibits the digestive organs.

Some drugs block specific receptors. For example, "beta-blockers" regulate the heart in cardiac disease by preventing β receptors from binding epinephrine, the neurotransmitter that increases the rate and strength of heart contractions.

Functions of the Autonomic Nervous System

Most organs are supplied by both sympathetic and parasympathetic fibers, and the two systems generally have opposite effects. The sympathetic system tends to act as an accelerator for those organs needed to meet a stressful situation. It promotes what is called the **fight-or-flight response** because in the most primitive terms, the person must decide to stay and "fight it out" with the enemy or to run away from danger. The times when the sympathetic nervous system comes into play can be summarized by the four Es, that is, times of emergency, excitement, embarrassment, and exercise. If you think of what happens to a person who is in any of these situations, you can easily remember the effects of the sympathetic nervous system:

- Increase in the rate and force of heart contractions

- Increase in blood pressure due partly to the more effective heartbeat and partly to constriction of small arteries in the skin and the internal organs

- Dilation of blood vessels to skeletal muscles, bringing more blood to these tissues

- Dilation of the bronchial tubes to allow more oxygen to enter

- Stimulation of the central portion of the adrenal gland. This produces hormones, including epinephrine, that prepare the body to meet emergency situations in many ways (see Chapter 12). The sympathetic nerves and hormones from the adrenal gland reinforce each other

- Increase in basal metabolic rate

- Dilation of the pupil and decrease in focusing ability (for near objects)

The sympathetic system also acts as a brake on those systems not directly involved in the stress response, such as the urinary and digestive systems. If you try to eat while you are angry, you may note that your saliva is thick and so small in amount that you can swallow only with difficulty. Under these circumstances, when food does reach the stomach, it seems to stay there longer than usual.

The parasympathetic system normally acts as a balance for the sympathetic system once a crisis has passed. It is the "rest and digest" system. It causes constriction of the pupils, slowing of the heart rate, and constriction of the bronchial tubes. However, the parasympathetic nervous system also stimulates certain activities needed for maintenance of homeostasis. Among other actions, it promotes

Disease in Context revisited

➤ Sue Learns About Her MS

"Sue, I can't really answer the question of why you developed multiple sclerosis," Dr. Jensen explained to her patient. "There is evidence that the disease has a genetic component but the environment, and perhaps even a virus, might be involved. We do know that multiple sclerosis affects women more frequently than men, and is more prevalent in areas like the northern United States and Canada. We also know that MS is an autoimmune disease. Normally, immune cells travel through the brain and spinal cord looking for pathogens. In multiple sclerosis, the immune cells make a mistake and cause inflammation in healthy nervous tissue. This inflammatory response damages neuroglial cells called oligodendrocytes. These cells form the myelin sheath that covers and insulates the axons of neurons much like the plastic covering on an electrical wire does. When the oligodendrocytes are damaged, they are unable to make this myelin sheath and the axons can't properly transmit nerve impulses. Right now, it appears that the largest areas of demyelination are in the white matter tracts of your spinal cord."

"Is there a medication I can take to stop the disease?" asked Sue.

"Unfortunately," replied the doctor, "there isn't a cure for MS yet. But, we can slow down the disease's progress using anti-inflammatory drugs and interferons to decrease the inflammation and depress the immune response."

During this case we saw that neurons carrying information to and from the central nervous system require myelin sheaths. Inflammation and subsequent damage of the myelin sheath in diseases like multiple sclerosis have profound effects on sensory and motor function. For more information about the inflammatory response and interferon, see Chapter 17. We'll visit Sue one last time in Chapter 24, Development and Birth, and learn how she copes with her disease while pregnant.

9

the formation and release of urine and activity of the digestive tract. Saliva, for example, flows more easily and profusely under its effects. These stimulatory actions are summarized by the acronym SLUDD: salivation, lacrimation (tear formation), urination, digestion, defecation.

Most body organs receive both sympathetic and parasympathetic stimulation, the effects of the two systems on a given organ generally being opposite. Table 9-4 shows some of the actions of these two systems.

CHECKPOINT 9-15 ➤ Which division of the ANS stimulates a stress response, and which division reverses the stress response?

Word Anatomy

Medical terms are built from standardized word parts (prefixes, roots, and suffixes). Learning the meanings of these parts can help you remember words and interpret unfamiliar terms.

WORD PART	MEANING	EXAMPLE
Role of the Nervous System		
soma-	body	The *somatic* nervous system controls skeletal muscles that move the body.
aut/o	self	The *autonomic* nervous system is automatically controlled and is involuntary.

WORD PART	MEANING	EXAMPLE
neur/i	nerve, nervous tissue	The *neurilemma* is the outer membrane of the myelin sheath around an axon.
-lemma	sheath	See preceding example.

The Nervous System at Work

de-	remove	*Depolarization* removes the charge on the plasma membrane of a cell.
re-	again, back	*Repolarization* restores the charge on the plasma membrane of a cell.
post-	after	The *postsynaptic* cell is located after the synapse and receives neurotransmitter from the presynaptic cell.

The Spinal Cord

myel/o	spinal cord	*Poliomyelitis* is an infectious disease that involves the spinal cord and other parts of the CNS.
-plegia	paralysis	*Monoplegia* is paralysis of one limb.
para-	beyond	*Paraplegia* is paralysis of both lower limbs.
hemi-	half	*Hemiplegia* is paralysis of one side of the body.
tetra-	four	*Tetraplegia* is paralysis of all four limbs.

Summary

I. **ROLE OF THE NERVOUS SYSTEM**
   A. Structural divisions—anatomic
      1. Central nervous system (CNS)—brain and spinal cord
      2. Peripheral nervous system (PNS)—spinal and cranial nerves
   B. Functional divisions—physiologic
      1. Somatic nervous system—voluntary; supplies skeletal muscles
      2. Autonomic (visceral) nervous system—involuntary; supplies smooth muscle, cardiac muscle, glands

II. **NEURONS AND THEIR FUNCTIONS**
   A. Structure of a neuron
      1. Cell body
      2. Cell fibers
         a. Dendrite—carries impulses to cell body
         b. Axon—carries impulses away from cell body
      3. Myelin sheath
         a. Covers and protects some axons
         b. Speeds conduction
         c. Made by Schwann cells in PNS; other cells in CNS
            (1) Neurilemma—outermost layer of Schwann cell; aids axon repair
         d. White matter—myelinated tissue; gray matter—unmyelinated tissue

   B. Types of neurons
      1. Sensory (afferent)—carry impulses toward CNS
      2. Motor (efferent)—carry impulses away from CNS
      3. Interneurons—in CNS
   C. Nerves and tracts—bundles of neuron fibers
      1. Nerve—in peripheral nervous system
         a. Held together by connective tissue
            (1) Endoneurium—around a single fiber
            (2) Perineurium—around each fascicle
            (3) Epineurium—around whole nerve
         b. Types of nerves
            (1) Sensory (afferent) nerve—contains only fibers that carry impulses toward the CNS (from a receptor)
            (2) Motor (efferent) nerve—contains only fibers that carry impulses away from the CNS (to an effector)
            (3) Mixed nerve—contains both sensory and motor fibers
      2. Tract—in central nervous system

III. **NEUROGLIA**
   A. Nonconducting cells
   B. Protect and support nervous tissue

IV. **THE NERVOUS SYSTEM AT WORK**
   A. Nerve impulse
      1. Potential—electrical charge on the plasma membrane of neuron

2. Action potential
   a. Depolarization—reversal of charge
   b. Repolarization—return to normal
   c. Involves changes in concentrations of Na$^+$ and K$^+$
3. Nerve impulse—spread of action potential along membrane
4. Myelin sheath speeds conduction
B. Synapse—junction between neurons
   1. Nerve impulse transmitted from presynaptic neuron to postsynaptic neuron
   2. Neurotransmitter—carries impulse across synapse
   3. Receptors—in postsynaptic membrane; pick up neurotransmitters
   4. Neurotransmitter removed by diffusion, destruction by enzyme, return to presynaptic cell (reuptake)
   5. Electrical synapses—in smooth muscle, cardiac muscle, CNS

V. SPINAL CORD
A. Location
   1. In vertebral column
   2. Ends between first and second lumbar vertebrae
B. Structure of the spinal cord
   1. H-shaped area of gray matter
   2. White matter around gray matter
      a. Ascending tracts—carry impulses toward brain
      b. Descending tracts—carry impulses away from brain
C. Reflex arc—pathway through the nervous system
   1. Components
      a. Receptor—detects stimulus
      b. Sensory neuron—receptor to CNS
      c. Central neuron—in CNS
      d. Motor neuron—CNS to effector
      e. Effector—muscle or gland that responds
   2. Reflex activities—simple reflex is rapid, automatic response using few neurons
      a. Examples—stretch reflex, eye blink, withdrawal reflex
      b. Spinal reflex—coordinated in spinal cord
D. Medical procedures involving the spinal cord
      a. Lumbar puncture
      b. Administration of drugs
E. Diseases and other disorders of the spinal cord
   1. Diseases—multiple sclerosis, amyotrophic lateral sclerosis, poliomyelitis

2. Tumors
3. Injuries

VI. SPINAL NERVES—31 PAIRS
A. Roots
   1. Dorsal (sensory)
   2. Ventral (motor)
B. Mixed nerves—combine sensory and motor fibers
C. Branches of the spinal nerves
   1. Plexuses—networks formed by anterior branches
      a. Cervical plexus
      b. Brachial plexus
      c. Lumbosacral plexus
   2. Dermatome—region of the skin supplied by a single spinal nerve
D. Disorders of the spinal nerves—peripheral neuritis, sciatica, herpes zoster, Guillain-Barré

VII. AUTONOMIC NERVOUS SYSTEM (VISCERAL NERVOUS SYSTEM)
A. Characteristics
   1. Involuntary
   2. Controls glands, smooth muscle, heart (cardiac) muscle
   3. Two motor neurons (preganglionic and postganglionic)
B. Divisions of the autonomic nervous system
   1. Sympathetic nervous system
      a. Thoracolumbar
      b. Adrenergic—uses adrenaline
      c. Synapses in sympathetic chains and three collateral ganglia (celiac, superior mesenteric, inferior mesenteric)
   2. Parasympathetic system
      a. Craniosacral
      b. Cholinergic—uses acetylcholine
      c. Synapses in terminal ganglia in or near effector organs
C. Cellular receptors
   1. Affect neurotransmitter's action
   2. Types
      a. Cholinergic—bind ACh
      b. Adrenergic—bind norepinephrine and epinephrine
D. Functions of the autonomic nervous system
   1. Divisions
      a. Sympathetic—stimulates fight-or-flight (stress) response
      b. Parasympathetic—returns body to normal
   2. Usually have opposite effects on an organ

9

Questions for Study and Review

BUILDING UNDERSTANDING

Fill in the blanks

1. The brain and spinal cord make up the _____ nervous system.

2. Action potentials are conducted away from the neuron cell body by the _____.

3. During an action potential, the flow of Na$^+$ into the cell causes _____.

4. In the spinal cord, sensory information travels in _____ tracts.

5. With few exceptions, the sympathetic nervous system uses the neurotransmitter _____ to act on effector organs.

Matching > Match each numbered item with the most closely related lettered item.

___ 6. Cells that carry impulses from the CNS

___ 7. Cells that carry impulses to the CNS

___ 8. Cells that carry impulses within the CNS

___ 9. Cells that detect a stimulus

___ 10. Cells that carry out a response to a stimulus

a. receptors

b. effectors

c. sensory neurons

d. motor neurons

e. interneurons

Multiple Choice

___ 11. Skeletal muscles are voluntarily controlled by the
  a. central nervous system
  b. somatic nervous system
  c. parasympathetic nervous system
  d. sympathetic nervous system

___ 12. The cells involved in most nervous system tumors are called
  a. motor neurons
  b. sensory neurons
  c. interneurons
  d. neuroglia

___ 13. The correct order of synaptic transmission is
  a. postsynaptic neuron, synapse, and presynaptic neuron
  b. presynaptic neuron, synapse, and postsynaptic neuron
  c. presynaptic neuron, postsynaptic neuron, and synapse
  d. postsynaptic neuron, presynaptic neuron, and synapse

___ 14. Afferent nerve fibers enter the part of the spinal cord called the
  a. dorsal horn
  b. ventral horn
  c. gray commissure
  d. central canal

___ 15. The "fight-or-flight" response is promoted by the
  a. sympathetic nervous system
  b. parasympathetic nervous system
  c. somatic nervous system
  d. reflex arc

UNDERSTANDING CONCEPTS

16. Differentiate between the terms in each of the following pairs:

    a. neurons and neuroglia
    b. vesicle and receptor
    c. gray matter and white matter
    d. nerve and tract

17. Describe an action potential. How does conduction along a myelinated fiber differ from conduction along an unmyelinated fiber?

18. Discuss the structure and function of the spinal cord.

19. Explain the reflex arc using stepping on a tack as an example.

20. Describe the anatomy of a spinal nerve. How many pairs of spinal nerves are there?

21. Define a *plexus*. Name the three main spinal nerve plexuses.

22. Compare and contrast multiple sclerosis and Guillain-Barré syndrome.

23. Differentiate between the functions of the sympathetic and parasympathetic divisions of the autonomic nervous system.

CONCEPTUAL THINKING

24. Clinical depression is associated with abnormal serotonin levels. Medications that block the removal of this neurotransmitter from the synapse can control the disorder. Based on this information, is clinical depression associated with increased or decreased levels of serotonin? Explain your answer.

25. Mr. Hayward visits his dentist for a root canal and is given Novocaine, a local anesthetic, at the beginning of the procedure. Novocaine reduces membrane permeability to Na^+. What effect does this have on action potential?

26. In Sue's case, her symptoms were caused by demyelination in her central nervous system. Would her symptoms be the same or different if her spinal nerves were involved? Explain why.

9

The Nervous System: The Brain and Cranial Nerves

Learning Outcomes

After careful study of this chapter, you should be able to:

1. Give the location and functions of the four main divisions of the brain
2. Name and describe the three meninges
3. Cite the function of cerebrospinal fluid and describe where and how this fluid is formed
4. Name and locate the lobes of the cerebral hemispheres
5. Cite one function of the cerebral cortex in each lobe of the cerebrum
6. Name two divisions of the diencephalon and cite the functions of each
7. Locate the three subdivisions of the brain stem and give the functions of each
8. Describe the cerebellum and cite its functions
9. Name some techniques used to study the brain
10. Cite the names and functions of the 12 cranial nerves
11. List some disorders that involve the brain, its associated structures, or the cranial nerves
12. Show how word parts are used to build words related to the nervous system (see Word Anatomy at the end of the chapter)

Selected Key Terms

The following terms and other boldface terms in the chapter are defined in the Glossary

aphasia
brain stem
cerebellum
cerebral cortex
cerebrospinal fluid (CSF)
cerebrum
concussion
diencephalon
electroencephalograph (EEG)
gyrus (pl. gyri)
hematoma
hypothalamus
medulla oblongata
meninges
midbrain
pons
stroke
sulcus (pl. sulci)
thalamus
ventricle

PASSport to Success

Visit *thePoint* or see the Student Resource CD in the back of this book for definitions and pronunciations of key terms as well as a pretest for this chapter.

Disease in Context

Frank's Case: Blood Clot in the Brain

Ross loved his job as a physiotherapist. He especially enjoyed his current position at the hospital where he was a member of the brain injury team. His responsibility was to design and implement rehabilitation programs for patients recovering from brain injury.

When Ross arrived at work there was a new medical chart waiting for him at his desk. He opened it and scanned its contents. Yesterday evening, Frank Carter, a 68-year-old African American, was transported by ambulance to the emergency room. According to Frank's wife, he had collapsed suddenly in their living room. Worried that he was having a heart attack, she called 911. At the hospital, Frank appeared confused and disoriented. His speech was slurred and he had difficulty forming words. He reported double-vision, dizziness, and a severe headache. He had a history of high blood pressure and, according to his wife, had smoked a pack of cigarettes per day for most of his adult life. The emergency room physician examined Frank and noted muscle weakness and a diminished sense of touch on the right side of his face and arm. Based upon his neurological findings, the physician ordered an emergency CT scan of Frank's brain. The results of the scan indicated that there was a blood clot blocking Frank's left middle cerebral artery, preventing blood flow to his left cerebral hemisphere. Frank wasn't having a heart attack—he was having a stroke. The emergency physician administered tissue plasminogen activator (tPA) to dissolve the clot and restore blood flow to his brain.

Frank's neurological symptoms are due to a lack of blood flow to a part of his brain called the cerebrum. In this chapter we'll learn about the structure and function of the brain. We'll also revisit Frank and look at Ross' assessment of his stroke symptoms.

The Brain

The brain occupies the cranial cavity and is covered by membranes, fluid, and the skull bones. Although the brain's various regions communicate and function together, the brain may be divided into distinct areas for ease of study (Fig. 10-1, Table 10-1):

- The **cerebrum** (SER-e-brum) is the largest part of the brain. It is divided into right and left **cerebral** (SER-e-bral) **hemispheres** by a deep groove called the **longitudinal fissure** (Fig. 10-2). Each hemisphere is further subdivided into lobes.

- The **diencephalon** (di-en-SEF-ah-lon) is the area between the cerebral hemispheres and the brain stem. It includes the thalamus and the hypothalamus.

- The **brain stem** connects the cerebrum and diencephalon with the spinal cord. The superior portion of the brain stem is the **midbrain**. Inferior to the midbrain is the **pons** (ponz), followed by the **medulla oblongata** (meh-DUL-lah ob-long-GAH-tah). The pons connects the midbrain with the medulla, whereas the medulla connects the brain with the spinal cord through a large opening in the base of the skull (foramen magnum).

- The **cerebellum** (ser-eh-BEL-um) is located immediately below the posterior part of the cerebral hemispheres

and is connected with the cerebrum, brain stem, and spinal cord by means of the pons. The word *cerebellum* means "little brain."

Each of these divisions is described in greater detail later in this chapter.

CHECKPOINT 10-1 ➤ What are the main divisions of the brain?

Protective Structures of the Brain and Spinal Cord

The **meninges** (men-IN-jez) are three layers of connective tissue that surround both the brain and spinal cord to form a complete enclosure (Fig. 10-3). The outermost of these membranes, the **dura mater** (DU-rah MA-ter), is the thickest and toughest of the meninges. (*Mater* is from the Latin meaning "mother," referring to the protective function of the meninges; *dura* means "hard.") Around the brain, the dura mater is in two layers, and the outer layer is fused to the cranial bones. In certain places, these two layers separate to provide venous channels, called **dural sinuses,** for the drainage of blood coming from the brain tissue.

The middle layer of the meninges is the **arachnoid** (ah-RAK-noyd). This membrane is loosely attached to the

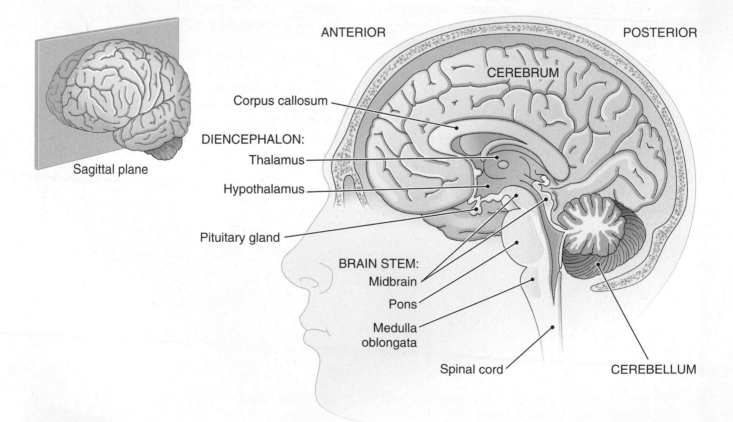

ANTERIOR   POSTERIOR

CEREBRUM

Corpus callosum

DIENCEPHALON:
　Thalamus
Hypothalamus

Pituitary gland

Sagittal plane

BRAIN STEM:
　Midbrain
　Pons
　Medulla oblongata

Spinal cord   CEREBELLUM

Figure 10-1 Brain, sagittal section. Main divisions are shown.

Table 10-1	Organization of the Brain	
Division	**Description**	**Functions**
Cerebrum	Largest and uppermost portion of the brain. Divided into two hemispheres, each subdivided into lobes	Cortex (outer layer) is site for conscious thought, memory, reasoning, and abstract mental functions, all localized within specific lobes
Diencephalon	Between the cerebrum and the brain stem. Contains the thalamus and hypothalamus	Thalamus sorts and redirects sensory input. Hypothalamus maintains homeostasis, controls autonomic nervous system and pituitary gland
Brain stem	Anterior region below the cerebrum	Connects cerebrum and diencephalon with spinal cord
Midbrain	Below the center of the cerebrum	Has reflex centers concerned with vision and hearing. Connects cerebrum with lower portions of the brain
Pons	Anterior to the cerebellum	Connects cerebellum with other portions of the brain. Helps to regulate respiration
Medulla oblongata	Between the pons and the spinal cord	Links the brain with the spinal cord. Has centers for control of vital functions, such as respiration and the heartbeat
Cerebellum	Below the posterior portion of the cerebrum. Divided into two hemispheres	Coordinates voluntary muscles. Maintains balance and muscle tone

10

deepest of the meninges by weblike fibers, allowing a space for the movement of cerebrospinal fluid (CSF) between the two membranes. (The arachnoid is named from the Latin word for spider because of its weblike appearance).

The innermost layer around the brain, the **pia mater** (PI-ah MA-ter), is attached to the nervous tissue of the brain and spinal cord and follows all the contours of these structures (see Fig. 10-3). It is made of a delicate connec-

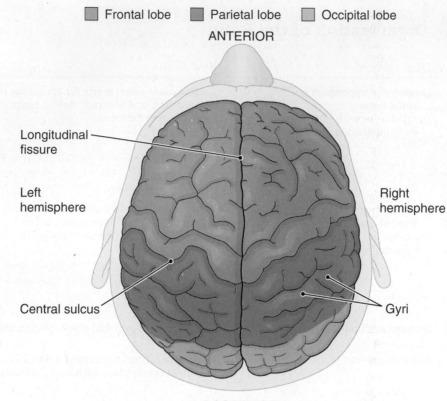

Frontal lobe   Parietal lobe   Occipital lobe

ANTERIOR

Longitudinal fissure

Left hemisphere

Right hemisphere

Central sulcus

Gyri

POSTERIOR

Figure 10-2 **External surface of the brain, superior view.** The division into two hemispheres and into lobes is visible.

Skin

Dural (venous) sinus

Periosteum

Skull

Arachnoid villus

Dura mater

Arachnoid

Meninges

Pia mater

Gray matter

White matter

Brain tissue

Figure 10-3 **Frontal (coronal) section of the top of the head.** The meninges and related parts are shown. **[ZOOMING IN ➤** What is located in the spaces where the dura mater divides into two layers? **]**

tive tissue (*pia* meaning "tender" or "soft"). The pia mater holds blood vessels that supply nutrients and oxygen to the brain and spinal cord.

CHECKPOINT 10-2 ➤ The meninges are protective membranes around the brain and spinal cord. What are the names of the three layers of the meninges from the outermost to the innermost?

Cerebrospinal Fluid

Cerebrospinal (ser-e-bro-SPI-nal) **fluid** is a clear liquid that circulates in and around the brain and spinal cord (Fig. 10-4). The function of the CSF is to support nervous tissue and to cushion shocks that would otherwise injure these delicate structures. This fluid also carries nutrients to the cells and transports waste products from the cells.

CSF flows freely through passageways in and around the brain and spinal cord and finally flows out into the subarachnoid space of the meninges. Much of the fluid then returns to the blood through projections called *arachnoid villi* in the dural sinuses (see Figs. 10-3 and 10-4).

VENTRICLES CSF forms in four spaces within the brain called **ventricles** (VEN-trih-klz) (Fig. 10-5). A vascular network in each ventricle, the **choroid** (KOR-oyd) **plexus**, forms CSF by filtration of the blood and by cellular secretion.

The four ventricles that produce CSF extend somewhat irregularly into the various parts of the brain. The largest are the lateral ventricles in the two cerebral hemispheres. Their extensions into the lobes of the cerebrum are called **horns**. These paired ventricles communicate with a midline space, the third ventricle, by means of openings called **interventricular foramina** (fo-RAM-in-ah). The third ventricle is surrounded by the diencephalon. Continuing down from the third ventricle, a small canal, the **cerebral aqueduct**, extends through the midbrain into the fourth ventricle, which is located between the brain stem and the cerebellum. This ventricle is continuous with the central canal of the spinal cord. In the roof of the fourth ventricle are three openings that allow the escape of CSF to the area that surrounds the brain and spinal cord.

Box 10-1, The Blood–Brain Barrier: Access Denied, presents information on protecting the brain.

CHECKPOINT 10-3 ➤ In addition to the meninges, CSF helps to support and protect the brain and spinal cord. Where is CSF produced?

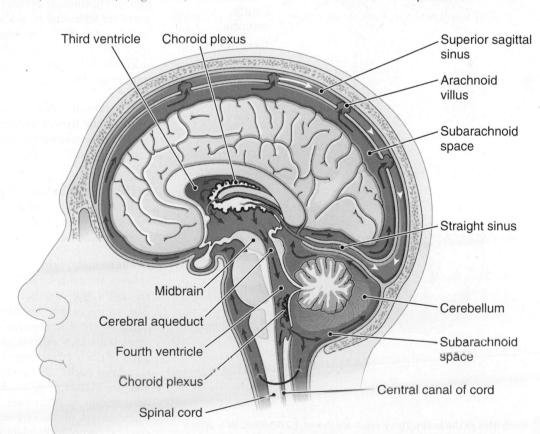

Figure 10-4 **Flow of cerebrospinal fluid (CSF).** Black arrows show the flow of CSF from the choroid plexuses and back to the blood in dural sinuses; white arrows show the flow of blood. (The actual passageways through which the CSF flows are narrower than those shown here, which have been enlarged for visibility.) **[ZOOMING IN ➤** Which ventricle is continuous with the central canal of the spinal cord? **]**

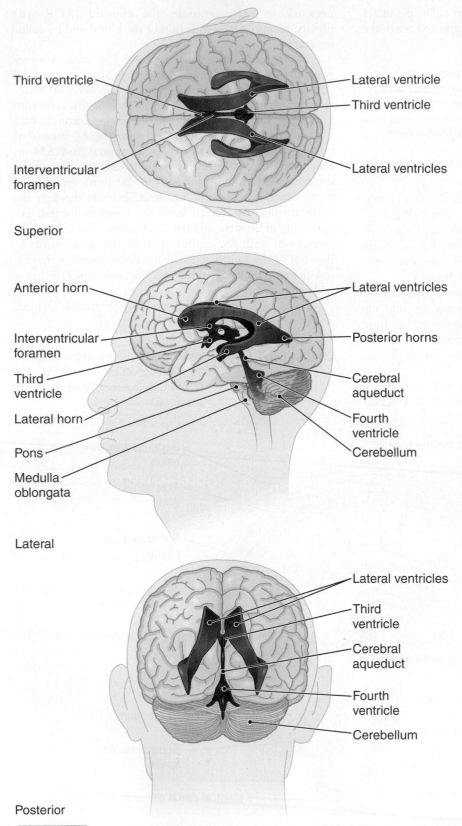

Third ventricle

Lateral ventricle

Third ventricle

Interventricular foramen

Lateral ventricles

Superior

Anterior horn

Lateral ventricles

Interventricular foramen

Posterior horns

Third ventricle

Cerebral aqueduct

Lateral horn

Fourth ventricle

Pons

Cerebellum

Medulla oblongata

Lateral

Lateral ventricles

Third ventricle

Cerebral aqueduct

Fourth ventricle

Cerebellum

Posterior

Figure 10-5 **Ventricles of the brain.** Three views are shown. [**ZOOMING IN ➤** Which are the largest ventricles?]

The Cerebral Hemispheres

Each cerebral hemisphere is divided into four visible **lobes** named for the overlying cranial bones. These are the frontal, parietal, temporal, and occipital lobes (Fig. 10-6). In addition, there is a small fifth lobe deep within each hemisphere that cannot be seen from the surface. Not much is known about this lobe, which is called the **insula** (IN-su-lah).

The outer nervous tissue of the cerebral hemispheres is gray matter that makes up the **cerebral cortex** (see Fig. 10-3). This thin layer of gray matter (2–4 mm thick) is the most highly evolved portion of the brain and is responsible for conscious thought, reasoning, and abstract mental functions. Specific functions are localized in the cortex of the different lobes, as described in greater detail later.

The cortex is arranged in folds forming elevated portions known as **gyri** (JI-ri), singular *gyrus*. These raised areas are separated by shallow grooves called **sulci** (SUL-si), singular *sulcus* (Fig. 10-7). Although there are many sulci, the following two are especially important landmarks:

- The **central sulcus**, which lies between the frontal and parietal lobes of each hemisphere at right angles to the longitudinal fissure (see Figs. 10-2 and 10-6)

- The **lateral sulcus**, which curves along the side of each hemisphere and separates the temporal lobe from the frontal and parietal lobes (see Fig. 10-6)

Internally, the cerebral hemispheres are made largely of white matter and a few islands of gray matter. The white matter consists of myelinated fibers that connect the cortical areas with each other and with other parts of the nervous system.

Basal nuclei, also called **basal ganglia**, are masses of gray matter located deep within each cerebral hemisphere. These groups of neurons work with the cerebral cortex to regulate body movement and the muscles of facial expression. The neurons of the basal nuclei secrete the neurotransmitter **dopamine** (DO-pah-mene).

Box 10-1   A Closer Look

The Blood–Brain Barrier: Access Denied

Neurons in the central nervous system (CNS) function properly only if the composition of the extracellular fluid bathing them is carefully regulated. The semipermeable blood–brain barrier helps maintain this stable environment by allowing some substances to cross it while blocking others. Whereas it allows glucose, amino acids, and some electrolytes to cross, it prevents passage of hormones, drugs, neurotransmitters, and other substances that might adversely affect the brain.

Structural features of CNS capillaries create this barrier. In most parts of the body, capillaries are lined with simple squamous epithelial cells that are loosely attached to each other. The small spaces between cells let materials move between the bloodstream and the tissues. In CNS capillaries, the simple squamous epithelial cells are joined by tight junctions that limit passage of materials between them. Astrocytes—specialized neuroglial cells that wrap around capillaries and limit their permeability—also contribute to this barrier.

The blood–brain barrier excludes pathogens, although some viruses, including poliovirus and herpesvirus, can bypass it by traveling along peripheral nerves into the CNS. Some streptococci also can breach the tight junctions. Disease processes, such as hypertension, ischemia (lack of blood supply), and inflammation, can increase the blood-brain barrier's permeability.

The blood–brain barrier is an obstacle to delivering drugs to the brain. Some antibiotics can cross it, whereas others cannot. Neurotransmitters also pose problems. In Parkinson disease, the neurotransmitter dopamine is deficient in the brain. Dopamine itself will not cross the barrier, but a related compound, L-dopa, will. L-dopa crosses the blood-brain barrier and is then converted to dopamine. Mixing a drug with a concentrated sugar solution and injecting it into the bloodstream is another effective delivery method. The solution's high osmotic pressure causes water to osmose out of capillary cells, shrinking them and opening tight junctions through which the drug can pass.

The **corpus callosum** (kah-LO-sum) is an important band of white matter located at the bottom of the longitudinal fissure (see Fig. 10-1). This band is a bridge between the right and left hemispheres, permitting impulses to cross from one side of the brain to the other.

The **internal capsule** is a compact band of myelinated fibers that carries impulses between the cerebral hemispheres and the brain stem. The vertical fibers that make up the internal capsule travel between the thalamus and some of the basal nuclei on each side and then radiate toward the cerebral cortex.

CHECKPOINT **10-4** ➤ What are the four surface lobes of each cerebral hemisphere?

Functions of the Cerebral Cortex

It is within the cerebral cortex, the layer of gray matter that forms the surface of

■ Frontal lobe   ■ Parietal lobe   ■ Temporal lobe   □ Occipital lobe

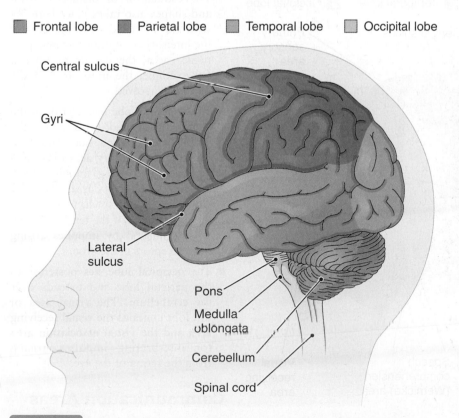

Figure 10-6 **External surface of the brain, lateral view.** The lobes and surface features of the cerebrum are visible. [**ZOOMING IN ➤** What structure separates the frontal from the parietal lobe?]

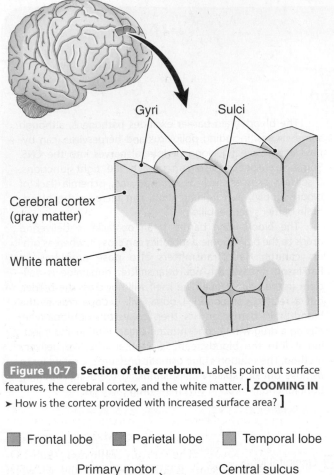

Figure 10-7 **Section of the cerebrum.** Labels point out surface features, the cerebral cortex, and the white matter. [**ZOOMING IN** ➤ How is the cortex provided with increased surface area?]

each cerebral hemisphere, that nerve impulses are received and analyzed. These activities form the basis of knowledge. The brain "stores" information, much of which can be recalled on demand by means of the phenomenon called *memory*. It is in the cerebral cortex that thought processes such as association, judgment, and discrimination take place. Conscious deliberation and voluntary actions also arise from the cerebral cortex.

Although the various brain areas act in coordination to produce behavior, particular functions are localized in the cortex of each lobe (Fig. 10-8). Some of these are described below:

■ The **frontal lobe**, which is relatively larger in humans than in any other organism, lies anterior to the central sulcus. The gyrus just anterior to the central sulcus in this lobe contains a **primary motor area**, which provides conscious control of skeletal muscles. Note that the more detailed the action, the greater the amount of cortical tissue involved (Fig. 10-9). The frontal lobe also contains two areas important in speech (the speech centers are discussed later).

■ The **parietal lobe** occupies the superior part of each hemisphere and lies posterior to the central sulcus. The gyrus just behind the central sulcus in this lobe contains the **primary sensory area**, where impulses from the skin, such as touch, pain, and temperature, are interpreted. The estimation of distances, sizes, and shapes also takes place here. As with the motor cortex, the greater the intensity of sensation from a particular area, the tongue or fingers, for example, the more area of the cortex is involved.

■ The **temporal lobe** lies inferior to the lateral sulcus and folds under the hemisphere on each side. This lobe contains the **auditory area** for receiving and interpreting impulses from the ear. The **olfactory area**, concerned with the sense of smell, is located in the medial part of the temporal lobe; it is stimulated by impulses arising from receptors in the nose.

■ The **occipital lobe** lies posterior to the parietal lobe and extends over the cerebellum. The visual area of this lobe contains the **visual receiving area** and the **visual association area** for interpreting impulses arising from the retina of the eye.

Communication Areas

The ability to communicate by written and verbal means is an interesting example of how areas of the cerebral cor-

Figure 10-8 **Functional areas of the cerebral cortex.** [**ZOOMING IN** ➤ What cortical area is posterior to the central sulcus? What area is anterior to the central sulcus?]

tongue, the soft palate, and the larynx are controlled here, in a region named the **motor speech area**, or **Broca** (bro-KAH) **area** (see Fig. 10-8). A person who suffers damage to this area may have difficulty in producing speech (motor aphasia). Similarly, the written speech center lies anterior to the cortical area that controls the arm and hand muscles. The ability to write words is usually one of the last phases in the development of learning words and their meanings.

- The **visual areas** of the occipital cortex are also involved in communication. Here, visual images of language are received. The visual area that lies anterior to the receiving cortex then interprets these visual impulses as words. The ability to read with understanding also develops in this area. You might *see* writing in the Japanese language, for example, but this would involve only the visual receiving area in the occipital lobe unless you could also *understand* the words.

There is a functional relation among areas of the brain. Many neurons must work together to enable a person to receive, interpret, and respond to verbal and written messages as well as to touch (tactile stimulus) and other sensory stimuli.

10

CHECKPOINT 10-5 ➤ Higher functions of the brain occur in a thin layer of gray matter on the surface of the cerebral hemispheres. What is the name of this outer layer of gray matter?

Memory and the Learning Process

Memory is the mental faculty for recalling ideas. In the initial stage of the memory process, sensory signals (e.g., visual, auditory) are retained for a very short time, perhaps only fractions of a second. Nevertheless, they can be used for further processing. **Short-term memory** refers to the retention of bits of information for a few seconds or perhaps a few minutes, after which the information is lost unless reinforced. **Long-term memory** refers to the storage of information that can be recalled at a later time. There is a tendency for a memory to become more fixed the more often a person repeats the remembered experience; thus, short-term memory signals can lead to long-term memories. Furthermore, the more often a memory is recalled, the more indelible it becomes; such a memory can be so deeply fixed in the brain that it can be recalled immediately.

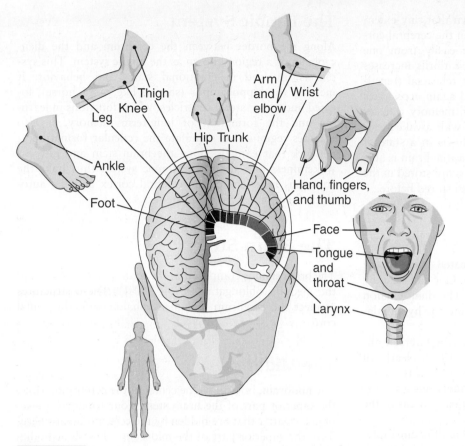

Figure 10-9 **Motor areas of the cerebral cortex (frontal lobe).** The amount of cortex involved in control of a body part is proportional to the degree of coordination needed in movement. The small figure indicates that control is contralateral. The right hemisphere controls the left side of the body and the left hemisphere controls the right side of the body.

tex are interrelated (see Fig. 10-8). The development and use of these areas are closely connected with the learning process.

- The **auditory areas** lie in the temporal lobe. One of these areas, the **auditory receiving area**, detects sound impulses transmitted from the environment, whereas the surrounding area, the **auditory association area**, interprets the sounds. Another region of the auditory cortex, the **speech comprehension area**, or **Wernicke** (VER-nih-ke) **area**, functions in speech recognition and the meaning of words. Someone who suffers damage in this region of the brain, as by a stroke, will have difficulty in understanding the meaning of speech. The beginnings of language are learned by hearing; thus, the auditory areas for understanding sounds are near the auditory receiving area of the cortex. Babies often appear to understand what is being said long before they do any talking themselves. It is usually several years before children learn to read or write words.

- The **motor areas** for spoken and written communication lie anterior to the most inferior part of the frontal lobe's motor cortex. The speech muscles in the

Careful anatomic studies have shown that tiny extensions called *fibrils* form at the synapses in the cerebral cortex, enabling impulses to travel more easily from one neuron to another. The number of these fibrils increases with age. Physiologic studies show that rehearsal (repetition) of the same information again and again accelerates and potentiates the degree of short-term memory transfer into long-term memory. A person who is wide awake memorizes far better than does a person who is in a state of mental fatigue. It has also been noted that the brain is able to organize information so that new ideas are stored in the same areas in which similar ones had been stored before.

The Diencephalon

The **diencephalon**, or interbrain, is located between the cerebral hemispheres and the brain stem. One can see it by cutting into the brain's central section. The diencephalon includes the **thalamus** (THAL-ah-mus) and the **hypothalamus** (Fig. 10-10).

The two parts of the thalamus form the lateral walls of the third ventricle (see Figs. 10-1 and 10-5). Nearly all sensory impulses travel through the masses of gray matter that form the thalamus. The role of the thalamus is to sort out the impulses and direct them to particular areas of the cerebral cortex.

The hypothalamus is located in the midline area inferior to the thalamus and forms the floor of the third ventricle. It helps to maintain homeostasis by controlling body temperature, water balance, sleep, appetite, and some emotions, such as fear and pleasure. Both the sympathetic and parasympathetic divisions of the autonomic nervous system are under hypothalamic control, as is the pituitary gland. The hypothalamus thus influences the heartbeat, the contraction and relaxation of blood vessels, hormone secretion, and other vital body functions.

CHECKPOINT 10-6 ➤ What are the two main portions of the diencephalon and what do they do?

Figure 10-10 **Regions of the diencephalon.** The figure shows the relationship among the thalamus, hypothalamus, and pituitary gland (hypophysis). **[ZOOMING IN ➤** To what part of the brain is the pituitary gland attached? **]**

Labels in figure:
Hypothalamus
Thalamus
Pituitary gland (hypophysis)
Diencephalon

The Limbic System

Along the border between the cerebrum and the diencephalon is a region known as the **limbic system**. This system is involved in emotional states and behavior. It includes the **hippocampus** (shaped like a sea horse), located under the lateral ventricles, which functions in learning and the formation of long-term memory. It also includes regions that stimulate the **reticular formation**, a network that extends along the brain stem and governs wakefulness and sleep. The limbic system thus links the conscious functions of the cerebral cortex and the automatic functions of the brain stem.

The Brain Stem

The brain stem is composed of the midbrain, the pons, and the medulla oblongata (see Fig. 10-1). These structures connect the cerebrum and diencephalon with the spinal cord.

The Midbrain

The **midbrain**, inferior to the center of the cerebrum, forms the superior part of the brain stem. Four rounded masses of gray matter that are hidden by the cerebral hemispheres form the superior part of the midbrain. These four bodies act as centers for certain reflexes involving the eye and the ear, for example, moving the eyes in order to track an image or to read. The white matter at the anterior of the midbrain conducts impulses between the higher centers of the cerebrum and the lower centers of the pons, medulla, cerebellum, and spinal cord. Cranial nerves III and IV originate from the midbrain.

The Pons

The **pons** lies between the midbrain and the medulla, anterior to the cerebellum (see Fig. 10-1). It is composed largely of myelinated nerve fibers, which connect the two halves of the cerebellum with the brain stem as well as with the cerebrum above and the spinal cord below. (Its name means "bridge.")

The pons is an important connecting link between the cerebellum and the rest of the nervous system, and it contains nerve fibers that carry impulses to and from the centers located above and below it. Certain reflex (involuntary) actions, such as some of those regulating respiration, are integrated in the pons. Cranial nerves V through VIII originate from the pons.

The Medulla Oblongata

The **medulla oblongata** of the brain stem is located between the pons and the spinal cord (see Fig. 10-1). It appears white externally because, like the pons, it contains many myelinated nerve fibers. Internally, it contains collections of cell bodies (gray matter) called **nuclei**, or *centers*. Among these are vital centers, such as the following:

■ The **respiratory center** controls the muscles of respiration in response to chemical and other stimuli.

■ The **cardiac center** helps regulate the rate and force of the heartbeat.

■ The **vasomotor** (vas-o-MO-tor) **center** regulates the contraction of smooth muscle in the blood vessel walls and thus controls blood flow and blood pressure.

The ascending sensory fibers that carry messages through the spinal cord up to the brain travel through the medulla, as do descending motor fibers. These groups of fibers form tracts (bundles) and are grouped together according to function.

The motor fibers from the motor cortex of the cerebral hemispheres extend down through the medulla, and most of them cross from one side to the other (decussate) while going through this part of the brain. The crossing of motor fibers in the medulla results in contralateral control—the right cerebral hemisphere controls muscles in the left side of the body and the left cerebral hemisphere controls muscles in the right side of the body, a characteristic termed *contralateral* (opposite side) *control*.

The medulla is an important reflex center; here, certain neurons end, and impulses are relayed to other neurons. The last four pairs of cranial nerves (IX through XII) are connected with the medulla.

CHECKPOINT 10-7 ➤ What are the three subdivisions of the brain stem?

The Cerebellum

The **cerebellum** is made up of three parts: the middle portion (vermis) and two lateral hemispheres, the left and right (Fig. 10-11). Like the cerebral hemispheres, the cerebellum has an outer area of gray matter and an inner portion that is largely white matter. However, the white matter is distributed in a treelike pattern. The functions of the cerebellum are as follows:

■ Help coordinate voluntary muscles to ensure smooth, orderly function. Disease of the cerebellum causes muscular jerkiness and tremors.

■ Help maintain balance in standing, walking, and sitting as well as during more strenuous activities. Messages from the internal ear and from sensory receptors in tendons and muscles aid the cerebellum.

■ Help maintain muscle tone so that all muscle fibers are slightly tensed and ready to produce changes in position as quickly as necessary.

CHECKPOINT 10-8 ➤ What are some functions of the cerebellum?

Brain Studies

Some of the imaging techniques used to study the brain are described in Box 1-2, Medical Imaging: Seeing Without Making a Cut, in Chapter 1. These techniques include:

■ CT (computed tomography) scan, which provides photographs of the bone, soft tissue, and cavities of the brain (Fig. 10-12A). Anatomic lesions, such as tumors or scar tissue accumulations, are readily seen.

■ MRI (magnetic resonance imaging), which gives more views of the brain than CT and may reveal tumors, scar tissue, and hemorrhaging not shown by CT (see Fig. 10-12B).

■ PET (positron emission tomography), which visualizes the brain in action (see Fig. 10-12C).

The Electroencephalograph

The interactions of the brain's billions of nerve cells give rise to measurable electric currents. These may be recorded using an instrument called the **electroencephalograph** (e-lek-tro-en-SEF-ah-lo-graf). Electrodes placed on the head pick up the electrical signals produced as the brain functions. These signals are then amplified and recorded to produce the tracings, or brain waves, of an electroencephalogram (EEG).

The electroencephalograph is used to study sleep patterns, to diagnose disease, such as epilepsy, to locate tumors, to study the effects of drugs, and to determine brain death. Figure 10-13 shows some typical normal and abnormal tracings.

Disorders of the Brain and Associated Structures

Infection and other factors can cause inflammation of the brain and its protective structures. **Meningitis** (men-in-JI-tis) is an inflammation of the meninges, the coverings of the brain and spinal cord. It is usually caused by bacteria that enter through the ear, nose, or throat, or are carried by the blood. In many cases, an injury, invasive procedure, septicemia (blood infection), or an adjoining infection allows the entry of pathogenic organisms. One of these organisms, the meningococcus (*Neisseria meningitidis*) is responsible for epidemics of meningitis among people living in close quarters. Other causative bacteria are *Haemophilus influenzae* (Hib), *Streptococcus pneumoniae*, and *Escherichia coli*. Some viruses, including the mumps virus, can cause meningitis, but usually produce mild forms of the disease that require no treatment.

Headache, stiff neck, nausea, and vomiting are common symptoms of meningitis. Diagnosis is by lumbar puncture and examination of the CSF for pathogens and white blood cells (pus). In cases of bacterial meningitis, early treatment with antibiotics can have good results.

10

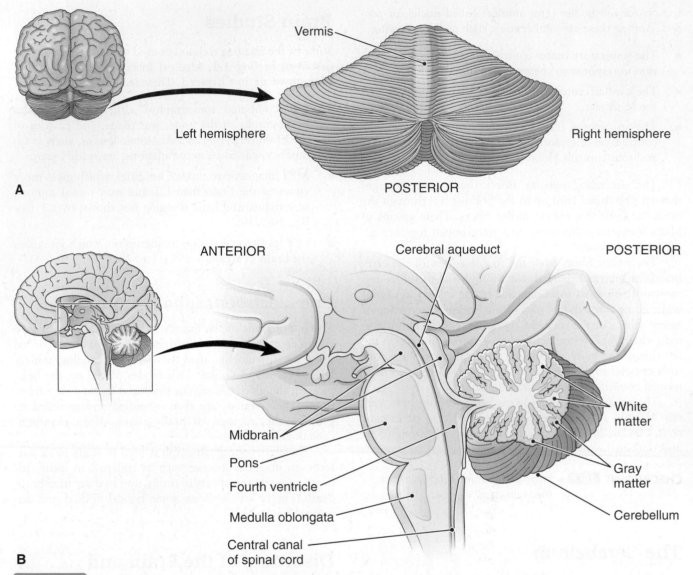

A

Vermis

Left hemisphere

Right hemisphere

POSTERIOR

ANTERIOR

Cerebral aqueduct

POSTERIOR

Midbrain

Pons

Fourth ventricle

Medulla oblongata

Central canal
of spinal cord

White
matter

Gray
matter

Cerebellum

B

Figure 10-11 **The cerebellum. (A)** Posterior view showing the two hemispheres. **(B)** Midsagittal section showing the distribution of gray and white matter. The three parts of the brain stem (midbrain, pons, and medulla oblongata) are also labeled.

Untreated cases have a high death rate. Vaccines are available against some of the bacteria that cause meningitis.

Inflammation of the brain is termed **encephalitis** (en-sef-ah-LI-tis), based on the scientific name for the brain, which is *encephalon*. Infectious agents that cause encephalitis include poliovirus, rabies virus, HIV (the cause of AIDS), insect-borne viruses, such as West Nile virus, and, rarely, the viruses that cause chickenpox and measles. Less frequently, exposure to toxic substances or reactions to certain viral vaccines can cause encephalitis. Brain swelling and diffuse nerve cell destruction accompany invasion of the brain by lymphocytes (white blood cells) in cases of encephalitis. Typical symptoms include fever, vomiting, and coma.

Hydrocephalus

An abnormal accumulation of CSF within the brain is termed **hydrocephalus** (hi-dro-SEF-ah-lus) (Fig. 10-14). It may result either from overproduction or impaired drainage of the fluid. As CSF accumulates in the ventricles or its transport channels, mounting pressure can squeeze the brain against the skull and destroy brain tissue. Possible causes include congenital malformations present during development, tumors, inflammation, or hemorrhage.

Hydrocephalus is more common in infants than in adults. Because the skull's fontanels have not closed in the developing infant, the cranium itself can become greatly enlarged. In contrast, in the adult, cranial enlargement cannot occur, so that even a slight increase in fluid results in symp-

Figure 10-12 **Imaging the brain. (A)** CT scan of a normal adult brain at the level of the fourth ventricle. **(B)** MRI of the brain showing a point of injury (arrows). **(C)** PET scan. (A and B, reprinted with permission from Erkonen WE. *Radiology 101*. Philadelphia: Lippincott Williams & Wilkins, 1998; C, Courtesy of Newport Diagnostic Center, Newport Beach, CA.)

toms of increased pressure within the skull and brain damage. Treatment of hydrocephalus involves the creation of a shunt (bypass) to drain excess CSF from the brain.

Stroke and Other Brain Disorders

Stroke, or **cerebrovascular** (ser-e-bro-VAS-ku-lar) **accident** (CVA), is by far the most common kind of brain disorder. The most common cause is a blood clot that blocks blood flow to an area of brain tissue. Another frequent cause is the rupture of a blood vessel resulting in **cerebral hemorrhage** (HEM-eh-rij) and destruction of

brain tissue. Stroke is most common among people older than 40 years of age and those with arterial wall damage, diabetes, or hypertension (high blood pressure). Smoking and excess alcohol consumption also increase the risk of stroke. Restoring blood flow to the affected area can reduce long-term damage. This can be done surgically or by administration of clot-dissolving medication, usually followed by medication to reduce brain swelling and minimize further damage.

A stroke's effect depends on the location of the artery and the extent of the involvement. Damage to the internal capsule's white matter in the inferior part of the cerebrum

10

Figure 10-13 **Electroencephalography. (A)** Normal brain waves. **(B)** Abnormal brain waves.

A   **B**

Figure 10-14 **Hydrocephalus. (A)** Congenital hydrocephalus causing pronounced enlargement of the head. **(B)** Coronal section of the brain showing marked enlargement of the lateral ventricles caused by a tumor that obstructed the flow of CSF. (Reprinted with permission from Rubin E, Farber JL. *Pathology*, 3rd ed. Philadelphia: Lippincott Williams & Wilkins, 1999.)

may cause extensive paralysis of the side opposite the affected area.

One possible aftereffect of stroke or other brain injury is **aphasia** (ah-FA-ze-ah), a loss or defect in language communication. Losses may involve the ability to speak or write (expressive aphasia) or to understand written or spoken language (receptive aphasia). The type of aphasia present depends on what part of the brain is affected. The lesion that causes aphasia in the right-handed person is likely to be in the left cerebral hemisphere.

Often, much can be done for stroke victims by care and retraining. The brain has tremendous reserves for adapting to different conditions. In many cases, some means of communication can be found even though speech areas are damaged.

Cerebral palsy (PAWL-ze) is a disorder caused by brain damage occurring before or during the birth process. Characteristics include diverse muscular disorders that vary in degree from only slight weakness of the lower extremity muscles to paralysis of all four extremities as well as the speech muscles. With muscle and speech training and other therapeutic approaches, children with cerebral palsy can be helped.

Epilepsy is a chronic disorder involving an abnormality of the brain's electrical activity with or without apparent changes in the nervous tissues. One manifestation of epilepsy is seizure activity, which may be so mild that it is hardly noticeable or so severe that it results in loss of consciousness. In most cases, the cause is not known. An EEG study of brain waves usually shows abnormalities and is helpful in both diagnosis and treatment (see Fig. 10-13B). Many people with epilepsy can lead normal, active lives with appropriate medical treatment.

Tumors of the brain may develop in people of any age but are somewhat more common in young and middle-aged

adults than in other groups (Fig. 10-15). Most brain tumors originate from the neuroglia (support tissue of the brain) and are called **gliomas** (gli-O-mas). Such tumors tend not to metastasize (spread to other areas), but they nevertheless can do harm by compressing brain tissue. The symptoms produced depend on the type of tumor, its location, and its degree of destructiveness. Involvement of the cerebrum's frontal portion often causes mental symptoms, such as changes in personality and in levels of consciousness.

Figure 10-15 **Brain tumor.** MRI shows a large tumor that arises from the cerebellum and pushes the brain stem forward. (Reprinted with permission from Erkonen WE. *Radiology 101*. Philadelphia: Lippincott Williams & Wilkins, 1998.)

Early surgery and radiation therapy offer hope of cure in some cases. The blood-brain barrier, however, limits the effectiveness of injected chemotherapeutic agents (see Box 10-1). A newer approach to chemotherapy for brain tumors is to implant timed-release drugs into a tumor site at the time of surgery.

CHECKPOINT 10-9 ➤ What is the common term for cerebrovascular accident (CVA)?

CHECKPOINT 10-10 ➤ What type of cells are commonly involved in brain tumors?

PASSport to Success
Visit *thePoint* or see the Student Resource CD in the back of this book to view the animation *Stroke*, which illustrates this disorder.

Injury

A common result of head trauma is bleeding into or around the meninges (Fig. 10-16). Damage to an artery from a skull fracture, usually on the side of the head, may result in bleeding between the dura mater and the skull, an **epidural hematoma** (he-mah-TO-mah). The rapidly accumulating blood puts pressure on blood vessels and interrupts blood flow to the brain. Symptoms include headache, partial paralysis, dilated pupils, and coma. If the pressure is not relieved within a day or two, death results.

A tear in the wall of a dural sinus causes a **subdural hematoma**. This often results from a blow to the front or back of the head that separates the dura from the arachnoid, as occurs when the moving head hits a stationary object. Blood gradually accumulates in the subdural space, putting pressure on the brain and causing headache, weakness, and confusion. Death results from continued bleeding. Bleeding into the brain tissue itself results in an intracerebral hematoma.

Cerebral **concussion** (kon-CUSH-on) results from a blow to the head or from sudden movement of the brain against the skull, as in violent shaking. The effects include loss of consciousness, headache, dizziness, vomiting, and even paralysis and impaired brain function. These vary in length and severity with the degree of damage.

Frequent observations of level of consciousness, pupil response, and extremity reflexes are important in the patient with a head injury (see Box 10-2, Brain Injury: A Heads-Up).

Degenerative Diseases

Alzheimer (ALZ-hi-mer) **disease** is a brain disorder resulting from an unexplained degeneration of the cerebral cortex and hippocampus (Fig. 10-17). The disorder develops gradually and eventually causes severe intellectual impairment with mood changes and confusion. Memory loss, especially for recent events, is a common early symptom. Dangers associated with Alzheimer disease are injury, infection, malnutrition, and inhalation of food or fluids into the lungs. Changes in the brain occur many years before noticeable signs of the disease appear. These changes include the development of amyloid, an abnormal protein, and a tangling of neuron fibers that prevents communication between cells.

At present, there is no cure, but several drugs have been developed that can delay the progression of early disease. In some tests, herbal extracts of *Ginkgo biloba*, the hormone estrogen, vitamin E, antiinflammatory drugs, and calcium channel blockers (drugs used primarily to regulate the heartbeat) have shown some signs of preventing or delaying the disease. Drugs also can control some of its physical and behavioral effects. Stress reduction is an important part of patient care.

Multi-infarct dementia (de-MEN-she-ah) represents the accumulation of brain damage resulting from chronic ischemia (is-KE-me-ah) (lack of blood supply), such as would be caused by a series of small strokes. There is a stepwise deterioration of function. People with multi-infarct dementia are troubled by progressive loss of memory, judgment, and cognitive function. Many people older than 80 years of age have some evidence of this disorder.

Epidural hematoma   Subdural hematoma   Intracerebral hematoma

Figure 10-16 Hematomas. Compare the locations of epidural, subdural, and intracerebral hematomas. (Reprinted with permission from Cohen BJ. *Medical Terminology*, 4th ed. Philadelphia: Lippincott Williams & Wilkins, 2004.)

Box 10-2 | **Clinical Perspectives**

Brain Injury: A Heads-Up

Traumatic brain injury is a leading cause of death and disability in the United States. Each year, approximately 1.5 million Americans sustain a brain injury, of whom about 50,000 will die and 80,000 will suffer long-term or permanent disability. The leading causes of traumatic brain injury are motor vehicle accidents, gunshot wounds, and falls. Other causes include shaken baby syndrome (caused by violent shaking of an infant or toddler) and second impact syndrome (when a second head injury occurs before the first has fully healed).

Brain damage occurs either from penetrating head trauma or acceleration-deceleration events where a head in motion suddenly comes to a stop. Nervous tissue, blood vessels, and possibly the meninges may be bruised, torn, lacerated, or ruptured, which may lead to swelling, hemorrhage, and hematoma. The best protection from brain injury is to prevent it. The following is a list of safety tips:

- Always wear a seat belt and secure children in approved car seats.
- Never drive after using alcohol or drugs or ride with an impaired driver.
- Always wear a helmet during activities such as biking, motorcycling, in-line skating, horseback riding, football, ice hockey, and batting and running bases in baseball and softball.
- Inspect playground equipment and supervise children using it. Never swing children around to play "airplane," nor vigorously bounce or shake them.
- Allow adequate time for healing after a head injury before resuming potentially dangerous activities.
- Prevent falls by using a nonslip bathtub or shower mat and using a step stool to reach objects on high shelves. Use a safety gate at the bottom and top of stairs to protect young children (and adults with dementia or other disorienting conditions).
- Keep unloaded firearms in a locked cabinet or safe and store bullets in a separate location.

For more information, contact the Brain Injury Association of America.

A   B

Figure 10-17 **Effects of Alzheimer disease. (A)** Normal brain. **(B)** Brain of a patient with Alzheimer disease shows atrophy of the cortex with narrow gyri and enlarged sulci. (Reprinted with permission from Rubin E, Farber JL. *Pathology*, 3rd ed. Philadelphia: Lippincott Williams & Wilkins, 1999.)

Parkinson disease is a progressive neurologic condition characterized by tremors, rigidity of limbs and joints, slow movement, and impaired balance. The disease usually arises from cell death in a part of the brain, the substantia nigra, that produces the neurotransmitter dopamine. The lack of dopamine results in overactivity of the basal nuclei, brain areas that control voluntary movement. The average age of onset is 55 years. Similar changes, together known as *parkinsonism*, may result from encephalitis or other brain diseases, exposure to certain toxins, or repeated head injury, as may occur in boxing.

The main therapy for Parkinson disease is administration of L-dopa, a substance that is capable of entering the brain and converting to dopamine (see Box 10-1). Drugs are now available that mimic the effects of dopamine, prevent its breakdown, or increase the effectiveness of L-dopa. Other approaches to treatment include implanting fetal cells that can do the missing cells' job and implanting a device that electrically stimulates the brain to control symptoms of Parkinson disease.

PASSport to Success

Speech therapists help to treat patients with language or communication problems from any cause. Visit *thePoint* or see the Student Resource CD in the back of this book for more information on this career.

Cranial Nerves

There are 12 pairs of cranial nerves (in this discussion, when a cranial nerve is identified, a pair is meant). They are numbered, usually in Roman numerals, according to their connection with the brain, beginning anteriorly and proceeding posteriorly (Fig. 10-18). Except for the first two pairs, all the cranial nerves arise from the brain stem. The first 9 pairs and the 12th pair supply structures in the head.

From a functional viewpoint, we may think of cranial nerve messages as belonging to one of four categories:

- **Special sensory impulses,** such as those for smell, taste, vision, and hearing, located in special sense organs in the head.

- **General sensory impulses,** such as those for pain, touch, temperature, deep muscle sense, pressure, and vibrations. These impulses come from receptors that are widely distributed throughout the body.

- **Somatic motor impulses** resulting in voluntary control of skeletal muscles.

- **Visceral motor impulses** producing involuntary control of glands and involuntary muscles (cardiac and smooth muscle). These motor pathways are part of the autonomic nervous system, parasympathetic division.

Names and Functions of the Cranial Nerves

A few of the cranial nerves (I, II, and VIII) contain only sensory fibers; some (III, IV, VI, XI, and XII) contain all or mostly motor fibers. The remainder (V, VII, IX, and X) contain both sensory and motor fibers; they are known as *mixed nerves*. All 12 nerves are listed below and summarized in Table 10-2:

I. The **olfactory nerve** carries smell impulses from receptors in the nasal mucosa to the brain.

II. The **optic nerve** carries visual impulses from the eye to the brain.

III. The **oculomotor nerve** is concerned with the contraction of most of the eye muscles.

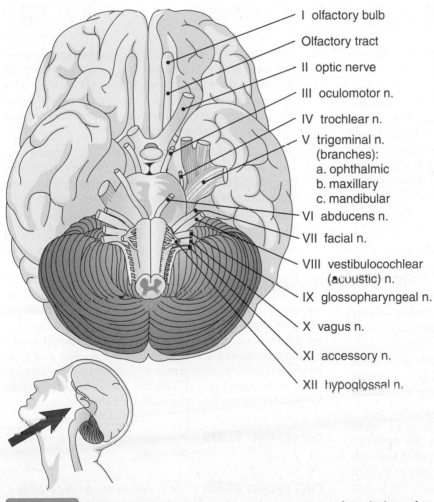

I olfactory bulb
   Olfactory tract
II optic nerve
III oculomotor n.
IV trochlear n.
V trigeminal n.
   (branches):
   a. ophthalmic
   b. maxillary
   c. mandibular
VI abducens n.
VII facial n.
VIII vestibulocochlear
   (acoustic) n.
IX glossopharyngeal n.
X vagus n.
XI accessory n.
XII hypoglossal n.

Figure 10-18 **Cranial nerves.** The 12 pairs of cranial nerves are seen from the base of the brain.

Table 10-2 The Cranial Nerves and Their Functions

Nerve (Roman numeral designation)	Name	Function
I	Olfactory	Carries impulses for the sense of smell toward the brain
II	Optic	Carries visual impulses from the eye to the brain
III	Oculomotor	Controls contraction of eye muscles
IV	Trochlear	Supplies one eyeball muscle
V	Trigeminal	Carries sensory impulses from eye, upper jaw, and lower jaw toward the brain
VI	Abducens	Controls an eyeball muscle
VII	Facial	Controls muscles of facial expression; carries sensation of taste; stimulates small salivary glands and lacrimal (tear) gland
VIII	Vestibulocochlear	Carries sensory impulses for hearing and equilibrium from the inner ear toward the brain
IX	Glossopharyngeal	Carries sensory impulses from tongue and pharynx (throat); controls swallowing muscles and stimulates the parotid salivary gland
X	Vagus	Supplies most of the organs in the thoracic and abdominal cavities; carries motor impulses to the larynx (voice box) and pharynx
XI	Accessory	Controls muscles in the neck and larynx
XII	Hypoglossal	Controls muscles of the tongue

IV. The **trochlear** (TROK-le-ar) **nerve** supplies one eyeball muscle.

V. The **trigeminal** (tri-JEM-in-al) **nerve** is the great sensory nerve of the face and head. It has three branches that transport general sense impulses (e.g., pain, touch, temperature) from the eye, the upper jaw, and the lower jaw. Motor fibers to the muscles of mastication (chewing) join the third branch. It is branches of the trigeminal nerve that a dentist anesthetizes to work on the teeth without causing pain.

VI. The **abducens** (ab-DU-senz) **nerve** is another nerve sending controlling impulses to an eyeball muscle.

VII. The **facial nerve** is largely motor. The muscles of facial expression are all supplied by branches from the facial nerve. This nerve also includes special sensory fibers for taste (anterior two-thirds of the tongue), and it contains secretory fibers to the smaller salivary glands (the submandibular and sublingual) and to the lacrimal (tear) gland.

VIII. The **vestibulocochlear** (ves-tib-u-lo-KOK-le-ar) **nerve** carries sensory impulses for hearing and equilibrium from the inner ear. This nerve was formerly called the auditory or acoustic nerve.

IX. The **glossopharyngeal** (glos-o-fah-RIN-je-al) **nerve** contains general sensory fibers from the posterior tongue and the pharynx (throat). This nerve also contains sensory fibers for taste from the posterior third of the tongue, secretory fibers that supply the largest salivary gland (parotid), and motor nerve fibers to control the swallowing muscles in the pharynx.

X. The **vagus** (VA-gus) **nerve** is the longest cranial nerve. (Its name means "wanderer.") It supplies most of the organs in the thoracic and abdominal cavities. This nerve also contains motor fibers to the larynx (voice box) and pharynx and to glands that produce digestive juices and other secretions.

XI. The **accessory nerve** (formerly called the *spinal accessory nerve*) is a motor nerve with two branches. One branch controls two muscles of the neck, the trapezius and sternocleidomastoid; the other supplies muscles of the larynx.

XII. The **hypoglossal nerve**, the last of the 12 cranial nerves, carries impulses controlling the tongue muscles.

It has been traditional in medical schools for students to use mnemonics (ne-MON-iks), or memory devices, to remember anatomic lists. As an aside, part of the tradition was that these devices be bawdy. The original mnemonic for the names of the cranial nerves no longer applies, as a few of the names have been changed. Can you and your classmates make up a mnemonic phrase using the first letter of each cranial nerve? You can also check the Internet for sites where medical mnemonics are shared.

CHECKPOINT 10-11 ➤ How many pairs of cranial nerves are there?

CHECKPOINT 10-12 ➤ The cranial nerves are classified as being sensory, motor, or mixed. What is a mixed nerve?

Disorders Involving the Cranial Nerves

Destruction of optic nerve (II) fibers may result from increased pressure of the eye's fluid on the nerves, as occurs in glaucoma, from the effect of poisons, and from some infections. Certain medications, when used in high doses over long periods, can damage the branch of the vestibulocochlear nerve responsible for hearing.

Injury to a nerve that contains motor fibers causes paralysis of the muscles supplied by these fibers. The oculomotor nerve (III) may be damaged by certain infections or various poisonous substances. Because this nerve supplies so many muscles connected with the eye, including the levator, which raises the eyelid, injury to it causes a paralysis that usually interferes with eye function.

Bell palsy is a facial paralysis caused by damage to the facial nerve (VII), usually on one side of the face. This injury results in facial distortion because of one-sided paralysis of the muscles of facial expression.

Neuralgia (nu-RAL-je-ah) in general means "nerve pain." A severe spasmodic pain affecting the fifth cranial nerve is known as **trigeminal neuralgia** or **tic douloureux** (tik du-lu-RU) (from French, meaning "painful twitch"). At first, the pain comes at relatively long intervals, but as time goes on, intervals between episodes usually shorten while pain durations lengthen. Treatments include microsurgery and high-frequency current.

Aging of the Nervous System

The nervous system is one of the first systems to develop in the embryo. By the beginning of the third week of development, the rudiments of the central nervous system have appeared. Beginning with maturity, the nervous system begins to undergo changes. The brain begins to decrease in size and weight due to a loss of cells, especially in the cerebral cortex, accompanied by decreases in synapses and neurotransmitters. The speed of processing information decreases, and movements are slowed. Memory diminishes, especially for recent events. Changes in the vascular system throughout the body with a narrowing of the arteries (atherosclerosis) reduce the brain's blood flow. Vascular degeneration increases the likelihood of stroke.

Much individual variation is possible, however, with regard to location and severity of changes. Although age might make it harder to acquire new skills, tests have shown that practice enhances skill retention. As with other body systems, the nervous system has vast reserves, and most elderly people are able to cope with life's demands.

10

Disease in Context revisited

➤ Frank's Stroke Recovery

"Good morning Mr. Carter. My name is Ross Baker and I'm a physiotherapist with the Brain Injury Team. My job is to assist your stroke recovery by helping you regain your strength, balance, and coordination. Before we continue, may I test your muscular and sensory functions?"

With Frank's permission, the physiotherapist began his assessment. He noted hemiplegia (muscle paralysis) in Frank's right arm and leg. Stroke damage to the primary motor area in the frontal lobe of Frank's *left* cerebral hemisphere had caused motor deficits in his *right* limbs. Loss of contralateral control is typical in stroke patients because most motor fibers from the cerebral cortex cross over (decussate) from one side of the medulla oblongata to the other before continuing down the spinal cord in descending tracts. For Frank, this meant that motor information from his damaged left cerebral hemisphere was not reaching the skeletal muscles of his right limbs.

The physiotherapist also noted a diminished sense of touch (hypesthesia) on Frank's right side, which suggested that the stroke had damaged the left parietal lobe's primary sensory area as well. Like motor deficits, contralateral sensory deficits are typical in stroke patients because sensory fibers that enter one side of the spinal cord immediately cross over to the opposite side before continuing up the cord in ascending pathways. As a result, sensory information from Frank's right side was not processed in his left cerebral cortex.

Ross used his understanding of brain and spinal cord anatomy to make sense of Frank's symptoms. Based on his assessment of Frank's motor and sensory deficits, Ross will devise and implement a rehabilitation plan for him. Other allied health professionals like occupational and speech therapists will also help Frank recover from his stroke. See *thePoint* or see the Student Resource CD in the back of this book for more information on these and other health professions careers.

Word Anatomy

Medical terms are built from standardized word parts (prefixes, roots, and suffixes). Learning the meanings of these parts can help you remember words and interpret unfamiliar terms.

WORD PART	MEANING	EXAMPLE
Protective Structures of the Brain and Spinal Cord		
cerebr/o	brain	*Cerebrospinal* fluid circulates around the brain and spinal cord.
chori/o	membrane	The *choroid* plexus is the vascular membrane in the ventricle that produces CSF.
gyr/o	circle	A *gyrus* is a circular raised area on the surface of the brain.
encephal/o	brain	The *diencephalon* is the part of the brain located between the cerebral hemispheres and the brain stem.
contra-	opposed, against	The cerebral cortex has *contralateral* control of motor function.
later/o	lateral, side	See preceding example.
Brain Studies		
tom/o	cut	*Tomography* is a method for viewing sections as if cut through the body.
Disorders of the Brain and Associated Structures		
cephal/o	head	*Hydrocephalus* is the accumulation of fluid within the brain.
-rhage	bursting forth	A cerebral *hemorrhage* is a sudden bursting forth of blood in the brain.
phasia	speech, ability to talk	*Aphasia* is a loss or defect in language communication.
Cranial Nerves		
gloss/o	tongue	The *hypoglossal* nerve controls muscles of the tongue.

Summary

I. **THE BRAIN**
  A. Main parts—cerebrum, diencephalon, brain stem, cerebellum

II. **PROTECTIVE STRUCTURES OF THE BRAIN AND SPINAL CORD**
  A. Meninges
    1. Dura mater—tough outermost layer
    2. Arachnoid—weblike middle layer
    3. Pia mater—vascular innermost layer
  B. Cerebrospinal fluid (CSF)
    1. Circulates around and within brain and spinal cord
    2. Cushions and protects
    3. Ventricles—four spaces within brain where CSF is produced
      a. Choroid plexus—vascular network in ventricle that produces CSF

III. **THE CEREBRAL HEMISPHERES**
  A. Structure
    1. Two hemispheres
    2. Lobes—frontal, parietal, temporal, occipital, insula
    3. Cortex—outer layer of gray matter
      a. In gyri (folds) and sulci (grooves)
      b. Specialized functions—interpretation, memory, conscious thought, judgment, voluntary actions
    4. Basal nuclei (ganglia)—regulate movement and facial expression
    5. Corpus callosum—band of white matter connecting cerebral hemispheres
    6. Internal capsule—connects each cerebral hemisphere to lower parts of brain
  B. Functions of the cerebral cortex
  C. Communication areas
  D. Memory and the learning process

IV. **DIENCEPHALON**—Area between cerebral hemispheres and brain stem
  A. Thalamus—directs sensory impulses to cortex
  B. Hypothalamus—maintains homeostasis, controls pituitary
  C. Limbic system
    1. Contains parts of cerebrum and diencephalon
    2. Controls emotion and behavior

V. **BRAIN STEM**
  A. Midbrain—involved in eye and ear reflexes
  B. Pons—connecting link for other divisions
  C. Medulla oblongata
    1. Connects with spinal cord
    2. Contains vital centers for respiration, heart rate, vasomotor activity

VI. **THE CEREBELLUM**—Regulates coordination, balance, muscle tone

VII. **BRAIN STUDIES**
  A. Imaging—computed tomography (CT), magnetic resonance imaging (MRI), positron emission tomography (PET)
  B. Electroencephalograph (EEG)—measures electrical waves produced as brain functions

VIII. **DISORDERS OF THE BRAIN AND ASSOCIATED STRUCTURES**
  A. Inflammation
    1. Meningitis—inflammation of the meninges
    2. Encephalitis—inflammation of the brain
  B. Hydrocephalus—abnormal accumulation of CSF
  C. Stroke and other brain disorders
    1. Cerebrovascular accident (CVA); stroke
      a. Causes—cerebral hemorrhage, blood clot
      b. Effects—paralysis, aphasia
    2. Cerebral palsy—cause is brain damage before or during birth
    3. Epilepsy—characterized by seizures
    4. Tumors—usually involve neuroglia (gliomas)
  D. Injury
    1. Often results in hematoma—accumulation of blood
    2. Concussion—caused by sudden blow
  E. Degenerative diseases
    1. Alzheimer disease—degeneration of cerebral cortex and hippocampus
    2. Multi-infarct dementia—caused by many small strokes
    3. Parkinson disease—deficiency of neurotransmitter dopamine

IX. **CRANIAL NERVES**
  A. 12 pairs attached to brain
  B. Functions
    1. Carry special and general sensory impulses
    2. Carry somatic and visceral motor impulses
  C. Types
    1. Sensory (I, II, VIII)
    2. Motor (III, IV, VI, XI, XII)
    3. Mixed (V, VII, IX, X)
  D. Disorders involving the cranial nerves
    1. Bell palsy—facial paralysis (cranial nerve VII)
    2. Trigeminal neuralgia—pain in cranial nerve V

X. **AGING OF THE NERVOUS SYSTEM**

10

Questions for Study and Review

BUILDING UNDERSTANDING

Fill in the blanks

1. The thickest and toughest layer of the meninges is the _____.

2. The third and fourth ventricles are connected by a small canal called the _____.

3. The muscles of speech are controlled by a region named _____.

4. Inflammation of the brain is termed _____.

5. The cells responsible for most brain tumors are _____.

Matching > Match each numbered item with the most closely related lettered item.

___ 6. The sensory nerve of the face

___ 7. The motor nerve of the muscles of facial expression

___ 8. The sensory nerve for hearing and equilibrium

___ 9. The motor nerve for swallowing

___ 10. The motor nerve for digestion

   a. trigeminal nerve

   b. facial nerve

   c. vestibulocochlear nerve

   d. glossopharyngeal nerve

   e. vagus nerve

Multiple Choice

___ 11. The cerebrum is divided into left and right hemispheres by the
   a. central sulcus
   b. lateral sulcus
   c. longitudinal fissure
   d. insula

___ 12. The primary sensory area interprets all of the following sensations except
   a. vision
   b. pain
   c. touch
   d. temperature

___ 13. An abnormal accumulation of CSF within the brain is called
   a. cerebral hemorrhage
   b. subdural hematoma
   c. hemiplegia
   d. hydrocephalus

___ 14. Tremors, limb rigidity, slow movement, and impaired balance are signs of
   a. meningitis
   b. Bell palsy
   c. Alzheimer disease
   d. Parkinson disease

___ 15. Pain messages are classified as
   a. special sensory impulses
   b. general sensory impulses
   c. somatic motor impulses
   d. visceral motor impulses

UNDERSTANDING CONCEPTS

16. Briefly describe the effects of injury to the following brain areas:
    a. cerebrum
    b. diencephalon
    c. brain stem
    d. cerebellum

17. A neurosurgeon has drilled a hole through her patient's skull and is preparing to remove a cerebral glioma. List, in order, the membranes she must cut through to reach the cerebral cortex.

18. Compare and contrast the functions of the following structures:
    a. frontal lobe and parietal lobe
    b. temporal lobe and occipital lobe
    c. thalamus and hypothalamus

19. What is the function of the limbic system? Describe the effect of damage to the hippocampus.

20. Compare and contrast the following nervous system disorders:
    a. meningitis and encephalitis
    b. epidural hematoma and subdural hematoma
    c. Alzheimer disease and multi-infarct dementia
    d. Bell palsy and trigeminal neuralgia

21. Describe Parkinson disease and therapies used to treat it.

22. The term cerebellum means "little cerebrum." Why is this an appropriate term?

23. Make a table of the 12 cranial nerves and their functions. According to your table, which ones are sensory, motor, or mixed?

CONCEPTUAL THINKING

24. The parents of Molly R. (2-month-old Caucasian female) are informed that their daughter requires a shunt to drain excess CSF from her brain. What disorder does Molly have? How would you explain this disorder to her parents? What would happen to Molly if the shunt was not put in place?

25. In the case story, Frank suffered a stroke. How would you explain the term "stroke" to his family? Why

were many of his symptoms isolated to the right side of his body?

26. In Frank's case, stroke damage was isolated to his cerebrum. Some strokes, though, can affect the brain stem. Why is damage to this part of the brain life-threatening?

10

The Sensory System

Learning Outcomes

After careful study of this chapter, you should be able to:

1. Describe the function of the sensory system
2. Differentiate between the special and general senses and give examples of each
3. Describe the structure of the eye
4. List and describe the structures that protect the eye
5. Define *refraction* and list the refractive parts of the eye
6. Differentiate between the rods and the cones of the eye
7. Compare the functions of the extrinsic and intrinsic muscles of the eye
8. Describe the nerve supply to the eye
9. Describe the three divisions of the ear
10. Describe the receptor for hearing and explain how it functions
11. Compare static and dynamic equilibrium and describe the location and function of these receptors
12. Explain the function of proprioceptors
13. List several methods for treatment of pain
14. Describe sensory adaptation and explain its value
15. List some disorders of the sensory system
16. Show how word parts are used to build words related to the sensory system (see Word Anatomy at the end of the chapter)

Selected Key Terms

The following terms and other boldface terms in the chapter are defined in the Glossary

accommodation
cataract
choroid
cochlea
conjunctiva
convergence
cornea
glaucoma
gustation
lacrimal apparatus
lens (crystalline lens)
olfaction
organ of Corti
ossicle
proprioceptor
refraction
retina
sclera
semicircular canal
sensory adaptation
sensory receptor
tympanic membrane
vestibule
vitreous body

PASSport to Success

Visit *thePoint* or see the Student Resource CD in the back of this book for definitions and pronunciations of key terms as well as a pretest for this chapter.

Disease
in Context

> ## Paul's Second Case: Seeing More of the Sun's Effects

Paul glanced once again at the postcard sitting on his entranceway table as he arrived home in the evening. He knew it said he was due for a checkup with his ophthalmologist, but after his run-in with skin cancer six months earlier, he was in no hurry to see the inside of a medical office. *Well, it's just routine, and I may need a slight change in my prescription, so I'll make the call*, he thought.

At the office, Dr. Gilbert greeted Paul and asked how he was feeling in general and if he thought there had been any change in his vision. "My vision sometimes seems a little blurry, especially when my eyes are tired, but no major changes," Paul replied. Dr. Gilbert proceeded with the eye exam, testing his visual acuity and checking on his astigmatism.

"You're right; not much change," said the ophthalmologist. "But, we'll give you a new prescription for your glasses. At 42, you're a little young for presbyopia—far-sightedness that develops with age—but we'll do the routine check for glaucoma. I know your father developed that condition, and it does have a hereditary factor." The doctor dilated Paul's eyes with drops and examined the fundus of each eye with an ophthalmoscope. In answer to Paul's query, he explained that in this way he could examine the health of the retina and the optic nerve and also look at the vessels at the back of the eye for any signs of diabetes or circulatory problems. In addition, he used a tonometer to test for glaucoma, a condition that can damage the eye with high fluid pressure. "I need to check on another patient," he told Paul. "Then I'll be back to explain what I've found. Just sit in the waiting room for a few minutes, please."

Dr. Gilbert uses his knowledge of the structure and function of the eye to diagnose medical conditions. In this chapter, you will learn about the eye and other sensory system organs. As well, we'll examine the consequences of Paul's sun-loving youth on his eyes and vision.

The Senses

The sensory system protects a person by detecting changes in the environment. An environmental change becomes a *stimulus* when it initiates a nerve impulse, which then travels to the central nervous system (CNS) by way of a sensory (afferent) neuron. A stimulus becomes a sensation—something we experience—only when a specialized area of the cerebral cortex interprets the nerve impulse received. Many stimuli arrive from the external environment and are detected at or near the body surface. Others, such as stimuli from the viscera, originate internally and help to maintain homeostasis.

Sensory Receptors

The part of the nervous system that detects a stimulus is the **sensory receptor.** In structure, a sensory receptor may be one of the following:

- The free dendrite of a sensory neuron, such as the receptors for pain and temperature
- A modified ending, or **end-organ,** on the dendrite of an afferent neuron, such as those for touch
- A specialized cell associated with an afferent neuron, such as the rods and cones of the eye's retina and the receptors in the other special sense organs

Receptors can be classified according to the type of stimulus to which they respond:

- Chemoreceptors, such as receptors for taste and smell, detect chemicals in solution.
- Photoreceptors, located in the retina of the eye, respond to light.
- Thermoreceptors detect change in temperature. Many of these receptors are located in the skin.
- Mechanoreceptors respond to movement, such as stretch, pressure, or vibration. These include pressure receptors in the skin, receptors that monitor body position, and the receptors of hearing and equilibrium in the ear, which are activated by the movement of cilia on specialized receptor cells.

Any receptor must receive a stimulus of adequate intensity, that is, at least a **threshold stimulus,** in order to respond and generate a nerve impulse.

Special and General Senses

Another way of classifying the senses is according to the distribution of their receptors. A **special sense** is localized in a special sense organ; a **general sense** is widely distributed throughout the body.

- Special senses
  - > **Vision** from receptors in the eye
  - > **Hearing** from receptors in the internal ear
  - > **Equilibrium** from receptors in the internal ear
  - > **Taste** from receptors in the tongue
  - > **Smell** from receptors in the upper nasal cavities
- **General senses**
  - > **Pressure, temperature, pain,** and **touch** from receptors in the skin and internal organs
  - > Sense of **position** from receptors in the muscles, tendons, and joints

The Eye and Vision

In the embryo, the eye develops as an outpocketing of the brain. It is a delicate organ, protected by a number of structures:

- The skull bones form the walls of the eye orbit (cavity) and protect the posterior part of the eyeball.
- The upper and lower eyelids aid in protecting the eye's anterior portion (Fig. 11-1). The eyelids can be closed to keep harmful materials out of the eye, and blinking helps to lubricate the eye. A muscle, the levator palpebrae, is attached to the upper eyelid. When this muscle contracts, it keeps the eye open. If the muscle becomes weaker with age, the eyelids may droop and interfere with vision, a condition called *ptosis.*
- The eyelashes and eyebrow help to keep foreign matter out of the eye.
- A thin membrane, the **conjunctiva** (kon-junk-TI-vah), lines the inner surface of the eyelids and covers the visible portion of the white of the eye (sclera). Cells

Figure 11-1   **The eye's protective structures.** (Reprinted with permission from Bickley LS. *Bates' Guide to Physical Examination and History Taking,* 8th ed. Philadelphia: Lippincott Williams & Wilkins, 2003.)

Figure 11-2 **The lacrimal apparatus.** The lacrimal (tear) gland and its associated ducts are shown.

within the conjunctiva produce mucus that aids in lubricating the eye. Where the conjunctiva folds back from the eyelid to the eye's anterior surface, a sac is formed. The lower portion of the conjunctival sac can be used to instill medication drops. With age, the conjunctiva often thins and dries, resulting in inflammation and enlarged blood vessels.

■ Tears, produced by the **lacrimal** (LAK-rih-mal) **glands** (Fig. 11-2), lubricate the eye and contain an enzyme that protects against infection. As tears flow across the eye from the lacrimal gland, located in the orbit's upper lateral part, they carry away small particles that may have entered the eye. The tears then flow into ducts near the eye's nasal corner where they drain into the nose by way of the **nasolacrimal** (na-zo-LAK-rih-

mal) **duct** (see Fig. 11-2). An excess of tears causes a "runny nose"; a greater overproduction of them results in the tears spilling onto the cheeks. With age, the lacrimal glands produce less secretion, but tears still may overflow onto the cheek if the nasolacrimal ducts become plugged.

> **PASSport to Success** Visit *thePoint* or see the Student Resource CD in the back of this book for an image of *ptosis*.

CHECKPOINT 11-1 ➤ What are some structures that protect the eye?

Coats of the Eyeball

The eyeball has three separate coats, or tunics (Fig. 11-3).

1. The outermost tunic, called the **sclera** (SKLE-rah), is made of tough connective tissue. It is commonly referred to as the *white of the eye*. It appears white because of the collagen it contains and because it has no blood vessels to add color. (Reddened or "bloodshot" eyes result from inflammation and swelling of blood vessels in the conjunctiva).

2. The second tunic of the eyeball is the **choroid** (KO-royd). This coat is composed of a delicate network of connective tissue interlaced with many blood vessels. It also contains much dark brown pigment. The choroid may be compared to the dull black lining of a camera in that it prevents incoming light rays from scattering and reflecting off the eye's inner surface. The blood vessels at the posterior, or fundus, of the eye can reveal signs of disease, and visualization of these vessels with an **ophthalmoscope** (of-THAL-mo-skope) is an important part of a medical examination.

3. The innermost tunic, the **retina** (RET-ih-nah), is the eye's actual receptor layer. It contains light-sensitive cells known as **rods** and **cones**, which generate the nerve impulses associated with vision.

CHECKPOINT 11-2 ➤ What are the names of the tunics of the eyeball?

Pathway of Light Rays and Refraction

As light rays pass through the eye toward the retina, they travel through a

Figure 11-3 **The eye.** Note the three tunics, the refractive parts of the eye (cornea, aqueous humor, lens, vitreous body), and other structures involved in vision.

series of transparent, colorless parts described below and seen in Figure 11-3. On the way, they undergo a process known as **refraction**, which is the bending of light rays as they pass from one substance to another substance of different density. (For a simple demonstration of refraction, place a spoon into a glass of water and observe how the handle appears to bend at the surface of the water.) Because of refraction, light from a very large area can be focused on a very small area of the retina. The eye's transparent refracting parts are listed here, according to the pathway of light traveling from exterior to interior:

1. The **cornea** (KOR-ne-ah) is an anterior continuation of the sclera, but it is transparent and colorless, whereas the rest of the sclera is opaque and white. The cornea is referred to frequently as the *window* of the eye. It bulges forward slightly and is the main refracting structure of the eye. The cornea has no blood vessels; it is nourished by the fluids that constantly wash over it.

2. The **aqueous** (A-kwe-us) **humor**, a watery fluid that fills much of the eyeball anterior to the lens, helps maintain the cornea's slight forward curve. The aqueous humor is constantly produced and drained from the eye.

3. The **lens**, technically called the *crystalline lens*, is a clear, circular structure made of a firm, elastic material. The lens has two bulging surfaces and is thus described as biconvex. The lens is important in light refraction because it is elastic and its thickness can be adjusted to focus light for near or far vision.

4. The **vitreous** (VIT-re-us) **body** is a soft jellylike substance that fills the entire space posterior to the lens (the adjective *vitreous* means "glasslike"). Like the aqueous humor, it is important in maintaining the shape of the eyeball as well as in aiding in refraction.

CHECKPOINT 11-3 ➤ What are the structures that refract light as it passes through the eye?

Function of the Retina

The retina has a complex structure with multiple layers of cells (Fig. 11-4). The deepest layer is a pigmented layer just anterior to the choroid. Next are the rods and cones, the receptor cells of the eye, named for their shape. Details on how these two types of cells differ are presented in Table 11-1. Anterior to the rods and cones are connecting neurons that carry impulses toward the optic nerve.

The rods are highly sensitive to light and thus function in dim light, but they do not provide a sharp image. They are more numerous than the cones and are distributed more toward the periphery (anterior portion) of the retina. (If you visualize the retina as the inside of a bowl, the rods would be located toward the bowl's lip). When you enter into dim light, such as a darkened movie theater, you cannot see for a short period. It is during this time that the rods are beginning to function, a change that is described as **dark adaptation**. When you are able to see again, images are blurred and appear only in shades of gray, because the rods are unable to differentiate colors.

The cones function in bright light, are sensitive to color, and give sharp images. The cones are localized at the retinal center, especially in a tiny depressed area near the optic nerve that is called the **fovea centralis** (FO-ve-ah sen-TRA-lis) (Fig. 11-5; see also Fig. 11-3). (Note that *fovea* is a general term for a pit or depression.) Because this area contains the highest concentration of cones, it is the point of sharpest vision. The fovea is contained within a yellowish spot, the **macula lutea** (MAK-u-lah LU-te-ah), an area that may show degenerative changes with age.

There are three types of cones, each sensitive to either red, green, or blue light. Color blindness results from a lack of retinal cones. People who completely lack cones are totally colorblind; those who lack one type of cone

LIGHT WAVES

Fibers to optic nerve

Connecting neurons

Retina

Photoreceptor cells

Rod   Cone

Pigmented layer

Choroid

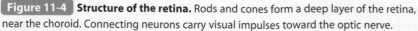

Figure 11-4 **Structure of the retina.** Rods and cones form a deep layer of the retina, near the choroid. Connecting neurons carry visual impulses toward the optic nerve.

Table 11-1	Comparison of the Rods and Cones of the Retina	
Characteristic	Rods	Cones
Shape	Cylindrical	Flask shaped
Number	About 120 million in each retina	About 6 million in each retina
Distribution	Toward the periphery (anterior) of the retina	Concentrated at the center of the retina
Stimulus	Dim light	Bright light
Visual acuity (sharpness)	Low	High
Pigments	Rhodopsin (visual purple)	Pigments sensitive to red, green, or blue
Color perception	None; shades of gray	Respond to color

are partially color blind. This disorder, because of its pattern of inheritance, occurs almost exclusively in males.

The rods and cones function by means of pigments that are sensitive to light. The rod pigment is **rhodopsin** (ro-DOP-sin), or visual purple. Vitamin A is needed for manufacture of these pigments. If a person is lacking in vitamin A, and thus rhodopsin, he or she may have difficulty seeing in dim light because the light is inadequate to activate the rods; this condition is termed **night blindness.** Nerve impulses from the rods and cones flow into sensory neurons that eventually merge to form the optic nerve (cranial nerve II) at the eye's posterior (see Figs. 11-3 and 11-5). The impulses travel to the visual center in the brain's occipital cortex.

When an **ophthalmologist** (of-thal-MOL-o-jist), a physician who specializes in treatment of the eye, examines the retina with an ophthalmoscope, he or she can see abnormalities in the retina and in the retinal blood vessels. Some of these changes may signal more widespread diseases that affect the eye, such as diabetes and high blood pressure (hypertension).

CHECKPOINT 11-4 ➤ What are the receptor cells of the retina?

PASSport to Success

Visit *thePoint* or see the Student Resource CD in the back of this book to view the animation *The Retina,* which illustrates the structure and function of this visual receptor.

Muscles of the Eye

Two groups of muscles are associated with the eye. Both groups are important in adjusting the eye so that a clear image can form on the retina.

THE EXTRINSIC MUSCLES The voluntary muscles attached to the eyeball's outer surface are the **extrinsic** (eks-TRIN-sik) **muscles.** The six ribbonlike extrinsic muscles connected with each eye originate on the orbital bones and insert on the surface of the sclera (Fig. 11-6). They are named

11

Figure 11-5 **The fundus (back) of the eye as seen through an ophthalmoscope.** (Reprinted with permission from Moore KL, Dalley AF. *Clinically Oriented Anatomy,* 4th ed. Baltimore: Lippincott Williams & Wilkins, 1999.)

Labels on figure: Blood vessels — Optic disk — Retina — Fovea centralis (in macula lutea)

■ The abducens nerve (cranial nerve VI) supplies the lateral rectus extrinsic eye muscle.

To summarize, the steps in vision are:

1. Light refracts.
2. The muscles of the iris adjust the pupil.
3. The ciliary muscle adjusts the lens (accommodation).
4. The extrinsic eye muscles produce convergence.
5. Light stimulates retinal receptor cells (rods and cones).
6. The optic nerve transmits impulses to the brain.
7. The occipital lobe cortex interprets the impulses.

CHECKPOINT `11-8` ➤ What is cranial nerve II and what does it do?

Errors of Refraction and Other Eye Disorders

Hyperopia (hi-per-O-pe-ah), or farsightedness, usually results from an abnormally short eyeball (Fig. 11-11A). In this situation, light rays focus behind the retina because they cannot bend sharply enough to focus on the retina. The lens can thicken only to a given limit to accommodate for near vision. If the need for refraction exceeds this limit, a person must move an object away from the eye to see it clearly. Glasses with convex lenses that increase light refraction can correct for hyperopia.

Myopia (mi-O-pe-ah), or nearsightedness, is another eye defect related to development. In this case, the eyeball is too long or the cornea bends the light rays too sharply, so that the focal point is in front of the retina (see Fig. 11-11B). Distant objects appear blurred and may appear clear only if brought near the eye. A concave lens corrects for myopia by widening the angle of refraction and moving the focal point backward. Nearsightedness in a young person becomes worse each year until the person reaches his or her 20s.

Another common visual defect, **astigmatism** (ah-STIG-mah-tizm), is caused by irregularity in the curvature of the cornea or the lens. As a result, light rays are incorrectly bent, causing blurred vision. Astigmatism is often found in combination with hyperopia or myopia, so a careful eye examination is needed to obtain an accurate prescription for corrective lenses. Surgical techniques are now available to correct some visual defects and eliminate the need for eyeglasses or contact lenses. Such refractive surgery can be used to correct nearsightedness, farsightedness, and astigmatism. In these procedures, the cornea is reshaped, often using a laser, to change the refractive angle of light as it passes through.

CHECKPOINT `11-9` ➤ What are some errors of refraction?

STRABISMUS Strabismus (strah-BIZ-mus) is a deviation of the eye that results from lack of eyeball muscle coordination. That is, the two eyes do not work together. In **convergent strabismus**, the eye deviates toward the nasal side, or medially. This disorder gives an appearance of being cross-eyed. In **divergent strabismus**, the affected eye deviates laterally.

If these disorders are not corrected early, the transmission and interpretation of visual impulses from the affected eye to the brain is decreased. The brain does not develop ways to "see" images from the eye. Loss of vision in a

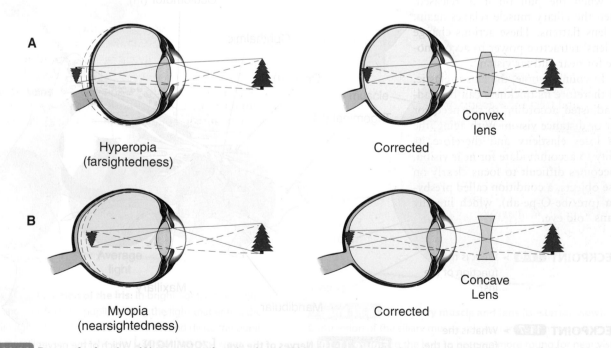

A
Hyperopia
(farsightedness)

Convex
lens
Corrected

B
Myopia
(nearsightedness)

Concave
Lens
Corrected

Figure 11-11 **Errors of refraction. (A)** Hyperopia (farsightedness). **(B)** Myopia (nearsightedness). A convex lens corrects for hyperopia; a concave lens corrects for myopia, as shown in the right column of the figure.

healthy eye because it cannot work properly with the other eye is termed **amblyopia** (am-ble-O-pe-ah). Care by an ophthalmologist as soon as the condition is detected may result in restoration of muscle balance. In some cases, eye exercises, eye glasses, and patching of one eye correct the defect. In other cases, surgery is required to alter muscle action.

INFECTIONS Inflammation of the conjunctiva is called **conjunctivitis** (kon-junk-tih-VI-tis). It may be acute or chronic and may be caused by a variety of irritants and pathogens. "Pinkeye" is a highly contagious acute conjunctivitis that is usually caused by cocci or bacilli. Sometimes, irritants such as wind and excessive glare cause an inflammation, which may in turn lead to susceptibility to bacterial infection.

Inclusion conjunctivitis is an acute eye infection caused by *Chlamydia trachomatis* (klah-MID-e-ah trah-KO-mah-tis). This same organism causes a sexually transmitted reproductive tract infection. In underdeveloped countries where this eye infection appears in chronic form, it is known as **trachoma** (trah-KO-mah). If not treated, scarring of the conjunctiva and cornea can cause blindness. The use of antibiotics and proper hygiene to prevent reinfection has reduced the incidence of blindness from this disorder in many parts of the world.

An acute eye infection of the newborn, caused by organisms acquired during passage through the birth canal, is called **ophthalmia neonatorum** (of-THAL-me-ah ne-o-na-TO-rum). The usual cause is gonococcus, chlamydia, or some other sexually transmitted organism. Preventive doses of an appropriate antiseptic or antibiotic solution are routinely administered into a newborn's conjunctiva just after birth.

The iris, choroid coat, ciliary body, and other parts of the eyeball may become infected by various organisms. Such disorders are likely to be serious; fortunately, they are not common. Syphilis spirochetes, tubercle bacilli, and a variety of cocci may cause these painful infections. They may follow a sinus infection, tonsillitis, conjunctivitis, or other disorder in which the infecting agent can spread from nearby structures. An ophthalmologist is trained to diagnose and treat these conditions.

INJURIES The most common eye injury is a laceration or scratch of the cornea caused by a foreign body. Injuries caused by foreign objects or by infection may result in corneal scar formation, leaving an area of opacity through which light rays cannot pass. If such an injury involves the central area anterior to the pupil, blindness may result.

Because the cornea lacks blood vessels, a person can receive a corneal transplant without danger of rejection. Eye banks store corneas obtained from donors, and corneal transplantation is a fairly common procedure.

Severe traumatic eye injuries, such as penetration of deeper structures, may not be subject to surgical repair. In such cases, an operation to remove the eyeball, a procedure called **enucleation** (e-nu-kle-A-shun), is performed.

It is important to prevent infection in cases of eye injury. Even a tiny scratch can become so seriously infected

that blindness may result. Injuries by pieces of glass and other sharp objects are a frequent cause of eye damage. The incidence of accidents involving the eye has been greatly reduced by the use of protective goggles.

CATARACT A **cataract** is an opacity (cloudiness) of the lens or the lens' outer covering. An early cataract causes a gradual loss of visual acuity (sharpness). An untreated cataract leads to complete vision loss. Surgical removal of the lens followed by implantation of an artificial lens is a highly successful procedure for restoring vision. Although the cause of cataracts is not known, age is a factor, as is excess exposure to ultraviolet rays. Diseases such as diabetes, as well as certain medications, are known to accelerate cataract development.

GLAUCOMA Glaucoma is a condition characterized by excess pressure of the aqueous humor. This fluid is produced constantly from the blood, and after circulation in the eye, it is reabsorbed into the bloodstream. Interference with this fluid's normal reentry into the bloodstream leads to an increase in pressure inside the eyeball.

The most common type of glaucoma usually progresses rather slowly, with vague visual disturbances being the only symptom. In most cases, the aqueous humor's high pressure causes destruction of some optic nerve fibers before the person is aware of visual change. Many glaucoma cases are diagnosed by the measurement of pressure in the eye, which should be part of a routine eye examination for people older than 35 years or for those with a family history of glaucoma. Early diagnosis and continuous treatment with medications to reduce pressure frequently result in the preservation of vision.

DISORDERS INVOLVING THE RETINA Diabetes as a cause of blindness is increasing in the United States. In **diabetic retinopathy** (ret-in-OP-ah-the), the retina is damaged by blood vessel hemorrhages and growth of new vessels. Other eye disorders directly related to diabetes include optic atrophy, in which the optic nerve fibers die; cataracts, which occur earlier and with greater frequency among diabetics than among nondiabetics; and retinal detachment.

In cases of **retinal detachment**, the retina separates from the underlying choroid layer as a result of trauma or an accumulation of fluid or tissue between the layers. This disorder may develop slowly or may occur suddenly. If it is left untreated, complete detachment can occur, resulting in blindness. Surgical treatment includes a sort of "spot welding" with an electric current or a weak laser beam. A series of pinpoint scars (connective tissue) develops to reattach the retina.

Macular degeneration is another leading cause of blindness. This name refers to the macula lutea, the yellow area of the retina that contains the fovea centralis. Changes in this area distort the center of the visual field. In one form of macular degeneration, material accumulates on the retina, causing gradual vision loss. In another form, abnormal blood vessels grow under the retina, causing it to detach. Laser surgery may stop the growth of these vessels and delay vision loss. Factors contributing to macular degeneration are smoking, exposure to sunlight, and a high cholesterol diet. Some forms are known to be hereditary. Box 11-1, Eye Surgery: A Glimpse of the Cutting Edge, provides information on new methods of treating eye disorders.

 PASSport to Success Visit *thePoint* or see the Student Resource CD in the back of this book for illustrations of the eye disorders described and also cataract surgery.

The Ear

The ear is the sense organ for both hearing and equilibrium (Fig. 11-12). It is divided into three main sections:

- The **outer ear** includes an outer projection and a canal ending at a membrane.
- The **middle ear** is an air space containing three small bones.
- The **inner ear** is the most complex and contains the sensory receptors for hearing and equilibrium.

The Outer Ear

The external portion of the ear consists of a visible projecting portion, the **pinna** (PIN-nah), also called the **auricle** (AW-rih-kl), and the **external auditory canal**, or **meatus** (me-A-tus), that leads into the ear's deeper parts. The pinna directs sound waves into the ear, but it is probably of little importance in humans. The external auditory canal extends medially from the pinna for about 2.5 cm or more, depending on which wall of the canal is measured. The skin lining this tube is thin and, in the first part of the canal, contains many wax-producing **ceruminous** (seh-RU-mih-nus) **glands**. The wax, or **cerumen** (seh-RU-men), may become dried and impacted in the canal and must then be removed. The same kinds of disorders that involve the skin elsewhere—atopic dermatitis, boils, and other infections—may also affect the skin of the external auditory canal.

The **tympanic** (tim-PAN-ik) **membrane**, or eardrum, is at the end of the external auditory canal. It is a boundary between this canal and the middle ear cavity, and it vibrates freely as sound waves enter the ear.

The Middle Ear and Ossicles

The middle ear cavity is a small, flattened space that contains three small bones, or **ossicles** (OS-ih-klz) (see Fig. 11-12). The three ossicles are joined in such a way that they amplify the sound waves received by the tympanic membrane as they transmit the sounds to the inner ear. The first bone is shaped like a hammer and is called the **malleus** (MAL-e-us) (Fig. 11-13). The handlike part of the malleus is attached to the tympanic membrane, whereas the headlike part is connected to the second bone, the **incus** (ING-kus). The incus is shaped like an anvil, an

---

Box 11-1 **Hot Topics**

Eye Surgery: A Glimpse of the Cutting Edge

Cataracts, glaucoma, and refractive errors are the most common eye disorders affecting Americans. In the past, cataract and glaucoma treatments concentrated on managing the diseases. Refractive errors were corrected using eyeglasses and, more recently, contact lenses. Today, laser and microsurgical techniques can remove cataracts, reduce glaucoma, and allow people with refractive errors to put their eyeglasses and contacts away. These cutting-edge procedures include:

- *Laser in situ keratomileusis (LASIK)* to correct refractive errors. During this procedure, a laser reshapes the cornea to allow light to refract directly on the retina, rather than in front of or behind it. A microkeratome (surgical knife) is used to cut a flap in the cornea's outer layer. A computer-controlled laser sculpts the middle layer of the cornea and then the flap is replaced. The procedure takes only a few minutes and patients recover their vision quickly and usually with little postoperative pain.

- *Laser trabeculoplasty* to treat glaucoma. This procedure uses a laser to help drain fluid from the eye and lower intraocular pressure. The laser is aimed at drainage canals located between the cornea and iris and makes several burns that are believed to open the canals and allow fluid to drain better. The procedure is typically painless and takes only a few minutes.

- *Phacoemulsification* to remove cataracts. During this surgical procedure, a very small incision (approximately 3 mm long) is made through the sclera near the cornea's outer edge. An ultrasonic probe is inserted through this opening and into the center of the lens. The probe uses sound waves to emulsify the lens' central core, which is then suctioned out. Then, an artificial lens is permanently implanted in the lens capsule. The procedure is typically painless, although the patient may feel some discomfort for 1 to 2 days afterward.

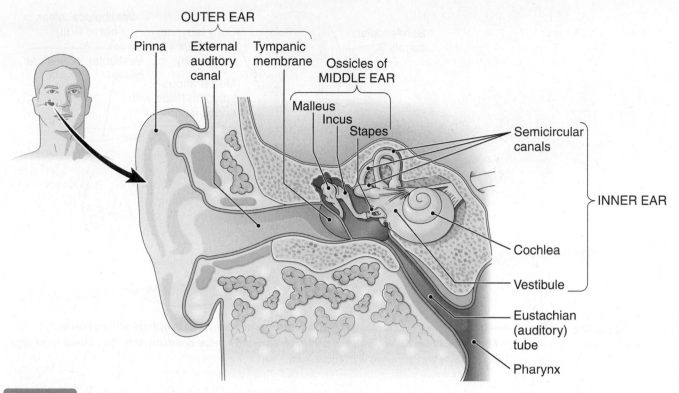

Figure 11-12 **The ear.** Structures in the outer, middle, and inner divisions are shown.

iron block used in shaping metal, as is used by a black-smith. The innermost ossicle is shaped somewhat like the stirrup of a saddle and is called the **stapes** (STA-peze). The base of the stapes is in contact with the inner ear.

CHECKPOINT 11-10 ➤ What are the ossicles of the ear and what do they do?

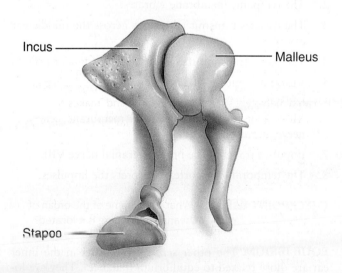

Incus ——

—— Malleus

Stapes ——

Figure 11-13 **The ossicles of the middle ear.** The handle of the malleus is in contact with the tympanic membrane, and the headlike part with the incus. The base of the stapes is in contact with the inner ear (×30). (Image provided by Anatomical Chart Co.)

THE EUSTACHIAN TUBE The **eustachian** (u-STA-shun) **tube** (auditory tube) connects the middle ear cavity with the throat, or pharynx (FAR-inks) (see Fig. 11-12). This tube opens to allow pressure to equalize on the two sides of the tympanic membrane. A valve that closes the tube can be forced open by swallowing hard, yawning, or blowing with the nose and mouth sealed, as one often does when experiencing pain from pressure changes in an airplane.

The mucous membrane of the pharynx is continuous through the eustachian tube into the middle ear cavity. At the posterior of the middle ear cavity is an opening into the mastoid air cells, which are spaces inside the temporal bone's mastoid process (see Fig. 7-5B).

The Inner Ear

The ear's most complicated and important part is the internal portion, which is described as a *labyrinth* (LAB-ih-rinth) because it has a complex mazelike construction. It consists of three separate areas containing sensory receptors. The skeleton of the inner ear is called the **bony labyrinth** (Fig. 11-14). It has three divisions:

■ The **vestibule** consists of two bony chambers that contain some of the receptors for equilibrium.

■ The **semicircular canals** are three projecting bony tubes located toward the posterior. Areas at the bases of the semicircular canals also contain receptors for equilibrium.

11

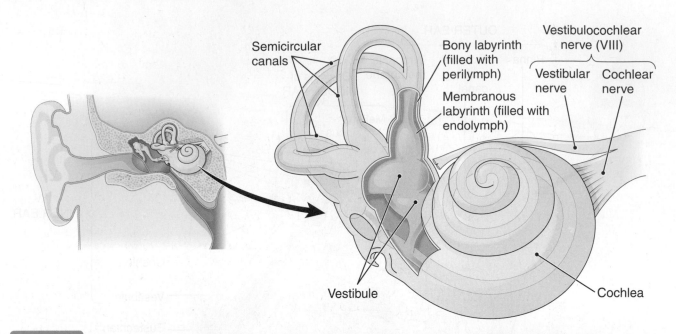

Semicircular canals

Bony labyrinth (filled with perilymph)

Membranous labyrinth (filled with endolymph)

Vestibulocochlear nerve (VIII)

Vestibular nerve

Cochlear nerve

Vestibule

Cochlea

Figure 11-14 **The inner ear.** The vestibule, semicircular canals, and cochlea are made of a bony shell (labyrinth) with an interior membranous labyrinth. Endolymph fills the membranous labyrinth and perilymph is around it in the bony labyrinth. The cochlea is the organ of hearing. The semicircular canals and vestibule are concerned with equilibrium.

■ The **cochlea** (KOK-le-ah) is coiled like a snail shell and is located toward the anterior. It contains the receptors for hearing.

All three divisions of the bony labyrinth contain a fluid called **perilymph** (PER-e-limf).

Within the bony labyrinth is an exact replica of this bony shell made of membrane, much like an inner tube within a tire. The tubes and chambers of this **membranous labyrinth** are filled with a fluid called **endolymph** (EN-do-limf) (see Fig. 11-14). The endolymph is within the membranous labyrinth, and the perilymph surrounds it. These fluids are important to the sensory functions of the inner ear.

HEARING The organ of hearing, called the **organ of Corti** (KOR-te), consists of ciliated receptor cells located inside the membranous cochlea, or **cochlear duct** (Fig. 11-15). Sound waves enter the external auditory canal and cause vibrations in the tympanic membrane. The ossicles amplify these vibrations and finally transmit them from the stapes to a membrane covering the **oval window** of the inner ear.

As the sound waves move through the fluids in these chambers, they set up vibrations in the cochlear duct. As a result, the tiny, hairlike cilia on the receptor cells (hair cells) begin to move back and forth against the **tectorial membrane** above them. (The membrane is named from a Latin word that means "roof.") This motion sets up nerve impulses that travel to the brain in the **cochlear nerve**, a branch of the eighth cranial nerve (formerly called the *auditory* or *acoustic nerve*). Sound waves ultimately leave the ear through another membrane-covered space in the bony labyrinth, the **round window**.

Hearing receptors respond to both the pitch (tone) of sound and its intensity (loudness). The various pitches stimulate different regions of the organ of Corti. Receptors detect higher-pitched sounds near the base of the cochlea and lower-pitched sounds near the top. Loud sounds stimulate more cells and produce more vibrations, sending more nerve impulses to the brain. Exposure to loud noises, such as very loud music, jet plane noise, or industrial noises, can damage the receptors for particular pitches of sound and lead to hearing loss for those tones.

The steps in hearing are:

1. Sound waves enter the external auditory canal.

2. The tympanic membrane vibrates.

3. The ossicles transmit vibrations across the middle ear cavity.

4. The stapes transmits the vibrations to the inner ear fluid.

5. Vibrations move cilia on hair cells of the organ of Corti in the cochlear duct.

6. Movement against the tectorial membrane generates nerve impulses.

7. Impulses travel to the brain in cranial nerve VIII.

8. The temporal lobe cortex interprets the impulses.

CHECKPOINT 11-11 ➤ What is the name of the organ of hearing and where is it located?

EQUILIBRIUM The other sensory receptors in the inner ear are those related to equilibrium (balance). They are located in the vestibule and the semicircular canals. Receptors for the sense of equilibrium are also ciliated cells or hair cells. As the head moves, a shift in the position of the cilia within the thick fluid around them generates a nerve impulse.

body when moving in a straight line, as in a moving vehicle or when tilting the head. This form of equilibrium is termed **static equilibrium**. Each receptor is called a **macula**. (There is also a macula in the eye, but *macula* is a general term that means "spot.") The fluid above the hair cells contains small crystals of calcium carbonate, called **otoliths** (O-to-liths), which add drag to the fluid around the receptor cells and increase the effect of gravity's pull (Fig. 11-16). Similar devices that help in balance are found in lower animals, such as fish and crustaceans.

The receptors for **dynamic equilibrium** function when the body is spinning or moving in different directions. The receptors, called **cristae** (KRIS-te), are located at the bases of the semicircular canals (Fig. 11-17). It's easy to remember what these receptors do, because the semicircular canals go off in different directions.

Nerve fibers from the vestibule and from the semicircular canals form the **vestibular** (ves-TIB-u-lar) **nerve**, which joins the cochlear nerve to form the vestibulocochlear nerve, the eighth cranial nerve.

CHECKPOINT 11-13 ➤ What are the two types of equilibrium?

Otitis and Other Disorders of the Ear

Infection and inflammation of the middle ear cavity, **otitis media** (o-TI-tis ME-de-ah), is relatively common. A variety of bacteria and viruses may cause otitis media, and it is a frequent complication of measles, influenza, and other infections, especially those of the pharynx. Pathogens are transmitted from the pharynx to the middle ear most often in children, partly because the eustachian tube is relatively short and horizontal in the child; in the adult, the tube is longer and tends to slant down toward the pharynx. Antibiotic drugs have reduced complications and have caused a marked reduction in the amount of surgery done to drain middle ear infections. In some cases, however, pressure from pus or exudate in the middle ear can be relieved only by cutting the tympanic membrane, a procedure called a **myringotomy** (mir-in-GOT-o-me). Placement of a **tympanostomy**

Figure 11-15 Cochlea and the organ of Corti. The arrows show the direction of sound waves in the cochlea.

CHECKPOINT 11-12 ➤ Where are the receptors for equilibrium located?

Receptors located in the vestibule's two small chambers sense the position of the head or the position of the

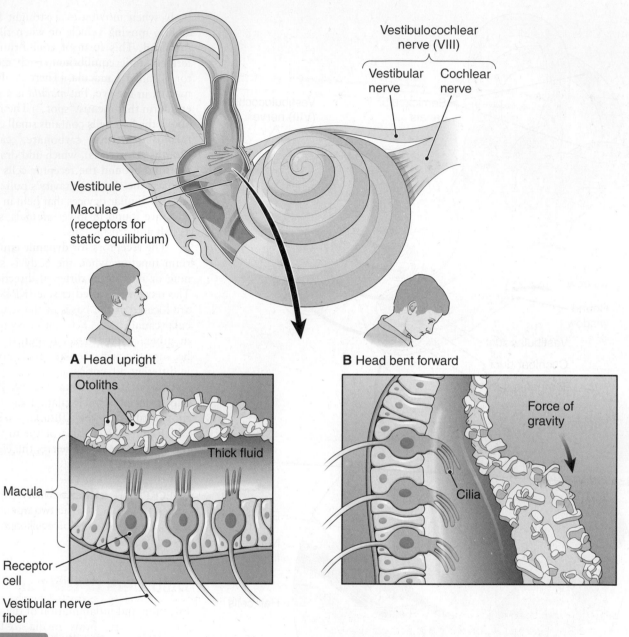

Figure 11-16 **Action of the receptors (maculae) for static equilibrium.** As the head moves, the thick fluid above the receptor cells (hair cells), weighted with otoliths, pulls on the cells' cilia, generating a nerve impulse. **[ZOOMING IN ➤** What happens to the cilia on the receptor cells when the fluid around them moves? **]**

(tim-pan-OS-to-me) **tube** in the eardrum allows pressure to equalize and prevents further damage to the eardrum.

Otitis externa is inflammation of the external auditory canal. Infections in this area may be caused by a fungus or bacterium. They are most common among those living in hot climates and among swimmers, leading to the alternate name "swimmer's ear."

HEARING LOSS Another disorder of the ear is hearing loss, which may be partial or complete. When the loss is complete, the condition is called **deafness.** The two main types of hearing loss are **conductive hearing loss** and **sensorineural hearing loss.**

Conductive hearing loss results from interference with the passage of sound waves from the outside to the inner ear. In this condition, wax or a foreign body may obstruct the external canal. Blockage of the eustachian tube prevents the equalization of air pressure on both sides of the tympanic membrane, thereby decreasing the membrane's ability to vibrate. Another cause of conductive hearing loss is damage to the tympanic membrane and ossicles resulting from chronic otitis media or from **otosclerosis** (o-to-skle-RO-sis), a hereditary bone disorder that prevents normal vibration of the stapes. Surgical removal of the diseased stapes and its replacement with an artificial device allows sound conduction from the ossicles to the cochlea.

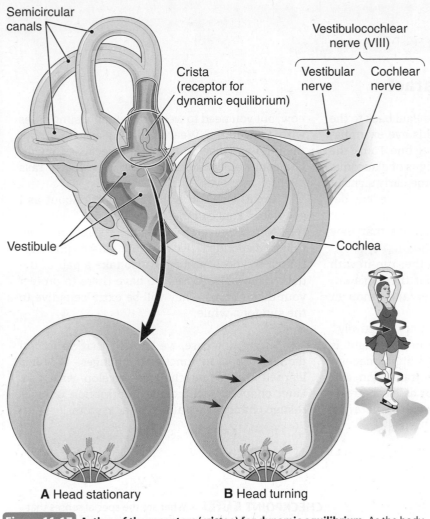

A Head stationary   **B** Head turning

Figure 11-17 **Action of the receptors (cristae) for dynamic equilibrium.** As the body spins or moves in different directions, the cilia bend as the head changes position, generating nerve impulses.

Sensorineural hearing loss may involve the cochlea, the vestibulocochlear nerve, or the brain areas concerned with hearing. It may result from prolonged exposure to loud noises, from the long-term use of certain drugs, or from exposure to various infections and toxins. People with severe hearing loss that originates in the inner ear may benefit from a cochlear implant. This prosthetic device stimulates the cochlear nerve directly, bypassing the receptor cells, and may restore hearing for medium to loud sounds.

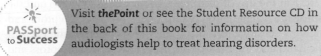

PASSport to Success Visit **thePoint** or see the Student Resource CD in the back of this book for information on how audiologists help to treat hearing disorders.

Presbycusis (pres-be-KU-sis) is a slowly progressive hearing loss that often accompanies aging. The condition involves gradual atrophy of the sensory receptors and cochlear nerve fibers. The affected person may experience a sense of isolation and depression, and may need psychological help. Because the ability to hear high-pitched sounds is usually lost first, it is important to address elderly people in clear, low-pitched tones.

Other Special Sense Organs

The sense organs of taste and smell are designed to respond to chemical stimuli.

Sense of Taste

The sense of taste, or **gustation** (gus-TA-shun), involves receptors in the tongue and two different nerves that carry taste impulses to the brain (Fig. 11-18). The taste receptors, known as **taste buds**, are located along the edges of small, depressed areas called **fissures**. Taste buds are stimulated only if the substance to be tasted is in solution or dissolves in the fluids of the mouth. Receptors for four basic tastes are localized in different regions, forming a "taste map" of the tongue (see Fig. 11-18B):

- **Sweet** tastes are most acutely experienced at the tip of the tongue (hence the popularity of lollipops and ice cream cones).

- **Salty** tastes are most acute at the anterior sides of the tongue.

- **Sour** tastes are most effectively detected by the taste buds located laterally on the tongue.

- **Bitter** tastes are detected at the tongue's posterior part.

Taste maps vary among people, but in each person certain tongue regions are more sensitive to a specific basic taste. Other tastes are a combination of these four with additional smell sensations. More recently, researchers have identified some other tastes besides these basic four: water, alkaline (basic), and metallic. Another is umami (u-MOM-e), a pungent or savory taste based on a response to the amino acid glutamate. Glutamate is found in MSG (monosodium glutamate), a flavor enhancer used in Asian food. Water taste receptors are mainly in the throat and may help to regulate water balance.

The nerves of taste include the facial and the glossopharyngeal cranial nerves (VII and IX). The interpretation of taste impulses is probably accomplished by the brain's lower frontal cortex, although there may be no sharply separate gustatory center.

11

Disease in Context revisited

▶ Early Signs of Cataract

D r. Gilbert's assistant called Paul back to the consultation room after his eye examination. "You seem to be doing fine, Paul," the ophthalmologist reported. "No signs of glaucoma. I am a little concerned about some early signs of cataract, though. These opacities of the lens develop with age in most people, and they're not hereditary, but there's firm evidence that they are influenced by sun exposure."

"Yikes!" Paul exploded. "Another run-in with the sun! I've already heard about the sun's unfriendly rays with my skin cancer, and I thought that's where it would end."

"Cataracts can be dealt with pretty effectively," said Dr. Gilbert, "but there's more. Sunlight is also a factor in a more serious condition, macular degeneration, which affects central vision and can lead to blindness. That's not as easily treatable at present. I don't see any signs of that right

now, but you need to wear good quality sunglasses with a UV filter. Wearing dark glasses without the filter is worse than nothing, because they dilate your pupils and allow more harmful UV rays to enter your eyes."

"Great! One more thing to worry about as I get older," Paul complained.

"Not a worry if you take precautions," Dr. Gilbert responded. "Pick up your glasses prescription at the desk, and Paul, also take a pair of the dark disposable glasses we have there to protect your dilated eyes. They will be extra-sensitive to the sun for a while."

During this case, we learned that structural damage leads to functional changes. We also learned that some changes develop with age. Later chapters will include information on age-related changes that affect other systems.

Sense of Smell

The importance of the sense of smell, or **olfaction** (ol-FAK-shun), is often underestimated. This sense helps to detect gases and other harmful substances in the environment and helps to warn of spoiled food. Smells can trigger memories and other psychological responses. Smell is also important in sexual behavior.

The receptors for smell are located in the epithelium of the nasal cavity's superior region (see Fig. 11-18). Again, the chemicals detected must be in solution in the fluids that line the nose. Because these receptors are high in the nasal cavity, one must "sniff" to bring odors upward in the nose.

The impulses from the smell receptors are carried by the olfactory nerve (I), which leads directly to the olfactory center in the brain's temporal cortex. The interpretation of smell is closely related to the sense of taste, but a greater variety of dissolved chemicals can be detected by smell than by taste. The smell of foods is just as important in stimulating appetite and the flow of digestive juices as is the sense of taste. When one has a cold, food often seems tasteless and unappetizing because nasal congestion reduces the ability to smell the food.

The olfactory receptors deteriorate with age and food may become less appealing. It is important when presenting food to elderly people that the food look inviting so as to stimulate their appetites.

CHECKPOINT 11-14 ▶ What are the special senses that respond to chemical stimuli?

The General Senses

Unlike the special sensory receptors, which are localized within specific sense organs, limited to a relatively small area, the general sensory receptors are scattered throughout the body. These include receptors for touch, pressure, heat, cold, position, and pain (Fig. 11-19).

Sense of Touch

The touch receptors, **tactile** (TAK-til) **corpuscles**, are found mostly in the dermis of the skin and around hair follicles. Touch sensitivity varies with the number of touch receptors in different areas. They are especially numerous and close together in the tips of the fingers and the toes. The lips and the tip of the tongue also contain many of these receptors and are very sensitive to touch. Other areas, such as the back of the hand and the back of the neck, have fewer receptors and are less sensitive to touch. Also included in this category are receptors in the walls of the large arteries that monitor blood pressure. Known as **baroreceptors** (bar-o-re-SEP-torz), these receptors trigger responses that control blood pressure as the vessels stretch (see Chapter 15).

Sense of Temperature

The temperature receptors are **free nerve endings**, receptors that are not enclosed in capsules but are merely branchings of nerve fibers. Temperature receptors are widely distributed in the skin, and there are separate receptors for heat and cold. A warm object stimulates only the heat receptors, and a cool object affects only the cold receptors. Internally, there are temperature receptors in the brain's hypothalamus, which help to adjust body temperature according to the temperature of the circulating blood.

Sense of Position

Receptors located in muscles, tendons, and joints relay impulses that aid in judging one's position and changes in the locations of body parts in relation to each other. They also inform the brain of the amount of muscle contraction and tendon tension. These rather widespread receptors, known as **proprioceptors** (pro-pre-o-SEP-tors), are aided in this function by the internal ear's equilibrium receptors.

Information received by these receptors is needed for the coordination of muscles and is important in such activities as walking, running, and many more complicated skills, such as playing a musical instrument. They help to provide a sense of body movement, known as **kinesthesia** (kin-es-THE-ze-ah). Proprioceptors play an important part in maintaining muscle tone and good posture. They also help to assess the weight of an object to be lifted so that the right amount of muscle force is used.

The nerve fibers that carry impulses from these receptors enter the spinal cord and ascend to the brain in the posterior part of the cord. The cerebellum is a main coordinating center for these impulses.

TASTE ZONES:
Sweet   Salty   Sour   Bitter

A

B

Figure 11-18 **Special senses that respond to chemicals. (A)** Organs of taste (gustation) and smell (olfaction). **(B)** A taste map of the tongue.

Sense of Pressure

Even when the skin is anesthetized, it can still respond to pressure stimuli. These sensory end-organs for deep pressure are located in the subcutaneous tissues beneath the skin and also near joints, muscles, and other deep tissues. They are sometimes referred to as *receptors for deep touch*.

CHECKPOINT 11-15 ➤ What are examples of general senses?

CHECKPOINT 11-16 ➤ What are proprioceptors and where are they located?

Labels in figure:
- Olfactory bulb
- Olfactory receptors
- Nostril
- Tongue with taste receptors
- Facial nerve (VII)
- Glossopharyngeal nerve (IX)
- Papillae

11

Pain
Touch
Cold
Heat
Pressure
Cell bodies
Dendrites
Axons
Synapses (in spinal cord)

Figure 11-19 **Sensory receptors in the skin.** Synapses are in the spinal cord.

Sense of Pain

Pain is the most important protective sense. The receptors for pain are widely distributed free nerve endings. They are found in the skin, muscles, and joints and to a lesser extent in most internal organs (including the blood vessels and viscera). Two pathways transmit pain to the CNS. One is for acute, sharp pain, and the other is for slow, chronic pain. Thus, a single strong stimulus produces the immediate sharp pain, followed in a second or so by the slow, diffuse, burning pain that increases in severity with time.

Referred pain is pain that is felt in an outer part of the body, particularly the skin, but actually originates in an internal organ located nearby. Liver and gallbladder disease often cause referred pain in the skin over the right shoulder. Spasm of the coronary arteries that supply the heart may cause pain in the left shoulder and arm. Infection of the appendix is felt as pain of the skin covering the lower right abdominal quadrant.

Apparently, some neurons in the spinal cord have the twofold duty of conducting impulses from visceral pain receptors in the chest and abdomen and from somatic pain receptors in neighboring areas of the skin, resulting in re-

ferred pain. The brain cannot differentiate between these two possible sources, but because most pain sensations originate in the skin, the brain automatically assigns the pain to this more likely place of origin. Knowing where visceral pain is referred to in the body is of great value in diagnosing chest and abdominal disorders.

Sometimes, the cause of pain cannot be remedied quickly, and occasionally it cannot be remedied at all. In the latter case, it is desirable to lessen the pain as much as possible. Some pain relief methods that have been found to be effective include:

- **Analgesic drugs.** An analgesic (an-al-JE-zik) is a drug that relieves pain. There are two main categories of such agents:

  > **Nonnarcotic analgesics** act locally to reduce inflammation and are effective for mild to moderate pain. Most of these drugs are commonly known as nonsteroidal antiinflammatory drugs (NSAIDs). Examples are ibuprofen (i-bu-PRO-fen) and naproxen (na-PROK-sen).

  > **Narcotics** act on the CNS to alter the perception and response to pain. Effective for severe pain, narcotics are administered by varied methods, including orally and by intramuscular injection. They are also effectively administered into the space surrounding the spinal cord. An example of a narcotic drug is morphine.

> **Anesthetics.** Although most commonly used to prevent pain during surgery, anesthetic injections are also used to relieve certain types of chronic pain.

> **Endorphins** (en-DOR-fins) are released naturally from certain brain regions and are associated with pain control. Massage, acupressure, and electric stimulation are among the techniques that are thought to activate this system of natural pain relief.

> **Applications of heat or cold** can be a simple but effective means of pain relief, either alone or in combination with medications. Care must be taken to avoid injury caused by excessive heat or cold.

> **Relaxation or distraction techniques** include several methods that reduce pain perception in the CNS. Relaxation techniques counteract the fight-or-flight response to pain and complement other pain-control methods.

Sensory Adaptation

When sensory receptors are exposed to a continuous stimulus, receptors often adjust themselves so that the sensation becomes less acute. The term for this phenomenon is **sensory adaptation**. For example, if you immerse your hand in very warm water, it may be uncomfortable; however, if you leave your hand there, soon the water will feel less hot (even if it has not cooled appreciably).

Receptors adapt at different rates. Those for warmth, cold, and light pressure adapt rapidly. In contrast, those for pain do not adapt. In fact, the sensations from the slow pain fibers tend to increase over time. This variation in receptors allows us to save energy by not responding to unimportant stimuli while always heeding the warnings of pain.

Word Anatomy

Medical terms are built from standardized word parts (prefixes, roots, and suffixes). Learning the meanings of these parts can help you remember words and interpret unfamiliar terms.

WORD PART	MEANING	EXAMPLE
The Eye and Vision		
ophthalm/o	eye	An *ophthalmologist* is a physician who specializes in treatment of the eye.
-scope	instrument for examination	An *ophthalmoscope* is an instrument used to examine the posterior of the eye.
lute/o	yellow	The macula *lutea* is a yellowish spot in the retina that contains the fovea centralis.
presby-	old	*Presbyopia* is farsightedness that occurs with age.
-opia	disorder of the eye or vision	*Hyperopia* is farsightedness.
ambly/o	dimness	*Amblyopia* is poor vision in a healthy eye that cannot work properly with the other eye.
e-	out	*Enucleation* is removal of the eyeball.
The Ear		
tympan/o	drum	The *tympanic* membrane is the eardrum.
equi-	equal	*Equilibrium* is balance (*equi-* combined with the Latin word *libra* meaning "balance").
ot/o	ear	*Otitis* is inflammation of the ear.
lith	stone	*Otoliths* are small crystals in the inner ear that aid in static equilibrium.
myring/o	tympanic membrane	*Myringotomy* is a cutting of the tympanic membrane to relieve pressure.
-stomy	creation of an opening between two structures	A *tympanostomy* tube creates a passageway through the tympanic membrane.
-cusis	hearing	*Presbycusis* is hearing loss associated with age.

11

WORD PART	MEANING	EXAMPLE
The General Senses		
propri/o-	own	*Proprioception* is perception of one's own body position.
kine	movement	*Kinesthesia* is a sense of body movement.
-esthesia	sensation	*Anesthesia* is loss of sensation, as of pain.
-alges/i	pain	An *analgesic* is a drug that relieves pain.
narc/o	stupor	A *narcotic* is a drug that alters the perception of pain.

Summary

I. **THE SENSES**
   A. Protect by detecting changes (stimuli) in the environment
   B. Sensory receptors—detect stimuli
      1. Structural types
         a. Free dendrite
         b. End-organ—modified dendrite
         c. Specialized cell—in special sense organs
      2. Types based on stimulus
         a. Chemoreceptors—respond to chemicals
         b. Thermoreceptors—respond to temperature
         c. Photoreceptors—respond to light
         d. Mechanoreceptors—respond to movement
   C. Special and general senses
      1. Special senses—vision, hearing, equilibrium, taste, smell
      2. General senses—touch, pressure, temperature, position, pain

II. **THE EYE AND VISION**
   A. Protection of the eyeball—bony orbit, eyelid, eyelashes, conjunctiva, lacrimal glands (produce tears)
   B. Coats of the eyeball
      1. Sclera—white of the eye
         a. Cornea—anterior
      2. Choroid—pigmented; contains blood vessels
      3. Retina—receptor layer
   C. Pathway of light rays and refraction
      1. Refraction—bending of light rays as they pass through substances of different density
      2. Refracting parts—cornea, aqueous humor, lens, vitreous body
   D. Function of the retina
      1. Cells
         a. Rods—cannot detect color; function in dim light
         b. Cones—detect color; function in bright light
      2. Pigments—sensitive to light; rod pigment is rhodopsin

   E. Muscles of the eye
      1. Extrinsic muscles—six move each eyeball
      2. Intrinsic muscles
         a. Iris—colored ring around pupil; regulates the amount of light entering the eye
         b. Ciliary muscle—regulates the thickness of the lens to accommodate for near vision
   F. Nerve supply to the eye
      1. Sensory nerves
         a. Optic nerve (II)—carries impulses from retina to brain
         b. Ophthalmic branch of trigeminal (V)
      2. Motor nerves—move eyeball
         a. Oculomotor (III), trochlear (IV), abducens (VI)
   G. Errors of refraction and other eye disorders
      1. Errors of refraction—hyperopia (farsightedness), myopia (nearsightedness), astigmatism
      2. Strabismus—deviation
      3. Infections—conjunctivitis, trachoma, ophthalmia neonatorum
      4. Injuries
      5. Cataract—opacity of the lens
      6. Glaucoma—damage caused by increased pressure
      7. Retinal disorders—retinopathy, retinal detachment, macular degeneration

III. **THE EAR**
   A. Outer ear—pinna, auditory canal (meatus), tympanic membrane (eardrum)
   B. Middle ear and ossicles
      1. Ossicles—malleus, incus, stapes
      2. Eustachian tube—connects middle ear with pharynx to equalize pressure
   C. Inner ear
      1. Bony labyrinth—contains perilymph
      2. Membranous labyrinth—contains endolymph
      3. Divisions
         a. Cochlea—contains receptors for hearing (organ of Corti)

b.   Vestibule—contains receptors for static equilibrium (maculae)

c.   Semicircular canals—contain receptors for dynamic equilibrium (cristae)

4.   Receptor (hair) cells function by movement of cilia

5.   Nerve—vestibulocochlear (auditory) nerve (VIII)

D.   Disorders of the ear

1.   Otitis (infection)—otitis media, otitis externa

2.   Hearing loss

a.   conductive

b.   sensorineural

IV.   OTHER SPECIAL SENSE ORGANS

A.   Sense of taste (gustation)

1.   Receptors—taste buds on tongue

2.   Basic tastes—sweet, salty, sour, bitter

3.   Nerves—facial (VII) and glossopharyngeal (IX)

B.   Sense of smell (olfaction)

1.   Receptors—in upper part of nasal cavity

2.   Nerve—olfactory nerve (I)

V.   GENERAL SENSES

A.   Sense of touch—tactile corpuscles

B.   Sense of pressure—receptors in skin deep tissue, large arteries

C.   Sense of temperature—receptors are free nerve endings

D.   Sense of position (proprioception)—receptors are proprioceptors in muscles, tendons, joints

1.   Kinesthesia—sense of movement

E.   Sense of pain—receptors are free nerve endings

1.   Referred pain—originates internally but felt at surface

2.   Relief of pain—analgesic drugs, anesthetics, endorphins, heat, cold, relaxation and distraction techniques

VI.   SENSORY ADAPTATION

A.   Adjustment of receptors so that sensation becomes less acute

B.   Receptors adapt at different rates; pain receptors do not adapt

Questions for Study and Review

BUILDING UNDERSTANDING

Fill in the blanks

1. The part of the nervous system that detects a stimulus is the _____.

2. The bending of light rays as they pass from air to fluid is called _____.

3. Nerve impulses are carried from the ear to the brain by the _____ nerve.

4. Information about the position of the knee joint is provided by _____.

5. A receptor's ability to decrease its sensitivity to a continuous stimulus is called _____.

Matching > Match each numbered item with the most closely related lettered item.

____ **6.** Slowly progressive hearing loss

____ **7.** Irregularity in the curvature of the cornea or lens

____ **8.** Deviation of the eye due to lack of coordination of the eyeball muscles

____ **9.** Increased pressure inside the eyeball

____ **10.** Loss of vision in a healthy eye because it cannot work properly with the other eye

a. glaucoma

b. amblyopia

c. presbycusis

d. astigmatism

e. strabismus

Multiple Choice

___ **11.** All of the following are special senses except
   a. smell
   b. taste
   c. equilibrium
   d. pain

___ **12.** From superficial to deep, the order of the eyeball's tunics is
   a. retina, choroid, and sclera
   b. sclera, retina, and choroid
   c. choroid, retina, and sclera
   d. sclera, choroid, and retina

___ **13.** The part of the eye most responsible for light refraction is the
   a. cornea
   b. lens
   c. vitreous body
   d. retina

___ **14.** Information from the retina is carried to the brain by the
   a. ophthalmic nerve
   b. optic nerve
   c. oculomotor nerve
   d. abducens nerve

___ **15.** Receptors in the vestibule sense
   a. muscle tension
   b. sound
   c. light
   d. equilibrium

UNDERSTANDING CONCEPTS

16. Differentiate between the terms in each of the following pairs:
   a. special sense and general sense
   b. aqueous humor and vitreous body
   c. rods and cones
   d. endolymph and perilymph
   e. static and dynamic equilibrium

17. Trace the path of a light ray from the outside of the eye to the retina.

18. Define *convergence* and *accommodation* and describe several disorders associated with them.

19. List in order the structures that sound waves pass through in traveling through the ear to the receptors for hearing.

20. Compare and contrast conductive hearing loss and sensorineural hearing loss.

21. Name the four basic tastes. Where are the taste receptors? Name the nerves of taste.

22. Trace the pathway of a nerve impulse from the olfactory receptors to the olfactory center in the brain.

23. Name several types of pain-relieving drugs. Describe several methods for relieving pain that do not involve drugs.

CONCEPTUAL THINKING

24. Maria M., a 4-year-old female, is taken to see the pediatrician because of a severe earache. Examination reveals that the tympanic membrane is red and bulging outward toward the external auditory canal. What disorder does Maria have? Why is the incidence of this disorder higher in children than in adults? What treatment options are available to Maria?

25. You and a friend have just finished riding the roller coaster at the amusement park. As you walk away from the ride, your friend stumbles and comments that the ride has affected her balance. How do you explain this?

26. In the case story, Paul discovered he might be developing an age-related eye disorder. What is a cataract? What are some other age-related disorders of the sensory system?

11

The Endocrine System: Glands and Hormones

Selected Key Terms

The following terms and other boldface terms in the chapter are defined in the Glossary

endocrine
hormone
hypothalamus
pituitary (hypophysis)
prostaglandin
receptor
steroid
target tissue

Learning Outcomes

After careful study of this chapter, you should be able to:

1. Compare the effects of the nervous system and the endocrine system in controlling the body
2. Describe the functions of hormones
3. Discuss the chemical composition of hormones
4. Explain how hormones are regulated
5. Identify the glands of the endocrine system on a diagram
6. List the hormones produced by each endocrine gland and describe the effects of each on the body
7. Describe how the hypothalamus controls the anterior and posterior pituitary
8. Describe the effects of hyposecretion and hypersecretion of the various hormones
9. List tissues other than the endocrine glands that produce hormones
10. List some medical uses of hormones
11. Explain how the endocrine system responds to stress
12. Show how word parts are used to build words related to the endocrine system (see Word Anatomy at the end of the chapter)

PASSport to Success

Visit *thePoint* or see the Student Resource CD in the back of this book for definitions and pronunciations of key terms as well as a pretest for this chapter.

Disease in Context

➤ Becky's Case: When an Endocrine Organ Fails

Becky stumbled down the stairs, wiping the sleep from her eyes, and hoping that Max hadn't finished all the pancakes that she could smell from the kitchen. "How was your sleep last night?" asked Becky's mother, who slid a plate across the table toward her. "Awful," sighed Becky, drowning her pancakes in a lake of syrup. "I woke up a bunch of times to go to the bathroom."

"Were you actually able to make it this time?" chimed Becky's little brother. Becky wished Max hadn't brought *that* up. She hoped he wasn't blabbing to his friends that she was wetting the bed again. "You know, if you didn't drink so much, you wouldn't have to pee so much," explained Max, as his sister gulped down her third glass of orange juice. Becky ate her pancakes and pretended that she didn't care about Max's comment. But, he was right. She was so thirsty—and hungry!

It was a long day when the bell finally rang and Becky boarded the bus for the ride home. Math class had been a disaster because she couldn't concentrate. During gym she was tired and had a stomach ache. And, she had to keep asking for permission to go to the bathroom! Now, she was exhausted and her head hurt. During breakfast, her mom mentioned she would make an appointment for Becky to see her doctor. Now, Becky thought that was a good idea.

Later that week, Becky's pediatrician weighed her, measured her height, and asked her a bunch of questions. "So, let me see if I've got this right, Becky," said Dr. Carter. "For the past week or so, you've felt lethargic and nau-seated and had a headache. You've been really thirsty and have needed to urinate frequently. You've also been really hungry. You've had some difficulty concentrating at school and have even felt fatigued when playing sports." Becky wasn't too sure what lethargic meant, but other than that he seemed to have gotten the facts right. So, Becky nodded her head yes.

Turning to Becky's mother, Dr. Carter said, "Checking her chart, it appears that she's lost several pounds since her last appointment—despite her appetite. I'm going to order a urine test and blood test. I'd like to see what her glucose levels are." Becky didn't enjoy the tests one bit. Having to pee in a cup was gross and as for the blood test, that was the worst!

A few days later, Dr. Carter called Becky's mother. "The urinalysis was positive for glucose and ketones, suggesting that Becky is not metabolizing glucose correctly. Her blood test revealed that she's hyperglycemic. In other words, her blood sugar is too high. We need to run a few more tests, but my diagnosis so far is that Becky has type 1 diabetes mellitus and needs insulin."

Dr. Carter suspects that Becky's pancreas, an important endocrine organ, does not produce sufficient amounts of the hormone insulin. Without insulin, Becky's cells cannot convert glucose into energy. As we will see later, Dr. Carter's diagnosis has a dramatic effect on Becky's health.

The endocrine system consists of a group of glands that produces regulatory chemicals called **hormones**. The endocrine system and the nervous system work together to control and coordinate all other body systems. The nervous system controls such rapid actions as muscle movement and intestinal activity by means of electrical and chemical stimuli. The effects of the endocrine system occur more slowly and over a longer period. They involve chemical stimuli only, and these chemical messengers have widespread effects on the body.

Although the nervous and endocrine systems differ in some respects, the two systems are closely related. For example, the activity of the pituitary gland, which in turn regulates other glands, is controlled by the brain's hypothalamus. The connections between the nervous system and the endocrine system enable endocrine function to adjust to the demands of a changing environment.

Hormones

Hormones are chemical messengers that have specific regulatory effects on certain cells or organs. Hormones from the endocrine glands are released, not through ducts, but directly into surrounding tissue fluids. Most then diffuse into the bloodstream, which carries them throughout the body. They regulate growth, metabolism, reproduction, and behavior. Some hormones affect many tissues, for example, growth hormone, thyroid hormone, and insulin. Others affect only specific tissues. For example, one pituitary hormone, thyroid-stimulating hormone (TSH), acts only on the thyroid gland; another, adrenocorticotropic hormone (ACTH), stimulates only the outer portion of the adrenal gland. Others act more locally, close to where they are secreted.

The specific tissue acted on by each hormone is the **target tissue**. The cells that make up these tissues have **receptors** in the plasma membrane or within the cytoplasm to which the hormone attaches. Once a hormone binds to a receptor on or in a target cell, it affects cell activities, regulating the manufacture of proteins, changing the permeability of the membrane, or affecting metabolic reactions.

Hormone Chemistry

Chemically, hormones fall into two main categories:

- **Amino acid compounds.** These hormones are proteins or related compounds also made of amino acids. All hormones except those of the adrenal cortex and the sex glands fall into this category.
- **Lipids.** These hormones are made of fatty acids. Most are **steroids**, derived from cholesterol. Steroid hormones are produced by the adrenal cortex and the sex glands. They can be recognized by the ending *–one*, as in progesterone, testosterone. Prostaglandins, described later in this chapter, are also in the lipid category.

CHECKPOINT 12-1 ➤ What are hormones and what are some effects of hormones?

Hormone Regulation

The amount of each hormone that is secreted is normally kept within a specific range. Negative feedback, described in Chapter 1, is the method most commonly used to regulate these levels. In negative feedback, the hormone itself (or the result of its action) controls further hormone secretion. Each endocrine gland tends to oversecrete its hormone, exerting more effect on the target tissue. When the target tissue becomes too active, there is a negative effect on the endocrine gland, which then decreases its secretory activity.

We can use as an example the secretion of thyroid hormones (Fig. 12-1). As described in more detail later in the chapter, a pituitary hormone, called *thyroid-stimulating hormone* (TSH), triggers hormone secretion from the thyroid gland located in the neck. As blood levels of these hormones rise under the effects of TSH, they act as negative feedback messengers to inhibit TSH release from the pituitary. With less TSH, the thyroid releases less hormone and blood levels drop. When hormone levels fall below the normal range, the pituitary can again begin to release TSH. This is a typical example of the kind of self-regulating system that keeps hormone levels within a set normal range.

Less commonly, some hormones are produced in response to positive feedback. In this case, response to a hormone promotes further hormone release. Examples are the action of oxytocin during labor, as described in Chapter 1, and the release of some hormones in the menstrual cycle, as described in Chapter 23.

Hormone release may fall into a rhythmic pattern. Hormones of the adrenal cortex follow a 24-hour cycle related to a person's sleeping pattern, with the secretion level greatest just before arising and least at bedtime. Hormones of the female menstrual cycle follow a monthly pattern.

CHECKPOINT 12-2 ➤ Hormone levels are normally kept within a specific range. What is the most common method used to regulate secretion of hormones?

The Endocrine Glands and Their Hormones

The remainder of this chapter deals with hormones and the tissues that produce them. Refer to Figure 12-2 to locate each of the endocrine glands as you study them. Table 12-1 summarizes the information on the endocrine glands and their hormones. Each section of the chapter also includes information on the effects of a hormone's hypersecretion (oversecretion) or hyposecretion (undersecretion), summarized in Table 12-2.

Hypothalamus

Low level of thyroid hormones stimulates release of TSH

Anterior pituitary

TSH

⊕ Stimulates

⊖ Inhibits

Thyroid gland

High level of thyroid hormones inhibits release of TSH

Figure 12-1 **Negative feedback control of thyroid hormones.** The anterior pituitary releases thyroid-stimulating hormone (TSH) when the blood level of thyroid hormones is low. A high level of thyroid hormones inhibits release of TSH and thyroid hormone levels fall.

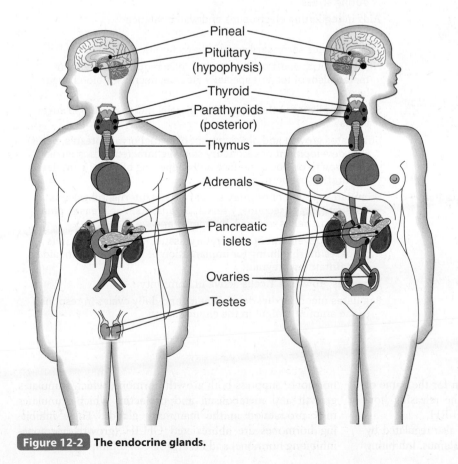

Pineal
Pituitary (hypophysis)
Thyroid
Parathyroids (posterior)
Thymus
Adrenals
Pancreatic islets
Ovaries
Testes

Figure 12-2 **The endocrine glands.**

Although most of the discussion centers on the endocrine glands, it is important to note that many tissues—other than the endocrine glands—also secrete hormones. That is, they produce substances that act on other tissues, usually at some distance from where they are produced. These tissues include the brain, digestive organs, and kidney. Some of these other tissues will be discussed later in the chapter.

The Pituitary

The **pituitary** (pih-TU-ih-tar-e), or **hypophysis** (hi-POF-ih-sis), is a small gland about the size of a cherry. It is located in a saddlelike depression of the sphenoid bone just posterior to the point where the optic nerves cross. It is surrounded by bone except where it connects with the brain's hypothalamus by a stalk called the **infundibulum** (in-fun-DIB-u-lum). The gland is divided into two parts, the **anterior lobe** and the **posterior lobe** (Fig. 12-3).

The pituitary is often called the *master gland* because it releases hormones that affect the working of other glands, such as the thyroid, gonads (ovaries and testes), and adrenal glands. (Hormones that stimulate other glands may be recognized by the ending *-tropin*, as in *thyrotropin*, which means "acting on the thyroid gland.") However, the pituitary itself is controlled by the hypothalamus, by means of secretions and nerve impulses sent to the pituitary through the infundibulum (see Fig. 12-3).

CONTROL OF THE PITUITARY

The hormones produced in the anterior pituitary are not released until chemical messengers called **releasing hormones** arrive from the hypothalamus. These releasing hormones travel to the anterior pituitary by way of a special type of circulatory pathway called a **portal system**. By this circulatory "detour," some of the blood that leaves the hypothalamus travels to capillaries in the anterior pituitary before returning to the heart. As the blood circulates through the capillaries, it delivers the hormones that stimulate the release of anterior pituitary secretions. Hypothalamic releasing hormones are indicated with the

12

Table 12-1	The Endocrine Glands and Their Hormones	
Gland	**Hormone**	**Principal Functions**
Anterior pituitary	GH (growth hormone)	Promotes growth of all body tissues
	TSH (thyroid-stimulating hormone)	Stimulates thyroid gland to produce thyroid hormones
	ACTH (adrenocorticotropic hormone)	Stimulates adrenal cortex to produce cortical hormones; aids in protecting body in stress situations (injury, pain)
	PRL (prolactin)	Stimulates milk secretion by mammary glands
	FSH (follicle-stimulating hormone)	Stimulates growth and hormone activity of ovarian follicles; stimulates growth of testes; promotes development of sperm cells
	LH (luteinizing hormone)	Causes development of corpus luteum at site of ruptured ovarian follicle in female; stimulates testosterone secretion in male
Posterior pituitary	ADH (antidiuretic hormone)	Promotes reabsorption of water in kidney tubules; at high concentration stimulates constriction of blood vessels
	Oxytocin	Causes contraction of uterine muscle; causes milk ejection from mammary glands
Thyroid	Thyroxine (T_4) and triiodothyronine (T_3)	Increase metabolic rate, influencing both physical and mental activities; required for normal growth
	Calcitonin	Decreases calcium level in blood
Parathyroids	PTH (parathyroid hormone)	Regulates exchange of calcium between blood and bones; increases calcium level in blood
Adrenal medulla	Epinephrine and norepinephrine	Increases blood pressure and heart rate; activates cells influenced by sympathetic nervous system plus many not affected by sympathetic nerves
Adrenal cortex	Cortisol (95% of glucocorticoids)	Aids in metabolism of carbohydrates, proteins, and fats; active during stress
	Aldosterone (95% of mineralocorticoids)	Aids in regulating electrolytes and water balance
	Sex hormones	May influence secondary sexual characteristics
Pancreatic islets	Insulin	Needed for transport of glucose into cells; required for cellular metabolism of foods, especially glucose; decreases blood sugar levels
	Glucagon	Stimulates liver to release glucose, thereby increasing blood sugar levels
Testes	Testosterone	Stimulates growth and development of sexual organs (testes, penis) plus development of secondary sexual characteristics, such as hair growth on body and face and deepening of voice; stimulates maturation of sperm cells
Ovaries	Estrogens (e.g., estradiol)	Stimulates growth of primary sexual organs (uterus, tubes) and development of secondary sexual organs, such as breasts, plus changes in pelvis to ovoid, broader shape
	Progesterone	Stimulates development of secretory tissue of mammary glands; prepares uterine lining for implantation of fertilized ovum; aids in maintaining pregnancy
Thymus	Thymosin	Promotes growth of T cells active in immunity
Pineal	Melatonin	Regulates mood, sexual development, and daily cycles in response to the amount of light in the environment

abbreviation *RH* added to an abbreviation for the name of the hormone stimulated. For example, the releasing hormone that controls growth hormone is GH-RH.

Two anterior pituitary hormones are also regulated by inhibiting hormones (IH) from the hypothalamus. Inhibiting hormones suppress both growth hormone, which stimulates growth and metabolism, and prolactin, which stimulates milk production in the mammary glands. These inhibiting hormones are abbreviated GH-IH (growth hormone-inhibiting hormone) and PIH (prolactin-inhibiting hormone).

Table 12-2 Disorders Associated with Endocrine Dysfunction

Hormone	Effects of Hypersecretion	Effects of Hyposecretion
Growth hormone	Gigantism (children), acromegaly (adults)	Dwarfism (children)
Antidiuretic hormone	Syndrome of inappropriate antidiuretic hormone (SIADH)	Diabetes insipidus
Aldosterone	Aldosteronism	Addison disease
Cortisol	Cushing syndrome	Addison disease
Thyroid hormone	Graves disease, thyrotoxicosis	Infantile hypothyroidism in children; myxedema in adults
Insulin	Hypoglycemia	Diabetes mellitus; hyperglycemia
Parathyroid hormone	Bone degeneration	Tetany (muscle spasms)

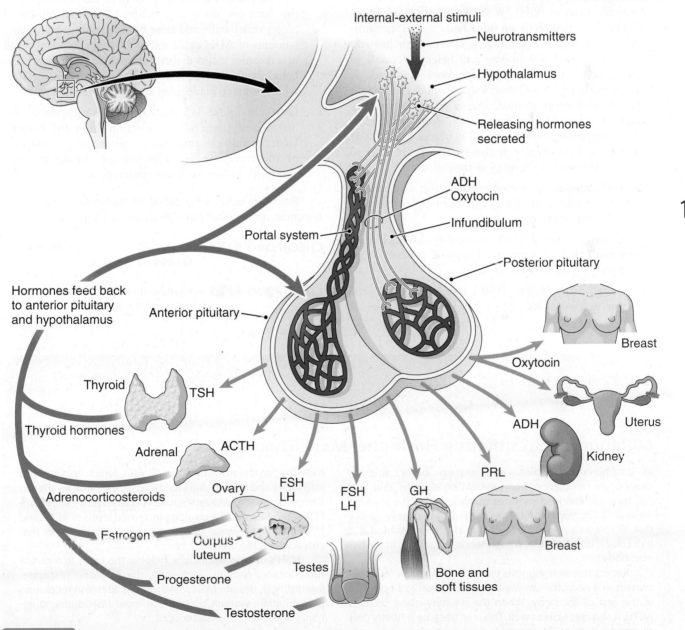

Figure 12-3 **The hypothalamus, pituitary gland, and target tissues.** Arrows indicate the hormones' target tissues and feedback pathways. [**ZOOMING IN ➤** What two structures does the infundibulum connect?]

The two hormones of the posterior pituitary (antidiuretic hormone, or ADH, and oxytocin) are actually produced in the hypothalamus and stored in the posterior pituitary. Their release is controlled by nerve impulses that travel over pathways (tracts) between the hypothalamus and the posterior pituitary.

 PASSport to Success   Visit *thePoint* or see the Student Resource CD in the back of this book for more details and illustrations of the disorders in Table 12-2.

CHECKPOINT 12-3 ➤ What part of the brain controls the pituitary?

ANTERIOR LOBE HORMONES

- **Growth hormone (GH)**, or **somatotropin** (so-mah-to-TRO-pin), acts directly on most body tissues, promoting protein manufacture that is essential for growth. GH causes increases in size and height to occur in youth, before the closure of long bone epiphyses. A young person with a GH deficiency will remain small, though well proportioned, unless treated with adequate hormone. GH is produced throughout life. It stimulates protein synthesis and is needed for cellular maintenance and repair. It also stimulates the liver to release fatty acids for energy in time of stress.

- **Thyroid-stimulating hormone (TSH)**, or **thyrotropin** (thi-ro-TRO-pin), stimulates the thyroid gland to produce thyroid hormones.

- **Adrenocorticotropic** (ad-re-no-kor-tih-ko-TRO-pik) **hormone (ACTH)** stimulates hormone production in the cortex of the adrenal glands.

- **Prolactin** (pro-LAK-tin) **(PRL)** stimulates milk production in the breasts.

- **Follicle-stimulating hormone (FSH)** stimulates the development of eggs in the ovaries and sperm cells in the testes.

- **Luteinizing** (LU-te-in-i-zing) **hormone (LH)** causes ovulation in females and sex hormone secretion in both males and females.

FSH and LH are classified as **gonadotropins** (gon-ah-do-TRO-pinz), hormones that act on the gonads to regulate growth, development, and reproductive function in both males and females.

POSTERIOR LOBE HORMONES

- **Antidiuretic** (an-ti-di-u-RET-ik) **hormone (ADH)** promotes the reabsorption of water from the kidney tubules and thus decreases water excretion. Large amounts of this hormone cause contraction of smooth muscle in blood vessel walls and raise blood pressure. Inadequate amounts of ADH cause excessive water loss and result in a disorder called **diabetes insipidus**. This type of diabetes should not be confused with diabetes mellitus, which is due to inadequate amounts of insulin.

- **Oxytocin** (ok-se-TO-sin) causes contractions of the uterus and triggers milk ejection from the breasts. Under certain circumstances, commercial preparations of this hormone are administered during or after childbirth to cause uterine contraction.

Box 12-1 offers information on melanocyte-stimulating hormone, another hormone produced in the pituitary gland.

CHECKPOINT 12-4 ➤ What are the hormones from the anterior pituitary?

CHECKPOINT 12-5 ➤ What hormones are released from the posterior pituitary?

Box 12-1   A Closer Look

Melanocyte-Stimulating Hormone: More Than a Tan?

In amphibians, reptiles, and certain other animals, melanocyte-stimulating hormone (MSH) darkens skin and hair by stimulating melanocytes to manufacture the pigment melanin. In humans, though, MSH levels are usually so low that its role as a primary regulator of skin pigmentation and hair color is questionable. What, then, is its function in the human body?

Recent research suggests that MSH is probably more important as a neurotransmitter in the brain than as a hormone in the rest of the body. When the pituitary gland secretes ACTH, it secretes MSH as well. This is so because pituitary cells do not produce ACTH directly but produce a large precursor

molecule, proopiomelanocortin (POMC), which enzymes cut into ACTH and MSH. In Addison disease, the pituitary tries to compensate for decreased glucocorticoid levels by increasing POMC production. The resulting increased levels of ACTH and MSH appear to cause the blotchy skin pigmentation that characterizes the disease.

MSH's other roles include helping the brain to regulate food intake, fertility, and even the immune response. Interestingly, despite MSH's relatively small role in regulating pigmentation, women do produce more MSH during pregnancy and often have darker skin.

TUMORS OF THE PITUITARY The effects of pituitary tumors depend on the cell types in the excess tissue. Some of these tumors contain an excessive number of the cells that produce growth hormone. A person who develops such a tumor in childhood will grow to an abnormally tall stature, a condition called **gigantism** (ji-GAN-tizm) (see Table 12-2). Although people with this condition are large, they are usually very weak.

If the GH-producing cells become overactive in the adult, a disorder known as **acromegaly** (ak-ro-MEG-ah-le) develops. In acromegaly, the bones of the face, hands, and feet widen. The fingers resemble a spatula, and the face takes on a coarse appearance: the nose widens, the lower jaw protrudes, and the forehead bones may bulge. Multiple body systems may be affected by acromegaly, including the cardiovascular and nervous systems.

Tumors may destroy the pituitary's secreting tissues so that signs of underactivity develop. Patients with this condition often become obese and sluggish and may exhibit signs of underactivity of other endocrine glands that are controlled by the pituitary, such as the ovaries, testes, or thyroid. Pituitary tumors also may involve the optic nerves and cause blindness.

Evidence of tumor formation in the pituitary gland may be obtained by radiographic examinations of the skull. The pressure of the tumor distorts the sella turcica, the saddlelike space in the sphenoid bone that holds the pituitary. Physicians also use computed tomography (CT) and magnetic resonance imaging (MRI) scans to diagnose pituitary abnormalities.

The Thyroid Gland

The **thyroid**, located in the neck, is the largest of the endocrine glands (Fig. 12-4). The thyroid has two roughly oval lateral lobes on either side of the larynx (voice box) connected by a narrow band called an **isthmus** (IS-mus). A connective tissue capsule encloses the entire gland.

HORMONES OF THE THYROID GLAND The thyroid produces two hormones that regulate metabolism. The principal hormone is **thyroxine** (thi-ROK-sin), which is symbolized as T_4, based on the four iodine atoms in each molecule. The other hormone, which contains three atoms of iodine, is **triiodothyronine** (tri-i-o-do-THI-ro-nene), or T_3. These hormones function to increase the metabolic rate in body cells. In particular, they increase energy metabolism and protein metabolism. Both thyroid hormones and growth hormone are needed for normal growth.

The thyroid gland needs an adequate iodine supply to produce its hormones. Iodine deficiency is rare now because of widespread availability of this mineral in iodized salt, vegetables, seafood, dairy products, and processed foods.

Another hormone produced by the thyroid gland is **calcitonin** (kal-sih-TO-nin), which is active in calcium metabolism. Calcitonin lowers the amount of calcium circulating in the blood by promoting the deposit of calcium in bone tissue. Calcitonin works with parathyroid hormone and with vitamin D to regulate calcium metabolism, as described below.

DISORDERS OF THE THYROID GLAND A **goiter** (GOY-ter) is an enlargement of the thyroid gland, which may or may not be associated with overproduction of hormone. A **simple goiter** is the uniform overgrowth of the thyroid gland, with a smooth surface appearance. An **adenomatous** (ad-eh-NO-mah-tus), or **nodular, goiter** is an irregular-appearing goiter accompanied by tumor formation.

> PASSport to Success Visit **thePoint** or see the Student Resource CD in the back of this book for a goiter illustration.

For various reasons, the thyroid gland may become either underactive or overactive. Thyroid underactivity, known as **hypothyroidism** (hi-po-THI-royd-izm), shows up as two characteristic states related to age:

- **Infantile hypothyroidism** is a condition resulting from hypothyroidism in infants and children. The usual cause is a failure of the thyroid gland to form during fetal development (congenital hypothyroidism). The infant suffers lack of physical growth and lack of mental development. Early and continuous treatment with replacement hormone can alter the outlook of this disease. By state law, all newborns are tested for hypothyroidism in the U.S.

- **Myxedema** (mik-seh-DE-mah) results from thyroid atrophy (wasting) in the adult. The patient becomes sluggish both mentally and physically and often feels cold. The hair becomes dry and the skin becomes dry and waxy. The tissues of the face swell. Because thyroid hormone can be administered orally, the patient with myxedema regains health easily, although treatment must be maintained throughout life.

Hyperthyroidism is the opposite of hypothyroidism, that is, overactivity of the thyroid gland with excessive

Figure 12-4 Thyroid gland (anterior view). The two lobes and isthmus of the thyroid are shown in relation to other structures in the throat. The epiglottis is a cartilage of the larynx. [**ZOOMING IN ▶** What structure is superior to the thyroid? Inferior to the thyroid?]

Epiglottis
Thyroid gland (right lobe)
Hyoid bone
Isthmus of thyroid gland
Larynx
Trachea

hormone secretion. A common form of hyperthyroidism is **Graves disease**, which is characterized by a goiter, a strained appearance of the face, intense nervousness, weight loss, a rapid pulse, sweating, tremors, and an abnormally quick metabolism. Another characteristic symptom is protrusion (bulging) of the eyes, known as **exophthalmos** (ek-sof-THAL-mos), which is caused by swelling of the tissue behind the eyes (Fig. 12-5). Treatment of hyperthyroidism may take the following forms:

- Suppression of hormone production with medication
- Destruction of thyroid tissue with radioactive iodine
- Surgical removal of part of the thyroid gland

An exaggerated form of hyperthyroidism with a sudden onset is called a **thyroid storm**. Untreated, it is usually fatal, but with appropriate care, most affected people can be saved.

Thyroiditis (thi-royd-I-tis) is a general term meaning inflammation of the thyroid. The cause may be infection or autoimmunity, that is, abnormal production of antibodies to the thyroid gland. **Hashimoto disease** is an autoimmune thyroiditis that may be hereditary and may also involve excess intake of iodine. The disease results in thyroid enlargement (goiter) and hypothyroidism. It is treated with thyroid hormone replacement and, in some cases, surgery.

CHECKPOINT 12-6 ➤ What is the effect of thyroid hormones on cells?

TESTS OF THYROID FUNCTION The most frequently used thyroid function tests are blood tests that measure the uptake of radioactive iodine added to a blood sample. These very sensitive tests are used to detect abnormal thyroid function and to monitor response to drug therapy. A test for the level of thyroid-stimulating hormone (from the pituitary) is frequently done at the same time. Further testing involves giving a person oral radioactive iodine and measuring the amount and distribution of radiation that accumulates in the thyroid gland.

The Parathyroid Glands

The four tiny **parathyroid glands** are embedded in the thyroid's posterior capsule (Fig. 12-6). The secretion of these glands, **parathyroid hormone** (**PTH**), promotes calcium release from bone tissue, thus increasing the amount of calcium circulating in the bloodstream. PTH also causes the kidney to conserve calcium. Low PTH, as may be caused by removal of the parathyroids, results in muscle spasms known as *tetany*.

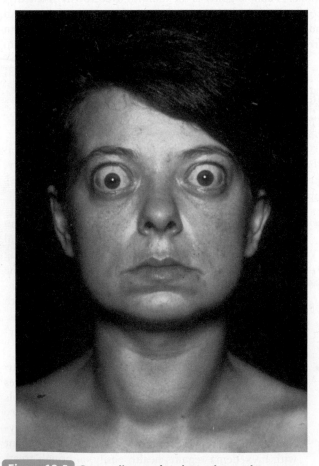

Figure 12-5 Graves disease showing goiter and exophthalmos. Goiter is enlargement of the thyroid; exophthalmos is bulging of the eyes. (Sandoz Pharmaceutical Corporation.)

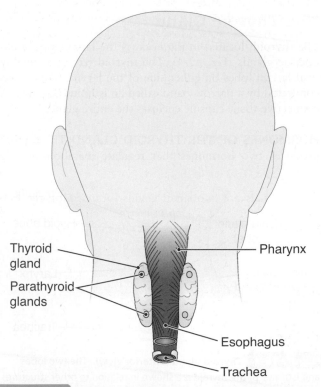

Figure 12-6 Parathyroid glands (posterior view). The four small parathyroid glands are embedded in the posterior surface of the thyroid.

PTH works with calcitonin from the thyroid gland to regulate calcium metabolism. These hormone levels are controlled by negative feedback based on the amount of calcium in the blood. When calcium is high, calcitonin is produced; when calcium is low, PTH is produced.

CALCIUM METABOLISM Calcium balance is required not only for the health of bones and teeth but also for the proper function of the nervous system and muscles. One other hormone is needed for calcium balance in addition to calcitonin and PTH. This is **calcitriol** (kal-sih-TRI-ol), technically called dihydroxycholecalciferol (di-hi-drok-se-ko-le-kal-SIF-eh-rol), the active form of vitamin D. Calcitriol is produced by modification of vitamin D in the liver and then the kidney. It increases intestinal absorption of calcium to raise blood calcium levels.

Calcitonin, PTH, and calcitriol work together to regulate the amount of calcium in the blood and provide calcium for bone maintenance and other functions.

DISORDERS OF THE PARATHYROID GLANDS Inadequate production of parathyroid hormone, as a result of removal or damage to the parathyroid glands, for example, causes a series of muscle contractions involving particularly the hands and face. These spasms result from a low concentration of blood calcium, and the condition is called **tetany** (TET-ah-ne). This low calcium tetany should not be confused with the infection called *tetanus* (lockjaw).

In contrast, if there is excess production of PTH, as may happen in parathyroid tumors, calcium is removed from its normal storage place in the bones and released into the bloodstream. The loss of calcium from the bones leads to fragile bones that fracture easily. Because the kidneys ultimately excrete the calcium, kidney stone formation is common in such cases.

CHECKPOINT 12-7 ➤ What mineral is regulated by calcitonin and parathyroid hormone (PTH)?

The Adrenal Glands

The **adrenals** are two small glands located atop the kidneys. Each adrenal gland has two parts that act as separate glands. The inner area is called the **medulla**, and the outer portion is called the **cortex** (Fig. 12-7).

HORMONES FROM THE ADRENAL MEDULLA The hormones of the adrenal medulla are released in response to stimulation by the sympathetic nervous system. The principal hormone produced by the medulla is **epinephrine**, also called **adrenaline**. Another hormone released from the adrenal medulla, **norepinephrine** (noradrenaline), is closely related chemically and is similar in its actions to epinephrine. These two hormones are referred to as the *fight-or-flight hormones* because of their effects during emergency situations. We have already learned about these hormones in studying the autonomic nervous system.

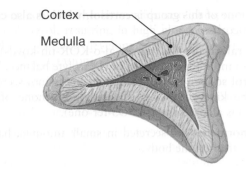

Figure 12-7 **The adrenal gland.** The medulla secretes epinephrine and norepinephrine. The cortex secretes steroid hormones. (Reprinted with permission from Gartner LP, Hiatt JL. *Color Atlas of Histology*, 3rd ed. Philadelphia: Lippincott Williams & Wilkins, 2000.) **[ZOOMING IN ➤** What is the outer region of the adrenal gland called? The inner region? **]**

When released from nerve endings instead of being released directly into the bloodstream, they function as neurotransmitters. Some of their effects are as follows:

- Stimulation of the involuntary muscle in the walls of the arterioles, causing these muscles to contract and blood pressure to rise accordingly
- Conversion of glycogen stored in the liver into glucose. The glucose pours into the blood and travels throughout the body, allowing the voluntary muscles and other tissues to do an extraordinary amount of work
- Increase in the heart rate
- Increase in the metabolic rate of body cells
- Dilation of the bronchioles, through relaxation of the smooth muscle in their walls

CHECKPOINT 12-8 ➤ The main hormone from the adrenal medulla also functions as a neurotransmitter in the sympathetic nervous system. What is the name of this hormone?

HORMONES FROM THE ADRENAL CORTEX There are three main groups of hormones secreted by the adrenal cortex:

- **Glucocorticoids** (glu-ko-KOR-tih-koyds) maintain the body's carbohydrate reserve by stimulating the liver to convert amino acids into glucose (sugar) instead of protein. The production of these hormones increases in times of stress to aid the body in responding to unfavorable conditions. They raise the level of nutrients in the blood, not only glucose, but also amino acids from tissue proteins and fatty acids from fats stored in adipose tissue. Glucocorticoids also have the ability to suppress the inflammatory response and are often administered as medication for this purpose. The major

HORMONES OF THE SEX GLANDS All male sex hormones are classified as **androgens** (AN-dro-jens). The main androgen produced by the testes is testosterone (tes-TOS-ter-one).

In the female, the hormones that most nearly parallel testosterone in their actions are the **estrogens** (ES-tro-jens), produced by the ovaries. Estrogens contribute to the development of the female secondary sex characteristics and stimulate mammary gland development, the onset of menstruation, and the development and functioning of the reproductive organs.

The other hormone produced by the ovaries, called **progesterone** (pro-JES-ter-one), assists in the normal development of pregnancy (gestation). All the sex hormones are discussed in more detail in Chapter 23.

CHECKPOINT 12-13 ➤ In addition to controlling reproduction, sex hormones confer certain features associated with male and female gender. What are these features called as a group?

The Thymus Gland

The **thymus gland** is a mass of lymphoid tissue that lies in the upper part of the chest superior to the heart. This gland is important in the development of immunity. Its hormone, **thymosin** (THI-mo-sin), assists in the maturation of certain white blood cells known as T cells (T lymphocytes) after they have left the thymus gland and taken up residence in lymph nodes throughout the body.

The Pineal Gland

The **pineal** (PIN-e-al) **gland** is a small, flattened, cone-shaped structure located posterior to the midbrain and connected to the roof of the third ventricle (see Fig. 12-2).

The pineal produces the hormone **melatonin** (mel-ah-TO-nin) during dark periods. Little hormone is produced during daylight hours. This pattern of hormone secretion influences the regulation of sleep–wake cycles. (See also Box 12-2, Seasonal Affective Disorder.) Melatonin also appears to delay the onset of puberty.

Other Hormone-Producing Tissues

Originally, the word *hormone* applied to the secretions of the endocrine glands only. The term now includes various body substances that have regulatory actions, either locally or at a distance from where they are produced. Many body tissues produce substances that regulate the local environment. Some of these other hormone-producing organs are the following:

- The stomach secretes a hormone that stimulates its own digestive activity.
- The small intestine secretes hormones that stimulate the production of digestive juices and help regulate the digestive process.
- The kidneys produce a hormone called **erythropoietin** (e-rith-ro-POY-eh-tin), which stimulates red blood cell production in the bone marrow. This hormone is produced when there is a decreased oxygen supply in the blood.
- The brain, as noted, secretes releasing hormones and release-inhibiting hormones that control the anterior pituitary, as well as ADH and oxytocin that are released from the posterior pituitary.
- The atria (upper chambers) of the heart produce a substance called **atrial natriuretic** (na-tre-u-RET-ik) **peptide** (ANP) in response to their increased filling

---

Box 12-2 **Clinical Perspectives**

Seasonal Affective Disorder: Seeing the Light

We all sense that long dark days make us blue and sap our motivation. Are these learned responses or is there a physical basis for them? Studies have shown that the amount of light in the environment does have a physical effect on behavior. Evidence that light alters mood comes from people who are intensely affected by the dark days of winter—people who suffer from **seasonal affective disorder**, aptly abbreviated SAD. When days shorten, these people feel sleepy, depressed, and anxious. They tend to overeat, especially carbohydrates. Research suggests that SAD has a genetic basis and may be associated with decreased levels of serotonin.

As light strikes the retina of the eye, it sends impulses that decrease the amount of melatonin produced by the pineal gland in the brain. Because melatonin depresses mood, the final effect of light is to elevate mood. Daily exposure to bright lights has been found to improve the mood of most people with SAD. Exposure for 15 minutes after rising in the morning may be enough, but some people require longer sessions both morning and evening. Other aids include aerobic exercise, stress management techniques, and antidepressant medications.

with blood. ANP increases sodium excretion by the kidneys and lowers blood pressure.

■ The **placenta** (plah-SEN-tah) produces several hormones during pregnancy. These cause changes in the uterine lining and, later in pregnancy, help to prepare the breasts for lactation. Pregnancy tests are based on the presence of placental hormones.

Prostaglandins

Prostaglandins (pros-tah-GLAN-dins) are a group of local hormones made by most body tissues. Their name comes from the fact that they were first discovered in male prostate glands. Prostaglandins are produced, act, and are rapidly inactivated in or close to their sites of origin. A bewildering array of functions has been ascribed to these substances. Some prostaglandins cause constriction of blood vessels, bronchial tubes, and the intestine, whereas others cause dilation of these same structures. Prostaglandins are active in promoting inflammation; certain antiinflammatory drugs, such as aspirin, act by blocking prostaglandin production. Some prostaglandins have been used to induce labor or abortion and have been recommended as possible contraceptive agents.

Overproduction of prostaglandins by the uterine lining (endometrium) can cause painful cramps of the uterine muscle. Treatment with prostaglandin inhibitors has been successful in some cases. Much has been written about these substances, and extensive research on them continues.

CHECKPOINT 12-14 ▸ What are some organs other than the endocrine glands that produce hormones?

Hormones and Treatment

Hormones used for medical treatment are obtained from several different sources. Some are extracted from animal tissues. Some hormones and hormonelike substances are available in synthetic form, meaning that they are manufactured in commercial laboratories. A few hormones are produced by the genetic engineering technique of recombinant DNA. In this method, a gene for the cellular manufacture of a given product is introduced in the laboratory into the common bacterium *Escherichia coli*. The organisms are then grown in quantity, and the desired substance is harvested and purified.

A few examples of natural and synthetic hormones used in treatment are:

■ **Growth hormone** is used for the treatment of children with a deficiency of this hormone. It is also used to strengthen bones and build body mass in the elderly. Adequate supplies are available from recombinant DNA techniques.

■ **Insulin** is used in the treatment of diabetes mellitus. Pharmaceutical companies now produce "human" insulin by recombinant DNA methods.

■ **Adrenal steroids**, primarily the glucocorticoids, are used for the relief of inflammation in such diseases as rheumatoid arthritis, lupus erythematosus, asthma, and cerebral edema; for immunosuppression after organ transplantation; and for relief of symptoms associated with circulatory shock.

■ **Epinephrine** (adrenaline) has many uses, including stimulation of the heart muscle when rapid response is required, treatment of asthmatic attacks by relaxation of the small bronchial tubes, and treatment of the acute allergic reaction called **anaphylaxis** (an-ah-fi-LAK-sis).

■ **Thyroid hormones** are used in the treatment of hypothyroid conditions (infantile hypothyroidism and myxedema) and as replacement therapy after surgical removal of the thyroid gland.

■ **Oxytocin** is used to cause uterine contractions and induce labor.

■ **Androgens**, including testosterone and androsterone, are used in severe chronic illness to aid tissue building and promote healing.

■ **Estrogen and progesterone** are used as oral contraceptives (birth control pills; "the pill"). They are highly effective in preventing pregnancy. Occasionally, they give rise to unpleasant side effects, such as nausea. More rarely, they cause serious complications, such as thrombosis (blood clots) or hypertension (high blood pressure). These adverse side effects are more common among women who smoke. Any woman taking birth control pills should have a yearly medical examination.

Estrogen and progesterone preparations have been used to treat symptoms associated with menopause and protect against adverse changes that occur after menopause. Recent studies on the most popular form of these hormones have raised questions about their benefits and revealed some risks associated with their use. This issue is still under study.

Hormones and Stress

Stress in the form of physical injury, disease, emotional anxiety, and even pleasure calls forth a specific physiologic response that involves both the nervous system and the endocrine system. The nervous system response, the "fight-or-flight" response, is mediated by parts of the brain, especially the hypothalamus, and by the sympathetic nervous system, which releases epinephrine. During stress, the hypothalamus also triggers the release of ACTH from the anterior pituitary. The hormones released from the adrenal cortex as a result of ACTH stimulation raise the levels of glucose and other nutrients in the blood and inhibit

12

inflammation. Growth hormone, thyroid hormones, sex hormones, and insulin are also released.

These hormones help the body meet stressful situations. Unchecked, however, they are harmful and may lead to such stress-related disorders as high blood pressure, heart disease, ulcers, insomnia, back pain, and headaches. Cortisones decrease the immune response, leaving the body more susceptible to infection.

Although no one would enjoy a life totally free of stress in the form of stimulation and challenge, unmanaged stress, or "distress," has negative physical effects. For this reason, techniques such as biofeedback and meditation to control stress are useful. The simple measures of setting priorities, getting adequate periods of relaxation, and getting regular physical exercise are important in maintaining total health.

CHECKPOINT 12-15 ➤ What are some hormones released in time of stress?

PASSport to Success

Visit **thePoint** or see the Student Resource CD in the back of this book for information on careers in exercise and fitness.

Aging and the Endocrine System

Some of the changes associated with aging, such as loss of muscle and bone tissue, can be linked to changes in the endocrine system. The main clinical conditions associated with the endocrine system involve the pancreas and the thyroid.

Many elderly people develop type 2 diabetes mellitus as a result of decreased insulin secretion, which is made worse by poor diet, inactivity, and increased body fat. Some elderly people also show the effects of decreased thyroid hormone secretion.

Sex hormones decline during the middle-age years in both males and females. These changes come from decreased activity of the gonads but also involve the more basic level of the pituitary gland and the secretion of gonadotropic hormones. Decrease in bone mass leading to osteoporosis is one result of these declines. With age, there is also a decrease in growth hormone levels and diminished activity of the adrenal cortex.

Thus far, the only commonly applied treatment for endocrine failure associated with age has been sex hormone replacement therapy for women at menopause. This supplementation has shown some beneficial effects on mucous membranes, the cardiovascular system, bone mass, and mental function.

Disease in Context revisited

➤ Becky's New "Normal"

Becky stumbled down the stairs wiping the sleep from her eyes as she made her way to the kitchen, hoping that Max hadn't finished all the pancakes that she could smell from down the hallway. "Good morning, sleepy-head," greeted her mother as she handed Becky the glucose monitor and lancet. "How was your sleep last night?"

"Great," yawned Becky as she lanced the side of her finger and squeezed a tiny drop of blood onto the monitor's test strip. After a few seconds, the monitor beeped and displayed her blood glucose concentration. "I'm normal," said Becky, half-expecting a wise-crack from her little brother, but he kept on eating.

Since Dr. Carter's diagnosis, Becky had been getting used to her new "normal." It wasn't easy being diabetic. She had to be really careful about what she ate and when. She had to measure her

glucose before meals and inject herself with insulin after. Monitoring her glucose wasn't too bad, but Becky didn't think she would ever get used to the needles. She was also a little worried about what the kids at school were saying about her and her disease. One unexpected benefit was that Max seemed to have a new-found respect for her and her ability to inject herself. "What a weirdo!" she thought as she carefully poured a little bit of syrup on her pancakes.

During this case, we saw that the lack of the hormone insulin had widespread effects on Becky's whole body. In later chapters, we will learn more about the endocrine system's role in regulating body function. We'll also check on how Becky is managing her diabetes in Chapter 20: Metabolism, Nutrition, and Body Temperature.

Word Anatomy

Medical terms are built from standardized word parts (prefixes, roots, and suffixes). Learning the meanings of these parts can help you remember words and interpret unfamiliar terms.

WORD PART	MEANING	EXAMPLE
The Endocrine Glands and Their Hormones		
trop/o	acting on, influencing	*Somatotropin* stimulates growth in most body tissues.
cortic/o	cortex	*Adrenocorticotropic* hormone acts on the adrenal cortex.
lact/o	milk	*Prolactin* stimulates milk production in the breasts.
ur/o	urine	*Antidiuretic* hormone promotes reabsorption of water in the kidneys and decreases excretion of urine.
oxy	sharp, acute	*Oxytocin* stimulates uterine contractions during labor.
toc/o	labor	See preceding example.
acr/o	end, extremity	*Acromegaly* causes enlargement of hands and feet.
-megaly	enlargement	See preceding example.
myx/o	mucus	In *myxedema,* the skin takes on a swollen, waxy appearance.
edem	swelling	See preceding example.
ren/o	kidney	The *adrenal* glands are near (ad-) the kidneys.
nephr/o	kidney	*Epinephrine* is another name for adrenaline.
insul/o	pancreatic islet, island	*Insulin* is a hormone produced by the pancreatic islets.
glyc/o	sugar, glucose	*Hyperglycemia* is high blood sugar.
andr/o	male	An *androgen* is any male sex hormone.
Other Hormone-Producing Tissues		
-poiesis	making, forming	*Erythropoietin* is a hormone from the kidneys that stimulates production of red blood cells.
natri	sodium (*L. natrium*)	Atrial *natriuretic* peptide stimulates release of sodium in the urine.

12

Summary

I. **HORMONES**
  A. Functions of hormones
     1. Affect other cells or organs—target tissue
     2. Widespread effects on growth, metabolism, reproduction
     3. Bind to receptors on target cells
  B. Hormone chemistry
     1. Amino acid compounds—proteins and related compounds
     2. Lipids—made from fatty acids
        a. Steroids

(1) Derived from cholesterol
(2) Produced by adrenal cortex and sex glands
        b. Prostaglandins
  C. Regulation of hormones—mainly negative feedback
II. **ENDOCRINE GLANDS AND THEIR HORMONES**
  A. Pituitary
     1. Regulated by hypothalamus
        a. Anterior pituitary
           (1) Releasing hormones (RH) sent through portal system

(2) Inhibiting hormones for GH and PRL

b. Posterior pituitary

(1) Stores hormones made by hypothalamus

(2) Released by nervous stimulation

2. Anterior lobe hormones

a. Growth hormone (GH)—stimulates growth, tissue repair

b. Thyroid-stimulating hormone (TSH)

c. Adrenocorticotropic hormone (ACTH)—acts on cortex of adrenal gland

d. Prolactin (PRL)—stimulates milk production in mammary glands

e. Follicle-stimulating hormone (FSH)—acts on gonads

f. Luteinizing hormone (LH)—acts on gonads

3. Posterior lobe hormones

a. Antidiuretic hormone (ADH)—promotes reabsorption of water in the kidneys

b. Oxytocin—stimulates uterine contractions

4. Pituitary tumors—may cause underactivity or overactivity of pituitary

B. Thyroid gland

1. Hormones of the thyroid gland

a. Thyroxine (T4) and triiodothyronine (T3) increase metabolic rate

b. Calcitonin—decreases blood calcium levels

2. Disorders of the thyroid gland

a. Goiter—enlarged thyroid

b. Hypothyroidism—causes infantile hypothyroidism or myxedema

c. Hyperthyroidism—e.g., Graves disease

d. Thyroiditis—inflammation of thyroid; e.g., Hashimoto thyroiditis

3. Thyroid function tests—radioactive iodine used

C. Parathyroid glands—secrete parathyroid hormone (PTH), which increases blood calcium levels

1. Calcium metabolism

2. Disorders of the parathyroid glands

D. Adrenal glands

1. Hormones of adrenal medulla (inner region)

a. Epinephrine and norepinephrine—act as neurotransmitters

2. Hormones of adrenal cortex (outer region)

a. Glucocorticoids—released during stress to raise nutrients in blood; e.g., cortisol

b. Mineralocorticoids—regulate water and electrolyte balance; e.g., aldosterone

c. Sex hormones—produced in small amounts

3. Disorders of the adrenal cortex

E. Pancreas—islet cells of pancreas secrete hormones

1. Insulin

a. Lowers blood glucose

b. Lack or poor cellular response causes diabetes mellitus

(1) Type 1 (T1DM)—autoimmune disease that requires insulin

(2) Type 2 (T2DM)—usually controlled with diet, exercise, weight loss

(3) Gestational—occurs curing pregnancy

2. Glucagon

a. Raises blood glucose

F. Sex glands—needed for reproduction and development of secondary sex characteristics

1. Testes—secrete testosterone

2. Ovaries—secrete estrogen and progesterone

G. Thymus gland—secretes thymosin, which aids in development of T lymphocytes

H. Pineal gland—secretes melatonin

1. Regulates sexual development and sleep–wake cycles

2. Controlled by environmental light

III. **OTHER HORMONE-PRODUCING TISSUES**

A. Stomach and small intestine—secrete hormones that regulate digestion

B. Kidneys—secrete erythropoietin, which increases production of red blood cells

C. Brain—releasing and inhibiting hormones, ADH, oxytocin

D. Atria of heart—ANP causes loss of sodium by kidney and lowers blood pressure

E. Placenta—secretes hormones that maintain pregnancy and prepare breasts for lactation

F. Prostaglandins—produced by cells throughout body; have varied effects

IV. **HORMONES AND TREATMENT**

A. Growth hormone—treatment of deficiency in children, in elderly for bone strength and body mass

B. Insulin—treatment of diabetes mellitus

C. Steroids—reduction of inflammation, suppression of immunity

D. Epinephrine—treatment of asthma, anaphylaxis, shock

E. Thyroid hormone—treatment of hypothyroidism

F. Oxytocin—contraction of uterine muscle

G. Androgens—promote healing

H. Estrogen and progesterone—contraception, symptoms of menopause

V. **HORMONES AND STRESS**

A. Body's response to stress involves nervous and endocrine systems, hormones

B. Fight-or-flight response mediated by brain: hypothalamus, sympathetic nervous system

C. Hormones help body to meet stressful situations

D. Unmanaged stress can be harmful; stress management techniques help maintain overall health

VI. **AGING AND THE ENDOCRINE SYSTEM**

A. Aging-associated changes linked with endocrine system changes—loss of muscle and bone tissue

B. Main clinical conditions associated with endocrine system involve pancreas, thyroid

1. Type 2 diabetes mellitus

2. Decline in sex hormones in males and females

a. Decreased bone mass—osteoporosis

C. Sex hormone replacement therapy for women at menopause—only common treatment for age-associated endocrine failure

Questions for Study and Review

BUILDING UNDERSTANDING

Fill in the blanks

1. Chemical messengers carried by the blood are called _____.

2. The part of the brain that regulates endocrine activity is the _____.

3. Red blood cell production in the bone marrow is stimulated by _____.

4. A hormone produced by the heart is _____.

5. Local hormones active in promoting inflammation are _____.

Matching > Match each numbered item with the most closely related lettered item.

___ 6. A disorder caused by overproduction of growth hormone in the adult.   **a.** hypoglycemia

___ 7. A disorder caused by underproduction of parathyroid hormone.   **b.** gigantism

___ 8. A disorder caused by overproduction of insulin.   **c.** tetany

___ 9. A disorder caused by overproduction of growth hormone in the child.   **d.** diabetes insipidus

___ 10. A disorder caused by underproduction of antidiuretic hormone.   **e.** acromegaly

Multiple Choice

___ 11. A target tissue responds to a hormone only if it has the appropriate
   a. amino acid
   b. transporter
   c. ion channel
   d. receptor

___ 12. Uterine contractions and milk ejection are promoted by
   a. prolactin
   b. oxytocin
   c. estrogen
   d. luteinizing hormone

___ 13. The principal hormone that increases the metabolic rate in body cells is
   a. thyroxine
   b. triiodothyronine
   c. aldosterone
   d. progesterone

___ 14. Epinephrine and norepinephrine are released by the
   a. adrenal cortex
   b. adrenal medulla
   c. kidneys
   d. pancreas

___ 15. Sleep-wake cycles are regulated by the
   a. pituitary
   b. thyroid
   c. thymus
   d. pineal

12

The Blood

Learning Outcomes

After careful study of this chapter, you should be able to:

1. List the functions of the blood
2. List the main ingredients in plasma
3. Describe the formation of blood cells
4. Name and describe the three types of formed elements in the blood and give the function of each
5. Characterize the five types of leukocytes
6. Define *hemostasis* and cite three steps in hemostasis
7. Briefly describe the steps in blood clotting
8. Define *blood type* and explain the relation between blood type and transfusions
9. List the possible reasons for transfusions of whole blood and blood components
10. Define *anemia* and list the causes of anemia
11. Define *leukemia* and name the two types of leukemia
12. Describe several forms of clotting disorders
13. Specify the tests used to study blood
14. Show how word parts are used to build words related to the blood (see Word Anatomy at the end of the chapter)

Selected Key Terms

The following terms and other boldface terms in the chapter are defined in the Glossary

agglutination

anemia

antigen

antiserum

centrifuge

coagulation

cryoprecipitate

erythrocyte

fibrin

hematocrit

hemoglobin

hemolysis

hemorrhage

hemostasis

leukemia

leukocyte

megakaryocyte

plasma

platelet (thrombocyte)

serum

thrombocytopenia

transfusion

PASSport to Success

Visit *thePoint* or see the Student Resource CD in the back of this book for definitions and pronunciations of key terms as well as a pretest for this chapter.

Disease in Context

➤ Cole's Case: A Hemoglobin Abnormality

Both baby Cole and his mother Jada were resting comfortably in the maternity ward. Although Cole was only a few hours old, he had already been bathed, fed, and thoroughly examined by a pediatrician. As part of the hospital's routine neonatal procedures, a sample of Cole's blood was collected and sent to the hematology laboratory.

When Cole's blood sample arrived in the laboratory, a technologist divided it into several portions for analysis. First, she tested for Cole's blood type. When she added anti-B serum to his blood, the erythrocytes in the sample clumped together. There was no reaction to the anti-A serum. Since the antibodies in the sera showed only B antigens on the red blood cells, the medical laboratory technologist knew that Cole's blood was type B. Next, she performed a blood cell count using an automated machine. Cole's platelet count was normal, suggesting that he did not suffer from thrombocytopenia, the most common clotting disorder. His leukocyte count was normal too, signifying that his immune system was healthy. His erythrocyte count was also within normal limits, indicating that his red bone marrow (the site of erythrocyte production) was functioning as well. As required by many hospitals in the United States, the technologist screened Cole's blood for the presence of abnormal hemoglobin in his erythrocytes. When the test result came back positive for abnormal hemoglobin, the technologist requested that a blood sample be drawn from both of Cole's parents. She needed to run some more sensitive blood tests to determine whether or not the infant suffered from sickle cell disease.

The medical laboratory technologist performed several tests on Cole's blood. In this chapter, you will study blood and learn about its constituents and functions. Later, we'll find out more about Cole's abnormal hemoglobin.

The circulating blood is of fundamental importance in maintaining homeostasis. This life-giving fluid brings nutrients and oxygen to the cells and carries away waste. The heart pumps blood continuously through a closed system of vessels. The heart and blood vessels are described in Chapters 14 and 15.

Blood is classified as a connective tissue because it consists of cells suspended in an intercellular background material, or matrix. Blood cells share many characteristics of origination and development with other connective tissues. However, blood differs from other connective tissues in that its cells are not fixed in position; instead, they move freely in the plasma, the blood's liquid portion.

Whole blood is a viscous (thick) fluid that varies in color from bright scarlet to dark red, depending on how much oxygen it is carrying. (It is customary in drawings to color blood high in oxygen as red and blood low in oxygen as blue.) The blood volume accounts for approximately 8% of total body weight. The actual quantity of circulating blood differs with a person's size; the average adult male, weighing 70 kg (154 pounds), has about 5 liters (5.2 quarts) of blood.

Functions of the Blood

The circulating blood serves the body in three ways: transportation, regulation, and protection.

Transportation

- **Gases.** Oxygen from inhaled air diffuses into the blood through thin membranes in the lungs and is carried by the circulation to all body tissues. Carbon dioxide, a waste product of cell metabolism, is carried from the tissues to the lungs, where it is breathed out.

- **Nutrients.** The blood transports nutrients and other needed substances, such as electrolytes (salts) and vitamins, to the cells. These materials enter the blood from the digestive system or are released into the blood from body reserves.

- **Waste.** The blood transports the waste products from the cells to sites where they are removed. For example, the kidney removes excess water, acid, electrolytes, and urea (a nitrogen-containing waste). The liver removes blood pigments, hormones, and drugs, and the lungs eliminate carbon dioxide.

- **Hormones.** The blood carries hormones from their sites of origin to the organs they affect.

Regulation

- **pH.** Buffers in the blood help keep the pH of body fluids steady at about 7.4. (The actual range of blood pH is 7.35 to 7.45.) Recall that pH is a measure of a solution's acidity or alkalinity. At an average pH of 7.4, blood is slightly alkaline (basic).

- **Fluid balance.** The blood regulates the amount of fluid in the tissues by means of substances (mainly proteins) that maintain the proper osmotic pressure. Recall that osmotic pressure is related to the concentration of dissolved and suspended materials in a solution. Proper osmotic pressure is needed for fluid balance, as described in Chapter 15.

- **Heat.** The blood transports heat that is generated in the muscles to other parts of the body, thus aiding in the regulation of body temperature.

Protection

- **Disease.** The blood is important in defense against disease. It carries the cells and antibodies of the immune system that protect against pathogens.

- **Blood loss.** The blood contains factors that protect against blood loss from the site of an injury. The process of blood coagulation, needed to prevent blood loss, is described later in this chapter.

CHECKPOINT 13-1 ➤ What are some substances transported in the blood?

CHECKPOINT 13-2 ➤ What is the pH range of the blood?

Visit *thePoint* or see the Student Resource CD in the back of this book for information on careers in hematology, the study of blood.

Blood Constituents

The blood is divided into two main components (Fig. 13-1). The liquid portion is the **plasma**. The **formed elements,** which include cells and cell fragments, fall into three categories, as follows:

- **Erythrocytes** (eh-RITH-ro-sites), from *erythro,* meaning "red," are the red blood cells, which transport oxygen.

- **Leukocytes** (LU-ko-sites), from *leuko,* meaning "white," are the several types of white blood cells, which protect against infection.

- **Platelets,** also called **thrombocytes** (THROM-bo-sites), are cell fragments that participate in blood clotting.

Table 13-1 summarizes information on the different types of formed elements. Figure 13-2 shows all the categories of formed elements in a blood smear, that is, a blood sample spread thinly over the surface of a glass slide, as viewed under a microscope.

CHECKPOINT 13-3 ➤ What are the two main components of blood?

Figure 13-1 **Composition of whole blood.** Percentages show the relative proportions of the different components of plasma and formed elements.

Blood Plasma

About 55% of the total blood volume is plasma. The plasma itself is 91% water. Many different substances, dissolved or suspended in the water, make up the other 9% by weight (see Fig. 13-1). The plasma content may vary somewhat because substances are removed and added as the blood circulates to and from the tissues. However, the body tends to maintain a fairly constant level of most substances. For example, the level of glucose, a simple sugar, is maintained at a remarkably constant level of about one-tenth of one percent (0.1%) in solution.

After water, the next largest percentage (about 8%) of material in the plasma is **protein**. The plasma proteins include the following:

- **Albumin** (al-BU-min), the most abundant protein in plasma, is important for maintaining the blood's osmotic pressure. This protein is manufactured in the liver.

- **Clotting factors**, necessary for blood coagulation, are also manufactured in the liver.

- **Antibodies** combat infection. Antibodies are made by certain white blood cells.

- **Complement** consists of a group of enzymes that helps antibodies in their fight against pathogens (see Chapter 17).

The remaining 1% of the plasma consists of nutrients, electrolytes, and other materials that must be transported. With regard to the nutrients, the principal carbohydrate found in the plasma is glucose. This simple sugar is absorbed from digested foods in the intestine. It is also stored as glycogen in the liver and skeletal muscles; this glucose can be released as needed to supply energy. Amino acids, the products of protein digestion, also circulate in the plasma. Lipids constitute a small percentage of blood plasma. Lipid components include fats, cholesterol, and lipoproteins, which are proteins bound to cholesterol.

The electrolytes in the plasma appear primarily as chloride, carbonate, or phosphate salts of sodium, potassium, calcium, and magnesium. These salts have a variety of functions, including the formation of bone (calcium and phosphorus), the production of certain hormones (such as iodine for the production of thyroid hormones), and the maintenance of the acid–base balance (such as sodium and potassium carbonates and phosphates present in buffers).

Other materials transported in plasma include vitamins, hormones, waste products, drugs, and dissolved gases, primarily oxygen and carbon dioxide.

13

Table 13-1 Formed Elements of Blood

Formed Element	Number per µL of Blood	Description	Function
Erythrocyte (red blood cell)	5 million	Tiny (7 µm diameter), biconcave disk without nucleus (anuclear)	Carries oxygen bound to hemoglobin; also carries some carbon dioxide and buffers blood
Leukocyte (white blood cell)	5,000 to 10,000	Larger than red cell with prominent nucleus that may be segmented (granulocyte) or unsegmented (agranulocyte); vary in staining properties	Protects against pathogens; destroys foreign matter and debris; some are active in the immune system; located in blood, tissues, and lymphatic system
Platelet	150,000 to 450,000	Fragment of large cell (megakaryocyte)	Hemostasis; forms a platelet plug and starts blood clot-

Platelet

Leukocyte

Erythrocytes

Figure 13-2 **Blood cells as viewed under the microscope.** All three types of formed elements are visible. [ZOOMING IN ➤ Which cells are the most numerous in the blood?]

Figure 13-3 **Red blood cells as seen under a scanning electron microscope.** This type of microscope provides a three-dimensional view of the cells. [ZOOMING IN ➤ Why are these cells described as biconcave?]

CHECKPOINT 13-4 ➤ Next to water, what is the most abundant type of substance in plasma?

The Formed Elements

All of the blood's formed elements are produced in red bone marrow, which is located in the ends of long bones and in the inner mass of all other bones. The ancestors of all the blood cells are called **hematopoietic** (blood-forming) **stem cells**. These cells have the potential to develop into any of the blood cell types produced within the red bone marrow.

In comparison with other cells, most blood cells are short lived. The need for constant blood cell replacement means that normal activity of the red bone marrow is absolutely essential to life.

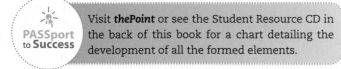

PASSport to Success   Visit ***thePoint*** or see the Student Resource CD in the back of this book for a chart detailing the development of all the formed elements.

CHECKPOINT 13-5 ➤ Where do blood cells form?

CHECKPOINT 13-6 ➤ What type of cell gives rise to all blood cells?

ERYTHROCYTES Erythrocytes, the red blood cells (RBCs, or red cells), measure about 7 μm in diameter. They are disk-shaped bodies with a depression on both sides. This biconcave shape creates a central area that is thinner than the edges (Fig. 13-3). Erythrocytes are different from other cells in that the mature form found in the circulating blood lacks a nucleus (is anuclear) and also lacks most of the other organelles commonly found in cells. As red cells mature, these components are lost, providing more space for the cells to carry oxygen. This vital gas is bound in the red cells to **hemoglobin** (he-mo-GLO-bin), a protein that contains iron (see Box 13-1,

Hemoglobin: Door-to-Door Oxygen Delivery). Hemoglobin, combined with oxygen, gives the blood its characteristic red color. The more oxygen carried by the hemoglobin, the brighter is the blood's red color. Therefore, the blood that goes from the lungs to the tissues is a bright red because it carries a great supply of oxygen; in contrast, the blood that returns to the lungs is a much darker red because it has given up much of its oxygen to the tissues.

Hemoglobin has two lesser functions in addition to the transport of oxygen. Hemoglobin that has given up its oxygen is able to carry hydrogen ions. In this way, hemoglobin acts as a buffer and plays an important role in acid–base balance (see Chapter 21). Hemoglobin also carries some carbon dioxide from the tissues to the lungs for elimination. The carbon dioxide is bound to a different part of the molecule than the part that holds oxygen, so that it does not interfere with oxygen transport.

Hemoglobin's ability to carry oxygen can be blocked by carbon monoxide. This odorless and colorless but harmful gas combines with hemoglobin to form a stable compound that can severely restrict the erythrocytes' ability to carry oxygen. Carbon monoxide is a byproduct of the incomplete burning of fuels, such as gasoline and other petroleum products and coal, wood, and other carbon-containing materials. It also occurs in cigarette smoke and automobile exhaust.

Erythrocytes are by far the most numerous of the blood cells, averaging from 4.5 to 5 million per microliter (μL or mcL) of blood. (A microliter is one millionth of a liter.) Because mature red cells have no nucleus and cannot divide, they must be replaced constantly. After leaving the bone marrow, they circulate in the bloodstream for about 120 days before their membranes deteriorate and they are destroyed by the liver and spleen. Red cell production is stimulated by the hormone **erythropoietin** (eh-rith-ro-POY-eh-tin) (**EPO**), which is released from the kidney in response to decreased oxygen. Constant red cell production requires an adequate supply of nutrients, particularly protein, the B vitamins B_{12} and folic acid, required for the production of DNA, and the minerals iron and copper for

Box 13-1	A Closer Look

Hemoglobin: Door-to-Door Oxygen Delivery

The hemoglobin molecule is a protein made of four amino acid chains (the globin part of the molecule), each of which holds an iron-containing heme group. Each of the four hemes can bind one molecule of oxygen.

Hemoglobin allows the blood to carry much more oxygen than it could were the oxygen simply dissolved in the plasma. A red blood cell contains about 250 million hemoglobins, each capable of binding four molecules of oxygen. So, a single red blood cell can carry about one billion oxygen molecules! Hemoglobin reversibly binds oxygen, picking it up in the lungs and releasing it in the body tissues. Active cells need more oxygen and also generate heat and acidity. These changing conditions promote the release of oxygen from hemoglobin into metabolically active tissues.

Immature red blood cells (erythroblasts) produce hemoglobin as they mature into erythrocytes in the red bone marrow. When the liver and spleen destroy old erythrocytes they break down the released hemoglobin. Some of its components are recycled, and the remainder leaves the body as a brown fecal pigment called stercobilin. In spite of some conservation, dietary protein and iron are still essential to maintain hemoglobin supplies.

Hemoglobin. This protein in red blood cells consists of four amino acid chains (globins), each with an oxygen-binding heme group.

the production of hemoglobin. Vitamin C is also important for the proper absorption of iron from the small intestine.

CHECKPOINT 13-7 ➤ Red cells are modified to carry a maximum amount of hemoglobin. What is the main function of hemoglobin?

LEUKOCYTES The **leukocytes**, or white blood cells (WBCs, or white cells), are different from the erythrocytes in appearance, quantity, and function. The cells themselves are round, but they contain prominent nuclei of varying shapes and sizes. Occurring at a concentration of 5,000 to 10,000 per microliter (μL) of blood, leukocytes are outnumbered by red cells by about 700 to 1. Although the red cells have a definite color, the leukocytes are colorless.

The different types of white cells are identified by their size, the shape of the nucleus, and the appearance of granules in the cytoplasm when the cells are stained. The stain commonly used for blood is Wright stain, which is a mixture of dyes that differentiates the various blood cells. The "granules" in the white cells are actually lysosomes and other secretory vesicles. They are present in all white blood cells, but they are more easily stained and more visible in some cells than in others. The relative percentage of the different types of leukocytes is a valuable clue in arriving at a medical diagnosis (Table 13-2).

The granular leukocytes, or **granulocytes** (GRAN-u-lo-sites), are so named because they show visible granules

13

Table 13-2	Leukocytes (White Blood Cells)	
Cell Type	**Relative Percentage (Adult)**	**Function**
Granulocytes		
Neutrophils	54%–62%	Phagocytosis
Eosinophils	1%–3%	Allergic reactions; defense against parasites
Basophils	<1%	Allergic reactions; inflammatory reactions
Agranulocytes		
Lymphocytes	25%–38%	Immunity (T cells and B cells)
Monocytes	3%–7%	Phagocytosis

in the cytoplasm when stained (see Fig. 13-4A–C). Each has a very distinctive, highly segmented nucleus. The different types of granulocytes are named for the type of dyes they take up when stained. They include the following:

- **Neutrophils** (NU-tro-fils) stain with either acidic or basic dyes and show lavender granules.

- **Eosinophils** (e-o-SIN-o-fils) stain with acidic dyes (eosin is one) and have beadlike, bright pink granules.

- **Basophils** (BA-so-fils) stain with basic dyes and have large, dark blue granules that often obscure the nucleus.

The neutrophils are the most numerous of the white cells, constituting approximately 60% of all leukocytes (see Table 13-2). Because the nuclei of the neutrophils have various shapes, these cells are also called **polymorphs** (meaning "many forms") or simply *polys*. Other nicknames are *segs*, referring to the segmented nucleus, and *PMNs*, an abbreviation of **polymorphonuclear neutrophils**. Before reaching full maturity and becoming segmented, a neutrophil's nucleus looks like a thick, curved band (Fig. 13-5). An increase in the number of these **band cells** (also called *stab* or *staff cells*) is a sign of infection and active neutrophil production.

The eosinophils and basophils make up a small percentage of the white cells but increase in number during allergic reactions.

The agranular leukocytes, or **agranulocytes**, are so named because they lack easily visible granules (see Fig. 13-4D,E). Their nuclei are round or curved and are not segmented. There are two types of agranular leukocytes:

- **Lymphocytes** (LIM-fo-sites) are the second most numerous of the white cells. Although lymphocytes originate in the red bone marrow, they develop to maturity in lymphoid tissue and can multiply in this tissue as well (see Chapter 16). They circulate in the lymphatic system and are active in immunity.

- **Monocytes** (MON-o-sites) are the largest in size. They average about 5% of the leukocytes.

Function of Leukocytes Leukocytes clear the body of foreign material and cellular debris. Most importantly, they destroy pathogens that may invade the body. Neutrophils and monocytes engage in **phagocytosis** (fag-o-si-TO-sis), the engulfing of foreign matter (Fig. 13-6). Whenever pathogens enter the tissues, as through a wound, phagocytes are attracted to the area. They squeeze between the cells of the capillary walls and proceed by ameboid (ah-ME-boyd), or amebalike, motion to the area of infection where they engulf the invaders. Lysosomes in the cytoplasm then digest the foreign organisms and the cells eliminate the waste products.

When foreign organisms invade, the bone marrow and lymphoid tissue go into emergency production of white cells, and their number increases enormously as a result.

Granulocytes

A Neutrophil — Nucleus, Erythrocyte

B Eosinophil — Erythrocyte, Granules, Nucleus

C Basophil — Nucleus, Granules

Agranulocytes

D Lymphocyte — Platelet, Nucleus, Erythrocyte

E Monocyte — Erythrocyte, Nucleus

Figure 13-4 **Granulocytes (A-C) and agranulocytes (D,E). (A)** The neutrophil has a large, segmented nucleus. **(B)** The eosinophil has many bright pink-staining granules. **(C)** The basophil has large dark blue-staining granules. **(D)** The lymphocyte has a large undivided nucleus. **(E)** The monocyte is the largest of the leukocytes. [**ZOOMING IN** ➤ Which group of leukocytes has segmented nuclei? Which specific type of leukocyte is largest in size? Smallest in size?]

A Mature neutrophil

B Band cell (immature neutrophil)

Figure 13-5 **Stages in neutrophil development.** **(A)** A mature neutrophil has a segmented nucleus. **(B)** An immature neutrophil is called a band cell because the nucleus is shaped like a thick, curved band. (×1325) (Reprinted with permission from Gartner LP, Hiatt JL. *Color Atlas of Histology*, 3rd ed. Philadelphia: Lippincott Williams & Wilkins, 2000.)

Detection of an abnormally large number of white cells in the blood is an indication of infection. In battling pathogens, leukocytes themselves may be destroyed. A mixture of dead and living bacteria, together with dead and living leukocytes, forms **pus**. A collection of pus localized in one area is known as an **abscess**.

Some monocytes enter the tissues, enlarge, and mature into **macrophages** (MAK-ro-faj-ez), which are highly active in disposing of invaders and foreign material. Although most circulating lymphocytes live only 6 to 8 hours, those that enter the tissues may survive for longer periods—days, months, or even years.

CHECKPOINT **13-8** ➤ What are the types of granular leukocytes? Of agranular leukocytes?

CHECKPOINT **13-9** ➤ What is the most important function of leukocytes?

Some lymphocytes become **plasma cells**, active in the production of circulating antibodies needed for immunity. The activities of the various white cells are further discussed in Chapter 17.

PLATELETS The **blood platelets** (thrombocytes) are the smallest of all the formed elements (Fig. 13-7A). These tiny structures are not cells in themselves but rather fragments constantly released from giant bone marrow cells called **megakaryocytes** (meg-ah-KAR-e-o-sites) (Fig. 13-7B). Platelets do not have nuclei or DNA, but they do contain active enzymes and mitochondria. The number of platelets in the circulating blood has been estimated to range from 150,000 to 450,000 per µL. They have a lifespan of about 10 days.

Platelets are essential to blood **coagulation** (clotting). When blood comes in contact with any tissue other than the smooth lining of the blood vessels, as in the case of injury, the platelets stick together and form a plug that seals the wound. The platelets then release chemicals that participate in the formation of a clot to stop blood loss. More details on these reactions follow.

CHECKPOINT **13-10** ➤ What is the function of blood platelets?

Hemostasis

Hemostasis (he-mo-STA-sis) is the process that prevents blood loss from the circulation when a blood vessel is ruptured by an injury. Events in hemostasis include the following:

1. **Contraction** of the smooth muscles in the blood vessel wall. This reduces blood flow and loss from the defect

13

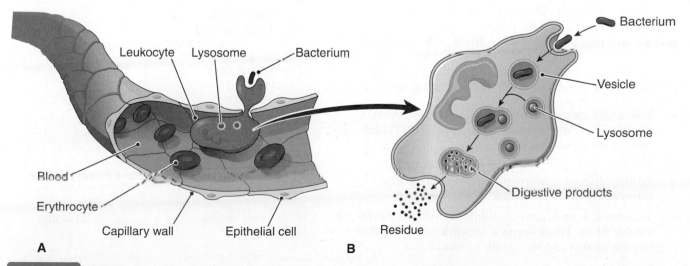

A   **B**

Figure 13-6 **Phagocytosis.** **(A)** A phagocytic leukocyte (white blood cell) squeezes through a capillary wall in the region of an infection and engulfs a bacterium. **(B)** The bacterium is enclosed in a vesicle and digested by a lysosome. [**ZOOMING IN** ➤ What type of epithelium makes up the capillary wall?]

A Platelets   **B** Megakaryocyte

Figure 13-7 **Platelets (thrombocytes).** **(A)** Platelets in a blood smear. **(B)** A megakaryocyte releases platelets. (B, Reprinted with permission from Gartner LP, Hiatt JL. *Color Atlas of Histology*, 3rd ed. Philadelphia: Lippincott Williams & Wilkins, 2000.)

in the vessel. The term for this reduction in a vessel's diameter is *vasoconstriction*.

2. Formation of a **platelet plug.** Activated platelets become sticky and adhere to the defect to form a temporary plug.

3. Formation of a **blood clot** (coagulation).

Blood Clotting

The many substances necessary for blood clotting, or coagulation, are normally inactive in the bloodstream. A balance is maintained between compounds that promote clotting, known as **procoagulants**, and those that prevent clotting, known as **anticoagulants**. In addition, there are chemicals in the circulation that dissolve any unnecessary and potentially harmful clots that may form. Under normal conditions, the substances that prevent clotting prevail. When an injury occurs, however, the procoagulants are activated, and a clot is formed.

The clotting process is a well-controlled series of separate events involving 12 different factors, each designated by a Roman numeral. The final step in these reactions is the conversion of a plasma protein called **fibrinogen** (fi-BRIN-o-jen) into solid threads of **fibrin**, which form the clot.

A few of the final steps involved in blood clot formation are described below and diagrammed in Figure 13-8:

■ Substances released from damaged tissues stimulate the formation of **prothrombinase** (pro-THROM-bih-nase), a substance that triggers the final clotting mechanism.

■ Prothrombinase converts prothrombin in the blood to **thrombin.** Calcium is needed for this step.

■ Thrombin, in turn, converts soluble fibrinogen into insoluble fibrin. **Fibrin** forms a network of threads that entraps plasma and blood cells to form a clot.

Blood clotting occurs in response to injury. Blood also clots when it comes into contact with some surface other than the lining of a blood vessel, for example, a glass or

plastic tube used for a blood specimen. In this case, the preliminary steps of clotting are somewhat different and require more time, but the final steps are the same as those described above.

The fluid that remains after clotting has occurred is called **serum** (plural, *sera*). Serum contains all the components of blood plasma *except* the clotting factors, as expressed in the formula:

Plasma = serum + clotting factors

Several methods used to measure the body's ability to coagulate blood are described later in this chapter.

> **PASSport to Success** Visit *thePoint* or see the Student Resource CD in the back of this book for a summary diagram and an animation on hemostasis.

CHECKPOINT 13-11 ➤ What happens when fibrinogen converts to fibrin?

Blood Types

If for some reason the amount of blood in the body is severely reduced, through **hemorrhage** (HEM-eh-rij) (excessive bleeding) or disease, the body cells suffer from lack of oxygen and nutrients. One possible measure to take in such an emergency is to administer blood from another person into the veins of the patient, a procedure called **transfusion.** Care must be taken in transferring blood from one person to another, however, because the patient's plasma may contain substances, called *antibodies* or *agglutinins*, that can cause the red cells of the donor's blood to

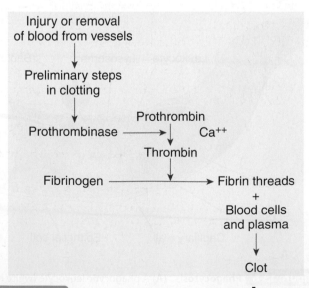

Figure 13-8 **Final steps in blood clot formation.** [ZOOMING IN ➤ What material in the blood forms a clot?]

rupture and release their hemoglobin. Such cells are said to be **hemolyzed** (HE-mo-lized), and the resulting condition can be dangerous.

Certain proteins, called **antigens** (AN-ti-jens) or *agglutinogens*, on the surface of the red cells cause these incompatibility reactions. There are many types of such proteins, but only two groups are particularly likely to cause a transfusion reaction, the so-called A and B antigens and the Rh factor.

The ABO Blood Type Group

There are four blood types involving the A and B antigens: A, B, AB, and O (Table 13-3). These letters indicate the type of antigen present on the red cells. If only the A antigen is present, the person has type A blood; if only the B antigen is present, he or she has type B blood. Type AB red cells have both antigens, and type O have neither. Of course no one has antibodies to his or her own blood type antigens, or their plasma would destroy their own cells. Each person does, however, develop antibodies that react with the AB antigens he or she is lacking. (The reason for the development of these antibodies is not totally understood, because people usually develop antibodies only when they have been exposed to an antigen.) It is these antibodies in the patient's plasma that can react with antigens on the donor's red cells to cause a transfusion reaction.

TESTING FOR BLOOD TYPE Blood sera containing antibodies to the A or B antigens are used to test for blood type. These antisera are prepared in animals using either the A or the B antigens to induce a response. Blood serum containing antibodies that can agglutinate and destroy red cells with A antigen is called **anti-A serum**; blood serum containing antibodies that can destroy red cells with B antigen is called **anti-B serum**. When combined with a blood sample in the laboratory, each antiserum causes the corresponding red cells to clump together in a process known as **agglutination** (ah-glu-tih-NA-shun). The blood's agglutination pattern when mixed *separately* with these two sera reveals its blood type (Fig. 13-9). Type A reacts with anti-A serum only; type B reacts with anti-B serum only. Type AB agglutinates with both, and type O agglutinates with neither A nor B.

A blood specimen from any person who has had a prior blood transfusion or a pregnancy is tested further for

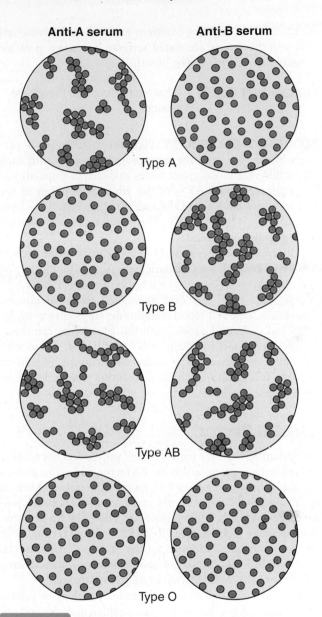

Figure 13-9 **Blood typing.** Labels at the top of each column denote the kind of antiserum added to the blood samples. Anti-A serum agglutinates (causes to clump) red cells in type A blood, but anti-B serum does not. Anti-B serum agglutinates red cells in type B blood, but anti-A serum does not. Both sera agglutinate type AB blood cells, and neither serum agglutinates type O blood. [**ZOOMING IN ➤** Can you tell from these reactions whether these cells are Rh positive or Rh negative?]

13

Table 13-3	The ABO Blood Group System				
Blood Type	Red Blood Cell Antigen	Reacts with Antiserum	Plasma Antibodies	Can Take From	Can Donate To
A	A	Anti-A	Anti-B	A, O	A, AB
B	B	Anti-B	Anti-A	B, O	B, AB
AB	A, B	Anti-A, Anti-B	None	AB, A, B, O	AB
O	None	None	Anti-A, Anti-B	O	O, A, B, AB

the presence of any less common antibodies. Both the red cells and the serum are tested separately for any possible cross-reactions with donor blood.

CHECKPOINT **13-12** ➤ What are the four ABO blood type groups?

BLOOD COMPATIBILITY Heredity determines a person's blood type, and the percentage of people with each of the different blood types varies in different populations. For example, about 45% of the white population of the United States have type O blood, 40% have A, 11% have B, and only 4% have AB. The percentages vary within other population groups.

In an emergency, type O blood can be given to any ABO type because the cells lack both A and B antigens and will not react with either A or B antibodies (see Table 13-3). People with type O blood are called *universal donors*. Conversely, type AB blood contains no antibodies to agglutinate red cells, and people with this blood type can therefore receive blood from any ABO type donor. Those with AB blood are described as *universal recipients*. Whenever possible, it is safest to give the same blood type as the recipient's blood.

The Rh Factor

More than 85% of the United States' population has another red cell antigen group called the **Rh factor**, named for *Rh*esus monkeys, in which it was first found. Rh is also known as the *D antigen*. People with this antigen are said to be **Rh positive**; those who lack this protein are said to be **Rh negative**. If Rh-positive blood is given to an Rh-negative person, he or she may produce antibodies to the "foreign" Rh antigens. The blood of this "Rh-sensitized" person will then destroy any Rh-positive cells received in a later transfusion.

Rh incompatibility is a potential problem in certain pregnancies. A mother who is Rh negative may develop antibodies to the Rh protein of an Rh-positive fetus (the fetus having inherited this factor from the father). Red cells from the fetus that enter the mother's circulation during pregnancy and childbirth evoke the response. In a subsequent pregnancy with an Rh-positive fetus, some of the anti-Rh antibodies may pass from the mother's blood into the blood of her fetus and destroy the fetus's red cells. This condition is called **hemolytic disease of the newborn** (HDN). An older name is *erythroblastosis fetalis*. HDN is now prevented by administration of immune globulin Rh$_o$(D), trade name RhoGAM, to the mother during pregnancy and shortly after delivery. These preformed antibodies clear the mother's circulation of Rh antigens and prevent stimulation of an immune response. In many cases, a baby born with HDN could be saved by a transfusion that replaces much of the baby's blood with Rh-negative blood.

CHECKPOINT **13-13** ➤ What are the blood antigens most often involved in incompatibility reactions?

Uses of Blood and Blood Components

Blood can be packaged and kept in blood banks for emergencies. To keep the blood from clotting, a solution such as citrate-phosphate-dextrose-adenine (CPDA-1) is added. The blood may then be stored for up to 35 days. The blood supplies in the bank are dated with an expiration date to prevent the use of blood in which red cells may have disintegrated. Blood banks usually have all types of blood and blood products available. It is important that there be an extra supply of type O, Rh-negative blood because in an emergency this type can be used for any patient. It is normal procedure to test the recipient and give blood of the same type.

A person can donate his or her own blood before undergoing elective (planned) surgery to be used during surgery if needed. This practice eliminates the possibility of incompatibility and of disease transfer as well. Such **autologous** (aw-TOL-o-gus) (self-originating) blood is stored in a blood bank only until the surgery is completed.

Whole Blood Transfusions

The transfer of whole human blood from a healthy person to a patient is often a life-saving process. Whole blood transfusions may be used for any condition in which there is loss of a large volume of blood, for example:

■ In the treatment of massive hemorrhage from serious mechanical injuries

■ For blood loss during internal bleeding, as from bleeding ulcers

■ During or after an operation that causes considerable blood loss

■ For blood replacement in the treatment of hemolytic disease of the newborn

Caution and careful evaluation of the need for a blood transfusion is the rule, however, because of the risk for transfusion reactions and the transmission of viral diseases, particularly hepatitis.

Use of Blood Components

Most often, when some blood ingredient is needed, it is not whole blood but a blood component that is given. Blood can be broken down into its various parts, which may be used for different purposes.

A common method for separating the blood plasma from the formed elements is by use of a **centrifuge** (SEN-trih-fuje), a machine that spins in a circle at high speed to separate a mixture's components according to density. When a container of blood is spun rapidly, all the blood's formed elements are pulled into a clump at the bottom of the container. They are thus separated from the plasma, which is less dense. The formed elements may be further separated and used for specific purposes, for example, packed red cells alone or platelets alone.

Blood losses to the donor can be minimized if the blood is removed, the desired components are separated, and the remainder is returned to the donor. The general term for this procedure is **hemapheresis** (hem-ah-fer-E-sis) (from the Greek word *apheresis* meaning "removal") If the plasma is removed and the formed elements returned to the donor, the procedure is called **plasmapheresis** (plas-mah-fer-E-sis).

USE OF PLASMA Blood plasma alone may be given in an emergency to replace blood volume and prevent circulatory failure (shock). Plasma is especially useful when blood typing and the use of whole blood are not possible, such as in natural disasters or in emergency rescues. Because the red cells have been removed from the plasma, there are no incompatibility problems; plasma can be given to anyone. Plasma separated from the cellular elements is usually further separated by chemical means into various components, such as plasma protein fraction, serum albumin, immune serum, and clotting factors.

The packaged plasma that is currently available is actually plasma protein fraction. Further separation yields serum albumin that is available in solutions of 5% or 25% concentration. In addition to its use in treatment of circulatory shock, these solutions are given when plasma proteins are deficient. They increase the blood's osmotic pressure and thus draw fluids back into circulation. The use of plasma proteins and serum albumin has increased because these blood components can be treated with heat to prevent transmission of viral diseases.

In emergency situations healthcare workers may administer fluids known as *plasma expanders*. These are cell-free isotonic solutions used to maintain blood fluid volume to prevent circulatory shock.

Fresh plasma may be frozen and saved. When frozen plasma is thawed, a white precipitate called **cryoprecipitate** (kri-o-pre-SIP-ih-tate) forms in the bottom of the container. Plasma frozen when it is less than 6 hours old contains all the factors needed for clotting. Cryoprecipitate is especially rich in clotting factor VIII and fibrinogen. These components may be given when there is a special need for these factors.

The plasma's gamma globulin fraction contains antibodies produced by lymphocytes when they come in contact with foreign agents, such as bacteria and viruses. Antibodies play an important role in the immune system (see Chapter 17). Commercially prepared immune sera are available for administration to patients in immediate need of antibodies, such as infants born to mothers with active hepatitis.

CHECKPOINT 13-14 ▶ How is blood commonly separated into its component parts?

Blood Disorders

Abnormalities involving the blood may be divided into three groups:

- **Anemia** (ah-NE-me-ah), a disorder in which there is an abnormally low level of hemoglobin or red cells in the blood and thus impaired delivery of oxygen to the tissues.
- **Leukemia** (lu-KE-me-ah), a neoplastic blood disease characterized by an increase in the number of white cells.
- **Clotting disorders**, conditions characterized by an abnormal tendency to bleed because of a breakdown in the body's clotting mechanism.

Anemia

Anemia may result from loss of red cells, as through excessive bleeding (hemorrhage), or from conditions that cause the cells to hemolyze (rupture). In other cases, bone marrow failure or nutritional deficiencies impede the production of red cells or hemoglobin.

 PASSport to Success Visit *thePoint* or see the Student Resource CD in the back of this book for summary diagrams of the erythrocyte life cycle and causes of anemia.

EXCESSIVE LOSS OR DESTRUCTION OF RED CELLS Red cells may form properly but be lost through injury or destroyed after they are formed.

Hemorrhagic anemia Hemorrhagic loss of red cells may be sudden and acute or gradual and chronic. The average adult has about 5 liters of blood. If a person loses as much as 2 liters suddenly, death usually results. If the loss is gradual, however, over a period of weeks, or months, the body can compensate and withstand the loss of as much as 4 or 5 liters. Possible causes of chronic blood loss include bleeding ulcers, excessive menstrual flow, and bleeding hemorrhoids (piles). If the cause of the blood loss can be corrected, the body is usually able to restore the blood to normal. This process can take as long as 6 months, and until the blood returns to normal, the affected person may have **hemorrhagic** (hem-eh-RAJ-ik) **anemia**.

Hemolytic anemia Anemia caused by excessive red cell destruction is called **hemolytic** (he-mo-LIH-tik) **anemia**. The spleen, along with the liver, normally destroys old red cells. Occasionally, an overactive spleen destroys the cells too rapidly, causing anemia. Infections may also cause red cell loss. For example, the malarial parasite multiplies in and destroys red cells, and certain bacteria, particularly streptococci, produce a toxin that causes hemolysis.

Certain inherited diseases that cause the production of abnormal hemoglobin may also result in hemolytic anemia. The hemoglobin in normal adult cells is of the A type and is designated *HbA*. In the inherited disease **sickle cell anemia**, the hemoglobin in many of the red cells is abnormal (HbS). When these cells give up their oxygen to the tissues, they are transformed from the normal disk shape into a sickle shape (Fig. 13-10). These sickle cells are fragile

13

Sickle-shaped cell

Figure 13-10 A blood smear in sickle cell anemia. Abnormal cells take on a crescent (sickle) shape when they give up oxygen. (Reprinted with permission from Rubin R, Strayer DS. *Rubin's Pathology: Clinicopathologic Foundations of Medicine*, 5th ed. Baltimore: Lippincott Williams & Wilkins, 2007.) [ZOOMING IN ➤ What kind of cell is in the upper left corner of this picture? What are the small dark bodies between the cells?]

and tend to break easily. Because of their odd shape, they also tend to become tangled in masses that can block smaller blood vessels. When obstruction occurs, there may be severe joint swelling and pain, especially in the fingers and toes, as well as abdominal pain. This aspect of sickle cell anemia is referred to as *sickle cell crisis*.

Sickle cell anemia occurs almost exclusively in black people. About 8% of African Americans have one of the genes for the abnormal hemoglobin and are said to have the **sickle cell trait**. It is only when the involved gene is transmitted from both parents that the clinical disease appears. About 1% of African Americans have two of these genes and thus have **sickle cell disease**. One drug has been found to reduce the frequency of painful crisis in certain adults. Hydroxyurea causes the body to make some hemoglobin of an alternate form (fetal hemoglobin) so that the red cells are not as susceptible to sickling. People taking hydroxyurea require blood tests every 2 weeks to assess for drug-induced bone marrow suppression.

PASSport to Success   Visit *thePoint* or see the Student Resource CD in the back of this book for a figure explaining and illustrating sickle cell disease in greater detail.

IMPAIRED PRODUCTION OF RED CELLS OR HEMOGLOBIN
Many factors can interfere with normal red cell production. Anemia that results from a deficiency of some nutrient is referred to as *nutritional anemia*. These conditions may arise from a deficiency of the specific nutrient in the diet, from an inability to absorb the nutrient, or from drugs that interfere with the body's use of the nutrient.

Deficiency Anemia The most common nutritional anemia is **iron-deficiency anemia**. Iron is an essential constituent of hemoglobin. The average diet usually provides

enough iron to meet the needs of the adult male, but this diet often is inadequate to meet the needs of growing children and women of childbearing age.

A diet deficient in proteins or vitamins can also result in anemia. Folic acid, one of the B complex vitamins, is necessary for blood cell production. Folic acid deficiency anemia occurs in people with alcoholism, in elderly people on poor diets, and in infants or others suffering from intestinal disorders that interfere with the absorption of this water-soluble vitamin.

Pernicious (per-NISH-us) **anemia** is characterized by a deficiency of vitamin B_{12}, a substance essential for proper red cell formation. The cause is a permanent deficiency of **intrinsic factor**, a gastric juice secretion that is responsible for vitamin B_{12} absorption from the intestine. Neglected pernicious anemia can bring about deterioration in the nervous system, causing difficulty in walking, weakness and stiffness in the extremities, mental changes, and permanent damage to the spinal cord. Early treatment, including the intramuscular injection of vitamin B_{12} and attention to a prescribed diet, ensures an excellent outlook. This treatment must be kept up for the rest of the patient's life to maintain good health.

Thalassemia (thal-ah-SE-me-ah) includes a group of hereditary blood deficiencies in which hemoglobin is normal but is not produced in adequate amounts. To compound the problem, erythrocytes may be destroyed in the bone marrow before they mature. The red cells are small and pale, as in iron deficiency anemia, but instead of having low iron reserves, these patients absorb too much iron from the digestive tract and have excess iron in the blood and bone marrow. Forms of thalassemia may vary from causing chronic, lifelong anemia to premature death. The two mains types are α (alpha) and β (beta), according to the part of the hemoglobin molecule affected. Severe β thalassemia is also called *Cooley anemia*. Thalassemia is found mostly in populations of Mediterranean descent (the name comes from the Greek word for "sea").

Bone Marrow Suppression Bone marrow suppression or failure also leads to decreased red cell production. One type of bone marrow failure, **aplastic** (a-PLAS-tik) **anemia**, may be caused by a variety of physical and chemical agents. Chemical substances that injure the bone marrow include certain prescribed drugs and toxic agents such as gold compounds, arsenic, and benzene. Physical agents that may injure the marrow include x-rays, atomic radiation, radium, and radioactive phosphorus.

The damaged bone marrow fails to produce either red or white cells, so that the anemia is accompanied by **leukopenia** (lu-ko-PE-ne-ah), a drop in the number of white cells. Removal of the toxic agent, followed by blood transfusions until the marrow is able to resume its activity, may result in recovery. Bone marrow transplantations have also been successful.

Bone marrow suppression also may develop in patients with certain chronic diseases, such as cancer, kidney or liver disorders, and rheumatoid arthritis. Some medications are now available to stimulate bone marrow production of specific types of blood cells. The hormone EPO made by recombinant methods (genetic engineering) can be given in cases of severe anemia to stimulate red cell production.

CHECKPOINT 13-15 ➤ What is anemia?

Leukemia

Leukemia is a neoplastic disease of blood-forming tissue. It is characterized by an enormous increase in the number of white cells. Although the cells are high in number, they are incompetent and cannot perform their normal jobs. They also crowd out the other blood cells.

As noted earlier, the white cells have two main sources: red marrow, also called *myeloid tissue,* and lymphoid tissue. If this wild proliferation of white cells stems from cancer of the bone marrow, the condition is called **myelogenous** (mi-eh-LOJ-en-us) **leukemia.** When the cancer arises in the lymphoid tissue, so that most of the abnormal cells are lymphocytes, the condition is called **lymphocytic** (lim-fo-SIT-ik) **leukemia.** Both types of leukemia appear in acute and chronic forms.

> ☀ **PASSport to Success** Visit *thePoint* or see the Student Resource CD in the back of this book for micrographs of leukemic blood.

The cause of leukemia is unknown. Both inborn factors and various environmental agents have been implicated. Among the latter are chemicals (such as benzene), x-rays, radioactive substances, and viruses.

Patients with leukemia exhibit the general symptoms of anemia because the white cells overwhelm the red cells. In addition, they have a tendency to bleed easily, owing to a lack of platelets. White cell failure lowers immunity, resulting in frequent infections. The spleen is greatly enlarged, and several other organs may be increased in size because of internal accumulation of white cells. Treatment consists of x-ray therapy and chemotherapy (drug treatment), but the disease is malignant and thus may be fatal. With new chemotherapeutic methods, the outlook is improving, and many patients survive for years.

A bone marrow transplant can sometimes restore the normal hematopoietic stem cells destroyed along with abnormal cells in leukemia treatment. Hematologists also use the procedure to treat sickle cell anemia, thalassemia, aplastic anemia, and some immune disorders. Most patients receive allogenic transplants of cells from a close relative's bone marrow. It is important that the donor marrow match the recipient's marrow as closely as possible to avoid rejection, so potential donors undergo blood tests to determine compatibility. Sometimes the patient's own bone marrow can be harvested, treated, and replaced in an autologous transplant, which eliminates rejection. After intravenous delivery of the transplant, the donor stem cells travel to the recipient's bone marrow where they begin to produce new blood cells. Recovery time is long, and during this period the patient is very susceptible to infection, but bone marrow transplants improve survival rates for patients with leukemia and certain other blood disorders.

CHECKPOINT 13-16 ➤ What is leukemia?

Clotting Disorders

Most clotting disorders involve a disruption of the coagulation process, which brings about abnormal bleeding. Alternately, the disturbance may originate with excess clotting.

Hemophilia (he-mo-FIL-e-ah) is a rare hereditary bleeding disorder, a disease that influenced history by its occurrence in some Russian and Western European royal families. All forms of hemophilia are characterized by a deficiency of a specific clotting factor, most commonly factor VIII. In those with hemophilia, any injury may cause excess bruising and serious abnormal bleeding. There is also spontaneous internal bleeding, especially in the digestive tract, brain, and other soft tissues. Bleeding into the joints, a common effect of hemophilia, is not only painful, but can lead to serious disability if untreated. The needed clotting factors are now available in purified concentrated form for treatment in cases of injury, preparation for surgery, or abnormal bleeding. Cryoprecipitate contains factor VIII, and clotting factors are also produced by recombinant (genetic engineering) methods.

Von Willebrand disease is another hereditary clotting disorder. It involves a shortage of von Willebrand factor, a plasma component that helps platelets to adhere (stick) to damaged tissue and also carries clotting factor VIII. This disorder is treated by administration of the appropriate clotting factor. In mild cases, a drug similar to the hormone ADH may work to prevent bleeding by raising the level of von Willebrand factor in the blood.

The most common clotting disorder is a deficient number of circulating platelets (thrombocytes). The condition, called **thrombocytopenia** (throm-bo-si-to-PE-ne-ah), results in hemorrhage in the skin or mucous membranes. The decrease in platelets may result from their decreased production or increased destruction. There are several possible causes of thrombocytopenia, including diseases of the red bone marrow, liver disorders, and various drug toxicities. When a drug causes the disorder, its withdrawal leads to immediate recovery.

Disseminated intravascular coagulation (DIC) is a serious clotting disorder involving excessive coagulation. This disease occurs in cases of tissue damage caused by massive burns, trauma, certain acute infections, cancer, and some disorders of childbirth. During the progress of DIC, platelets and various clotting factors are used up faster than they can be produced, and serious hemorrhaging may result.

CHECKPOINT 13-17 ➤ What blood components are low in cases of thrombocytopenia?

13

Disease in Context revisited

➤ Sickle Cell Anemia

Dr. Kepron, a pediatric hematologist, carefully read Cole Armstrong's medical chart. Cole, now 2 days old, was positive for the presence of Hemoglobin S. Blood tests from his parents, Jada and Darryl, confirmed Cole's diagnosis—sickle cell anemia.

Later that afternoon, Dr. Kepron met with Cole's parents. "Cole has been diagnosed with sickle cell anemia," explained the doctor. "The disease is caused by a mutation in the gene that directs the manufacture of a blood protein called hemoglobin." Dr. Kepron told Darryl and Jada that they each carried two versions of the gene, one normal and one abnormal, but they did not express the disease because the normal gene masked the effect of the abnormal one. Cole had inherited a copy of the abnormal hemoglobin gene from each of his parents and thus expressed the disease.

"Hemoglobin is found in red blood cells," continued the doctor. "It's the protein that transports oxygen from the lungs to other tissues in the body. Normally, the red blood cells are round and flexible, which lets them bend and twist as they pass through the narrow capillaries in the body. Cole's abnormal hemoglobin causes the red blood cells to become stiff and sickle-shaped. As a result, the cells can become stuck in the capillaries, blocking blood flow and the delivery of oxygen to tissues and organs. I'm going to work with you to manage Cole's disease—if we monitor him carefully we should be able to minimize organ and tissue damage."

During this case we saw that sickle cell anemia is an inherited disease. To learn more about heredity and hereditary diseases, see Chapter 25.

Blood Studies

Many kinds of studies can be done on blood, and some of these have become a standard part of a routine physical examination. The tests included in a **complete blood count** (**CBC**) are shown in Appendix 4-2. Machines that are able to perform several tests at the same time have largely replaced manual procedures, particularly in large institutions. Standard blood tests are listed in Tables 2 and 3 of Appendix 4.

The Hematocrit

The **hematocrit** (he-MAT-o-krit) (Hct), the volume percentage of red cells in whole blood, is determined by spinning a blood sample in a high-speed centrifuge for 3 to 5 minutes to separate the cellular elements from the plasma (Fig. 13-11).

The hematocrit is expressed as the volume of packed red cells per unit volume of whole blood. For example, "hematocrit, 38%" in a laboratory report means that the patient has 38 mL red cells per dL (100 mL) of blood; red cells comprise 38% of the total blood volume. For adult men, the normal range is 42% to 54%, whereas for adult women the range is slightly lower, 36% to 46%. These normal ranges, like all normal ranges for humans, may vary depending on the method used and the interpretation of the results by an individual laboratory. Hematocrit values much below or much above these figures point to an abnormality requiring further study.

Hemoglobin Tests

A sufficient amount of hemoglobin in red cells is required for adequate oxygen delivery to the tissues. To measure its level, the hemoglobin is released from the red cells, and the color of the blood is compared with a known color scale.

Figure 13-11 Hematocrit. The tube on the left shows a normal hematocrit. The middle tube shows that the percentage of red blood cells is low, indicating anemia. The tube on the right shows an excessively high percentage of red cells, as seen in polycythemia. (Reprinted with permission from Cohen BJ. *Medical Terminology*, 4th ed. Philadelphia: Lippincott Williams & Wilkins, 2004.)

Hemoglobin (Hb) is expressed in grams per dL of whole blood. Normal hemoglobin concentrations for adult males range from 14 to 17 g per 100 mL blood. Values for adult women are in a somewhat lower range, at 12 to 15 g per 100 mL blood. The hemoglobin reading can also be expressed as a percentage of a given standard, usually the average male normal of 15.6 g Hb/dL. Thus, a reading of 90% would mean 90% of 15.6 or 14 g Hb/dL. A decrease in hemoglobin to below normal levels signifies anemia.

Normal and abnormal types of hemoglobin can be separated and measured by the process of **electrophoresis** (e-lek-tro-fo-RE-sis). In this procedure, an electric current is passed through the liquid that contains the hemoglobin to separate different components based on their electrical charge. This test is useful in the diagnosis of sickle cell anemia and other disorders caused by abnormal types of hemoglobin.

Blood Cell Counts

Most laboratories use automated methods for obtaining the data for blood counts. Visual counts are sometimes done using a **hemocytometer** (he-mo-si-TOM-eh-ter), a ruled slide used to count the cells in a given volume of blood under the microscope.

RED CELL COUNTS The normal red cell count varies from 4.5 to 5.5 million cells per μL (mcL) of blood. An increase in the red cell count is called **polycythemia** (pol-e-si-THE-me-ah). People who live at high altitudes develop polycythemia, as do patients with the disease **polycythemia** (pol-e-si-THE-me-ah) **vera**, a disorder of the bone marrow.

WHITE CELL COUNTS The leukocyte count varies from 5,000 to 10,000 cells per μL of blood. In **leukopenia**, the white count is below 5,000 cells per μL. This condition indicates depressed bone marrow or a bone marrow neoplasm. In **leukocytosis** (lu-ko-si-TO-sis), the white cell count exceeds 10,000 cells per μL. This condition is characteristic of most bacterial infections. It may also occur after hemorrhage, in cases of gout (a type of arthritis), and in uremia, the presence of nitrogenous waste in the blood as a result of kidney disease.

PLATELET COUNTS It is difficult to count platelets visually because they are so small. Laboratories can obtain more accurate counts with automated methods. These counts are necessary for the evaluation of platelet loss (thrombocytopenia) such as occurs after radiation therapy or cancer chemotherapy. The normal platelet count ranges from 150,000 to 450,000 per μL of blood, but counts may fall to 100,000 or less without causing serious bleeding problems. If a count is very low, a platelet transfusion may be given.

The Blood Slide (Smear)

In addition to the above tests, a CBC includes the examination of a stained blood slide (see Fig. 13-2). In this procedure, a drop of blood is spread thinly and evenly over a glass slide, and a special stain (Wright) is applied to differentiate the otherwise colorless white cells. The slide is then studied under the microscope. The red cells are examined for abnormalities in size, color, or shape and for variations in the percentage of immature forms, known as reticulocytes (see Box 13-2 to learn about reticulocytes and how their counts are used to diagnose disease). The number of platelets is estimated. Parasites, such as the malarial organism and others, may be found. In addition, a **differential white count** is done. This is an estimation of the percentage of each white cell type in the smear. Because each type has a specific function, changes in their proportions can be a valuable diagnostic aid (see Table 13-2).

CHECKPOINT 13-18 ➤ The hematocrit is a common blood test. What is a hematocrit?

Blood Chemistry Tests

Batteries of tests on blood serum are often done by machine. One machine, the Sequential Multiple Analyzer (SMA), can run some 20 tests per minute. Tests for electrolytes, such as sodium, potassium, chloride, and bicarbonate, may be performed at the same time along with tests for blood glucose, and nitrogenous waste products, such as blood urea nitrogen (BUN), and **creatinine** (kre-AT-in-in).

Other tests check for enzymes. Increased levels of **CK** (creatine kinase), **LDH** (lactic dehydrogenase), and other enzymes indicate tissue damage, such as damage that may occur in heart disease. An excess of **alkaline phosphatase** (FOS-fah-tase) could indicate a liver disorder or metastatic cancer involving bone (see Table 3 in Appendix 4).

Blood can be tested for amounts of lipids, such as cholesterol, triglycerides (fats), and lipoproteins, or for amounts of plasma proteins. These tests help to diagnose and evaluate diseases. For example, the presence of more than the normal amount of glucose in the blood indicates unregulated diabetes mellitus. The list of blood chemistry tests is extensive and is constantly increasing. We may now obtain values for various hormones, vitamins, antibodies, and toxic or therapeutic drug levels.

Coagulation Studies

Before surgery and during treatment of certain diseases, hemophilia for example, it is important to know that coagulation will take place within normal time limits. Because clotting is a complex process involving many reactants, a delay may result from a number of different causes, including lack of certain hormonelike substances, calcium salts, or vitamin K. The amounts of the various clotting factors are evaluated by percentage to aid in the diagnosis and treatment of bleeding disorders.

Additional tests for coagulation include tests for bleeding time, clotting time, capillary strength, and platelet function.

Box 13-2 Clinical Perspectives

Counting Reticulocytes to Diagnose Disease

As erythrocytes mature in the red bone marrow, they go through a series of stages in which they lose their nucleus and most other organelles, maximizing the space available to hold hemoglobin. In one of the last stages of development, small numbers of ribosomes and some rough endoplasmic reticulum remain in the cell and appear as a network, or reticulum, when stained. Cells at this stage are called **reticulocytes**. Reticulocytes leave the red bone marrow and enter the bloodstream where they become fully mature erythrocytes in about 24 to 48 hours. The average number of red cells maturing through the reticulocyte stage at any given time is about 1% to 2%. Changes in these numbers can be used in diagnosing certain blood disorders.

When erythrocytes are lost or destroyed, as from chronic bleeding or some form of hemolytic anemia, red blood cell production is "stepped up" to compensate for the loss. Greater numbers of reticulocytes are then released into the blood before reaching full maturity, and counts increase above normal. On the other hand, a decrease in the number of circulating reticulocytes suggests a problem with red

blood cell production, as in cases of deficiency anemias or suppression of bone marrow activity.

Reticulocytes. Some ribosomes and rough ER appear as a network in a late stage of erythrocyte development. (Reprinted with permission from Cormack DH. *Essential Histology*, 2nd ed. Philadelphia: Lippincott Williams & Wilkins, 2001.)

Bone Marrow Biopsy

A special needle is used to obtain a small sample of red marrow from the sternum, sacrum, or iliac crest in a procedure called a **bone marrow biopsy**. If marrow is taken from the sternum, the procedure may be referred to as a **sternal puncture**. Examination of the cells gives valuable information that can aid in the diagnosis of bone marrow disorders, including leukemia and certain kinds of anemia.

Word Anatomy

Medical terms are built from standardized word parts (prefixes, roots, and suffixes). Learning the meanings of these parts can help you remember words and interpret unfamiliar terms.

WORD PART	MEANING	EXAMPLE
Blood Constituents		
erythr/o	red, red blood cell	An *erythrocyte* is a red blood cell.
leuk/o	white, colorless	A *leukocyte* is a white blood cell.
thromb/o	blood clot	A *thrombocyte* is a cell fragment that is active in blood clotting.
hemat/o	blood	*Hematopoietic* stem cells form (-poiesis) all of the blood cells.
hemo	blood	*Hemoglobin* is a protein the carries oxygen in the blood.

WORD PART	MEANING	EXAMPLE
morph/o	shape	The nuclei of *polymorphs* have many shapes.
lymph/o	lymph, lymphatic system	*Lymphocytes* are white blood cells that circulate in the lymphatic system.
mon/o	single, one	A *monocyte* has a single, unsegmented nucleus.
phag/o	eat, ingest	Certain leukocytes take in foreign matter by the process of *phagocytosis*.
macr/o	large	A *macrophage* takes in large amounts of foreign matter by phagocytosis.
kary/o	nucleus	A *megakaryocyte* has a very large nucleus.

Hemostasis

-gen	producing, originating	*Fibrinogen* converts to fibrin in the formation of a blood clot.
pro-	before, in front of	Prothrombinase is an enzyme (-ase) that converts *prothrombin* to thrombin.

Blood Types

-lysis	loosening, dissolving, separating	A recipient's antibodies to donated red cells can cause *hemolysis* of the cells.

Uses of Blood and Blood Components

cry/o	cold	*Cryoprecipitate* forms when blood plasma is frozen and then thawed.

Blood Disorders

–emia (from –hemia)	blood	*Anemia* is a lack (an-) of red cells or hemoglobin.
–penia	lack of	*Leukopenia* is a lack of white cells.

Summary

13

I. **FUNCTIONS OF THE BLOOD**
  A. Transportation—of oxygen, carbon dioxide, nutrients, minerals, vitamins, hormones, waste
  B. Regulation—of pH, fluid balance, body temperature
  C. Protection—against foreign organisms, blood loss

II. **BLOOD CONSTITUENTS**
  A. Plasma—liquid component
    1. Water—main ingredient
    2. Proteins—albumin, clotting factors, antibodies, complement
    3. Nutrients—carbohydrates, lipids, amino acids
    4. Electrolytes (minerals)
    5. Waste products
    6. Gases—oxygen and carbon dioxide
    7. Hormones and other materials
  B. The formed elements—produced in red bone marrow from hematopoietic stem cells

    1. Erythrocytes (red cells)—carry oxygen bound to hemoglobin
    2. Leukocytes (white cells)—destroy invading organisms and remove waste
      a. Granulocytes—neutrophils (polymorphs, segs, PMNs), eosinophils, basophils
      b. Agranulocytes—lymphocytes, monocytes
    3. Platelets (thrombocytes)
      a. Fragments of megakaryocytes
      b. Participate in blood clotting

III. **HEMOSTASIS—PREVENTION OF BLOOD LOSS**
  A. Steps
    1. Contraction of blood vessels
    2. Formation of platelet plug
    3. Formation of blood clot
  B. Blood Clotting
    1. Regulators
      a. Procoagulants—promote clotting

b.   Anticoagulants—prevent clotting
2.   12 clotting factors
3.   Final steps in blood clotting
a.   Prothrombinase converts prothrombin to thrombin
b.   Thrombin converts fibrinogen to solid threads of fibrin
c.   Threads form clot
4.   Serum—fluid that remains after blood has clotted

IV.   **BLOOD TYPES**
A.   ABO blood type group—types A, B, AB, and O
1.   Tested by mixing blood sample with antisera to different antigens
2.   Incompatible transfusions cause destruction of donor red cells
B.   Rh factor—positive or negative

V.   **USES OF BLOOD AND BLOOD COMPONENTS**
A.   Blood banks—store blood
1.   Autologous blood—donated for a person's own use
B.   Whole blood transfusions—used only to replace large blood losses
C.   Use of blood components—formed elements separated by centrifugation
D.   Use of plasma
1.   Protein fractions
2.   Cryoprecipitate—obtained by freezing; contains clotting factors
3.   Gamma globulin—contains antibodies

VI.   **BLOOD DISORDERS**
A.   Anemia—lack of hemoglobin or red cells

1.   Loss or destruction of cells
a.   Hemorrhage
b.   Hemolysis (e.g., sickle cell anemia)
2.   Impaired production of cells
a.   Deficiency anemia (e.g., nutritional anemia, thalassemia)
b.   Pernicious anemia
c.   Bone marrow suppression
B.   Leukemia—excess production of white cells
1.   Myelogenous leukemia—cancer of bone marrow
2.   Lymphocytic leukemia—cancer of lymphoid tissue
C.   Clotting disorders
1.   Hemophilia, von Willebrand disease—hereditary lack of clotting factors
2.   Thrombocytopenia—lack of platelets
3.   Disseminated intravascular coagulation (DIC)

VII.   **BLOOD STUDIES**
A.   Hematocrit—measures percentage of packed red cells in whole blood
B.   Hemoglobin tests—color test, electrophoresis
C.   Blood cell counts
D.   Blood slide (smear)
E.   Blood chemistry tests—electrolytes, waste products, enzymes, glucose, hormones
F.   Coagulation studies—clotting factor assays, bleeding time, clotting time, capillary strength, platelet function
G.   Bone marrow biopsy

Questions for Study and Review

BUILDING UNDERSTANDING

Fill in the blanks

1.   The liquid portion of blood is called _____.
2.   The ancestors of all blood cells are called _____cells.
3.   Platelets are produced by certain giant cells called _____.

4.   Some monocytes enter the tissues and mature into phagocytic cells called _____.
5.   Erythrocytes have a lifespan of approximately _____ days.

Matching > Match each numbered item with the most closely related lettered item.

____   **6.** an increased erythrocyte count
____   **7.** a decreased erythrocyte count
____   **8.** an increased leukocyte count
____   **9.** a decreased leukocyte count
____   **10.** a decreased platelet count

a. thrombocytopenia
b. anemia
c. leukopenia
d. leukocytosis
e. polycythemia

Multiple choice

___ **11.** Red blood cells transport oxygen that is bound to
  a. erythropoietin
  b. complement
  c. hemoglobin
  d. thrombin

___ **12.** All of the following are granulocytes except
  a. lymphocytes
  b. neutrophils
  c. eosinophils
  d. basophils

___ **13.** Antibodies are produced by
  a. erythrocytes
  b. macrophages
  c. plasma cells
  d. band cells

___ **14.** The correct sequence of hemostatic events is
  a. vessel contraction, plug formation, blood clot
  b. blood clot, plug formation, vessel contraction
  c. plug formation, blood clot, vessel contraction
  d. vessel contraction, blood clot, plug formation

___ **15.** If one wanted to measure the number of eosinophils in a blood sample, he or she would conduct the following test:
  a. hematocrit
  b. electrophoresis
  c. complete blood cell count
  d. differential white blood cell count

UNDERSTANDING CONCEPTS

16. List the three main functions of blood. What is the average volume of circulating blood in the body?

17. Compare and contrast the following:
  a. formed elements and plasma
  b. erythrocyte and leukocyte
  c. hemorrhage and transfusion
  d. hemapheresis and plasmapheresis

18. List four main types of proteins in blood plasma and state their functions. What are some other substances carried in blood plasma?

19. Describe the structure and function of erythrocytes. State the normal blood cell count for erythrocytes.

20. Construct a chart that compares the structure and function of the five types of leukocytes. State the normal blood cell count for leukocytes.

21. Diagram the three final steps in blood clot formation.

22. Name the four blood types in the ABO system. What antigens and antibodies (if any) are found in each type?

23. Compare and contrast the following disease conditions:
  a. hemolytic anemia and aplastic anemia
  b. myelogenous leukemia and lymphocytic leukemia
  c. hemophilia and von Willebrand disease

CONCEPTUAL THINKING

24. J. Regan, a 40-year-old firefighter, has just had his annual physical. He is in excellent health, except for his red blood cell count, which is elevated. How might Mr. Regan's job explain his polycythemia?

25. If leukemia is associated with an elevated white blood cell count, why is it also associated with an increased risk of infection?

26. In Cole's case, he was diagnosed with sickle cell disease. Increased risk of infection is one consequence of the disease. Explain why a hemoglobin abnormality increases the risk of infection.

13

CHAPTER 14

The Heart and Heart Disease

Learning Outcomes

After careful study of this chapter, you should be able to:

1. Describe the three layers of the heart wall
2. Describe the structure of the pericardium and cite its functions
3. Compare the functions of the right and left sides of the heart
4. Name the four chambers of the heart and compare their functions
5. Name the valves at the entrance and exit of each ventricle and cite the function of the valves
6. Briefly describe blood circulation through the myocardium
7. Briefly describe the cardiac cycle
8. Name and locate the components of the heart's conduction system
9. Explain the effects of the autonomic nervous system on the heart rate
10. List and define several terms that describe variations in heart rates
11. Explain what produces the two main heart sounds
12. Describe several common types of heart disease
13. List five actions that can be taken to minimize the risk of heart disease
14. Briefly describe four methods for studying the heart
15. Describe several approaches to the treatment of heart disease
16. Show how word parts are used to build words related to the heart (see Word Anatomy at the end of the chapter)

Selected Key Terms

The following terms and other boldface terms in the chapter are defined in the Glossary

arrhythmia
atherosclerosis
atrium
bradycardia
coronary
coronary thrombosis
diastole
echocardiograph
electrocardiograph
endocardium
epicardium
fibrillation
infarct
ischemia
murmur
myocardium
pacemaker
pericardium
plaque
septum
stenosis
systole
tachycardia
valve
ventricle

PASSport to Success

Visit *thePoint* or see the Student Resource CD in the back of this book for definitions and pronunciations of key terms as well as a pretest for this chapter.

Disease in Context

Jim's Second Case: A Coronary Emergency

The emergency room's dispatch radio echoed from the triage desk. "This is Medic 5 en route with Jim, a 46-year-old Caucasian male. Suspected acute myocardial infarction while playing basketball. Cardiopulmonary resuscitation was initiated on scene. Patient was defibrillated in ambulance twice. Portable ECG indicates S-T interval depression and an inverted T wave. Patient is receiving oxygen through nasal cannulae. ETA approximately 10 minutes."

When Jim arrived at the ER, the emergency team rushed to stabilize him. A trauma nurse measured Jim's vital signs—he was hypertensive with tachycardia—while another inserted an IV needle into Jim's arm and placed an oxygen mask over his nose and mouth. Meanwhile, a phlebotomist drew blood from Jim's other arm for testing in the lab. A cardiology technician attached ECG leads to Jim's chest and began to record his cardiac muscle's electrical activity. The emergency doctor looked at the printout from the electrocardiograph and confirmed that Jim was having a heart attack. The doctor knew that one or more of the coronary arteries feed-

ing Jim's heart muscle was blocked with a thrombus (blood clot). He administered several medications in an attempt to restore blood flow to the heart and minimize myocardial damage. Aspirin, which prevents platelets from adhering to each other, was given to inhibit the formation of any more thrombi. Nitroglycerin, a potent vasodilator, was given to widen Jim's coronary arteries and thus increase blood flow to the heart. Morphine was given to manage Jim's pain and lower his cardiac output in order to reduce the heart's workload. Lastly, tissue plasminogen activator was administered to dissolve the thrombi present in Jim's coronary arteries.

Thanks to the quick action of the paramedics and emergency team, Jim was resting comfortably in the intensive care unit a few hours after thrombolytic treatment—he was lucky to be alive! Later in the chapter, we'll visit Jim again and learn how cardiac surgeons repair coronary arteries to prevent future infarctions.

Circulation and the Heart

The next two chapters investigate how the blood delivers oxygen and nutrients to the cells and carries away the waste products of cellular metabolism. The continuous one-way circuit of blood through the blood vessels is known as the **circulation**. The prime mover that propels blood throughout the body is the **heart**. This chapter examines the heart's structure and function as a foundation for the detailed discussion of blood vessels that follows.

The heart's importance has been recognized for centuries. Strokes (the contractions) of this pump average about 72 per minute and are carried on unceasingly for a whole lifetime. The beating of the heart is affected by the emotions, which may explain the frequent references to it in song and poetry. However, the heart's vital functions and its disorders are of more practical concern.

Location of the Heart

The heart is slightly bigger than a person's fist. This organ is located between the lungs in the center and a bit to the left of the body's midline (Fig. 14-1). It occupies most of the mediastinum, the central region of the thorax. The heart's **apex**, the pointed, inferior portion, is directed toward the left. The broad, superior **base** is the area of attachment for the large vessels carrying blood into and out of the heart. See Appendix 7 for a dissection photograph of the heart in position in the thorax.

Structure of the Heart

The heart is a hollow organ, with walls formed of three different layers. Just as a warm coat might have a smooth lining, a thick and bulky interlining, and an outer layer of a third fabric, so the heart wall has three tissue layers (Fig. 14-2, Table 14-1). Starting with the innermost layer, these are as follows:

- The **endocardium** (en-do-KAR-de-um) is a thin, smooth layer of epithelial cells that lines the heart's interior. The endocardium provides a smooth surface for easy flow as blood travels through the heart. Extensions of this membrane cover the flaps (cusps) of the heart valves.

- The **myocardium** (mi-o-KAR-de-um), the heart muscle, is the thickest layer and pumps blood through the vessels. Cardiac muscle's unique structure is described in more detail next.

- The **epicardium** (ep-ih-KAR-de-um) is a serous membrane that forms the thin, outermost layer of the heart wall.

The Pericardium

The **pericardium** (per-ih-KAR-de-um) is the sac that encloses the heart (Fig. 14-2, Table 14-2). The formation of the pericardial sac was described and illustrated in Chapter 4 under a discussion of membranes (see Fig. 4-9). This sac's outermost and heaviest layer is the fibrous pericardium. Connective tissue anchors this pericardial layer to the diaphragm, located inferiorly; the sternum, located anteriorly; and to other structures surrounding the heart, thus holding the heart in place. A serous membrane lines this fibrous sac and folds back at the base to cover the heart's surface. Anatomically, the outer layer of this serous membrane is called the parietal layer, and the inner layer is the visceral layer, also known as the epicardium, as previously noted. A thin film of fluid between these two layers reduces friction as the heart moves within the pericardium. Normally the visceral and parietal layers are very close together, but fluid may accumulate in the region between them, the pericardial cavity, under certain disease conditions.

Special Features of the Myocardium

Cardiac muscle cells are lightly striated (striped) based on alternating actin and myosin filaments, as seen in skeletal muscle cells (see Chapter 8). Unlike skeletal muscle cells, however, cardiac muscle cells have a single nucleus instead of multiple nuclei. Also, cardiac muscle tissue is involuntarily controlled. There are specialized partitions between cardiac muscle cells that show faintly under a microscope (Fig. 14-3). These **intercalated** (in-TER-cah-la-ted) **disks** are actually modified plasma

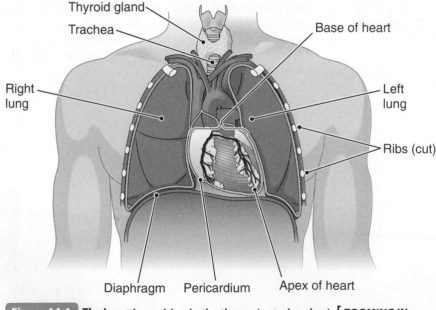

Thyroid gland
Trachea
Base of heart
Right lung
Left lung
Ribs (cut)
Diaphragm   Pericardium   Apex of heart

Figure 14-1   **The heart in position in the thorax (anterior view). [ZOOMING IN ➤** Why is the left lung smaller than the right lung? **]**

Another feature of cardiac muscle tissue is the branching of the muscle fibers (cells). These fibers are interwoven so that the stimulation that causes the contraction of one fiber results in the contraction of a whole group. The intercalated disks and the branching cellular networks allow cardiac muscle cells to contract in a coordinated manner.

Divisions of the Heart

Healthcare professionals often refer to the *right heart* and the *left heart*, because the human heart is really a double pump (Fig. 14-4). The right side pumps blood low in oxygen to the lungs through the **pulmonary circuit.** The left side pumps oxygenated blood to the remainder of the body through the **systemic circuit.** Each side of the heart is divided into two chambers. See Appendix 7 for a photograph of the human heart showing the chambers and the vessels that connect to the heart.

FOUR CHAMBERS The upper chambers on the right and left sides, the **atria** (A-tre-ah), are mainly blood-receiving chambers (Fig. 14-5, Table 14-3). The lower chambers on the right and left side, the **ventricles** (VEN-trih-klz) are forceful pumps. The chambers, listed in the order in which blood flows through them, are as follows:

1. The **right atrium** (A-tre-um) is a thin-walled chamber that receives the blood returning from the body tissues. This blood, which is low in oxygen, is carried in veins, the blood vessels leading back to the heart. The superior vena cava brings blood from the head, chest, and arms; the inferior vena cava delivers blood from the trunk and legs. A third vessel that opens into the

Heart wall

Epicardium (visceral pericardium)

Myocardium

Endocardium

Visceral pericardium

Pericardial cavity

Parietal pericardium

Fibrous pericardium

Serous pericardium

Figure 14-2 **Layers of the heart wall and pericardium.** The serous pericardium covers the heart and lines the fibrous pericardium. **[ZOOMING IN ➤** Which layer of the heart wall is the thickest? **]**

membranes that firmly attach adjacent cells to each other but allow for rapid transfer of electrical impulses between them. The adjective *intercalated* is from Latin and means "inserted between."

CHECKPOINT 14-1 ➤ What are the names of the innermost, middle, and outermost layers of the heart?

CHECKPOINT 14-2 ➤ What is the name of the sac that encloses the heart?

14

Table 14-1	Layers of the Heart Wall		
Layer	Location	Description	Function
Endocardium	Innermost layer of the heart wall	Thin, smooth layer of epithelial cells	Lines the interior of the chambers and covers the heart valves
Myocardium	Middle layer of the heart wall	Thick layer of cardiac muscle	Contracts to pump blood into the arteries
Epicardium	Outermost layer of the heart wall	Thin serous membrane	Covers the heart and forms the visceral layer of the serous pericardium

Table 14-2	Layers of the Pericardium		
Layer	**Location**	**Description**	**Function**
Fibrous pericardium	Outermost layer	Fibrous sac	Encloses and protects the heart; anchors heart to surrounding structures
Serous pericardium	Between the fibrous pericardium and the myocardium	Doubled membranous sac with fluid between layers	Fluid reduces friction within the pericardium as the heart functions
Parietal layer	Lines the fibrous pericardium	Serous membrane	Forms the outer layer of the serous pericardium
Visceral layer	Surface of the heart	Serous membrane	Forms the inner layer of the serous pericardium; also called the epicardium

right atrium brings blood from the heart muscle itself, as described later in this chapter.

2. The **right ventricle** pumps the venous blood received from the right atrium to the lungs. It pumps into a large pulmonary trunk, which then divides into right and left pulmonary arteries. Branches of these arteries carry blood to the lungs. An artery is a vessel that takes blood from the heart to the tissues. Note that the pulmonary arteries in Figure 14-5 are colored blue because they are carrying deoxygenated blood, unlike other arteries, which carry oxygenated blood.

3. The **left atrium** receives blood high in oxygen content as it returns from the lungs in pulmonary veins. Note that the pulmonary veins in Figure 14-5 are colored red because they are carrying oxygenated blood, unlike other veins, which carry deoxygenated blood.

4. The **left ventricle**, which is the chamber with the thickest wall, pumps oxygenated blood to all parts of the body. This blood goes first into the aorta (a-OR-tah), the largest artery, and then into the branching sys-

temic arteries that take blood to the tissues. The heart's apex, the lower pointed region, is formed by the wall of the left ventricle (see Fig. 14-2).

The heart's chambers are completely separated from each other by partitions, each of which is called a **septum**. The **interatrial** (in-ter-A-tre-al) **septum** separates the two atria, and the **interventricular** (in-ter-ven-TRIK-u-lar) **septum** separates the two ventricles. The septa, like the heart wall, consist largely of myocardium.

CHECKPOINT **14-3** ➤ The heart is divided into four chambers. What is the upper receiving chamber on each side called? What is the lower pumping chamber called?

FOUR VALVES One-way valves that direct blood flow through the heart are located at the entrance and exit of each ventricle (Fig. 14-6, Table 14-4). The entrance valves are the **atrioventricular** (a-tre-o-ven-TRIK-u-lar) (AV) **valves**, so named because they are between the atria and ventricles. The exit valves are the **semilunar** (sem-e-LU-nar) **valves**, so named because each flap of these valves resembles a half-moon. Each valve has a specific name, as follows:

- The **right atrioventricular** (AV) **valve** is also known as the **tricuspid** (tri-KUS-pid) **valve** because it has three cusps, or flaps, that open and close. When this valve is open, blood flows freely from the right atrium into the right ventricle. When the right ventricle begins to contract, however, the valve is closed by blood squeezed backward against the cusps. With the valve closed, blood cannot return to the right atrium but must flow forward into the pulmonary arterial trunk.

- The **left atrioventricular** (AV) **valve** is the bicuspid valve, but it is commonly referred to as the **mitral** (MI-tral) **valve** (named for a miter, the pointed, two-sided hat worn by bishops). It has two heavy cusps

Intercalated disk

Nucleus

Figure 14-3 **Cardiac muscle tissue viewed under the microscope (×540).** The sample shows light striations (arrowheads), intercalated disks, and branching fibers (arrow). (Reprinted with permission from Gartner LP, Hiatt JL. *Color Atlas of Histology*, 3rd ed. Philadelphia: Lippincott Williams & Wilkins, 2000.)

that permit blood to flow freely from the left atrium into the left ventricle. The cusps close when the left ventricle begins to contract; this closure prevents blood from returning to the left atrium and ensures the forward flow of blood into the aorta. Both the right and left AV valves are attached by means of thin fibrous threads to columnar muscles, called *papillary muscles*, in the walls of the ventricles. The function of these threads, called the **chordae tendineae** (KOR-de ten-DIN-e-e) (see Fig. 14-6), is to stabilize the valve flaps when the ventricles contract so that the blood's force will not push them up into the atria. In this manner, they help to prevent a backflow of blood when the heart beats.

■ The **pulmonary** (PUL-mon-ar-e) **valve**, also called the *pulmonic valve*, is a semilunar valve located between the right ventricle and the pulmonary trunk that leads to the lungs. As soon as the right ventricle begins to relax from a contraction, pressure in that chamber drops. The higher pressure in the pulmonary artery, described as *back pressure*, closes the valve and prevents blood from returning to the ventricle.

■ The **aortic** (a-OR-tik) **valve** is a semilunar valve located between the left ventricle and the aorta. After contraction of the left ventricle, back pressure closes the aortic valve and prevents the back flow of blood from the aorta into the ventricle.

Figure 14-7 traces a drop of blood as it completes a full circuit through the heart's chambers. Note that blood passes through the heart twice in making a trip from the heart's right side through the pulmonary circuit to the lungs and back to the heart's left side to start on its way through the systemic circuit. Although Figure 14-7 follows the path of a single drop of blood in sequence through the heart, the heart's two sides function in unison to pump blood through both circuits at the same time.

> *PASSport to Success* — Visit **thePoint** or see the Student Resource CD in the back of this book for a detailed picture of the chordae tendineae and for the animations *Blood Circulation* and *The Cardiac Cycle*.

CHECKPOINT 14-4 ➤ What is the purpose of valves in the heart?

Figure 14-4 **The heart as a double pump.** The right side of the heart pumps blood through the pulmonary circuit to the lungs to be oxygenated; the left side of the heart pumps blood through the systemic circuit to all other parts of the body. [**ZOOMING IN ➤** What vessel carries blood into the systemic circuit?]

Blood Supply to the Myocardium

Only the endocardium comes into contact with the blood that flows through the heart chambers. Therefore, the myocardium must have its own blood vessels to provide oxygen and nourishment and to remove waste products. Together, these blood vessels provide the **coronary** (KOR-o-na-re) **circulation**. The main arteries that supply blood to the heart muscle are the right and left coronary arteries (Fig. 14-8), named because they encircle the heart like a crown. These arteries, which are the first to branch off the aorta, arise just above the cusps of the aortic valve and branch to all regions of the heart muscle. They receive blood when the heart relaxes because the aortic valve must be closed to expose the entrance to these vessels (Fig. 14-9). After passing through capillaries in the myocardium, blood drains into a system of cardiac veins that brings blood back toward the right atrium. Blood finally collects *ultrasound cardiography*, high-frequency sound waves are sent to the heart from a small instrument on the chest surface. The ultrasound waves bounce off the heart and are recorded as they return, showing the heart in action. Movement of the echoes is traced on an electronic instrument called an *oscilloscope* and recorded on film. (The same principle is employed by submarines to detect ships.) The method is safe and painless, and it does not use x-rays. It provides information on the size and shape of heart structures, on cardiac function, and on possible heart defects.

CHECKPOINT 14-14 ➤ What do ECG and EKG stand for?

Treatment of Heart Disease

Heart specialists employ medical and surgical approaches, often in combination, in treating heart disease.

Medications

One of the oldest drugs for heart treatment, and still the most important drug for many patients, is **digitalis** (dij-ih-TAL-is). This agent, which slows and strengthens heart muscle contractions, is obtained from the leaf of the foxglove, a plant originally found growing wild in many parts of Europe. Foxglove is now cultivated to ensure a steady supply of digitalis for medical purposes.

Several forms of **nitroglycerin** are used to relieve angina pectoris. This drug dilates (widens) the vessels in the coronary circulation and improves the heart's blood supply.

Beta-adrenergic blocking agents ("beta-blockers") control sympathetic stimulation of the heart. They reduce the rate and strength of heart contractions, thus reducing the heart's oxygen demand. Propranolol is one example.

Antiarrhythmic agents (e.g., quinidine) are used to regulate the rate and rhythm of the heartbeat.

Slow calcium-channel blockers aid in the treatment of coronary heart disease and hypertension by several mechanisms. They may dilate vessels, control the force of heart contractions, or regulate conduction through the atrioventricular node. Their actions are based on the fact that calcium ions must enter muscle cells before contraction can occur.

Anticoagulants (an-ti-ko-AG-u-lants) are valuable drugs for some heart patients. They may be used to prevent clot formation in patients with damage to heart valves or blood vessels or in patients who have had a myocardial in-

farction. **Aspirin** (AS-pir-in), chemically known as acetyl-salicylic (a-SE-til-sal-ih-sil-ik) acid (ASA), is an inexpensive and time-tested drug for pain and inflammation that reduces blood clotting by interfering with platelet activity. A small daily dose of aspirin is recommended for patients with angina pectoris, those who have suffered a myocardial infarction, and those who have undergone surgery to open or bypass narrowed coronary arteries. It is contraindicated for people with bleeding disorders or gastric ulcers, because aspirin irritates the stomach lining.

Correction of Arrhythmias

If the SA node fails to generate a normal heartbeat or there is some failure in the cardiac conduction system, an electric, battery-operated **artificial pacemaker** can be employed (Fig. 14-17). This device, implanted under the skin, supplies regular impulses to stimulate the heartbeat. The implantation site is usually in the left chest area. A pacing wire (lead) from the pacemaker is then passed into the heart through a vessel and lodged in the heart. The lead may be fixed in an atrium or a ventricle (usually on the right side). A dual chamber pacemaker has a lead in each chamber to coordinate beats between the atrium and ventricle. Some pacemakers operate at a set rate; others can be set to stimulate a beat only when the heart fails to do so on its own. Another type of pacemaker adjusts its pacing rate

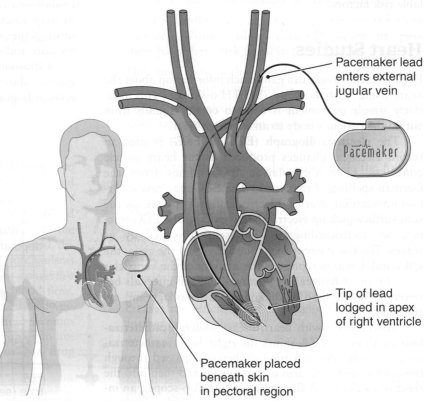

Pacemaker lead enters external jugular vein

Pacemaker

Tip of lead lodged in apex of right ventricle

Pacemaker placed beneath skin in pectoral region

Figure 14-17 **Placement of an artificial pacemaker.** The lead is placed in an atrium or ventricle (usually on the right side). A dual chamber pacemaker has leads in both chambers. (Reprinted with permission from Cohen BJ. *Medical Terminology*, 5th ed. Philadelphia: Lippincott Williams & Wilkins, 2008.)

in response to changing activity, as during exercise. This rather simple device has saved many people whose hearts cannot beat effectively alone. In an emergency, a similar stimulus can be supplied to the heart muscle through electrodes placed externally on the chest wall.

In cases of chronic ventricular fibrillation, a battery-powered device can be implanted in the chest to restore a normal rhythm. The device detects a rapid abnormal rhythm and delivers a direct shock to the heart. The restoration of a normal heartbeat either by electric shock or drugs, is called *cardioversion*, and this device is known as an implantable cardioverter-defibrillator (ICD). A lead wire from the defibrillator is placed in the right ventricle through the pulmonary artery. In cases of severe tachycardia, tissue that is causing the disturbance can be destroyed (ablated) by surgery or catheterization.

Heart Surgery

The heart-lung machine makes possible many operations on the heart and other thoracic organs. There are several types of machines in use, all of which serve as temporary substitutes for the patient's heart and lungs. The machine siphons off the blood from the large vessels entering the heart on the right side, so that no blood passes through the heart and lungs. While in the machine, the blood is oxygenated, and carbon dioxide is removed chemically. The blood is also "defoamed," or rid of air bubbles, which could fatally obstruct blood vessels. The machine then pumps the processed blood back into the general circulation through a large artery. Modern advances have enabled cardiac surgeons to perform certain procedures without bypassing the circulation, partially immobilizing the heart while it continues to beat.

Coronary artery bypass graft (CABG) to relieve obstruction in the coronary arteries is a common and often successful treatment (Fig. 14-18). While the damaged coronary arteries remain in place, healthy segments of blood vessels from other parts of the patient's body are grafted onto the vessels to bypass any obstructions. Usually, parts of the saphenous vein (a superficial vein in the leg) or the mammary artery in the chest are used.

Sometimes, as many as six or seven segments are required to establish an adequate blood supply. The mortality associated with this operation is low, and most patients are able to return to a nearly normal lifestyle after recovery from the surgery. The effectiveness of this procedure diminishes over a period of years, however, owing to blockage of the replacement vessels.

Less invasive surgical procedures include the technique of **angioplasty** (AN-je-o-plas-te), which is used to open restricted arteries in the heart and other areas of the body. In coronary angioplasty, a fluoroscope is used to guide a catheter with a balloon to the affected area (Fig. 14-19). There, the balloon is inflated to break up the blockage in the coronary artery, thus restoring effective circulation to the heart muscle. To prevent repeated blockage, a small tube called a **stent** may be inserted in the vessel to keep it open (Fig. 14-20). Modern stents are coated with drugs that prevent reocclusion.

Diseased valves may become so deformed and scarred from endocarditis that they are ineffective and often obstructive. In most cases, there is so much damage that **valve replacement** is the best treatment. Substitute valves made of a variety of natural and artificial materials have been used successfully.

The news media have given considerable attention to the **surgical transplantation** of human hearts and sometimes of lungs and hearts together. This surgery is done in specialized centers and is available to some patients with degenerative heart disease who are otherwise in good health. Tissues of the recently deceased donor and of the recipient must be as closely matched as possible to avoid rejection.

Efforts to replace a damaged heart with a completely artificial heart have not met with long-term success so far. There are devices available, however, to assist a damaged heart in pumping during recovery from heart attack or while a patient is awaiting a donor heart. The ventricular assist device (VAD) draws blood from a ventricle and pumps it into the aorta (on the left) or the pulmonary artery (on the right). Medical researchers are also testing a fully implantable artificial heart to use for the same purpose.

CHECKPOINT 14-15 ➤ What technique is used to open a restricted coronary artery with a balloon catheter?

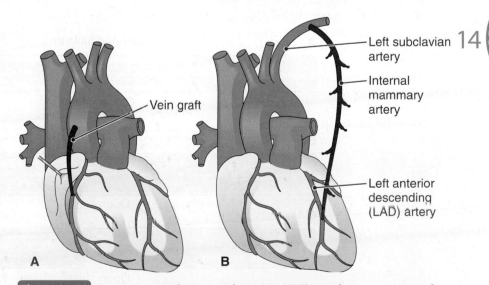

Vein graft

Left subclavian artery

Internal mammary artery

Left anterior descending (LAD) artery

A   B

Figure 14-18 **Coronary artery bypass graft (CABG). (A)** This graft uses a segment of the saphenous vein to carry blood from the aorta to a part of the right coronary artery that is distal to the occlusion. **(B)** The mammary artery is grafted to bypass an obstruction in the left anterior descending (LAD) artery. (Reprinted with permission from Cohen BJ. *Medical Terminology*, 5th ed. Philadelphia: Lippincott Williams & Wilkins, 2008.)

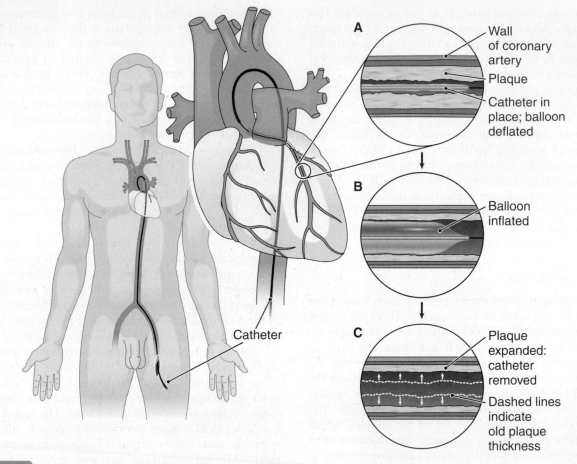

Figure 14-19 **Coronary angioplasty (PTCA).** **(A)** A guide catheter is threaded into the coronary artery. **(B)** A balloon catheter is inserted through the occlusion and inflated. **(C)** The balloon is inflated and deflated until plaque is flattened and the vessel is opened. (Reprinted with permission from Cohen BJ. *Medical Terminology*, 5th ed. Philadelphia: Lippincott Williams & Wilkins, 2008.)

Figure 14-20 **Arterial Stent. (A)** Stent closed, before balloon inflation. **(B)** Stent open, balloon inflated. The stent will remain expanded after balloon is deflated and removed. **(C)** Stent open, balloon removed. (Reprinted with permission from Cohen BJ. *Medical Terminology*, 5th ed. Philadelphia: Lippincott Williams & Wilkins, 2008.)

Disease in Context revisited

Jim's Heart Surgery

Several weeks after his heart attack, Jim was back in the hospital for his coronary bypass surgery. Even though his cardiologist had fully explained the procedure to him, Jim was still nervous—in a couple of hours a surgeon would literally have Jim's heart in his hands!

Jim was brought to the operating room and given general anesthesia. While the cardiac surgeon sawed through Jim's sternum, the saphenous vein was harvested from Jim's leg. Having split the sternum and retracted the ribs, the cardiac surgeon made an incision through the tough fibrous pericardium surrounding Jim's heart. Next, the surgeon inserted a cannula into Jim's right atrium and another one into his aorta. The doctor connected the cannulae to the heart-lung machine and stopped Jim's heart from beating. Now, venous blood from Jim's right atrium flowed through the heart-lung machine where it was oxygenated before being pumped into Jim's aorta. Then, the surgeon prepared the left coronary artery for bypass. He made a small incision through the arterial wall and carefully sutured the cut end of the harvested vein to the opening. Next, he sutured the other end of the vein to a small opening that he made in the aorta, bypassing the occluded portion of the coronary artery. He repeated this procedure two more times in different parts of Jim's obstructed coronary arteries—giving Jim a "triple bypass." The surgeon disconnected Jim from the heart-lung machine and restarted his heart. Blood flowed through the vein grafts to Jim's myocardium, bypassing the diseased parts of Jim's coronary arteries. Jim's surgery was a success!

Although this chapter concentrates on medical terms related to the heart, Jim's case also contains terminology about blood vessels. In Chapter 15, Blood Vessels and Blood Circulation, you will examine these terms in more detail.

Word Anatomy

Medical terms are built from standardized word parts (prefixes, roots, and suffixes). Learning the meanings of these parts can help you remember words and interpret unfamiliar terms.

WORD PART	MEANING	EXAMPLE
Structure of the Heart		
cardi/o	heart	The *myocardium* is the heart muscle.
pulmon/o	lung	The *pulmonary* circuit carries blood to the lungs.
Function of the Heart		
sin/o	sinus	The *sinoatrial* node is in a space (sinus) in the wall of the right atrium.
brady-	slow	*Bradycardia* is a slow heart rate.
tachy-	rapid	*Tachycardia* is a rapid heart rate.
Heart Disease		
cyan/o	blue	*Cyanosis* is a bluish discoloration of the skin due to lack of oxygen.
sten/o	narrowing, closure	*Stenosis* is a narrowing of a structure, such as a valve.
scler/o	hard	In *atherosclerosis*, vessels harden with fatty, gruel-like (ather/o) material that deposits on vessel walls.

14

WORD PART	MEANING	EXAMPLE
isch-	suppression	Narrowing of blood vessels leads to ischemia, a lack of blood (-emia) supply to tissues.

Heart Studies

steth/o	chest	A *stethoscope* is used to listen to body sounds, such as those heard through the wall of the chest.

Treatment of Heart Disease

angi/o	vessel	*Angioplasty* is used to reshape vessels that are narrowed by disease.
-plasty	molding, surgical formation	See preceding example.

Summary

I. **CIRCULATION AND THE HEART**
   A. Heart contractions drive blood through the blood vessels
   B. Location of the heart
      1. In mediastinum
      2. Slightly left of the midline; apex pointed toward left

II. **STRUCTURE OF THE HEART**
   A. Layers
      1. Endocardium—thin inner layer of epithelium
      2. Myocardium—thick muscle layer
      3. Epicardium—thin outer layer of serous membrane
         a. Also called visceral pericardium
   B. Pericardium
      1. Sac that encloses the heart
      2. Outer layer fibrous
      3. Inner layers—parietal and visceral serous membranes
   C. Special features of myocardium
      1. Lightly striated
      2. Intercalated disks
      3. Branching of fibers
   D. Divisions of the heart
      1. Two sides divided by septa
      2. Four chambers
         a. Atria—left and right receiving chambers
         b. Ventricles—left and right pumping chambers
      3. Four valves—prevent backflow of blood
         a. Right atrioventricular (AV) valve—tricuspid
         b. Left atrioventricular valve—mitral or bicuspid
         c. Pulmonary (semilunar) valve—at entrance to pulmonary artery
         d. Aortic (semilunar) valve—at entrance to aorta
   E. Blood supply to the myocardium
      1. Coronary arteries—first branches of aorta; fill when heart relaxes
      2. Coronary sinus—collects venous blood from heart and empties into right atrium

III. **FUNCTION OF THE HEART**
   A. Cardiac cycle
      1. Diastole—relaxation phase
      2. Systole—contraction phase
   B. Cardiac output
      1. Definition—volume pumped by each ventricle per minute
      2. Stroke volume—amount pumped with each beat
      3. Heart rate—number of beats per minute
   C. Heart's conduction system
      1. Sinoatrial node (pacemaker)—at top of right atrium
      2. Atrioventricular node—between atria and ventricles
      3. Atrioventricular bundle (bundle of His)—at top of interventricular septum
         a. Bundle branches—right and left, on either side of septum
         b. Purkinje fibers—branch through myocardium of ventricles
   D. Control of the heart rate
      1. Autonomic nervous system
         a. Sympathetic system—speeds heart rate
         b. Parasympathetic system—slows heart rate through vagus nerve
      2. Others—hormones, ions, drugs
      3. Variations in heart rates
         a. Bradycardia—slower rate than normal; less than 60 beats/minute

b. Tachycardia—faster rate than normal; more than 100 beats/minute

c. Sinus arrhythmia—related to breathing changes

d. Premature beat—extrasystole

E. Heart sounds

1. Normal

a. S_1 ("lub")—occurs at closing of atrioventricular valves

b. S_2 ("dup")—occurs at closing of semilunar valves

2. Abnormal—murmur

IV. **HEART DISEASE**

A. Classification of heart disease

1. Anatomic classification—endocarditis, myocarditis, pericarditis

2. Causal classification

B. Congenital heart diseases—present at birth

1. Failure of fetal lung bypasses to close

a. Atrial septal defect

b. Patent ductus arteriosus

2. Ventricular septal defect

3. Narrowing of aorta or pulmonary artery

4. Tetralogy of Fallot

C. Rheumatic heart disease—results from a type of streptococcal infection

1. Mitral stenosis—valve cusps do not open

2. Mitral regurgitation—valve cusps do not close

D. Coronary artery disease

1. Characteristics

a. Atherosclerosis—thickening and hardening of arteries with plaque

b. Ischemia—lack of blood to area fed by blocked arteries

c. Coronary occlusion—closure of coronary arteries, as by a thrombus (clot)

d. Infarct—area of damaged tissue

e. Angina pectoris—pain caused by lack of blood to heart muscle

f. Abnormal rhythm—arrhythmia

(1) Flutter—rapid, coordinated beats

(2) Fibrillation—rapid, uncoordinated contractions of heart muscle

(3) Heart block—interruption of electric conduction

2. Diagnosis

a. ECG

b. Substances in blood—creatine kinase MB, troponin

3. Treatment of heart attacks—CPR, defibrillation, thrombolytic drugs, monitoring, good health habits

E. Heart failure—due to hypertension, disease, malnutrition, anemia, age

V. **THE HEART IN THE ELDERLY**

A. Individual variations in how heart ages

B. Common variations include:

1. Decrease in heart size, strength of muscle contraction, flexibility of values, cardiac output

2. Abnormal rhythms, temporary failure of conduction system

VI. **PREVENTION OF HEART DISEASE**

A. Risk factors

B. Preventive measures—physical examination, proper diet, quitting smoking, regular exercise, control of chronic illness

VII. **HEART STUDIES**

A. Stethoscope—used to listen to heart sounds

B. Electrocardiograph (ECG, EKG)—records electrical activity as waves

C. Catheterization—thin tube inserted into heart for blood samples, pressure readings, and other tests

D. Fluoroscope—examines deep tissue with x-rays; used to guide catheter

E. Echocardiography—uses ultrasound to record pictures of heart in action

VIII. **TREATMENT OF HEART DISEASE**

A. Medications—examples are digitalis, nitroglycerin, beta-adrenergic blocking agents, antiarrhythmic agents, slow channel calcium-channel blockers, anticoagulants

B. Correction of arrhythmia

1. Artificial pacemakers—electronic devices implanted under skin to regulate heartbeat

2. Implantable cardioverter-defibrillator (ICD)

3. Destruction of abnormal tissue

C. Heart surgery

1. Bypass—vessels grafted to detour blood around blockage

2. Angioplasty—balloon catheter used to open blocked arterics

a. Stents used to keep vessels open

3. Valve replacement

4. Heart transplantation

5. Ventricular assist devices

6. Artificial hearts

14

Questions for Study and Review

BUILDING UNDERSTANDING

Fill in the blanks

1. The central thoracic region that contains the heart is the _____.

2. The layer of the heart responsible for pumping blood is called the_____.

3. The heart beat is initiated by electrical impulses from the_____.

4. Lack of blood to a tissue fed by blocked arteries is called _____.

5. Pain caused by lack of blood to heart muscle is called _____.

Matching > Match each numbered item with the most closely related lettered item.

___ 6. receives deoxygenated blood from the body

___ 7. receives oxygenated blood from the lungs

___ 8. sends deoxygenated blood to the lungs

___ 9. sends oxygenated blood to the body

a. right atrium

b. left atrium

c. right ventricle

d. left ventricle

Multiple choice

___ 10. Rapid transfer of electrical signals between cardiac muscle cells is promoted by
   a. the striated nature of the cells
   b. branching of the cells
   c. the abundance of mitochondria within the cells
   d. intercalated disks between the cells

___ 11. The upper chambers of the heart are separated by the
   a. intercalated disk
   b. interatrial septum
   c. interventricular septum
   d. ductus arteriosus

___ 12. One complete sequence of heart contraction and relaxation is called the
   a. systole
   b. diastole
   c. cardiac cycle
   d. cardiac output

___ 13. A medication that reduces the rate and strength of heart contractions by lowering sympathetic tone is called a(n)
   a. anticoagulant
   b. antiarrhythmic agent
   c. slow calcium-channel blocker
   d. beta-adrenergic blocking agent

___ 14. The ductus arteriosus shunts blood away from the
   a. lungs and towards the aorta
   b. lungs and towards the superior vena cava
   c. aorta and towards the lungs
   d. away from the superior vena cava and towards the lungs

___ 15. A regular variation in heart rate due to changes in the rate and depth of breathing is called a
   a. murmur
   b. cyanosis
   c. sinus arrhythmia
   d. stent

UNDERSTANDING CONCEPTS

16. Differentiate between the terms in each of the following pairs:
    a. pulmonary and systemic circuit
    b. coronary artery and coronary sinus
    c. serous pericardium and fibrous pericardium
    d. systole and diastole

17. Explain the purpose of the four heart valves and describe their structure and location. What prevents the valves from opening backwards?

18. Trace a drop of blood from the superior vena cava to the lungs and then from the lungs to the aorta.

19. Describe the order in which electrical impulses travel through the heart. What is an interruption of these impulses in the heart's conduction system called?

20. Compare the effects of the sympathetic and parasympathetic nervous systems on heart function.

21. Compare and contrast the following disease conditions:
    a. endocarditis and pericarditis
    b. tachycardia and bradycardia
    c. functional murmur and organic murmur
    d. flutter and fibrillation
    e. atrial and ventricular septal defect

22. What part does infection play in rheumatic heart disease?

23. List some age-related changes to the heart.

CONCEPTUAL THINKING

24. In the case story, Jim suffered a massive myocardial infarction. What can Jim do to lower his risk of having it happen again? What risk factors can he not change? Apply your knowledge of these factors to your own life or the life of someone you know.

25. Three-month-old Hannah R. is brought to the doctor by her parents. They have noticed that when she cries she becomes breathless and turns blue. The doctor examines Hannah and notices that she is lethargic, small for her age, and has a loud mitral valve murmur. With this information, explain the cause of Hannah's symptoms.

14

CHAPTER 15

Blood Vessels and Blood Circulation

Learning Outcomes

After careful study of this chapter, you should be able to:

1. Differentiate among the five types of blood vessels with regard to structure and function
2. Compare the pulmonary and systemic circuits relative to location and function
3. Name the four sections of the aorta and list the main branches of each section
4. Define *anastomosis*, cite its function, and give several examples
5. Compare superficial and deep veins and give examples of each type
6. Name the main vessels that drain into the superior and inferior venae cavae
7. Define *venous sinus* and give several examples of venous sinuses
8. Describe the structure and function of the hepatic portal system
9. Explain the forces that affect exchange across the capillary wall
10. Describe the factors that regulate blood flow
11. Define *pulse* and list factors that affect pulse rate
12. List the factors that affect blood pressure
13. Explain how blood pressure is commonly measured
14. List reasons why hypertension should be controlled
15. List some disorders that involve the blood vessels
16. List steps in first aid for hemorrhage
17. List four types of shock
18. Show how word parts are used to build words related to the blood vessels and circulation (see Word Anatomy at the end of the chapter)

Selected Key Terms

The following terms and other boldface terms in the chapter are defined in the Glossary

anastomosis
aneurysm
aorta
arteriole
artery
atherosclerosis
baroreceptor
capillary
embolus
endarterectomy
endothelium
hemorrhage
hypertension
hypotension
ischemia
phlebitis
pulse
shock
sinusoid
sphygmomanometer
thrombus
varicose vein
vasoconstriction
vasodilation
vein
vena cava
venous sinus
venule

PASSport to Success

Visit *thePoint* or see the Student Resource CD in the back of this book for definitions and pronunciations of key terms as well as a pretest for this chapter.

Disease in Context

➤ Reggie's Second Case: Embolytic Emergency

"And now, news from the Sports Desk. Yesterday, wide receiver Reggie Wilson was side-lined with a femoral fracture. Team doctors don't expect him to return until later in the season." Reggie pressed the off button on the hospital's television remote and closed his eyes for a moment. The last 24 hours had been a whirlwind—first the injury, then the surgery, and now the prospect of a long road to recovery. Well, *I've made it through tough situations before*, Reggie thought as he fell asleep.

Inside Reggie's thigh, his femur was beginning to repair itself, but a more dangerous situation lurked in the femoral vein that lay beside the fractured bone. During the accident, the vein's thin inner wall had been injured. Even though Reggie had received heparin (an anticoagulant) after his surgery, blood platelets had adhered to the damaged vein and formed a tiny clot on the inner lining of the vessel. Now that Reggie's thigh was immobile, blood flowed much more slowly through the femoral vein. This venous stasis allowed more and more platelets to stick together at the site of the clot until finally his vein was completely obstructed. Reggie had developed deep vein thrombosis. Blood continued to flow into Reggie's thigh through his femoral artery, but now, it could not flow out through the vein. Reggie's thigh began to swell and turn red because of the build up of blood within it. Although still asleep, Reggie felt some discomfort from the swelling in his leg and shifted his weight to relieve it. That slight movement caused a small piece of the clot to break away from the thrombus and be carried away toward his heart. Now, Reggie had developed an embolism!

A blood clot is traveling through Reggie's systemic veins toward his heart and lungs. In this chapter, we'll examine the important role the vascular system plays in carrying blood to and from the tissues. Later in the chapter, we'll see how Reggie's medical team manages his new emergency.

The blood vessels, together with the four chambers of the heart, form a closed system in which blood is carried to and from the tissues. Although whole blood does not leave the vessels, components of the plasma and tissue fluids can be exchanged through the walls of the tiniest vessels, the capillaries.

The vascular system is easier to understand if you refer to the appropriate illustrations in this chapter as the vessels are described. When this information is added to what you already know about the blood and the heart, a picture of the cardiovascular system as a whole will emerge.

Blood Vessels

Blood vessels may be divided into five groups, named below according to the sequence of blood flow from the heart:

1. **Arteries** carry blood away from the heart and toward the tissues. The heart's ventricles pump blood into the arteries.

2. **Arterioles** (ar-TE-re-olz) are small subdivisions of the arteries. They carry blood into the capillaries.

3. **Capillaries** are tiny, thin-walled vessels that allow for exchanges between systems. These exchanges occur between the blood and the body cells and between the blood and the air in the lung tissues. The capillaries connect the arterioles and venules.

4. **Venules** (VEN-ulz) are small vessels that receive blood from the capillaries and begin its transport toward the heart.

5. **Veins** are vessels formed by the merger of venules. They continue the transport of blood until it is returned to the heart

CHECKPOINT 15-1 ➤ What are the five types of blood vessels?

Blood Circuits

The vessels together may be subdivided into two groups, or circuits: pulmonary and systemic. Figure 15-1 diagrams blood flow in a closed system and the vessels in these two circuits. The true anatomic relation of these circuits to the heart is shown in Chapter 14, Figure 14-4.

THE PULMONARY CIRCUIT The **pulmonary circuit** delivers blood to the lungs, where carbon dioxide is eliminated and oxygen is replenished. The pulmonary vessels that carry blood to and from the lungs include the following:

1. The pulmonary trunk and its arterial branches, which carry blood from the right ventricle to the lungs

2. The capillaries in the lungs, through which gases are exchanged

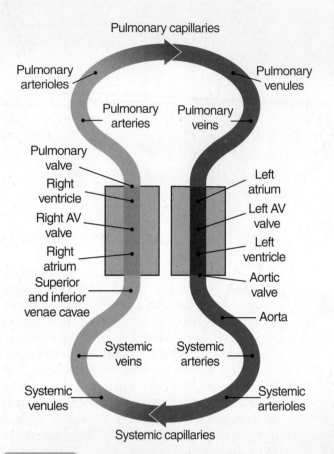

Figure 15-1 **Blood flow in a closed system of vessels.** Oxygen content changes as blood flows through the capillaries. **[ZOOMING IN ➤** Judging from color coding, which vessels pick up oxygen? Which vessels release oxygen? **]**

3. The pulmonary veins, which carry blood back to the left atrium

The pulmonary vessels differ from those in the systemic circuit in that the pulmonary arteries carry blood that is *low* in oxygen, and the pulmonary veins carry blood that is *high* in oxygen. All the remaining arteries carry highly oxygenated blood, and all remaining veins carry blood that is low in oxygen.

THE SYSTEMIC CIRCUIT The **systemic** (sis-TEM-ik) **circuit** serves the rest of the body. These vessels supply nutrients and oxygen to all the tissues and carry waste materials away from the tissues for disposal. The systemic vessels include the following:

1. The **aorta** (a-OR-tah), which receives blood from the left ventricle and then branches into the systemic arteries carrying blood to the tissues

2. The systemic capillaries, through which materials are exchanged

3. The systemic veins, which carry blood back toward the heart. The venous blood flows into the right atrium of the heart through the superior vena cava and inferior vena cava.

CHECKPOINT **15-2** ➤ What are the two blood circuits and what areas does each serve?

Vessel Structure

The arteries have thick walls because they must be strong enough to receive blood pumped under pressure from the heart's ventricles (Fig. 15-2). The three tunics (coats) of the arteries resemble the three tissue layers of the heart. Named from internal to external, they are:

1. The innermost membrane of simple, flat epithelial cells makes up the **endothelium** (en-do-THE-le-um), forming a smooth surface over which the blood flows easily.

2. The middle and thickest layer is made of smooth (involuntary) muscle, which is under the control of the autonomic nervous system.

3. An outer tunic is made of a supporting connective tissue.

Elastic tissue between the layers of the arterial wall allows these vessels to stretch when receiving blood and then return to their original size. The amount of elastic tissue diminishes as the arteries branch and become smaller.

The small subdivisions of the arteries, the arterioles, have thinner walls in which there is little elastic connective tissue but relatively more smooth muscle. The autonomic nervous system controls this involuntary muscle. The vessels become narrower (constrict) when the muscle contracts and widen (dilate) when the muscle relaxes. In this manner, the arterioles regulate the amount of blood that enters the various tissues at a given time. Change in the diameter of the arterioles is also a major factor in blood pressure control.

The microscopic capillaries that connect arterioles and venules have the thinnest walls of any vessels: one cell layer. The capillary walls are transparent and are made of smooth, squamous epithelial cells that are a continuation of the arterial lining. The thinness of these walls allows for exchanges between the blood and the body cells and between the lung tissue and the outside air. The capillary boundaries are the most important center of activity for the entire circulatory system. Their function is explained later in this chapter (see also Box 15-1, Capillaries).

PASSport to Success — Visit **thePoint** or see the Student Resource CD in the back of this book for micrographs of capillaries in longitudinal and cross sections.

Figure 15-2 **Sections of small blood vessels.** Drawings show the thick wall of an artery, the thin wall of a vein, and the single-layered wall of a capillary. A venous valve also is shown. The arrow indicates the direction of blood flow. **[ZOOMING IN ➤** Which vessels have valves that control blood flow? **]**

15

Box 15-1 · A Closer Look

Capillaries: The Body's Free Trade Zones

The exchange of substances between body cells and the blood occurs along about 50,000 miles (80,000 kilometers) of capillaries. Exchange rates vary because, based on their structure, different types of capillaries vary in permeability.

Continuous capillaries are the most common type and are found in muscle, connective tissue, the lungs, and the central nervous system (CNS). These capillaries are composed of a continuous layer of endothelial cells. Adjacent cells are loosely attached to each other, with small openings called intercellular clefts between them. Although continuous capillaries are the least permeable, water and small molecules can diffuse easily through their walls. Large molecules, such as plasma proteins and blood cells, cannot. In certain body regions, like the CNS, adjacent endothelial cells are joined tightly together, making the capillaries impermeable to many substances (see Box 10-1, The Blood-Brain Barrier, in Chapter 10 on the blood-brain barrier).

Fenestrated (FEN-es-tra-ted) capillaries are much more permeable than continuous capillaries, because they have many holes, or fenestrations, in the endothelium. These sieve-like capillaries are permeable to water and solutes as large as peptides. In the digestive tract, fenestrated capillaries permit rapid absorption of water and nutrients into the bloodstream. In the kidneys, they permit rapid filtration of blood plasma, the first step in urine formation.

Discontinuous capillaries, or sinusoids, are the most permeable. In addition to fenestrations, they have large spaces between endothelial cells that allow the exchange of water, large solutes, such as plasma proteins, and even blood cells. Sinusoids are found in the liver and red bone marrow, for example. Albumin, clotting factors, and other proteins formed in the liver enter the bloodstream through sinusoids. In red bone marrow, newly formed blood cells travel through sinusoids to join the bloodstream.

The smallest veins, the venules, are formed by the union of capillaries, and their walls are only slightly thicker than those of the capillaries. As the venules merge to form veins, the smooth muscle in the vessel walls becomes thicker and the venules begin to acquire the additional layers found in the larger vessels.

The walls of the veins have the same three layers as those of the arteries. However, the middle smooth muscle tunic is relatively thin in the veins. A vein wall is much thinner than the wall of a comparably sized artery. These vessels also have less elastic tissue between the layers. As a result, the blood within the veins is carried under much lower pressure. Because of their thinner walls, the veins are easily collapsed. Only slight pressure on a vein by a tumor or other mass may interfere with return blood flow.

Most veins are equipped with one-way valves that permit blood to flow in only one direction: toward the heart (see Fig. 15-2). Such valves are most numerous in the veins of the extremities. Figure 15-3 is a cross-section of an artery and a vein as seen through a microscope.

CHECKPOINT 15-3 ➤ What type of tissue makes up the middle layer of arteries and veins, and how is this tissue controlled?

CHECKPOINT 15-4 ➤ How many cell layers make up the wall of a capillary?

Systemic Arteries

The systemic arteries begin with the aorta, the largest artery, which measures about 2.5 cm (1 inch) in diameter.

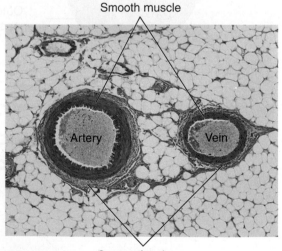

Smooth muscle

Artery

Vein

Connective tissue

Figure 15-3 **Cross-section of an artery and vein.** The smooth muscle and connective tissue of the vessels are visible in this photomicrograph. (Reprinted with permission from Cormack DH. *Essential Histology*, 2nd ed. Philadelphia: Lippincott Williams & Wilkins, 2001.) [**ZOOMING IN** ➤ Which type of vessel shown has a thicker wall?]

This vessel receives blood from the left ventricle, then travels downward through the body, branching to all organs. (See Appendix 7 for a dissection photograph showing the major arteries of the trunk.)

The Aorta and Its Parts

The aorta ascends toward the right from the left ventricle. Then it curves posteriorly and to the left. It continues downward posterior to the heart and just anterior to the vertebral column, through the diaphragm, and into the abdomen (Figs. 15-4 and 15-5). The aorta is one continuous artery, but it may be divided into sections:

1. The **ascending aorta** is near the heart and inside the pericardial sac.

2. The **aortic arch** curves from the right to the left and also extends posteriorly.

3. The **thoracic aorta** lies just anterior to the vertebral column posterior to the heart and in the space behind the pleura.

4. The **abdominal aorta** is the longest section of the aorta, spanning the abdominal cavity.

The thoracic and abdominal aorta together make up the descending aorta.

BRANCHES OF THE ASCENDING AORTA AND AORTIC ARCH The aorta's first, or ascending, part has two branches near the heart, called the **left** and **right coronary arteries**, which supply the heart muscle. These form a crown around the heart's base and give off branches to all parts of the myocardium.

The aortic arch, located immediately beyond the ascending aorta, divides into three large branches.

1. The **brachiocephalic** (brak-e-o-seh-FAL-ik) **artery** is a short vessel that supplies the arm and the head on the right side. After extending upward somewhat less than 5 cm (2 inches), it divides into the **right subclavian** (sub-KLA-ve-an) **artery**, which extends under the right clavicle (collar bone) and supplies the right upper extremity (arm), and the **right common carotid** (kah-ROT-id) **artery**, which supplies the right side of the neck, head, and brain. Note that the brachiocephalic artery is unpaired.

2. The **left common carotid artery** extends upward from the highest part of the aortic arch. It supplies the left side of the neck and the head.

3. The **left subclavian artery** extends under the left clavicle and supplies the left upper extremity. This is the aortic arch's last branch.

BRANCHES OF THE DESCENDING AORTA The thoracic aorta supplies branches to the chest wall and **esophagus** (e-SOF-ah-gus), the bronchi (subdivisions of the trachea), and their treelike subdivisions in the lungs. There are usually 9 to 10 pairs of **intercostal** (in-ter-KOS-tal) **arteries** that extend between the ribs, sending branches to the muscles and other structures of the chest wall.

The abdominal aorta has unpaired branches extending anteriorly

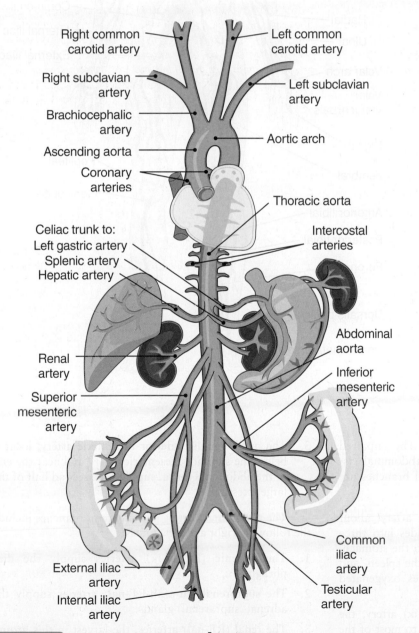

Right common carotid artery
Right subclavian artery
Brachiocephalic artery
Ascending aorta
Coronary arteries
Celiac trunk to:
Left gastric artery
Splenic artery
Hepatic artery
Renal artery
Superior mesenteric artery
External iliac artery
Internal iliac artery

Left common carotid artery
Left subclavian artery
Aortic arch
Thoracic aorta
Intercostal arteries
Abdominal aorta
Inferior mesenteric artery
Common iliac artery
Testicular artery

Figure 15-4 **The aorta and its branches. [ZOOMING IN ➤** How many brachiocephalic arteries are there? **]**

15

Figure 15-5 **Principal systemic arteries.**

and paired branches extending laterally. The unpaired vessels are large arteries that supply the abdominal viscera. The most important of these visceral branches are as follows:

1. The **celiac** (SE-le-ak) **trunk** is a short artery, about 1.25 cm (1/2 inch) long, that subdivides into three branches: the **left gastric artery** goes to the stomach, the **splenic** (SPLEN-ik) **artery** goes to the spleen, and the **hepatic** (heh-PAT-ik) **artery** carries oxygenated blood to the liver.

2. The **superior mesenteric** (mes-en-TER-ik) **artery,** the largest of these branches, carries blood to most of the small intestine and to the first half of the large intestine.

3. The much smaller **inferior mesenteric artery,** located below the superior mesenteric artery and near the end of the abdominal aorta, supplies the second half of the large intestine.

The abdominal aorta's paired lateral branches include the following right and left vessels:

1. The **phrenic** (FREN-ik) **arteries** supply the diaphragm.

2. The **suprarenal** (su-prah-RE-nal) **arteries** supply the adrenal (suprarenal) glands.

3. The **renal** (RE-nal) **arteries,** the largest in this group, carry blood to the kidneys.

4. The **ovarian** arteries in females and **testicular** (tes-TIK-u-lar) **arteries** in males (formerly called the spermatic arteries) supply the sex glands.

5. Four pairs of **lumbar** (LUM-bar) **arteries** extend into the musculature of the abdominal wall.

CHECKPOINT 15-5 ➤ What are the subdivisions of the aorta, the largest artery?

The Iliac Arteries and Their Subdivisions

The abdominal aorta finally divides into two **common iliac** (IL-e-ak) **arteries**. These vessels, which are about 5 cm (2 inches) long, extend into the pelvis, where each subdivides into an **internal** and an **external iliac artery** (see Fig. 15-5). The internal iliac vessels then send branches to the pelvic organs, including the urinary bladder, the rectum, and some reproductive organs.

Each external iliac artery continues into the thigh as the **femoral** (FEM-or-al) **artery**. This vessel gives rise to branches in the thigh and then becomes the **popliteal** (pop-LIT-e-al) **artery**, which subdivides below the knee. The subdivisions include the posterior and anterior **tibial arteries** and the **dorsalis pedis** (dor-SA-lis PE-dis), which supply the leg and the foot.

Arteries That Branch to the Arm and Head

Each common carotid artery travels along the trachea enclosed in a sheath with the internal jugular vein and the vagus nerve. Just anterior to the angle of the mandible (lower jaw) it branches into the **external** and **internal carotid arteries** (see Fig. 15-5). You can feel the pulse of the carotid artery just anterior to the large sternocleidomastoid muscle in the neck and below the jaw. The internal carotid artery travels into the head and branches to supply the eye, the anterior portion of the brain, and other structures in the cranium. The external carotid artery branches to the thyroid gland and to other structures in the head and upper part of the neck.

The **subclavian** (sub-KLA-ve-an) **artery** supplies blood to the arm and hand. Its first branch, however, is the **vertebral** (VER-the-bral) **artery**, which passes though the transverse processes of the first six cervical vertebrae and supplies blood to the posterior brain. The subclavian artery changes names as it travels through the arm and branches to the arm and hand. It first becomes the **axillary** (AK-sil-ar-e) **artery** in the axilla (armpit). The longest part of this vessel, the **brachial** (BRA-ke-al) **artery**, is in the arm proper. The brachial artery subdivides into two branches near the elbow: the **radial artery**, which continues down the thumb side of the forearm and wrist, and the **ulnar artery**, which extends along the medial or little finger side into the hand.

Just as the larger branches of a tree divide into limbs of varying sizes, so the arterial tree has a multitude of sub-divisions. Hundreds of names might be included. We have mentioned only some of them.

CHECKPOINT 15-6 ➤ What arteries are formed by the final division of the abdominal aorta?

CHECKPOINT 15-7 ➤ What areas are supplied by the brachiocephalic artery?

Anastomoses

A communication between two vessels is called an **anastomosis** (ah-nas-to-MO-sis). By means of arterial anastomoses, blood reaches vital organs by more than one route. Some examples of such end-artery unions are as follows:

- The **circle of Willis** (Fig. 15-6) receives blood from the two internal carotid arteries and from the **basilar** (BAS-il-ar) **artery**, which is formed by the union of the two vertebral arteries. This arterial circle lies just under the brain's center and sends branches to the cerebrum and other parts of the brain.

- The **superficial palmar arch** is formed by the union of the radial and ulnar arteries in the hand. It sends branches to the hand and the fingers.

- The **mesenteric** arches are made of communications between branches of the vessels that supply blood to the intestinal tract.

- **Arterial arches** are formed by the union of tibial artery branches in the foot. There are similar anastomoses in other parts of the body.

Arteriovenous anastomoses are blood shunts found in a few areas, including the external ears, the hands, and the feet. In this type of shunt, a small vessel known as a **metarteriole** (met-ar-TE-re-ole) or *thoroughfare channel*, connects the arterial system directly with the venous system, bypassing the capillaries (Fig. 15-7). This pathway provides a more rapid flow and a greater blood volume to these areas, thus protecting these exposed parts from freezing in cold weather.

CHECKPOINT 15-8 ➤ What is an anastomosis?

Systemic Veins

Whereas most arteries are located in protected and rather deep areas of the body, many of the principal systemic veins are found near the surface (Fig. 15-8). The most important of the **superficial veins** are in the extremities, and include the following:

- The veins on the back of the hand and at the front of the elbow. Those at the elbow are often used for drawing blood for test purposes, as well as for intravenous injections. The largest of this venous group are the **cephalic** (seh-FAL-ik), the **basilic** (bah-SIL-ik), and the **median cubital** (KU-bih-tal) **veins**.

15

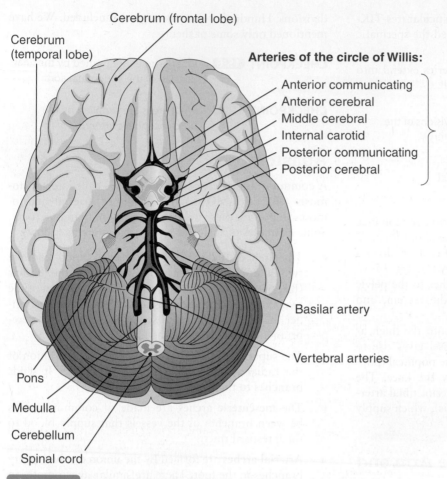

Cerebrum (temporal lobe)

Cerebrum (frontal lobe)

Arteries of the circle of Willis:

Anterior communicating
Anterior cerebral
Middle cerebral
Internal carotid
Posterior communicating
Posterior cerebral

Basilar artery

Vertebral arteries

Pons

Medulla

Cerebellum

Spinal cord

Figure 15-6 **Arteries that supply the brain.** The bracket at right groups the arteries that make up the circle of Willis.

- The **saphenous** (sah-FE-nus) **veins** of the lower extremities, which are the body's longest veins. The great saphenous vein begins in the foot and extends up the medial side of the leg, the knee, and the thigh. It finally empties into the femoral vein near the groin.

The **deep veins** tend to parallel arteries and usually have the same names as the corresponding arteries. Examples of these include the **femoral** and the external and internal **iliac** vessels of the lower body, and the **brachial, axillary,** and **subclavian** vessels of the upper extremities. Exceptions are found in the veins of the head and the neck. The two **jugular** (JUG-u-lar) **veins** on each side of the neck drain the areas supplied by the carotid arteries (*jugular* is from a Latin word meaning "neck"). The larger of the two veins, the internal jugular, receives blood from the large veins (cranial venous sinuses) that drain the head and also from regions of the face and neck. The smaller external jugular drains the areas supplied by the external carotid artery. Both veins empty directly into a subclavian vein. A **brachiocephalic vein** is formed on each side by the union of the subclavian and the jugular veins (see Fig. 15-8). (Remember, there is only *one* brachiocephalic artery.)

The Venae Cavae and Their Tributaries

Two large veins receive blood from the systemic vessels and empty directly into the heart's right atrium. The veins of the head, neck, upper extremities, and chest all drain into the **superior vena cava** (VE-nah KA-vah). This vessel is formed by the union of the right and left brachiocephalic veins, which drain the head, neck, and upper extremities. The unpaired **azygos** (AZ-ih-gos) **vein** drains the veins of the chest wall and empties into the superior vena cava just before the latter empties into the heart (see Fig. 15-8) (*azygous* is from a Greek word meaning "unpaired").

The **inferior vena cava,** which is much longer than the superior vena cava, returns blood from areas below the diaphragm. It begins in the lower abdomen with the union of the two common iliac veins. It then ascends along the abdomen's posterior wall, through a groove in the posterior part of the liver, through the diaphragm, and finally through the lower thorax to empty into the heart's right atrium.

Drainage into the inferior vena cava is more complicated than drainage into the superior vena cava. The large veins below the diaphragm may be divided into two groups:

- The right and left veins that drain paired parts and organs. They include the **iliac** veins from near the groin; four pairs of **lumbar veins** from the dorsal trunk and from the spinal cord; the **testicular veins** from the male testes and the **ovarian veins** from the female ovaries; the **renal** and **suprarenal veins** from the kidneys and adrenal glands near the kidneys; and finally the large **hepatic veins** from the liver. For the most part, these vessels empty directly into the inferior vena cava. The left testicular in the male and the left ovarian in the female empty into the left renal vein, which then takes this blood to the inferior vena cava; these veins thus constitute exceptions to the rule that the paired veins empty directly into the vena cava.

- Unpaired veins that drain the spleen and parts of the digestive tract (stomach and intestine) empty into a vein called the **hepatic portal vein.** Unlike other lower veins, which empty into the inferior vena cava, the hepatic portal vein is part of a special system that enables blood to circulate through the liver before returning to the heart. This system, the hepatic portal system, will be described in more detail later.

Other important venous sinuses are the **cranial venous sinuses**, which are located inside the skull and drain the veins from all over the brain (Fig. 15-9). The largest of the cranial venous sinuses are the following:

- The two **cavernous sinuses**, situated behind the eyeballs, drain the eyes' **ophthalmic** (of-THAL-mik) **veins**. They give rise to the **petrosal** (peh-TRO-sal) **sinuses**, which drain into the jugular veins.

- The **superior sagittal** (SAJ-ih-tal) **sinus** is a single long space located in the midline above the brain and in the fissure between the two cerebral hemispheres. It ends in an enlargement called the **confluence** (KON-flu-ens) **of sinuses**.

- The two **transverse sinuses**, also called the **lateral sinuses**, are large spaces between the layers of the dura mater (the outermost membrane around the brain). They begin posteriorly from the confluence of sinuses and then extend laterally. As each sinus extends around the skull's interior, it receives additional blood, including blood draining through the inferior sagittal sinus and straight sinus. Nearly all of the blood leaving the brain eventually empties into one of the transverse sinuses. Each sinus extends anteriorly to empty into an internal jugular vein, which then passes through a channel in the skull to continue downward in the neck.

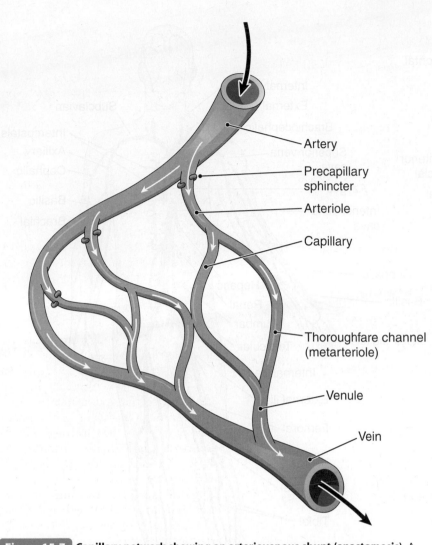

Figure 15-7 **Capillary network showing an arteriovenous shunt (anastomosis).** A connecting vessel, known as a thoroughfare channel or metarteriole, carries blood directly from an arteriole to a venule, bypassing the capillaries.

Artery
Precapillary sphincter
Arteriole
Capillary
Thoroughfare channel (metarteriole)
Venule
Vein

CHECKPOINT **15-9** ➤ Veins are described as superficial or deep. What does superficial mean?

CHECKPOINT **15-10** ➤ What two large veins drain the systemic blood vessels and empty into the right atrium?

Venous Sinuses

The word *sinus* means "space" or "hollow." A **venous sinus** is a large channel that drains deoxygenated blood, but does not have the usual tubular structure of the veins. One example of a venous sinus is the **coronary sinus**, which receives most of the blood from the heart wall (see Fig. 14-8 in Chapter 14). It lies between the left atrium and left ventricle on the heart's posterior surface, and empties directly into the right atrium, along with the two venae cavae.

CHECKPOINT **15-11** ➤ What is a venous sinus?

The Hepatic Portal System

Almost always, when blood leaves a capillary bed, it flows directly back to the heart. In a portal system, however, blood circulates through a second capillary bed, usually in a second organ, before it returns to the heart. A portal system is a kind of detour in the pathway of venous return that transports materials directly from one organ to another. Chapter 12 described the small local portal system that carries secretions from the hypothalamus to the pituitary gland. A much larger portal system is the **hepatic portal system**, which carries blood from the abdominal organs to the liver (Fig. 15-10).

The hepatic portal system includes the veins that drain blood from capillaries in the spleen, stomach, pancreas, and intestine. Instead of emptying their blood di-

Frontal
Superficial temporal
Occipital
External jugular
Internal jugular
Anterior facial
Lingual

Internal jugular
External jugular
Brachiocephalic
Superior vena cava
Azygos
Inferior vena cava
Median cubital
Cephalic
Basilic
Volar digitals
Subclavian
Intercostals
Axillary
Cephalic
Basilic
Brachial
Hepatic
Renal
Lumbar
Testicular
Internal iliac
External iliac
Femoral
Saphenous
Popliteal
Tibial
Venous arch
Dorsal digitals

Figure 15-8 **Principal systemic veins.** [ZOOMING IN ➤ How many brachiocephalic veins are there?]

rectly into the inferior vena cava, they deliver it through the hepatic portal vein to the liver. The portal vein's largest tributary is the **superior mesenteric vein**, which drains blood from the proximal portion of the intestine. It is joined by the **splenic vein** just under the liver. Other tributaries of the portal circulation are the **gastric, pancreatic**, and **inferior mesenteric veins**. As it enters the liver, the portal vein divides and subdivides into ever smaller branches.

Eventually, the portal blood flows into a vast network of sinuslike vessels called **sinusoids** (SI-nus-oyds). These enlarged capillary channels allow liver cells close contact with the blood coming from the abdominal organs. (Similar blood channels are found in the spleen and endocrine glands, including the thyroid and adrenals.)

After leaving the sinusoids, blood is finally collected by the hepatic veins, which empty into the inferior vena cava.

The purpose of the hepatic portal system is to transport blood from the digestive organs and the spleen to the liver sinusoids, so that the liver cells can carry out their functions. For example, when food is digested, most of the end products are absorbed from the small intestine into the bloodstream and transported to the liver by the portal system. In the liver, these nutrients are processed, stored, and released as needed into the general circulation.

CHECKPOINT 15-12 ➤ The hepatic portal system takes blood from the abdominal organs to what organ?

Superior sagittal sinus

Straight sinus

Confluence

Transverse sinus

Petrosal sinuses

Inferior sagittal sinus

Cavernous sinus

Ophthalmic vein

Internal jugular vein

Figure 15-9 **Cranial venous sinuses.** The inset shows the paired transverse sinuses, which carry blood from the brain to the jugular veins.

Circulation Physiology

Circulating blood might be compared to a bus that travels around the city, picking up and delivering passengers at each stop on its route. For example, as blood flows through capillaries surrounding the air sacs in the lungs, it picks up oxygen and unloads carbon dioxide. Later, when this oxygenated blood is pumped to capillaries in other parts of the body, it unloads the oxygen and picks up carbon dioxide and other substances generated by the cells (Fig. 15-11). The microscopic capillaries are of fundamental importance in these activities. It is only through the cells of these thin-walled vessels that the necessary exchanges can occur.

All living cells are immersed in a slightly salty liquid called **tissue fluid, or interstitial fluid.** Looking again at Figure 15-11, one can see how this fluid serves as "middle-man" between the capillary membrane and the neighboring cells. As water, oxygen, and other necessary cellular materials pass through the capillary walls, they enter the tissue fluid. Then, these substances make their way by diffusion to the cells. At the same time, carbon dioxide and

other metabolic end products leave the cells and move in the opposite direction. These substances enter the capillaries and are carried away in the bloodstream for processing in other organs or elimination from the body.

Capillary Exchange

Diffusion is the main process by which substances move between the cells and the capillary blood. Recall that diffusion is the movement of a substance from an area where it is in higher concentration to an area where it is in lower concentration. Diffusion does not require transporters or cellular energy.

An additional force that moves materials from the blood into the tissues is the pressure of the blood as it flows through the capillaries. Blood pressure is the force that filters, or "pushes," water and dissolved materials out of the capillary into the tissue fluid. Fluid is drawn back into the capillary by osmotic pressure, the "pulling force" of substances dissolved and suspended in the blood. Osmotic pressure is maintained by plasma proteins (mainly albumin), which are too large to go through the capillary wall. These processes result in the constant exchange of fluids across the capillary wall.

The movement of blood through the capillaries is relatively slow, owing to the much larger cross-sectional area of the capillaries compared with that of the vessels from which they branch. This slow progress through the capillaries allows time for exchanges to occur.

Note that even when the capillary exchange process is most efficient, some water is left behind in the tissues. Also, some proteins escape from the capillaries into the tissues. The lymphatic system, discussed in Chapter 16, collects this extra fluid and protein and returns them to the circulation (see Fig. 15-11).

CHECKPOINT 15-13 ➤ As materials diffuse back and forth between the blood and tissue fluid across the capillary wall, what force helps to push materials out of the capillary? What force helps to draw materials into the capillary?

The Dynamics of Blood Flow

Blood flow is carefully regulated to supply tissue needs without unnecessary burden on the heart. Some organs, such as the brain, liver, and kidneys, require large quanti-

15

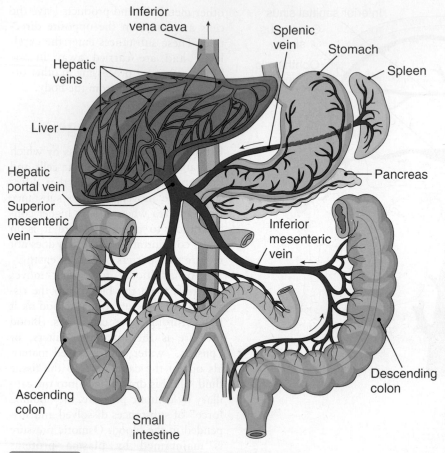

Figure 15-10 Hepatic portal system. Veins from the abdominal organs carry blood to the hepatic portal vein leading to the liver. Arrows show the direction of blood flow.
[**ZOOMING IN ➤** What vessel do the hepatic veins drain into?]

ties of blood even at rest. The requirements of some tissues, such as the skeletal muscles and digestive organs, increase greatly during periods of activity. For example, the blood flow in muscle can increase 25 times during exercise. The volume of blood flowing to a particular organ can be regulated by changing the size of the blood vessels supplying that organ.

An increase in a blood vessel's diameter is called **vasodilation**. This change allows for the delivery of more blood to an area. **Vasoconstriction** is a decrease in a blood vessel's diameter, causing a decrease in blood flow. These *vasomotor activities* result from the contraction or relaxation of smooth muscle in the walls of the blood vessels, mainly the arterioles. A **vasomotor center** in the medulla of the brain stem regulates vasomotor activities, sending its messages through the autonomic nervous system.

Blood flow into an individual capillary is regulated by a **precapillary sphincter** of smooth muscle that encircles the entrance to the capillary (see Fig. 15-7). This sphincter widens to allow more blood to enter when tissues need more oxygen.

CHECKPOINT 15-14 ➤ Name the two types of vasomotor changes.

CHECKPOINT 15-15 ➤ Where are vasomotor activities regulated?

BLOOD'S RETURN TO THE HEART

Blood leaving the capillary networks returns in the venous system to the heart, and even picks up some speed along the way, despite factors that work against its return. Blood flows in a closed system and must continually move forward as the heart contracts. However, by the time blood arrives in the veins, little force remains from the heart's pumping action. Also, because the veins expand easily under pressure, blood tends to pool in the veins. Considerable amounts of blood are normally stored in these vessels. Finally, the force of gravity works against upward flow from regions below the heart. Several mechanisms help to overcome these forces and promote blood's return to the heart in the venous system. These are:

- **Contraction of skeletal muscles.** As skeletal muscles contract, they compress the veins and squeeze blood forward (Fig. 15-12).

- **Valves** in the veins prevent back flow and keep blood flowing toward the heart.

- **Breathing.** Pressure changes in the abdominal and thoracic cavities during breathing also promote blood return in the venous system. During inhalation, the diaphragm flattens and puts pressure on the large abdominal veins. At the same time, chest expansion causes pressure to drop in the thorax. Together, these actions serve to both push and pull blood through these cavities and return it to the heart.

As evidence of these effects, if a person stands completely motionless, especially on a hot day when the superficial vessels dilate, enough blood can accumulate in the lower extremities to cause fainting from insufficient oxygen to the brain.

The Pulse

The ventricles regularly pump blood into the arteries about 70 to 80 times a minute. The force of ventricular contraction starts a wave of increased pressure that begins at the heart and travels along the arteries. This wave, called the **pulse**, can be felt in any artery that is relatively close to the surface, particularly if the vessel can be pressed down against a bone. At the wrist, the radial artery passes

Body cell   Leukocyte

Lymphatic capillary

Tissue (interstitial) fluid

Artery

Arteriole

Lymphatic vessel

Venule

Vein

Blood capillary

CO_2 O_2

Figure 15-11 **Connection between small blood vessels through capillaries.** The blood delivers oxygen (O_2) to the tissues and picks up carbon dioxide (CO_2) for transport to the lungs. Note the lymphatic capillaries, which aid in tissue drainage.

15

over the bone on the forearm's thumb side, and the pulse is most commonly obtained here. Other vessels sometimes used for taking the pulse are the carotid artery in the neck and the dorsalis pedis on the top of the foot.

Normally, the pulse rate is the same as the heart rate, but if a heartbeat is abnormally weak, or if the artery is obstructed, the beat may not be detected as a pulse. In checking another person's pulse, it is important to use your second or third finger. If you use your thumb, you may be feeling your own pulse. When taking a pulse, it is important to gauge the strength as well as the regularity and rate.

PULSE RATE Various factors may influence the pulse rate. We describe just a few here:

- The pulse is somewhat faster in small people than in large people and usually is slightly faster in women than in men.

- In a newborn infant, the rate may be from 120 to 140 beats/minute. As the child grows, the rate tends to become slower.

- Muscular activity influences the pulse rate. During sleep, the pulse may slow down to 60 beats/minute, whereas during strenuous exercise, the rate may go up to well over 100 beats/minute. For a person in good condition, the pulse does not go up as rapidly as it does in an inactive person, and it returns to a resting rate more quickly after exercise.

- Emotional disturbances may increase the pulse rate.

- In many infections, the pulse rate increases with the increase in temperature.

- Excessive secretion of thyroid hormone may cause a rapid pulse.

CHECKPOINT **15-16** ➤ What is the definition of *pulse*?

A   **B**

Figure 15-12 **Role of skeletal muscles and valves in blood return.** **(A)** Contracting skeletal muscle compresses the vein and drives blood forward, opening the proximal valve, while the distal valve closes to prevent backflow of blood. **(B)** When the muscle relaxes again, the distal valve opens, and the proximal valve closes until blood moving in the vein forces it open again. [**ZOOMING IN** ➤ Which of the two valves shown is closer to the heart?]

Blood Pressure

Blood pressure is the force exerted by the blood against the walls of the vessels. Blood pressure is determined by the heart's output and resistance to blood flow in the vessels. If either of these factors changes and there are no compensating changes, blood pressure will change (Fig. 15-13).

CARDIAC OUTPUT As described in Chapter 14, the output of the heart, or cardiac output (CO), is the volume of

blood pumped out of each ventricle in one minute. Cardiac output is the product of two factors:

- **Heart rate,** the number of times the heart beats each minute. The basic heart rate is set internally by the SA node, but can be influenced by the autonomic nervous system, hormones, and other substances circulating in the blood, such as ions.

- **Stroke volume,** the volume of blood ejected from the ventricle with each beat. The sympathetic nervous system can stimulate more forceful heart contractions to increase blood ejection. Also, if more blood returns to the heart in the venous system, stretching of the heart muscle will promote more forceful contractions.

RESISTANCE TO BLOOD FLOW
Resistance is opposition to blood flow owing to friction generated as blood slides along the vessel walls. Because the effects of resistance are seen mostly in small arteries and arterioles that are at a distance from the heart and large vessels, this factor is often described as *peripheral resistance*. Resistance in the vessels is affected by the following factors:

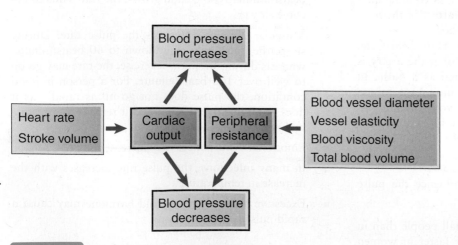

Figure 15-13 **Factors that influence blood pressure.**

- **Vasomotor changes.** A narrow vessel offers more resistance to blood flow than a wider vessel, just as it is harder to draw fluid through a narrow straw than through a wide straw. Thus, vasoconstriction increases resistance to flow and vasodilation lowers resistance.

  The medulla's vasomotor center, which controls vessel diameter, responds mainly to impulses from sensory receptors in the large vessels. The carotid arteries and the aorta have **baroreceptors** (bar-o-re-SEP-torz) in their walls that respond to changes in pressure. When they are stretched by increased blood pressure, they transmit signals that result in vasodilation. At the same time, central controls slow the heart rate to reduce cardiac output. With less stretching, the sympathetic nervous system causes the vessels to constrict and causes the heart rate to increase.

- **Elasticity of blood vessels.** Arteries normally expand to receive blood and then return to their original size. If vessels lose elasticity, as by atherosclerosis, they offer more resistance to blood flow. You've probably experienced this phenomenon if you've tried to blow up a firm, new balloon. More pressure is generated as you blow, and the balloon is a lot harder to inflate than a softer balloon, which expands more easily under pressure. Blood vessels lose elasticity with aging, thus increasing resistance and blood pressure.

- **Viscosity,** or thickness of the blood. Just as a milkshake is harder to suck through a straw than milk is, increased blood viscosity will increase blood pressure. Increased numbers of red blood cells, as in polycythemia, or a loss of plasma volume, as by dehydration, will increase blood viscosity. The hematocrit test described in Chapter 13 is one measure of blood viscosity; it measures the relative percentage of packed cells in whole blood.

- **Total blood volume,** the total amount of blood that is in the vascular system at a given time. A loss of blood volume, as by hemorrhage, will lower blood pressure. An increase in blood volume will generate more pressure within the vessels. It will also increase cardiac output by increasing venous return of blood to the heart.

To summarize, all of these relationships are expressed together by the following equation:

$$\text{Blood pressure} = \text{cardiac output} \times \text{peripheral resistance}$$

MEASUREMENT OF BLOOD PRESSURE The measurement and careful interpretation of blood pressure may prove a valuable guide in the care and evaluation of a person's health. Because blood pressure decreases as the blood flows from arteries into capillaries and finally into veins, healthcare providers ordinarily measure arterial pressure only, most commonly in the brachial artery of the arm. They use an instrument called a **sphygmomanometer** (sfig-mo-mah-NOM-eh-ter) (Fig. 15-14), more simply called a blood pressure cuff or blood pressure apparatus. This instrument measures two variables:

- **Systolic pressure,** which occurs during heart muscle contraction

- **Diastolic pressure,** which occurs during relaxation of the heart muscle

The sphygmomanometer is an inflatable cuff attached to a pressure gauge. Pressure is expressed in millimeters mercury (mm Hg), that is, the height to which the pressure can push a column of mercury in a tube. The examiner

A

B

Figure 15-14 **Measurement of blood pressure. (A)** A sphygmomanometer, or blood pressure cuff. **(B)** Once the cuff is inflated, the examiner releases the pressure and listens for sounds in the vessels with a stethoscope. (A, Reprinted with permission from Bickley LS. *Bates' Guide to Physical Examination and History Taking,* 8th ed. Philadelphia: Lippincott Williams & Wilkins, 2003; B, reprinted with permission from Taylor C, Lillis C, LeMone P. *Fundamentals of Nursing,* 5th ed. Philadelphia: Lippincott Williams & Wilkins, 2004.)

15

wraps the cuff around the patient's upper arm and inflates it with air until the brachial artery is compressed and the blood flow is cut off. Then, listening with a stethoscope, he or she slowly lets air out of the cuff until the first pulsations are heard. At this point, the pressure in the cuff is equal to the systolic pressure, and this pressure is read. Then, more air is let out gradually until a characteristic muffled sound indicates that the vessel is open and the diastolic pressure is read. Original-style sphygmomanometers display readings on a graduated column of mercury, but newer types display them on a dial or measure blood pressure electronically and give a digital reading. A typical normal systolic pressure is 120 mm Hg; a typical normal diastolic pressure is 80 mm Hg. Blood pressure is reported as systolic pressure first, then diastolic pressure, separated by a slash, such as 120/80.

Considerable experience is required to ensure an accurate blood pressure reading. Often it is necessary to repeat measurements. Note also that blood pressure varies throughout the day and under different conditions, so a single reading does not give a complete picture. Some people typically have a higher reading in a doctor's office because of stress. People who experience such "white coat hypertension" may need to take their blood pressure at home while relaxed to get a more accurate reading. A physician might recommend treatment for mild hypertension. Box 15-2 explains how cardiac catheterization is used to measure blood pressure with high accuracy.

CHECKPOINT 15-17 ➤ What is the definition of blood pressure?

CHECKPOINT 15-18 ➤ What two components of blood pressure are measured?

ABNORMAL BLOOD PRESSURE Lower-than-normal blood pressure is called **hypotension** (hi-po-TEN-shun). Because of individual variations in normal pressure levels, however, what would be a low pressure for one person might be normal for someone else. For this reason, hypotension is best evaluated in terms of how well the body tissues are being supplied with blood. A person whose systolic blood pressure drops to below his or her normal range may experience fainting episodes because of inadequate blood flow to the brain. The sudden lowering of blood pressure to below a person's normal level is one sign of shock; it may also occur in certain chronic diseases and in heart block.

Hypertension (hi-per-TEN-shun), or high blood pressure, has received a great deal of attention in medicine. Hypertension normally occurs temporarily as a result of excitement or exertion. However, it may persist in a number of conditions, including the following:

- Kidney disease and uremia (excess nitrogenous waste in the blood) or other toxic conditions

- Endocrine disorders, such as hyperthyroidism and acromegaly

- Arterial disease, including hardening of the arteries (atherosclerosis), which reduces vacular elasticity

- Tumors of the adrenal medulla (central portion) with the release of excess epinephrine

Hypertension that has no apparent medical cause is called **essential hypertension**. Excess of an enzyme called **renin** (RE-nin), produced in the kidney, appears to play a role in the severity of essential hypertension. Renin raises blood pressure by causing blood vessels to constrict and by promoting the kidney's retention of salt and water.

Box 15-2 Clinical Perspectives

Cardiac Catheterization: Measuring Blood Pressure from Within

Because arterial blood pressure decreases as blood flows farther away from the heart, measurement of blood pressure with a simple inflatable cuff around the arm is only a reflection of the pressure in the heart and pulmonary arteries. Precise measurement of pressure in these parts of the cardiovascular system is useful in diagnosing certain cardiac and pulmonary disorders.

More accurate readings can be obtained using a catheter (thin tube) inserted directly into the heart and large vessels. One type commonly used is the pulmonary artery catheter (also known as the Swan-Ganz catheter), which has an inflatable balloon at the tip. This device is threaded into the right side of the heart through a large vein. Typically, the right internal jugular vein is used because it is the shortest and most

direct route to the heart, but the subclavian and femoral veins may be used instead. The catheter's position in the heart is confirmed by a chest x-ray and, when appropriately positioned, the atrial and ventricular blood pressures are recorded. As the catheter continues into the pulmonary artery, pressure in this vessel can be read. When the balloon is inflated, the catheter becomes wedged in a branch of the pulmonary artery, blocking blood flow. The reading obtained is called the **pulmonary capillary wedge (PCW) pressure**. It gives information on pressure in the heart's left side and on resistance in the lungs. Combined with other tests, cardiac catheterization can be used to diagnose cardiac and pulmonary disorders such as shock, pericarditis, congenital heart disease, and heart failure.

It is important to treat even mild hypertension because this condition can eventually:

- Weaken vessels and lead to saclike bulges (aneurysms) in vessel walls that are likely to rupture. In the brain, vessel rupture is one cause of stroke. Rupture of a vessel in the eye may lead to blindness.
- Stress the heart by causing it to work harder to pump blood into the arterial system. In response to this greater effort, the heart enlarges, but eventually it weakens and becomes less efficient.
- Stress the kidneys and damage renal vessels.
- Damage the lining of vessels, predisposing to atherosclerosis.

PASSport to Success

Visit *thePoint* or see the Student Resource CD in the back of this book for an animation on hypertension.

Although medical caregivers often place emphasis on the systolic blood pressure, in many cases, the diastolic pressure is even more important. The total fluid volume in the vascular system and the condition of small arteries may have a greater effect on diastolic pressure. Table 15-1 lists degrees of hypertension as compared with normal blood pressure values.

TREATMENT OF HYPERTENSION Even though there is much individual variation in blood pressure, physicians have established guidelines for the diagnosis and treatment of hypertension. The first stage of hypertension begins at 140/90 mm Hg. Treatment at this point should be based on diet, exercise, and weight loss, if necessary. Drug therapy should be added to this regimen for people with pressure readings above 159/99 mm Hg. Drugs used to treat hypertension include the following:

- Diuretics, which promote water loss
- Drugs that limit production of renin
- Drugs that relax blood vessels

CHECKPOINT 15-19 ➤ What is meant by *hypertension* and *hypotension*?

Arterial Degeneration and Other Vascular Disorders

As a result of age or other degenerative changes, materials may be deposited within the arterial walls. These deposits cause an irregular thickening of the wall at the expense of the lumen (space inside the vessel), as well as a loss of elasticity. In some cases, calcium salts and scar tissue may cause this hardening of the arteries, technically called **arteriosclerosis** (ar-te-re-o-skle-RO-sis). The most common form of this disorder is **atherosclerosis** (ath-er-o-skle-RO-sis) (Fig. 15-15), in which areas of yellow, fatlike material, called **plaque** (PLAK), accumulate in the vessels and separate the muscle and elastic tissue. Sometimes, the arterial lining is also damaged, leading to possible blood clot (thrombus) formation and partial or complete obstruction of the vessel, as occurs in coronary thrombosis. Atherosclerosis begins with microscopic damage to the arterial endothelium caused by direct contact with LDL (the "bad" cholesterol), oxidizing chemicals, such as free-radicals, and some proteins. Lipids begin to accumulate in the arterial wall, followed by aggregation of platelets and macrophages, and plaque formation. The arterial wall soon bulges into the lumen and obstructs blood flow. Arteries in the heart, brain, kidneys, and the extremities seem to be especially vulnerable to this process.

Atherosclerosis and its complications (heart disease, stroke, and thrombosis) account for 40% of all deaths in the United States! A diet high in fats, particularly saturated fats, is known to contribute to atherosclerosis. Cigarette smoking also increases the extent and severity of this disorder. Arterial damage may be present for years without causing any noticeable symptoms. As the thickening of the wall continues and the lumen's diameter decreases, limiting blood flow, a variety of symptoms can appear. The nature of these disturbances varies with the area affected and with the extent of the arterial changes. Some examples are as follows:

- Leg cramps, pain, and sudden lameness while walking may be caused by insufficient blood supply to the lower extremities resulting from arterial damage.
- Headaches, dizziness, and mental disorders may be the result of cerebral artery sclerosis.
- Hypertension may result from a decrease in lumen size within many arteries throughout the body. Although hypertension may be present in young people with no apparent arterial damage, and atherosclerosis may be present without causing hypertension, the two are often found together in elderly people.

Table 15-1 Blood Pressure

Blood Pressure Classification (Adults)*

Category	Systolic (mm Hg)	Diastolic (mm Hg)
Optimal	<120	<80
Normal	<130	<85
High normal	130–139	85–89
Hypertension		
Stage 1 (mild)	140–159	90–99
Stage 2 (moderate)	160–179	100–109
Stage 3 (severe)	≥180	≥110

When the systolic and diastolic pressures are in different categories, the higher category is used.

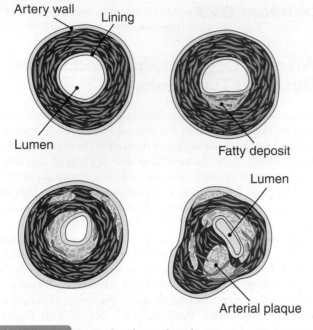

Figure 15-15 **Stages in atherosclerosis.**

angina pectoris may follow the lack of oxygen and the myocardial damage associated with sclerosis of the vessels that supply the heart.

■ An increase in the amount of urine with the appearance of albumin. Albumin is a normal plasma protein usually found in the urine only if there is kidney damage. Other symptoms referable to the kidneys may be caused by renal artery damage.

■ Ulceration and tissue necrosis (death) as a result of ischemia (lack of blood supply), especially in the extremities. If the dead tissue is invaded by bacteria, the result is **gangrene** (GANG-grene). The arterial damage that is caused by diabetes, for example, often leads to gangrene in the extremities of elderly diabetic patients.

PASSport to Success — Visit *thePoint* or see the Student Resource CD in the back of this book for illustrations of atherosclerosis development and its clinical effects.

TREATMENT FOR ARTERIAL DEGENERATION Balloon catheterization and bypass grafts used to treat arterial disease were discussed with reference to the heart in Chapter 14. Stents, small tubes inserted to keep vessels open, also discussed in relation to the heart, are used for other vessels as well. An additional treatment approach is **endarterectomy** (end-ar-ter-EK-to-me), removal of a ves-

■ Palpitations, dyspnea (difficulty in breathing), paleness, weakness, and other symptoms may be the result of coronary artery arteriosclerosis. The severe pain of

Disease in Context revisited

▶ Reggie's Pulmonary Embolism

As soon as the blood clot broke free in Reggie's femoral vein, it began its journey to the heart. The clot (now called an embolus) traveled within the right femoral vein, which entered the abdominal cavity and widened, becoming the external iliac vein. The embolus flowed into the large right common iliac vein, mixing with pelvic blood from the internal iliac vein. Then, the embolus was carried toward the even larger inferior vena cava. As the embolus traveled superiorly toward the heart, it joined with blood from the kidneys and intestines. The inferior vena cava carried the embolus through the diaphragm into the thoracic cavity and into the right atrium of the heart. The embolus flowed past the tricuspid valve into the right ventricle, which contracted and propelled the embolus past the pulmonary valve and into the pulmonary trunk. The embolus entered the left pulmonary artery and then traveled through successively

smaller arterial branches until finally it became wedged in one of the small arteries supplying blood to his left lung. Reggie had developed a pulmonary embolism!

Reggie felt a sharp crushing pain in his chest and woke with a start. He knew something was terribly wrong and pressed the panic button clipped to his hospital bed. Reggie's nurse rushed to his bedside and recognized that Reggie was in life-threatening danger. He received immediate treatment of tissue plasminogen activator (tPA) to dissolve the clots in his pulmonary artery and femoral vein and several doses of heparin to prevent more clots from forming. Reggie had survived his second medical emergency!

In this case, we followed an embolus as it traveled from Reggie's femoral vein to his pulmonary artery. Using the diagrams in this chapter, can you trace its pathway?

sel's thickened, atheromatous lining. Common sites for this procedure are the carotid artery or vertebral artery leading to the brain and the common iliac or femoral arteries leading to the lower limbs. Surgeons can remove a blockage by direct incision of a vessel. More commonly, to remove plaque, they use a cutting tool inserted with a catheter through the vessel opening.

ANEURYSM An **aneurysm** (AN-u-rizm) is a bulging sac in a blood vessel's wall caused by a localized weakness in that part of the vessel (Fig. 15-16). The aorta and vessels in the brain are common aneurysm sites. The damage to the wall may be congenital or a result of arteriosclerosis. Whatever the cause, the aneurysm may continue to grow in size. As it swells, it may cause some derangement of other structures, in which case definite symptoms are present. If undiagnosed, the weakened area eventually yields to the pressure, and the aneurysm bursts like a balloon, usually causing death. Surgical replacement of the damaged segment with a synthetic graft may be lifesaving.

 PASSport to Success Visit *thePoint* or see the Student Resource CD in the back of this book for a photograph of an aortic aneurysm.

Hemorrhage

A profuse escape of blood from the vessels is known as **hemorrhage** (HEM-or-ij), a word that means "a bursting forth of blood." Such bleeding may be external or internal, from vessels of any size, and may involve any part of the body. Capillary oozing usually is stopped by the normal process of clot formation.

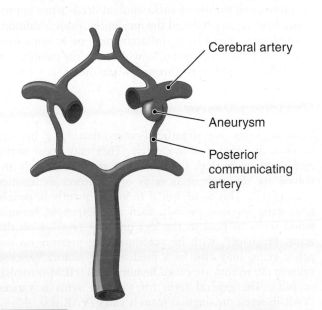

Cerebral artery

Aneurysm

Posterior communicating artery

Figure 15-16 A cerebral aneurysm in the circle of Willis. (Reprinted with permission from Cohen BJ. *Medical Terminology*, 4th ed. Philadelphia: Lippincott Williams & Wilkins, 2004.)

FIRST AID FOR HEMORRHAGE The loss of a small amount of blood will cause no problem for a healthy adult, but loss of one liter or more of blood is life-threatening. The first step to control bleeding is the application of direct pressure to the wound using a clean cloth. An assisting person should wear gloves to protect from blood-borne diseases. A bleeding extremity should be elevated above the heart level. In cases of severe, persistent bleeding, application of pressure where a local artery can be pressed against a bone slows the bleeding. The most important of these "pressure points" are the following:

- The **facial artery**, which may be pressed against the lower jaw for hemorrhage around the nose, mouth, and cheek. One can feel the pulse of the facial artery in the depression about 1 inch anterior to the lower jaw's angle.

- The **temporal artery**, which may be pressed against the side of the skull just anterior to the ear to stop hemorrhage on the side of the face and around the ear.

- The **common carotid artery** in the neck, which may be pressed back against the spinal column for bleeding in the neck and the head.

- The **subclavian artery**, which may be pressed against the first rib by a downward push with the thumb to stop bleeding from the shoulder or arm.

- The **brachial artery**, which may be pressed against the humerus (arm bone) by a push inward along the natural groove between the arm's two large muscles. This stops hand, wrist, and forearm hemorrhage.

- The **femoral artery** (in the groin), which may be pressed to avoid serious hemorrhage of the lower extremity.

It is important not to leave the pressure on too long, as this may cause damage to tissues supplied by arteries past the pressure point.

15

Shock

The word **shock** has a number of meanings. In terms of the circulating blood, it refers to a life-threatening condition in which there is inadequate blood flow to the body tissues. A wide range of conditions that reduce effective circulation can cause shock. The exact cause is often not known. However, a widely used classification is based on causative factors, the most important of which include the following:

- **Cardiogenic** (kar-de-o-JEN-ik) **shock**, sometimes called *pump failure*, is often a complication of heart muscle damage, as occurs in myocardial infarction. It is the leading cause of shock death.

- **Septic shock** is second only to cardiogenic shock as a cause of shock death. It is usually the result of an overwhelming bacterial infection.

■ **Hypovolemic** (hi-po-vo-LE-mik) **shock** is caused by a decrease in the volume of circulating blood and may follow severe hemorrhage or burns.

■ **Anaphylactic** (an-ah-fih-LAK-tik) **shock** is a severe allergic reaction to foreign substances to which the person has been sensitized (see Chapter 17 on Immunity).

When the cause is not known, shock is classified according to its severity.

In **mild shock**, regulatory mechanisms relieve the circulatory deficit. Signs are often subtle changes in heart rate and blood pressure. Constriction of small blood vessels and the detouring of blood away from certain organs increase the effective circulation. Mild shock may develop into a severe, life-threatening circulatory failure.

Severe shock is characterized by poor circulation, which causes further damage and deepening of the shock. Late shock symptoms include clammy skin, anxiety, low blood pressure, rapid pulse, and rapid, shallow breathing. Heart contractions are weakened, owing to the decrease in the heart's blood supply. The vascular walls also are weakened, so that the vessels dilate. The capillaries become more permeable and lose fluid, owing to the accumulation of metabolic wastes.

The victim of shock should first be placed in a horizontal position and covered with a blanket. If there is bleeding, it should be stopped. The patient's head should be kept turned to the side to prevent aspiration (breathing in) of vomited material, an important cause of death in shock cases. Further treatment of shock depends largely on treatment of the causative factors. For example, shock resulting from fluid loss, as in hemorrhage or burns, is best treated with blood products or plasma expanders (intravenous fluids). Shock caused by heart failure should be treated with drugs that improve heart muscle contractions. In any case, all measures are aimed at supporting the circulation and improving the cardiac output. Oxygen is frequently administered to improve oxygen delivery to the tissues.

CHECKPOINT `15-20` ➤ With regard to the circulation, what is meant by shock?

Thrombosis

Formation of a blood clot in a vessel is **thrombosis** (throm-BO-sis). A blood clot in a vein, termed *deep venous thrombosis* (DVT), most commonly develops in the deep veins of the calf muscle, although it may appear elsewhere. Thromboses typically occur in people who are recovering from surgery, injury, or childbirth or those who are bedridden. Clot formation may also be associated with some diseases, with obesity, and with certain drugs, such as hormonal medications. Symptoms are pain and swelling, often with warmth and redness below or around

Figure 15-17 **Varicose veins.** (Reprinted with permission from Bickley LS. *Bates' Guide to Physical Examination and History Taking*, 8th ed. Philadelphia: Lippincott Williams & Wilkins, 2003.)

the clot. Thrombosis can be diagnosed with ultrasound or with magnetic resonance imaging (MRI).

A dangerous complication of thrombosis is formation of an **embolus** (EM-bo-lus), a piece of the clot that becomes loose and floats in the blood. An embolus is carried through the circulatory system until it lodges in a vessel. If it reaches the lungs, sudden death from **pulmonary embolism** (EM-bo-lizm) may result. Prevention of infections, early activity to promote circulation after an injury or an operation, and the use of anticoagulant drugs when appropriate have greatly reduced the incidence of this condition.

Phlebitis (fleh-BI-tis), inflammation of a vein, may contribute to clot formation, in which case the condition is called **thrombophlebitis** (throm-bo-fleh-BI-tis).

Varicose Veins

Varicose veins are superficial veins that have become swollen, distorted, and ineffective. They may occur in the esophagus or rectum, but the veins most commonly involved are the saphenous veins of the lower extremities (Fig. 15-17). This condition is found frequently in people who stand for long periods, such as salespeople, because blood tends to pool in the legs and put pressure on the veins. Pregnancy, with its accompanying pressure on the pelvic veins, may also be a predisposing factor. Varicose veins in the rectum are called **hemorrhoids** (HEM-o-royds), or *piles*. The general term for varicose veins is **varices** (VAR-ih-seze); the singular form is **varix** (VAR-iks).

Word Anatomy

Medical terms are built from standardized word parts (prefixes, roots, and suffixes). Learning the meanings of these parts can help you remember words and interpret unfamiliar terms.

WORD PART	MEANING	EXAMPLE
Systemic Arteries		
brachi/o	arm	The *brachiocephalic* artery supplies blood to the arm and head on the right side.
cephal/o	head	See preceding example.
clav/o	clavicle	The *subclavian* artery extends under the clavicle on each side.
cost/o	rib	The *intercostal* arteries are between the ribs.
celi/o	abdomen	The *celiac* trunk branches to supply blood to the abdominal organs.
gastr/o	stomach	The *gastric* artery goes to the stomach.
splen/o	spleen	The *splenic* artery goes to the spleen.
hepat/o	liver	The *hepatic* artery supplies blood to the liver.
enter/o	intestine	The *mesenteric* arteries supply blood to the intestines.
phren/o	diaphragm	The *phrenic* artery supplies blood to the diaphragm.
ped/o	foot	The dorsalis *pedis* artery supplies blood to the foot.
stoma	mouth	An *anastomosis* is a communication between two vessels.
Circulation Physiology		
bar/o	pressure	A *baroreceptor* responds to changes in pressure.
sphygm/o	pulse	A *sphygmomanometer* is used to measure blood pressure.
man/o	pressure	See preceding example.
Arterial Degeneration and Other Vascular Disorders		
-ectomy	surgical removal	*Endarterectomy* is a procedure for removing plaque from the lining of a vessel.
phleb/o	vein	*Phlebitis* is inflammation of a vein.

15

Summary

I. BLOOD VESSELS
    A. Categories
        1. Arteries—carry blood away from heart
        2. Arterioles—small arteries
        3. Capillaries—allow for exchanges between blood and tissues, or blood and air in lungs; connect arterioles and venules
        4. Venules—small veins
        5. Veins—carry blood toward heart
    B. Blood circuits
        1. Pulmonary circuit—carries blood to and from lungs
        2. Systemic circuit—carries blood to and from rest of body
    C. Vessel structure
        1. Artery walls—layers (tunics)
            a. Innermost—single layer of flat epithelial cells (endothelium)
            b. Middle—thicker layer of smooth muscle and elastic connective tissue
            c. Outer—connective tissue
        2. Arterioles—thinner walls, less elastic tissue, more smooth muscle
        3. Capillaries—only endothelium; single layer of cells
        4. Venules—wall slightly thicker than capillary wall
        5. Veins—all three layers; thinner walls than arteries, less elastic tissue

II. SYSTEMIC ARTERIES
    A. The aorta and its parts
        1. Largest artery
        2. Divisions
            a. Ascending aorta
                (1) Left and right coronary arteries
            b. Aortic arch
                (1) Brachiocephalic artery—branches to arm and head on right
                (2) Left common carotid artery—supplies left side of neck and the head
                (3) Left subclavian artery—supplies left arm
            c. Descending aorta
                (1) Thoracic aorta—branches to chest wall, esophagus, bronchi
                (2) Abdominal aorta—supplies abdominal viscera
    B. Iliac arteries and their subdivisions
        1. Final divisions of aorta
        2. Branch to pelvis and legs
    C. Arteries that branch to the arm and head—common carotid, subclavian, brachial
    D. Anastomoses—communications between vessels

III. SYSTEMIC VEINS
    A. Location
        1. Superficial—near surface
        2. Deep—usually parallel to arteries with same names as corresponding arteries
    B. The venae cavae and their tributaries
        1. Superior vena cava—drains upper body
            a. Jugular veins drain head and neck
            b. Brachiocephalic veins empty into superior vena cava
        2. Inferior vena cava—drains lower body
    C. Venous sinuses—enlarged venous channels
    D. Hepatic portal system—carries blood from abdominal organs to liver, where it is processed before returning to heart

IV. CIRCULATION PHYSIOLOGY
    A. Capillary exchange
        1. Primary method—diffusion
        2. Medium—tissue fluid
        3. Blood pressure—drives fluid into tissues
        4. Osmotic pressure—pulls fluid into capillary
    B. Dynamics of blood flow
        1. Vasomotor activities
            a. Vasodilation—increase in diameter of blood vessel
            b. Vasoconstriction—decrease in diameter of blood vessel
            c. Vasomotor center—in medulla; controls contraction and relaxation of smooth muscle in vessel wall
        2. Precapillary sphincter—regulates blood flow into capillary
        3. Return of blood to heart
            a. Pumping action of heart
            b. Pressure of skeletal muscles on veins
            c. Valves in veins
            d. Breathing—changes in pressure move blood toward heart
    C. The pulse
        1. Wave of pressure that travels along arteries as ventricles contract
        2. Rate affected by size, age, gender, activity, and other factors
    D. Blood pressure
        1. Force exerted by blood against vessel walls

2. Factors
   a. Cardiac output—stroke volume x heart rate
   b. Resistance to blood flow—vessel diameter, vessel elasticity, blood viscosity, blood volume
      (1) Baroreceptors in large arteries respond to changes in pressure
      (2) Activate vasomotor center in medulla
3. Measured in arm with sphygmomanometer
   a. Systolic pressure
      (1) Occurs during heart contraction
      (2) Averages 120 mm Hg
   b. Diastolic pressure
      (1) Occurs during heart relaxation
      (2) Averages 80 mm Hg
4. Abnormal blood pressure
   a. Hypotension—low blood pressure
   b. Hypertension—high blood pressure
      (1) Essential hypertension—has no apparent medical cause
      (2) May involve renin, enzyme released from kidneys
      (3) May lead to aneurysm, stroke, stress on heart and kidneys, atherosclerosis
5. Treatment of hypertension—diuretics, reduction of renin, relaxation of blood vessels

V. **ARTERIAL DEGENERATION AND OTHER VASCULAR DISORDERS**
A. Arteriosclerosis—hardening of arteries with scar tissue, calcium salts, or fatty deposits
   1. Atherosclerosis—deposits of fatty material (plaque) in vessels
   2. Possible results—pain, breathing problems, angina pectoris, thrombosis (blood clot), tissue necrosis, gangrene
B. Aneurysm—weakness and bulging of a vessel; may burst
C. Hemorrhage
   1. Profuse loss of blood
   2. First aid measures: direct pressure, elevation of limb, pressure on artery
D. Shock—inadequate blood flow to tissues
E. Thrombosis—formation of blood clot in a vessel
   1. Embolus—piece of a clot traveling in circulation
      a. Pulmonary embolism—clot lodged in lung
   2. Phlebitis—inflammation of a vein; may lead to thrombophlebitis
      a. Varicose veins—swelling and loss of function in superficial veins, usually in legs and rectum (hemorrhoids)

Questions for Study and Review

BUILDING UNDERSTANDING

Fill in the blanks

1. Capillaries receive blood from vessels called _____.
2. The specific part of the brain that regulates blood pressure is the _____.
3. The flow of blood into an individual capillary is regulated by a(n) _____.
4. Lower-than-normal blood pressure is called _____.
5. Inflammation of a vein is called_____.

Matching > Match each numbered item with the most closely related lettered item.

___ **6.** Lack of blood supply to a tissue or organ

___ **7.** Bulging sac in the wall of a vessel

___ **8.** Loss of blood

___ **9.** An immobile blood clot within a vessel

___ **10.** A mobile blood clot within a vessel

a. embolus

b. thrombus

c. ischemia

d. aneurysm

e. hemorrhage

Multiple choice

___ **11.** The innermost layer of a blood vessel is composed of

    a. smooth muscle

    b. epithelium

    c. connective tissue

    d. nervous tissue

___ **12.** The largest artery in the body is the

    a. aorta

    b. brachiocephalic trunk

    c. splenic artery

    d. superior mesenteric artery

___ **13.** The main process by which substances move between the cells and the capillary blood is

    a. endocytosis

    b. exocytosis

    c. osmosis

    d. diffusion

___ **14.** The stomach, spleen, and liver receive blood via the

    a. hepatic portal system

    b. superior mesenteric artery

    c. inferior mesenteric artery

    d. celiac trunk

___ **15.** The medical term describing the deposition of material within arterial walls is

    a. shock

    b. gangrene

    c. arteriosclerosis

    d. stasis

UNDERSTANDING CONCEPTS

16. Differentiate between the terms in each of the following pairs:

    a. artery and vein

    b. arteriole and venule

    c. anastomosis and venous sinus

    d. vasoconstriction and vasodilation

    e. systolic and diastolic pressure

17. How does the structure of the blood vessels correlate with their function?

18. Trace a drop of blood from the left ventricle to the:

    a. right side of the head and neck

    b. lateral surface of the left hand

    c. right foot

    d. liver

    e. small intestine

19. Trace a drop of blood from capillaries in the wall of the small intestine to the right atrium. What is the purpose of going through the liver on this trip?

20. What physiological factors influence blood pressure?

21. Describe three mechanisms that promote the return of blood to the heart in the venous system.

22. What are some symptoms of arteriosclerosis and how are these produced?

23. What is shock and why is it so dangerous? Name some symptoms of shock and identify the types of shock based on (a) cause and (b) severity.

CONCEPTUAL THINKING

24. Kidney disease usually results in the loss of protein from the blood into the urine. One common sign of kidney disease is edema. Based on this information and your understanding of capillary exchange, explain why edema is often associated with kidney disease.

25. Cliff C., a 49-year-old self-described "couch potato," has a blood pressure of 162/100 mm Hg. What is Cliff's diagnosis? What can this disorder lead to? If you were Cliff's doctor, what treatments might you discuss with him?

26. In Reggie's case, an embolus traveled from his femoral vein to his pulmonary artery. Describe the pathway the embolus would take if it traveled from his femoral vein to the middle cerebral artery supplying blood to his left frontal lobe. What deficits would you suspect to see from this brain stroke? (*Hint*: consult Chapter 10!)

15

The Lymphatic System and Lymphoid Tissue

Selected Key Terms

The following terms and other boldface terms in the chapter are defined in the Glossary

adenoids
chyle
lacteal
lymph
lymphadenitis
lymphadenopathy
lymphangitis
lymphatic duct
lymph node
spleen
thymus
tonsil

Learning Outcomes

After careful study of this chapter, you should be able to:

1. List the functions of the lymphatic system
2. Explain how lymphatic capillaries differ from blood capillaries
3. Name the two main lymphatic ducts and describe the area drained by each
4. List the major structures of the lymphatic system and give the locations and functions of each
5. Describe the composition and function of the reticuloendothelial system
6. Describe the major lymphatic system disorders
7. Show how word parts are used to build words related to the lymphatic system (see Word Anatomy at the end of the chapter)

PASSport to Success

Visit *thePoint* or see the Student Resource CD in the back of this book for definitions and pronunciations of key terms as well as a pretest for this chapter.

Disease
in Context

> ## Mike's Second Case: Emergency Splenectomy

Alek, a 4th-year medical student, slumped into a chair in the lounge and closed his eyes. It was only a few hours into his shift, but he was already exhausted. Then, Alek's pager buzzed—*get to the operating room immediately!* Minutes later, he donned a sterile gown and gloves and entered the operating room, which buzzed with activity as the surgical team prepped the patient for emergency abdominal surgery. Alek listened carefully to the surgeon as she explained the case to the team. "Patient's name is Mike. He's 21 years old and was in a car accident about an hour ago. Paramedics noted significant bruising of the left upper quadrant, tachycardia, and hypotension." The surgeon glanced at the medical student and asked, "Alek, what does that suggest to you?"

Alek thought quickly and answered, "The location of the injury and cardiovascular problems suggest a ruptured spleen."

"That's exactly what the emergency team thought," replied the surgeon. "OK folks, let's open Mike up and see if Alek's right." Using a scalpel, the surgeon made a midsagittal incision through Mike's abdominal wall. Then, she made a transverse incision to open the left side of his abdominal cavity and suctioned out the blood that filled it. She located the purple-colored spleen in the left hypochondriac region and noted a large tear in the connective tissue capsule surrounding it. "You're right, Alek. We've got a ruptured spleen here, which we'll have to remove." The surgeon searched for the splenic artery supplying blood to the damaged organ and when she found it, tied it shut, and cut it. Then, she cut the ligaments that suspended the spleen between the stomach and transverse colon. Finally, she tied and cut the splenic vein and removed Mike's spleen. "OK," said the surgeon, "Let's close him up and get him to intensive care. Alek, good job today."

Mike's spleen, a lymphoid organ, was injured during a car accident and had to be removed. In this chapter, you will learn about the spleen and other organs that make up the lymphatic system. Later, we'll check in on Mike and learn about splenectomy's long-term consequences.

The Lymphatic System

The lymphatic system is a widespread system of tissues and vessels. Its organs are not in continuous order, but are scattered throughout the body, and it services almost all regions. Only bone tissue, cartilage, epithelium, and the central nervous system are not in direct communication with this system.

Functions of the Lymphatic System

The lymphatic system's functions are just as varied as its locations. These functions fall into three categories:

■ **Fluid balance.** As blood circulates through the capillaries in the tissues, water and dissolved substances are constantly exchanged between the bloodstream and the interstitial (in-ter-STISH-al) fluids that bathe the cells. Ideally, the volume of fluid that leaves the blood should be matched by the amount that returns to the blood. However, there is always a slight excess of fluid left behind in the tissues. In addition, some proteins escape from the blood capillaries and are left behind. This fluid and protein would accumulate in the tissues if not for a second drainage pathway through lymphatic vessels (Fig. 16-1).

In addition to the blood-carrying capillaries, the tissues also contain microscopic lymphatic capillaries. These small vessels pick up excess fluid and protein left behind in the tissues (Fig. 16-2). The capillaries then drain into larger vessels, which eventually return these materials to the venous system near the heart.

The fluid that circulates in the lymphatic system is called **lymph** (limf), a clear fluid similar in composi-

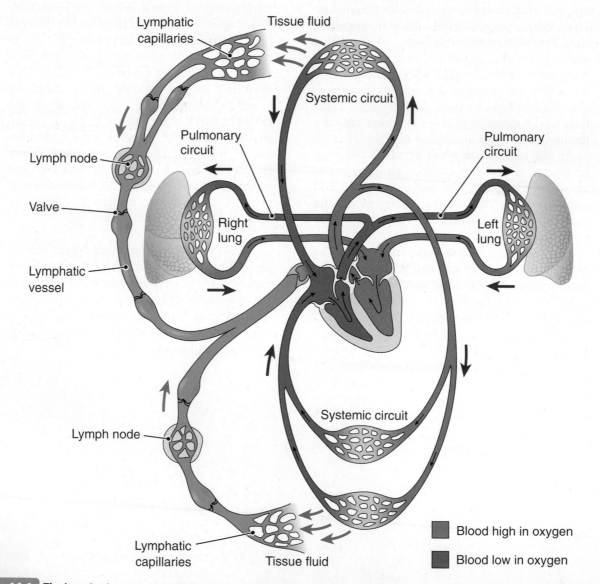

Lymphatic capillaries
Tissue fluid
Systemic circuit
Lymph node
Pulmonary circuit
Pulmonary circuit
Valve
Right lung
Left lung
Lymphatic vessel
Systemic circuit
Lymph node
Lymphatic capillaries
Tissue fluid

Blood high in oxygen
Blood low in oxygen

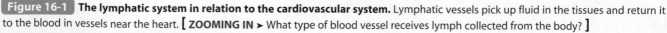

Figure 16-1 **The lymphatic system in relation to the cardiovascular system.** Lymphatic vessels pick up fluid in the tissues and return it to the blood in vessels near the heart. [**ZOOMING IN ➤** What type of blood vessel receives lymph collected from the body?]

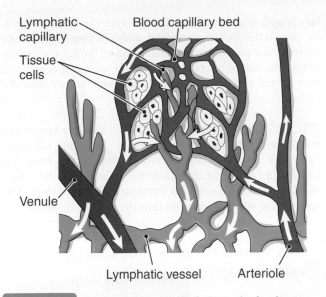

Figure 16-2 **Pathway of lymphatic drainage in the tissues.** Lymphatic capillaries are more permeable than blood capillaries and can pick up fluid and proteins left in the tissues as blood leaves the capillary bed to travel back toward the heart.

tion to interstitial fluid. Although lymph is formed from the components of blood plasma, it differs from the plasma in that it has much less protein.

■ **Protection from infection.** The lymphatic system is an important component of the immune system, which fights infection. One group of white blood cells, the lymphocytes, can live and multiply in the lymphatic system, where they attack and destroy foreign organisms. Lymphoid tissue scattered throughout the body filters out pathogens, other foreign matter, and cellular debris in body fluids. More will be said about the lymphocytes and immunity in Chapter 17.

■ **Absorption of fats.** Following the chemical and mechanical breakdown of food in the digestive tract, most nutrients are absorbed into the blood through intestinal capillaries. Many digested fats, however, are too large to enter the blood capillaries and are instead absorbed into lymphatic capillaries. These fats are added to the blood when lymph joins the bloodstream. The topic of digestion is covered in Chapter 19.

CHECKPOINT 16-1 ➤ What are three functions of the lymphatic system?

Lymphatic Circulation

Lymph travels through a network of small and large channels that are in some ways similar to the blood vessels. However, the system is not a complete circuit. It is a one-way system that begins in the tissues and ends when the lymph joins the blood (see Fig. 16-1).

Lymphatic Capillaries

The walls of the lymphatic capillaries resemble those of the blood capillaries in that they are made of one layer of flattened (squamous) epithelial cells. This thin layer, also called *endothelium*, allows for easy passage of soluble materials and water (Fig. 16-3). The gaps between the endothelial cells in the lymphatic capillaries are larger than those of the blood capillaries. The lymphatic capillaries are thus more permeable, allowing for easier entrance of relatively large protein molecules. The proteins do not move back out of the vessels because the endothelial cells overlap slightly, forming one-way valves to block their return.

Unlike the blood capillaries, the lymphatic capillaries arise blindly; that is, they are closed at one end and do not form a bridge between two larger vessels. Instead, one end simply lies within a lake of tissue fluid, and the other communicates with a larger lymphatic vessel that transports the lymph toward the heart (see Figs. 16-1 and 16-2).

Some specialized lymphatic capillaries located in the small intestine's lining absorb digested fats. Fats taken into these **lacteals** (LAK-te-als) are transported in the lymphatic vessels until the lymph is added to the blood. More information on the lymphatic system's role in digestion is found in Chapter 19.

CHECKPOINT 16-2 ➤ What are two differences between blood capillaries and lymphatic capillaries?

Lymphatic Vessels

The lymphatic vessels are thin-walled and delicate and have a beaded appearance because of indentations where valves are located (see Fig. 16-1). These valves prevent back flow in the same way as do those found in some veins.

Figure 16-3 **Structure of a lymphatic capillary.** Fluid and proteins can enter the capillary with ease through gaps between the endothelial cells. Overlapping cells act as valves to prevent the material from leaving.

16

Lymphatic vessels (Fig. 16-4) include **superficial** and **deep** sets. The surface lymphatics are immediately below the skin, often lying near the superficial veins. The deep vessels are usually larger and accompany the deep veins.

Lymphatic vessels are named according to location. For example, those in the breast are called **mammary** lymphatic vessels, those in the thigh are called **femoral** lymphatic vessels, and those in the leg are called **tibial** lymphatic vessels. At certain points, the vessels drain through lymph nodes, small masses of lymphatic tissue that filter the lymph. The nodes are in groups that serve a particular region. For example, nearly all the lymph from the upper extremity and the breast passes through the **axil-**

lary lymph nodes, whereas lymph from the lower extremity passes through the **inguinal nodes.** Lymphatic vessels carrying lymph away from the regional nodes eventually drain into one of two terminal vessels, the right lymphatic duct or the thoracic duct, both of which empty into the bloodstream.

THE RIGHT LYMPHATIC DUCT The **right lymphatic duct** is a short vessel, approximately 1.25 cm (1/2 inch) long, that receives only the lymph that comes from the body's superior right quadrant: the right side of the head, neck, and thorax, as well as the right upper extremity. The right lymphatic duct empties into the right subclavian vein

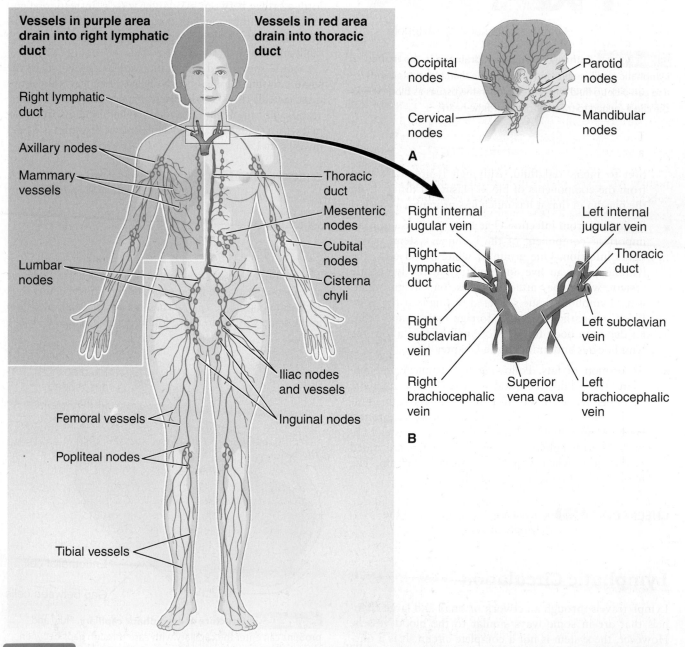

Figure 16-4 **Vessels and nodes of the lymphatic system. (A)** Lymph nodes and vessels of the head. **(B)** Drainage of right lymphatic duct and thoracic duct into subclavian veins.

near the heart (see Fig. 16-4B). Its opening into this vein is guarded by two pocket-like semilunar valves to prevent blood from entering the duct. The rest of the body is drained by the thoracic duct.

THE THORACIC DUCT The **thoracic duct**, or left lymphatic duct, is the larger of the two terminal vessels, measuring approximately 40 cm (16 inches) in length. As shown in Figure 16-4, the thoracic duct receives lymph from all parts of the body except those superior to the diaphragm on the right side. This duct begins in the posterior part of the abdominal cavity, inferior to the attachment of the diaphragm. The duct's first part is enlarged to form a cistern, or temporary storage pouch, called the **cisterna chyli** (sis-TER-nah KI-li). **Chyle** (kile) is the milky fluid that drains from the intestinal lacteals; it is formed by the combination of fat globules and lymph. Chyle passes through the intestinal lymphatic vessels and the lymph nodes of the mesentery (membrane around the intestines), finally entering the cisterna chyli. In addition to chyle, all the lymph from below the diaphragm empties into the cisterna chyli, passing through the various clusters of lymph nodes. The thoracic duct then carries this lymph into the bloodstream.

The thoracic duct extends upward through the diaphragm and along the posterior thoracic wall into the base of the neck on the left side. Here, it receives the left jugular lymphatic vessels from the head and neck, the left subclavian vessels from the left upper extremity, and other lymphatic vessels from the thorax and its parts. In addition to the valves along the duct, there are two valves at its opening into the left subclavian vein to prevent the passage of blood into the duct.

CHECKPOINT 16-3 ➤ What are the two main lymphatic vessels?

Movement of Lymph

The segments of lymphatic vessels located between the valves contract rhythmically, propelling the lymph forward. The contraction rate is related to the fluid volume in the vessel—the more fluid, the more rapid the contractions.

Lymph is also moved by the same mechanisms that promote venous return of blood to the heart. As skeletal muscles contract during movement, they compress the lymphatic vessels and drive lymph forward. Changes in pressures within the abdominal and thoracic cavities caused by breathing aid lymphatic movement during passage through these body cavities. Box 16-1, Lymphedema, describes what happens when lymph does not flow properly.

PASSport to Success

Massage therapy can improve lymphatic drainage and blood circulation as well as benefit muscles. Visit *thePoint* or see the Student Resource CD in the back of this book for more information about this field.

Lymphoid Tissue

Lymphoid (LIM-foyd) **tissue** is distributed throughout the body and makes up the lymphatic system's specialized organs. The lymph nodes have already been described rela-

---

Box 16-1   Clinical Perspectives

16

Lymphedema: When Lymph Stops Flowing

The body's fluid balance requires appropriate fluid distribution among the cardiovascular system, lymphatic system, and the tissues. **Edema** occurs when the balance is tipped toward excess fluid in the tissues. Often, edema is due to heart failure. However, blockage of lymphatic vessels (and the resulting fluid accumulation in the subcutaneous tissues) can cause another form of edema called **lymphedema**. The clinical hallmark of lymphedema is chronic swelling of an arm or leg, whereas heart failure usually causes swelling of both legs.

Lymphedema may be either primary or secondary. Primary lymphedema is a rare congenital condition caused by abnormal development of lymphatic vessels. Secondary lymphedema, or acquired lymphedema, can develop as a result of trauma to a limb, surgery, radiation therapy, or infection of the lymphatic vessels (lymphangitis). One of lymphedema's most common causes is the removal of axillary lymph nodes during mastectomy (breast removal), which disrupts lymph flow from the adjacent arm. Lymphedema may also occur following prostate surgery.

Therapies that encourage flow through the lymphatic vessels are useful in treating lymphedema. These therapies may include elevation of the affected limb, manual lymphatic drainage through massage, light exercise, and firm wrapping of the limb to apply compression. In addition, changes in daily habits can lessen lymphedema's effects. For example, further blockage of lymph drainage can be prevented by wearing loose-fitting clothing and jewelry, carrying a purse or handbag on the unaffected arm, and sitting with legs uncrossed. Lymphangitis requires the use of appropriate antibiotics. Prompt treatment is necessary because, in addition to swelling, other complications include poor wound healing, skin ulcers, and increased risk of infection.

tive to describing lymphatic circulation, but these tissues and other lymphatic system components are discussed in greater detail in the next section.

Lymph Nodes

The lymph nodes, as noted, are designed to filter the lymph once it is drained from the tissues (Fig. 16-5). They are also sites where lymphocytes of the immune system multiply and work to combat foreign organisms. The lymph nodes are small, rounded masses varying from pinhead size to as long as 2.5 cm (1 inch). Each has a fibrous connective tissue capsule from which partitions (trabeculae) extend into the node's substance. At various points in the node's surface, afferent lymphatic vessels pierce the capsule to carry lymph into the node. An indented area called the **hilum** (HI-lum) is the exit point for efferent lymphatic vessels carrying lymph out of the node. At this region, other structures, including blood vessels and nerves, connect with the node.

Each node is subdivided into lymph-filled spaces (sinuses) and cords of lymphatic tissue. Pulplike nodules in the outer region, or cortex, have germinal centers where certain immune lymphocytes multiply. The inner region, the medulla, has populations of immune cells, including lymphocytes and macrophages (phagocytes), along open channels that lead into the efferent vessels.

Lymph nodes are seldom isolated. As a rule, they are massed together in groups, varying in number from 2 or 3 to well over 100. Some of these groups are placed deeply, whereas others are superficial. The main groups include the following:

- **Cervical nodes**, located in the neck in deep and superficial groups, drain various parts of the head and neck. They often become enlarged during upper respiratory infections.

- **Axillary nodes**, located in the axillae (armpits), may become en-

larged after infections of the upper extremities and the breasts. Cancer cells from the breasts often metastasize (spread) to the axillary nodes.

- **Tracheobronchial** (tra-ke-o-BRONG-ke-al) **nodes** are found near the trachea and around the larger bronchial tubes. In people living in highly polluted areas, these nodes become filled with air contaminants.

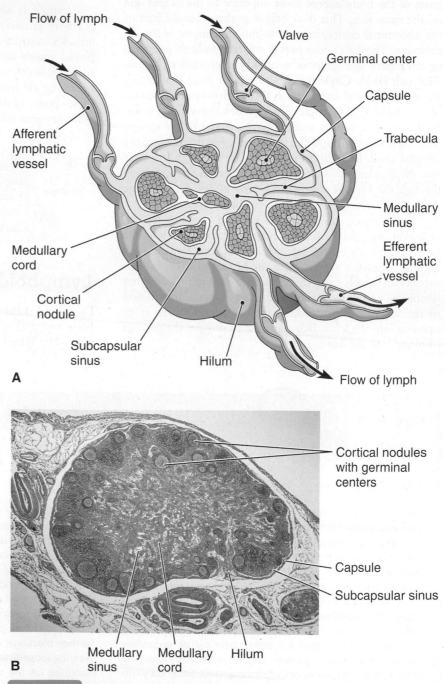

Figure 16-5 **Structure of a lymph node. (A)** Arrows indicate the flow of lymph through the node. **(B)** Section of a lymph node as seen under the microscope (low power). (B, Reprinted with permission from Cormack DH. *Essential Histology*, 2nd ed. Philadelphia: Lippincott Williams & Wilkins, 2001.) **[ZOOMING IN ➤** What type of lymphatic vessel carries lymph into a node? What type of lymphatic vessel carries lymph out of a node? **]**

- **Mesenteric** (mes-en-TER-ik) **nodes** are found between the two layers of peritoneum that form the mesentery. There are some 100 to 150 of these nodes.
- **Inguinal nodes**, located in the groin region, receive lymph drainage from the lower extremities and from the external genital organs. When they become enlarged, they are often referred to as **buboes** (BU-bose), from which bubonic plague got its name.

Box 16-2 explains the role of lymph node biopsy in the treatment of cancer.

CHECKPOINT 16-4 ➤ What is the function of the lymph nodes?

The Spleen

The spleen is an organ that contains lymphoid tissue designed to filter blood. It is located in the superior left hypochondriac region of the abdomen, high up under the dome of the diaphragm, and normally is protected by the lower part of the rib cage (Fig. 16-6). The spleen is a soft, purplish, and somewhat flattened organ, measuring approximately 12.5 to 16 cm (5 to 6 inches) long and 5 to 7.5 cm (2 to 3 inches) wide. The spleen's capsule, as well as its framework, is more elastic than that of the lymph nodes. It contains involuntary muscle, which enables the splenic capsule to contract and also to withstand some swelling.

Considering its size, the spleen has an unusually large blood supply. The organ is filled with a soft pulp that filters the blood. It also harbors phagocytes and lympho-

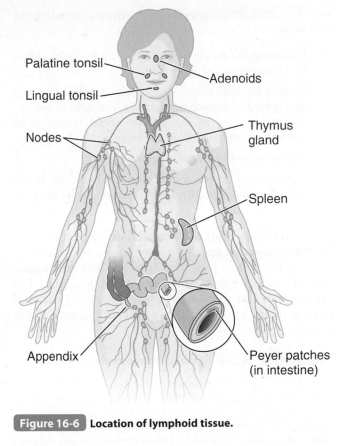

Figure 16-6 **Location of lymphoid tissue.**

Palatine tonsil
Adenoids
Lingual tonsil
Nodes
Thymus gland
Spleen
Appendix
Peyer patches (in intestine)

cytes, which are active in immunity. The spleen is classified as part of the lymphatic system because it contains prominent masses of lymphoid tissue. However, it has wider

Box 16-2 **Hot Topics**

Sentinel Node Biopsy: Finding Cancer Before It Spreads

Ordinarily, the lymphatic system is one of the body's primary defenses against disease. In cancer, though, it can be a vehicle for the spread (metastasis) of disease. When cancer cells enter the lymphatic vessels, they travel to other parts of the body, where they may establish new tumors. Along the way, some cancer cells become lodged in the lymph nodes.

In breast cancer, the degree of invasion of nearby lymph nodes helps determine what treatments are required after surgical removal of the tumor. Until recently, a mastectomy often included the removal of nearby lymphatic vessels and nodes (a procedure called axillary lymph node dissection). Biopsy of the nodes determined whether or not they contained cancerous cells. If they did, radiation treatment or chemotherapy was required. In many women with early-stage breast cancer, however, the axillary bodies do not contain cancerous cells. In addition, about 20% of the women

whose lymphatic vessels and nodes have been removed suffer impaired lymph flow, resulting in lymphedema, pain, disability, and an increased risk of infection.

Sentinel node biopsy is a diagnostic procedure that may minimize the need to perform axillary lymph node dissection, while still detecting metastasis. Surgeons use radioactive tracers to identify the first nodes that receive lymph from the area of a tumor. Biopsy of only these "sentinel nodes" reveals whether tumor cells are present, providing the earliest indication of metastasis. Research shows that sentinel lymph node biopsy is associated with less pain, fewer complications, and faster recovery than axillary lymph node dissection. However, clinical trials are ongoing to determine whether sentinel node biopsy is as successful as axillary dissection in finding cancer before it spreads.

functions than other lymphatic structures, including the following:

■ Cleansing the blood of impurities and cellular debris by filtration and phagocytosis.

■ Destroying old, worn-out red blood cells. The iron and other breakdown products of hemoglobin are carried to the liver by the hepatic portal system to be reused or eliminated from the body.

■ Producing red blood cells before birth.

■ Serving as a reservoir for blood, which can be returned to the bloodstream in case of hemorrhage or other emergency.

Splenectomy (sple-NEK-to-me), or surgical removal of the spleen, is usually a well-tolerated procedure. Although the spleen is the body's largest lymphoid organ, other lymphoid tissues can take over its functions. The human body has thousands of lymphoid structures, and the loss of any one or any group ordinarily is not a threat to life.

CHECKPOINT 16-5 ➤ What is filtered by the spleen?

The Thymus

Because of its appearance under a microscope, the **thymus** (THI-mus), located in the superior thorax deep to the sternum, traditionally has been considered part of the lymphoid system (see Fig. 16-6). Recent studies, however, suggest that this structure has a much wider function than other lymphoid tissue. It appears that the thymus plays a key role in immune system development before birth and during the first few months of infancy. Certain lymphocytes must mature in the thymus gland before they can perform their functions in the immune system (see Chapter 17). These T cells (T lymphocytes) develop under the effects of the thymus gland hormone called **thymosin** (THI-mo-sin), which also promotes lymphocyte growth and lymphoid tissue activity throughout the body. Removal of the thymus causes a generalized decrease in the production of T cells, as well as a decrease in the size of the spleen and of lymph nodes throughout the body.

The thymus is most active during early life. After puberty, the tissue undergoes changes; it shrinks in size and is replaced by connective tissue and fat.

CHECKPOINT 16-6 ➤ What kind of immune system cells develop in the thymus?

The Tonsils

The **tonsils** are unencapsulated masses of lymphoid tissue located in the vicinity of the pharynx (throat) where they remove contaminants from materials that are inhaled or swallowed (Fig. 16-7). The tonsils have deep grooves lined with lymphatic nodules. Lymphocytes attack pathogens

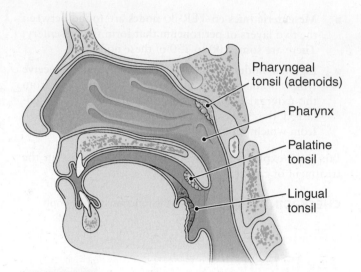

Figure 16-7   Location of the tonsils. All are in the vicinity of the pharynx (throat).

trapped in these grooves. The tonsils are located in three areas:

■ The **palatine** (PAL-ah-tine) **tonsils** are oval bodies located at each side of the soft palate. These are generally what is meant when one refers to "the tonsils."

■ The single **pharyngeal** (fah-RIN-je-al) **tonsil** is commonly referred to as the **adenoids** (from a general term that means "gland-like"). It is located behind the nose on the posterior wall of the upper pharynx.

■ The **lingual** (LING-gwal) **tonsils** are little mounds of lymphoid tissue at the posterior of the tongue.

Any of these tonsils may become so loaded with bacteria that they become reservoirs for repeated infections and their removal is advisable. In children, a slight enlargement of any of them is not an indication for surgery, however, because all lymphoid tissue masses tend to be larger in childhood. A physician must determine whether these masses are abnormally enlarged, taking the patient's age into account, because the tonsils function in immunity during early childhood. Surgery is considered if there is recurrent infection or if the enlarged tonsils make swallowing or breathing difficult. Their removal may also help children suffering from otitis media, because bacteria infecting the tonsils may travel to the middle ear. The surgery to remove the palatine tonsils is a tonsillectomy; an adenoidectomy is removal of the adenoids. Often these two procedures are done together and abbreviated as T & A. Most tonsillectomies are performed by electrocautery, which uses an electric current to burn the tissue away. A newer technique, which allows faster recovery and fewer complications, uses radiowaves to break down the tonsillar tissue.

CHECKPOINT 16-7 ➤ Tonsils filter tissue fluid. What is the general location of the tonsils?

Other Lymphoid Tissue

The **appendix** (ah-PEN-diks) is a fingerlike tube of lymphatic tissue, measuring approximately 8 cm (3 inches) long. It is attached, or "appended" to the first portion of the large intestine (see Fig. 16-6). Like the tonsils, it seems to be noticed only when it becomes infected, causing appendicitis. The appendix may, however, figure in the development of immunity, as do the tonsils.

In the mucous membranes lining portions of the digestive, respiratory, and urogenital tracts, there are areas of lymphatic tissue that help destroy outside contaminants. By means of phagocytosis and production of antibodies, substances that counteract infectious agents, this **mucosal-associated lymphoid tissue**, or MALT, prevents microorganisms from invading deeper tissues.

Peyer (PI-er) **patches** are part of the MALT system. These clusters of lymphoid nodules are located in the mucous membranes lining the distal small intestine. Peyer patches, along with the tonsils and appendix, are included in the specific network known as GALT, or **gut-associated lymphoid tissue**. All of these lymphatic tissues associated with mucous membranes are now recognized as an important first barrier against invading microorganisms.

The Reticuloendothelial System

The **reticuloendothelial** (reh-tik-u-lo-en-do-THE-le-al) **system** consists of related cells responsible for the destruction of worn-out blood cells, bacteria, cancer cells, and other foreign substances that are potentially harmful. Included among these cells are monocytes, relatively large white blood cells (see Fig. 13-4E in Chapter 13) that are formed in the bone marrow and then circulate in the bloodstream to various areas. Upon entering the tissues, monocytes develop into **macrophages** (MAK-ro-faj-ez), a term that means "big eaters."

Macrophages in some organs are given special names; **Kupffer** (KOOP-fer) cells, for example, are located in the lining of the liver sinusoids (blood channels). Other parts of the reticuloendothelial system are found in the spleen, bone marrow, lymph nodes, and brain. Some macro-phages are located in the lungs, where they are called *dust cells* because they ingest solid particles that enter the lungs; others are found in soft connective tissues all over the body.

This widely distributed protective system has been called by several other names, including tissue macrophage system, mononuclear phagocyte system, and monocyte-macrophage system. These names describe the type of cells found within this system.

Disorders of the Lymphatic System and Lymphoid Tissue

Lymphangitis (lim-fan-JI-tis), which is inflammation of lymphatic vessels, usually begins in the region of an infected and neglected injury and can be seen as red streaks extending along an extremity. Such inflamed vessels are a sign that bacteria have spread into the lymphatic system. If the lymph nodes are not able to stop the infection, pathogens may enter the bloodstream, causing **septicemia** (sep-tih-SE-me-ah), or blood poisoning. Streptococci often are the invading organisms in such cases.

In **lymphadenitis** (lim-fad-en-I-tis), or inflammation of the lymph nodes, the nodes become enlarged and tender. This condition reflects the body's attempt to combat an infection. Cervical lymphadenitis occurs during measles, scarlet fever, septic sore throat, diphtheria, and, frequently, the common cold. Chronic lymphadenitis may be caused by the bacillus that causes tuberculosis. Infections of the upper extremities cause enlarged axillary nodes, as does breast cancer. Infections of the external genitals or the lower extremities may cause enlargement of the inguinal lymph nodes.

Lymphedema

Edema is tissue swelling due to excess fluid. The condition has a variety of causes, but edema due to obstruction of lymph flow is called **lymphedema** (lim-feh-DE-mah). Possible causes of lymphedema include infection of the lymphatic vessels, a malignant growth that obstructs lymph flow, or loss of lymphatic vessels and nodes as a result of injury or surgery. Areas affected by lymphedema are more prone to infection because the lymphatic system's filtering activity is diminished. Mechanical methods to improve drainage and drugs to promote water loss are possible treatments for lymphedema (see Box 16-1, Lymphedema).

As mentioned in Chapter 5, **elephantiasis** is a great enlargement of the lower extremities resulting from lymphatic vessel blockage by small worms called **filariae** (fi-LA-re-e). These tiny parasites, carried by insects such as flies and mosquitoes, invade the tissues as embryos or immature forms. They then grow in the lymph channels and obstruct lymphatic flow. The swelling of the legs or, as sometimes happens in men, the scrotum, may be so great that the victim becomes incapacitated. This disease is especially common in certain parts of Asia and in some of the Pacific islands. No cure is known.

Lymphadenopathy

Lymphadenopathy (lim-fad-en-OP-ah-the) is a term meaning "disease of the lymph nodes." Enlarged lymph nodes are a common symptom in a number of infectious and cancerous diseases. For example, generalized lymphadenopathy is an early sign of infection with HIV (human immunodeficiency virus), the virus that causes AIDS (acquired immunodeficiency syndrome). **Infectious mononucleosis** (mon-o-nu-kle-O-sis) is an acute viral infection, the hallmark of which is a marked enlargement of the cervical lymph nodes. Mononucleosis is fairly common among college students. Enlarged lymph nodes are commonly referred to as glands, as in "swollen glands." However, they do not produce secretions and are not glands.

16

Visit *thePoint* or see the Student Resource CD in the back of this book for a picture of cervical lymphadenopathy.

Figure 16-8 **Reed-Sternberg cell characteristic of Hodgkin disease.** A typical cell has two nuclei with large, dark-staining nucleoli. (Reprinted with permission from Rubin E, Farber JL. *Pathology*, 3rd ed. Philadelphia: Lippincott Williams & Wilkins, 1999.)

Splenomegaly

Enlargement of the spleen, known as **splenomegaly** (spleno-MEG-ah-le), accompanies certain acute infectious diseases, including scarlet fever, typhus fever, typhoid fever, and syphilis. Many tropical parasitic diseases cause splenomegaly. A certain blood fluke (flatworm) that is fairly common among workers in Japan and other parts of Asia causes marked splenic enlargement.

Splenic anemia is characterized by enlargement of the spleen, hemorrhages from the stomach, and fluid accumulation in the abdomen. In this and other similar diseases, splenectomy appears to constitute a cure.

Lymphoma

Lymphoma (lim-FO-mah) is any tumor, benign or malignant, that occurs in lymphoid tissue. Two examples of malignant lymphoma are described next.

Hodgkin disease is a chronic malignant disease of lymphoid tissue, especially the lymph nodes. The incidence of this disease rises in two age groups: in the early 20s among both men and women, and again after age 50, more commonly among men. The cause is unknown, but in some cases may involve a viral infection. Hodgkin disease appears as painless enlargement of a lymph node or close group of nodes, often in the neck, but also in the armpit, thorax, and groin. It may spread throughout the lymphatic system and eventually to other systems if not controlled by treatment. Early signs are weight loss, fever, night sweats, fatigue, anemia, and decline in immune defenses. A clear sign of the disease is the presence of Reed-Sternberg cells in lymph node biopsy tissue (Fig. 16-8). Chemotherapy and radiotherapy, either separately or in combination, have been used with good results, affording patients many years of life.

Non-Hodgkin lymphoma is more common than Hodgkin disease. It appears mostly in older adults and patients with deficient immune systems, such as those with AIDS. Enlargement of the lymph nodes (lymphadenopathy), especially in the cervical region, is an early sign in many cases. It is more widespread through the lymphatic system than Hodgkin disease and spreads more readily to other tissues, such as the liver. Like Hodgkin disease, it may be related to a viral infection. It shares many of the same symptoms as are seen in Hodgkin disease, but there are no Reed-Sternberg cells on biopsy. The current cure rate with chemotherapy and radiation is approximately 50%.

CHECKPOINT 16-8 ➤ What is lymphadenopathy?

CHECKPOINT 16-9 ➤ What is lymphoma and what are two examples of malignant lymphoma?

Disease in Context revisited

▶ Mike's Splenectomy

Mike lay in his hospital bed thinking about the past couple of days. After the surgery, his doctor had explained that removal of his spleen had been necessary because it had ruptured during the car accident. He was still coming to terms with what that meant. In fact, until today, he wasn't even sure what the spleen was!

Earlier in the morning, Mike's physician came by to check in on him. During their conversation, Mike learned that the spleen is a bean-shaped purple organ about the size of a large bar of soap. It is normally located underneath the diaphragm in the upper left part of the abdomen. Given how little he knew about it, Mike was surprised to learn that one of the spleen's functions is to filter foreign substances from the blood and remove worn-out red blood cells. "You mean it's like an oil filter on a car?" asked Mike. "Sort of,"

replied the doctor. "But don't worry, other parts of your circulatory system will help clean your blood now."

Mike also learned that the spleen acts like a large lymph node, detecting and fighting disease-causing organisms. "So, now that my spleen is gone, am I going to be sick all the time?" asked Mike. "Well," answered the doctor, "As you recover, you'll need to take antibiotics to reduce the risk of infection. In the long term, if you have a fever or any sign of illness, come see me right away. In addition, make sure that you get your yearly flu vaccinations."

During this case, we saw that the spleen filters blood and protects the body from harmful organisms. In Chapter 17, we'll learn more about how certain blood cells and the lymphatic system protect us from disease.

Word Anatomy

Medical terms are built from standardized word parts (prefixes, roots, and suffixes). Learning the meanings of these parts can help you remember words and interpret unfamiliar terms.

16

WORD PART	MEANING	EXAMPLE
Lymphoid Tissue		
–oid	like, resembling	*Lymphoid* tissue makes up the specialized organs of the lymphatic system.
aden/o	gland	The *adenoids* are gland-like tonsils.
lingu/o	tongue	The *lingual* tonsils are at the back of the tongue.
Disorders of the Lymphatic System and Lymphoid Tissue		
-pathy	any disease	*Lymphadenopathy* is any disease of the lymph nodes.
-megaly	excessive enlargement	*Splenomegaly* is excessive enlargement of the spleen.

Summary

I. **LYMPHATIC SYSTEM**
   A. Functions
      1. Fluid balance—drains excess fluid and proteins from the tissues and returns them to the blood
      2. Protection from infection
         a. Lymphocytes fight foreign organisms
         b. Lymphoid tissue filters body fluids
      3. Absorption of fats—lacteals absorb digested fats from small intestine

II. **LYMPHATIC CIRCULATION**
   A. Lymphatic capillaries
      1. Made of endothelium (simple squamous epithelium)
      2. More permeable than blood capillaries
      3. Overlapping cells form one-way valves
   B. Lymphatic vessels
      1. Superficial and deep sets
      2. Right lymphatic duct
         a. Drains upper right part of body
         b. Empties into right subclavian vein
      3. Thoracic duct
         a. Drains remainder of body
         b. Empties into left subclavian vein
   C. Movement of lymph
      1. Valves in vessels
      2. Contraction of vessels
      3. Skeletal muscle contraction
      4. Breathing

III. **LYMPHOID TISSUE**
   A. Lymph nodes
      1. Along path of lymphatic vessels
      2. Filter lymph
   B. Spleen
      1. Filtration of blood
      2. Destruction of old red cells
      3. Production of red cells before birth
      4. Storage of blood
   C. Thymus
      1. Processing of T lymphocytes (T cells)
      2. Secretion of thymosin—stimulates T lymphocytes in lymphoid tissue

   D. Tonsils
      1. Filter swallowed and inhaled material
      2. Located near pharynx (throat)
         a. Palatine—near soft palate
         b. Pharyngeal (adenoids)—behind nose
         c. Lingual—back of tongue
   E. Other
      1. Appendix—attached to large intestine
      2. Mucosal—associated lymphoid tissue (MALT)
         a. Gut-associated lymphoid tissue (GALT)
            (1) Example—Peyer patches in lining of small intestine

IV. **THE RETICULOENDOTHELIAL SYSTEM**
   A. Cells throughout body that remove impurities
   B. Macrophages
      1. From monocytes
      2. Localize and given special names—e.g., Kuppfer cells, dust cells

V. **DISORDERS OF THE LYMPHATIC SYSTEM AND LYMPHOID TISSUE**
   A. Inflammations
      1. Lymphangitis—inflammation of lymphatic vessels
      2. Lymphadenitis—inflammation of lymph nodes that occurs during infection
   B. Lymphedema—swelling due to obstruction of lymph flow
      1. Removal of lymph nodes and vessels by injury, surgery
      2. Infection—e.g., elephantiasis caused by filariae (parasitic worms)
   C. Lymphadenopathy—disease of lymph nodes
   D. Splenomegaly—enlargement of the spleen
   E. Lymphoma—tumor of lymphoid tissue
      1. Hodgkin disease—chronic malignancy with enlarged lymph nodes
      2. Non-Hodgkin lymphoma—more common in older adults

Questions for Study and Review

BUILDING UNDERSTANDING

Fill in the blanks

1. The fluid that circulates in the lymphatic system is called _____.

2. Digested fats enter the lymphatic circulation through vessels called_____.

3. Fat globules and lymph combine to form a milky fluid called _____.

4. Surgical removal of the spleen is termed _____.

5. When filariae block lymphatic vessels they cause the disease called _____.

Matching > Match each numbered item with the most closely related lettered item.

___ 6. Inflammation of lymphatic vessels

___ 7. Inflammation of lymph nodes

___ 8. Fluid retention due to obstruction of lymph vessels

___ 9. Tumor that occurs in lymphoid tissue

a. lymphoma

b. lymphangitis

c. lymphedema

d. lymphadenitis

Multiple choice

___ 10. Compared to plasma, lymph contains much less
  a. fat
  b. protein
  c. carbohydrate
  d. water

___ 11. Lymph from the lower extremities returns to the cardiovascular system via the
  a. cisterna chyli
  b. right lymphatic duct
  c. thymus
  d. thoracic duct

___ 12. Macrophages and monocytes found throughout the body make up the
  a. tonsils
  b. Peyer patches
  c. reticuloendothelial system
  d. appendix

___ 13. The hallmark clinical sign of infectious mononucleosis is:
  a. splenomegaly
  b. lymphadenopathy
  c. lymphangitis
  d. edema

UNDERSTANDING CONCEPTS

14. How does the structure of lymphatic capillaries correlate with their function? List some differences between lymphatic and blood capillaries.

15. Describe three mechanisms that propel lymph through the lymphatic vessels.

16. Trace a globule of fat from a lacteal in the small intestine to the right atrium.

17. Describe the structure of a typical lymph node.

18. State the location of the spleen and list several of its functions.

19. Describe two forms of lymphoma.

CONCEPTUAL THINKING

20. Explain the absence of arteries in the lymphatic circulatory system.

21. In Mike's second case, he presented with hypotension and tachycardia due to a ruptured spleen. Explain how a ruptured spleen can cause these disorders.

22. In the case story, why was Mike treated with antibiotics and vaccinated for influenza following his splenectomy?

16

CHAPTER 17

Body Defenses, Immunity, and Vaccines

Learning Outcomes

After careful study of this chapter, you should be able to:

1. List the factors that determine the occurrence of infection
2. Differentiate between nonspecific and specific body defenses and give examples of each
3. Briefly describe the inflammatory reaction
4. List several types of innate immunity
5. Define *antigen* and *antibody*
6. Compare T cells and B cells with respect to development and type of activity
7. Explain the role of macrophages in immunity
8. Describe some protective effects of an antigen–antibody reaction
9. Differentiate between natural and artificial adaptive immunity
10. Differentiate between active and passive immunity
11. Define the term *vaccine* and give several examples of vaccines
12. Define the term *immune serum* and give several examples of immune sera
13. List several disorders of the immune system
14. Explain the possible role of the immune system in preventing cancer
15. Explain the role of the immune system in tissue transplantation
16. Show how word parts are used to build words related to body defenses, immunity, and vaccines (see Word Anatomy at the end of the chapter)

Selected Key Terms

The following terms and other boldface terms in the chapter are defined in the Glossary

allergy
anaphylaxis
antibody
antigen
antiserum
attenuated
autoimmunity
B cell
complement
gamma globulin
immunity
immunization
immunodeficiency
inflammation
interferon
interleukin
lymphocyte
macrophage
plasma cell
T cell
toxin
toxoid
transplantation
vaccine

PASSport to Success

Visit *thePoint* or see the Student Resource CD in the back of this book for definitions and pronunciations of key terms as well as a pretest for this chapter.

Disease in Context

▶ Maria's Second Case: Fighting Back Against Disease

"Hi there," the receptionist called out, as Maria Sanchez entered the senior personal care facility where she worked. "You've been out a while."

"Yes," said Maria, "over a week; a run-in with the flu."

"I suppose you're still on antibiotics then," added the receptionist.

"No," Maria replied. "Antibiotics don't work against viruses. It was just the old rest, fluids, and aspirin solution for me." Maria hung up her coat, changed out of her boots, and moved on toward the activities center to resume her duties as coordinator. Her assistant, Anna, was already there.

"So good to have you back, Maria. The residents say that things aren't the same without you," declared Anna. "You look a little pale, though. Are you feeling okay?"

"Pretty good, said Maria, "but I hope I don't have to go through that flu again."

"Well, the staff doctor is coming in this afternoon to give the residents their flu shots. Why don't you ask him about getting one yourself this time?" Anna suggested.

Later that day, the physician agreed that Maria should be included in the group getting immunized against the flu. "I've already had the flu. Aren't I immune now?" Maria asked.

"Not necessarily," replied Dr. Andrews. "Because there are many strains of the influenza virus around, you could still pick up an infection with another variety. You're not allergic to eggs are you?"

"No, but why do you ask?" Maria wanted to know.

"Well," explained Dr. Andrews, "even though newer methods of producing the vaccine are under development, the vaccine we're using now is still made the old-fashioned way by growing the virus in fertilized chicken eggs. There's another form of the vaccine given as a nasal spray, but in the older population, we still use the injectable one."

"Okay," said Maria, "shoot."

In Chapter 5 we followed the path of Maria's influenza virus infection. Later in this chapter, we'll learn how her body responds to the flu vaccine and how well the vaccine will protect her from another bout of the disease.

365

Chapter 5 presents a rather frightening list of harmful organisms that surround us in our environment. Fortunately, most of us survive contact with these invaders and even become more resistant to disease in the process. The job of protecting us from these harmful agents belongs in part to certain blood cells and to the lymphatic system, which together make up our **immune system**.

The immune system is part of our general body defenses against disease. Some of these defenses are **nonspecific**; that is, they are effective against any harmful agent that enters the body. Other defenses are referred to as **specific**; that is, they act only against a certain agent and no others.

Why Do Infections Occur?

Although the body is constantly exposed to pathogenic invasion, many conditions determine whether an infection will actually occur. Pathogens have a decided preference for certain body tissues and must have access to these tissues. The polio virus, for example, may be inhaled or swallowed in large numbers and at first may come into direct contact with the mucous membranes lining the respiratory and digestive tracts. However, it causes no apparent disorder of these tissues but goes on to attack only nervous tissue. In contrast, the viruses that cause influenza and the common cold do attack the respiratory mucous membranes. HIV, the virus that causes AIDS, attacks a certain type of T cell (T-lymphocyte) which has surface receptors for the virus.

The **portal of entry** is an important condition influencing infection. The respiratory tract is a common entrance route for pathogens. Other important entry points include the digestive system and the tubes that open into the urinary and reproductive systems. Any break in the skin or in a mucous membrane allows organisms such as staphylococci easy access to deeper tissues and may lead to infection, whereas unbroken skin or mucous membranes are usually not affected.

The **virulence** (VIR-u-lens) of an organism, or the organism's power to overcome its host's defenses, is another important factor. Virulence has two aspects: one may be thought of as "aggressiveness," or invasive power; the other is the organism's ability to produce **toxins** (poisons) that damage the body. Different organisms vary in virulence. A specific organism's virulence also can change; variants of the influenza virus, for example, can be more dangerous in some years than in others. Organisms may gain virulence as they pass from one infected host to another.

The **dose** (number) of pathogens that invade the body also is a determining factor in whether or not an infection develops. Even if the virulence of a particular organism happens to be low, infection may occur if a large number enter the body.

Finally, an individual's condition, or **predisposition**, to infection is also important. Disease organisms are around us all the time. Why does a person only occasion-ally get a cold, flu, or other infection? Part of the answer lies in the person's condition, as influenced by general physical and emotional health, nutrition, living habits, and age.

CHECKPOINT 17-1 ➤ What are some factors that influence the occurrence of infection?

Nonspecific Defenses

The features that protect the body against disease are usually considered as successive "lines of defense," beginning with the relatively simple or outer barriers and proceeding through progressively more complicated responses until the ultimate defense mechanism—immunity—is reached.

PASSport to Success — Visit *thePoint* or see the Student Resource CD in the back of this book for illustrations of nonspecific defenses.

Chemical and Mechanical Barriers

The first line of defense against invaders includes:

- The skin serves as a mechanical barrier as long as it remains intact. A serious danger to burn victims, for example, is the risk of infection as a result of skin destruction.

- The mucous membranes that line the passageways leading into the body also act as barriers, trapping foreign material in their sticky secretions. The cilia in membranes in the upper respiratory tract help to sweep impurities out of the body.

- Body secretions, such as tears, perspiration, and saliva, wash away microorganisms and may contain acids, enzymes, or other chemicals that destroy invaders. Digestive juices destroy many ingested bacteria and their toxins.

- Certain reflexes aid in the removal of pathogens. Sneezing and coughing, for instance, tend to remove foreign matter, including microorganisms, from the upper respiratory tract. Vomiting and diarrhea are ways in which toxins and bacteria may be expelled.

CHECKPOINT 17-2 ➤ What tissues constitute the first line of defense against the invasion of pathogens?

Phagocytosis

Phagocytosis is part of the second line of defense against invaders. In the process of phagocytosis, white blood cells take in and destroy waste and foreign material (see Fig. 13-6 in Chapter 13). Neutrophils and macrophages are the main phagocytic white blood cells. Neutrophils are a type of granular leukocyte. Macrophages are derived from monocytes, a type of agranular leukocyte. Both kinds of cells travel in the blood to infection sites. Some of the macrophages remain fixed in the tissues, for example, in the skin, liver, lungs, lymphoid tissue, and bone marrow, to fight infection and remove debris. Macrophages were mentioned in Chapter 16 as part of the reticuloendothelial system.

Natural Killer Cells

The **natural killer (NK) cell** is a type of lymphocyte different from those active in specific immunity, which are described later. NK cells can recognize body cells with abnormal membranes, such as tumor cells and cells infected with virus, and, as their name indicates, can destroy them on contact. NK cells are found in the lymph nodes, spleen, bone marrow, and blood. They destroy abnormal cells by secreting a protein that breaks down the cell membrane, but the way in which they find their targets is not yet completely understood.

Inflammation

Inflammation is a nonspecific defensive response to a tissue-damaging irritant. Any irritant can cause inflammation: friction, x-rays, fire, extreme temperatures, and wounds, as well as caustic chemicals and contact with allergens—all can be classified as irritants. Often, however, inflammation results from irritation caused by infection. With the entrance and multiplication of pathogens, a whole series of defensive processes begins. This **inflammatory reaction** is accompanied by four classic symptoms: heat, redness, swelling, and pain, as described below.

When tissues are injured, damaged cells release **histamine** (HIS-tah-mene) and other substances that cause the small blood vessels to dilate (widen). They also release attractant substances that bring a variety of white blood cells to the area, including granulocytes, macrophages, and **mast cells**, which are similar to basophils but reside in the tissues. These cells also secrete vasodilators and other substances that promote and prolong the inflammatory response. Increased blood flow causes heat, redness, and swelling in the tissues. Some of these substances also irritate pain receptors.

The cellular secretions then cause the epithelial cells in the capillary walls to contract, thus widening the gaps between the cells and increasing permeability. As blood flows through the vessels, leukocytes move through these altered walls and into the tissue, where they can reach the irritant directly. Fluid from the blood plasma also leaks out of the vessels into the tissues and begins to clot, thus limiting the spread of infection to other areas. The mixture of leukocytes and fluid, the **inflammatory exudate**, contributes to swelling and puts pressure on nerve endings, adding to the pain of inflammation.

Phagocytes are destroyed in large numbers as they work, and dead cells gradually accumulate in the area.

The mixture of exudate, living and dead white blood cells, pathogens, and destroyed tissue cells is **pus**.

Meanwhile, the lymphatic vessels begin to drain fluid from the inflamed area and carry it toward the lymph nodes for filtration. The regional lymph nodes become enlarged and tender, a sign that they are performing their protective function by working overtime to produce phagocytic cells that "clean" the lymph flowing through them.

> **PASSport to Success**
>
> Visit **thePoint** or see the Student Resource CD in the back of this book for a diagram summarizing the events in inflammation and for the animation *Acute Inflammation*.

Fever

An increase in body temperature above the normal range can be a sign that body defenses are active. When phagocytes are exposed to infecting organisms, they release substances that raise body temperature. Fever boosts the immune system in several ways. It stimulates phagocytes, increases metabolism, and decreases certain disease organisms' ability to multiply.

A common misperception is that fever is a dangerous symptom that should always be eliminated. Control of fever in itself does little to alter the course of an illness. Healthcare workers, however, should always be alert to fever development as a possible sign of a serious disorder and should recognize that an increased metabolic rate may have adverse effects on a weak patient's heart.

Interferon

Certain cells infected with a virus release a substance that prevents nearby cells from producing more virus. This substance was first found in cells infected with influenza virus, and it was called **interferon** because it "interferes" with multiplication and spread of the virus. Interferon is now known to be a group of substances. Each is abbreviated IFN with a Greek letter, alpha (α), beta (β), or gamma (γ), to indicate the category of interferon and additional letters or numbers to indicate more specific types, such as α2a or β1b.

Pure interferons are now available in adequate quantities for treatment because they are produced by genetic engineering in microorganisms. They are used to treat certain viral infections, such as hepatitis. Interferons are also of interest because they act nonspecifically on cells of the immune system. They have been used with varying success to boost the immune response in the treatment of malignancies, such as melanoma, leukemia, and Kaposi sarcoma, a cancer associated with AIDS. Interestingly, interferon β is used to treat the autoimmune disorder multiple sclerosis (MS), because it stimulates cells that depress the immune response.

CHECKPOINT 17-3 ➤ What are some nonspecific factors that help to control infection?

Immunity

Immunity is the final line of defense against disease. Immunity to disease can be defined as an individual's power to resist or overcome the effects of a *particular* disease agent or its harmful products. In a broader sense, the immune system will recognize *any* foreign material and attempt to get rid of it, as occurs in tissue transplantation from one individual to another. Immunity is a selective process; that is, immunity to one disease does not necessarily cause immunity to another. This selective characteristic is called **specificity** (spes-ih-FIS-ih-te).

There are two main categories of immunity:

■ **Innate immunity** is inborn and is inherited along with other characteristics in a person's genes.

■ **Adaptive immunity** develops after birth. Adaptive immunity may be acquired by **natural** or **artificial** means; in addition, it may be either **active** or **passive**.

Figure 17-1 summarizes the different types of immunity. Refer to this diagram as we investigate each category in turn.

Innate Immunity

Both humans and animals have what is called a **species immunity** to many of each other's diseases. Although certain diseases found in animals may be transmitted to humans, many infections, such as chicken cholera, hog cholera, distemper, and other animal diseases, do not affect human beings. However, the constitutional differences that make human beings immune to these disorders also make them susceptible to others that do not affect different species. Such infections as measles, scarlet fever, and diphtheria do not appear to affect animals who come in contact with infected humans.

Some members of a given group have a more highly developed **individual immunity** to specific diseases. For example, some people are prone to cold sores (fever blisters) caused by herpes virus, whereas others have never shown signs of this infection. Newspapers and magazines sometimes feature the advice of an elderly person who is asked to give his or her secret for living to a ripe old age. Some elderly people may say that they lived a carefully regulated life with the right amount of rest, exercise, and work, whereas others may boast of drinking alcohol, smoking, not exercising, and other kinds of unhealthy behavior. However, it is possible that the latter group resisted infection and maintained health despite their habits, rather than because of them, thanks to inherited resistance factors.

 PASSport to Success Visit **thePoint** or see the Student Resource CD in the back of this book for the animation *Immune Response*, which illustrates the following reactions.

Adaptive Immunity

Unlike innate immunity, which is due to inherited factors, adaptive immunity develops during a person's lifetime as that person encounters various specific harmful agents.

If the following description of the immune system seems complex, bear in mind that from infancy on, your immune system is able to protect you from millions of foreign substances, even synthetic substances not found in nature. All the while, the system is kept in check, so that it does not usually overreact to produce allergies or mistakenly attack and damage your own body tissues.

CHECKPOINT 17-4 ➤ What is the difference between innate and adaptive immunity?

ANTIGENS An **antigen** (AN-te-jen) (**Ag**) is any foreign substance that enters the body and induces an immune response. (The word is formed from *anti*body + *gen* because an antigen stimulates antibody production.) Most antigens are large protein molecules, but carbohydrates and some lipids may act as antigens. Antigens may be found on the surface of pathogenic organisms,

Figure 17-1 Types of immunity.

on the surface of red blood cells and tissue cells, on pollens, in toxins, and in foods. The critical feature of any substance described as an antigen is that it stimulates the activity of certain lymphocytes classified as T or B cells.

T CELLS Both T and B cells come from hematopoietic (blood-forming) stem cells in bone marrow, as do all blood cells. The T and B cells differ, however, in their development and their method of action. Some of the immature stem cells migrate to the thymus and become T cells, which constitute about 80% of the lymphocytes in the circulating blood. While in the thymus, these T lymphocytes multiply and become capable of combining with specific foreign antigens, at which time they are described as **sensitized**. These thymus-derived cells produce an immunity that is said to be **cell-mediated** immunity.

There are several types of T cells, each with different functions. The different types and some of their functions are as follows:

- **Cytotoxic T cells** (T_c) destroy foreign cells directly.

- **Helper T cells** (T_h) release substances known as **interleukins** (in-ter-LU-kinz) (IL) that stimulate other lymphocytes and macrophages and thereby assist in the destruction of foreign cells. (These substances are so named because they act between white blood cells). There are several subtypes of these helper T cells, one of which is infected and destroyed by the AIDS virus (HIV). The HIV-targeted T cells have a special surface receptor (CD_4) to which the virus attaches.

- **Regulatory T cells** (T_{reg}) suppress the immune response in order to prevent overactivity. These T cells may inhibit or destroy active lymphocytes.

- **Memory T cells** remember an antigen and start a rapid response if that antigen is contacted again.

The T cell portion of the immune system is generally responsible for defense against cancer cells, certain viruses, and other pathogens that grow within cells (intracellular parasites), as well as for the rejection of tissue transplanted from another person.

The Role of Macrophages Macrophages are phagocytic white blood cells derived from monocytes (their name means "big eater"). They act as processing centers for foreign antigens. They ingest foreign proteins, such as disease organisms, and break them down within phagocytic vesicles (Fig. 17-2). They then insert fragments of the foreign antigen into their plasma membrane. The foreign antigens are displayed on the macrophage's surface in combination with antigens that a T cell can recognize as belonging to the "self." Self-antigens are known as MHC (major histocompatibility complex) antigens because of their importance in cross-matching for tissue transplantation. They are also known as HLAs (human leukocyte antigens), because white blood cells are used in testing tissues for compatibility. Macrophages and other cells that present antigens to T cells are known as APCs (antigen-presenting cells).

For a T cell to react with a foreign antigen, that antigen must be presented to the T cell along with the MHC proteins. A special receptor on the T cell must bind with both the MHC protein and the foreign antigen fragment (see Fig. 17-2). The activated T_h then produces interleukins (ILs), which stimulate other leukocytes, such as B cells. There are many different types of interleukins, and they participate at different points in the immune response. They are produced by white cells and also by fibroblasts (cells in connective tissue that produce fibers) and by epithelial cells. Because ILs stimulate the cells active in immunity, they are used medically to boost the immune system.

CHECKPOINT 17-5 ➤ What is an antigen?

CHECKPOINT 17-6 ➤ List four types of T cells.

B CELLS AND ANTIBODIES An **antibody** (Ab), also known as an **immunoglobulin** (Ig), is a substance produced in response to an antigen. Antibodies are manufactured by B

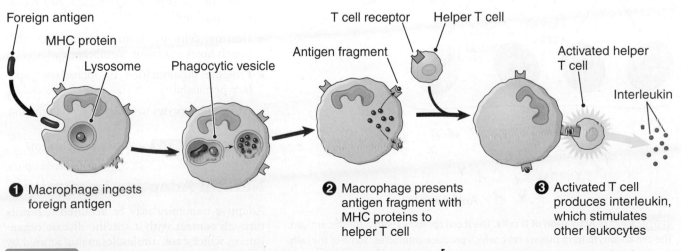

① Macrophage ingests foreign antigen
② Macrophage presents antigen fragment with MHC proteins to helper T cell
③ Activated T cell produces interleukin, which stimulates other leukocytes

Figure 17-2 **Activation of a helper T cell by a macrophage (antigen-presenting cell).** [**ZOOMING IN** ➤ What is contained in the lysosome that joins the phagocytic vesicle?]

cells (B lymphocytes), another type of lymphocyte active in the immune system. These cells must mature in the fetal liver or in lymphoid tissue before becoming active in the blood.

B cells have surface receptors that bind with a specific type of antigen (Fig. 17-3). Exposure to the antigen stimulates the cells to multiply rapidly and produce large numbers (clones) of **plasma cells**. These mature cells produce antibodies against the original antigen and release them into the blood, providing the form of immunity described as **humoral immunity** (the term *humoral* refers to body fluids).

Humoral immunity generally protects against circulating antigens and bacteria that grow outside the cells (extracellular pathogens). All antibodies are contained in a portion of the blood plasma called the **gamma globulin** fraction. Box 17-1, Antibodies, provides further information about the different types of antibodies.

Some antibodies produced by B cells remain in the blood to give long-term immunity. In addition, some of the activated B cells do not become plasma cells but, like certain T cells, become memory cells. On repeated contact with an antigen, these cells are ready to produce antibodies immediately. Because of this "immunologic memory," one is usually immune to a childhood disease after having it.

CHECKPOINT 17-7 ➤ What is an antibody?

CHECKPOINT 17-8 ➤ What type of cells produce antibodies?

The Antigen–Antibody Reaction

The antibody that is produced in response to a specific antigen, such as a bacterial cell or a toxin, has a shape that matches some part of that antigen, much in the same way that a key's shape matches the shape of its lock. The antibody can bind specifically to the antigen that caused its production and thereby destroy or inactivate it. Antigen–antibody interactions are illustrated and their protective effects are described in Table 17-1.

COMPLEMENT The destruction of foreign cells sometimes requires the enzymatic activity of a group of nonspecific proteins in the blood, together called **complement**. Complement proteins are always present in the blood, but they must be activated by antigen–antibody complexes or by foreign cell surfaces. Complement is so named because it assists with immune reactions. Some of complement's actions are to:

- Coat foreign cells to help phagocytes recognize and engulf them
- Destroy cells by forming complexes that punch holes in plasma membranes
- Promote inflammation by increasing capillary permeability
- Attract phagocytes to an area of inflammation

CHECKPOINT 17-9 ➤ What is complement?

Natural Adaptive Immunity

Adaptive immunity may be acquired naturally through contact with a specific disease organism, in which case, antibodies manufactured by the infected person's cells act against the infecting agent or its toxins. The infection that trig-

B cell with specific antigen receptors

B cell binds to antigen

Activated B cell multiples

B memory cells

Plasma cells

Antibodies

Figure 17-3 **Activation of B cells.** The B cell combines with a specific antigen. The cell divides to form plasma cells, which produce antibodies. Some of the cells develop into memory cells, which protect against reinfection. [**ZOOMING IN** ➤ What two types of cells develop from activated B cells?]

Box 17-1	A Closer Look

Antibodies: A Protein Army That Fights Disease

Antibodies are proteins secreted by plasma cells (activated B cells) in response to specific antigens. They are all contained in a fraction of the blood plasma known as gamma globulin. Because the plasma contains other globulins as well, antibodies have become known as immunoglobulins (Ig). Immunologic studies have shown that there are several classes of immunoglobulins that vary in molecular size and in function (see below). Studies of these antibody fractions can be helpful in making a diagnosis. For example, high levels of IgM antibodies, because they are the first to be produced in an immune response, indicate a recent infection.

Class	Abundance	Characteristics and Function
IgG	75%	Found in the blood, lymph, and intestines Enhances phagocytosis, neutralizes toxins, and activates complement Crosses the placenta and confers passive immunity from mother to fetus
IgA	15%	Found in glandular secretions such as sweat, tears, saliva, mucus, and digestive juices Provides local protection in mucous membranes against bacteria and viruses Also found in breast milk, providing passive immunity to newborn
IgM	5%–10%	Found in the blood and lymph The first antibody to be secreted after infection Stimulates agglutination and activates complement
IgD	<1%	Located on the surface of B cells
IgE	<0.1%	Located on basophils and mast cells Active in allergic reactions and parasitic infections

gers the immunity may be so mild as to cause no symptoms (is subclinical). Nevertheless, it stimulates the host's cells to produce an active immunity.

Each time a person is invaded by disease organisms, his or her cells manufacture antibodies that provide immunity against the infection. Such immunity may last for years, and in some cases for life. Because the host is actively involved in the production of antibodies, this type of immunity is called **active immunity**. See Box 17-2, Too Much Stress, for information on how stress affects the immune system.

Adaptive immunity also may be acquired naturally by the passage of antibodies from a mother to her fetus through the placenta. Because these antibodies come from an outside source, this type of immunity is called **passive immunity**. The antibodies obtained in this way do not last as long as actively produced antibodies, but they do help protect the infant for about 6 months, at which time the child's own immune system begins to function. Nursing an infant can lengthen this protective period because the mother's specific antibodies are present in her breast milk and colostrum (the first breast secretion). These are the only known examples of naturally acquired passive immunity.

CHECKPOINT 17-10 ➤ What is the difference between the active and passive forms of natural adaptive immunity?

Artificial Adaptive Immunity

A person who has not been exposed to repeated small doses of a particular organism has no antibodies against that organism and may be defenseless against infection. Therefore, medical personnel may use artificial measures to cause a person's immune system to manufacture antibodies. The administration of virulent pathogens obviously would be dangerous. Instead, laboratory workers treat the harmful agent to reduce its virulence before it is administered. In this way, the immune system is made to produce antibodies without causing a serious illness. This protective process is known as **vaccination** (vak-sin-A-shun), or **immunization**, and the solution used is called a **vaccine** (vak-SENE). Ordinarily, the administration of a vaccine is a preventive measure designed to provide protection in anticipation of invasion by a certain disease organism.

Originally, the word *vaccination* meant inoculation against smallpox. (The term even comes from the Latin word for *cow*, referring to cowpox, which is used to vaccinate against smallpox.) According to the World Health Organization, however, smallpox has now been eliminated as a result of widespread immunization programs. Mandatory vaccination has been discontinued because the chance of adverse side effects from the vaccine is thought

17

Table 17-1	Antigen–Antibody Interactions and Their Effects	
Interaction	**Effects**	
Prevention of attachment 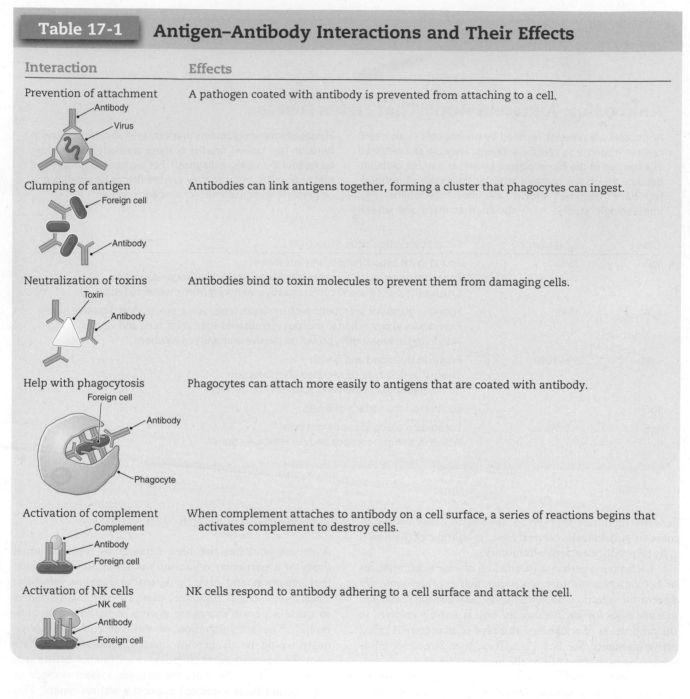	A pathogen coated with antibody is prevented from attaching to a cell.	
Clumping of antigen	Antibodies can link antigens together, forming a cluster that phagocytes can ingest.	
Neutralization of toxins	Antibodies bind to toxin molecules to prevent them from damaging cells.	
Help with phagocytosis	Phagocytes can attach more easily to antigens that are coated with antibody.	
Activation of complement	When complement attaches to antibody on a cell surface, a series of reactions begins that activates complement to destroy cells.	
Activation of NK cells	NK cells respond to antibody adhering to a cell surface and attack the cell.	

to be greater than the probability of contracting the disease.

All vaccines carry a risk of adverse side effects and may be contraindicated in some cases. People who are immunosuppressed, for example, should not be given vaccines that contain live virus. Also, pregnant women should not receive live virus vaccine because the virus could cross the placenta and harm the fetus.

TYPES OF VACCINES Vaccines can be made with live organisms or with organisms killed by heat or chemicals. If live organisms are used, they must be nonvirulent for humans, such as the cowpox virus used for smallpox immunization, or they must be treated in the laboratory to

weaken them as human pathogens. An organism weakened for use in vaccines is described as **attenuated**. In some cases, just an antigenic component of the pathogen is used as a vaccine. Another type of vaccine is made from the toxin produced by a disease organism. The toxin is altered with heat or chemicals to reduce its harmfulness, but it can still function as an antigen to induce immunity. Such an altered toxin is called a **toxoid**.

The newest types of vaccines are produced from antigenic components of pathogens or by genetic engineering. By techniques of recombinant DNA, the genes for specific disease antigens are inserted into the genetic material of harmless organisms. The antigens produced by these organisms are extracted and purified and used for

Box 17-2 Clinical Perspectives

Too Much Stress Makes the Immune System Sick

The impact of stress on the immune system is the most wide-ranging and significant of its many effects on the body. Stressors such as trauma, infection, debilitating disease, surgery, pain, extreme environmental conditions, and emotional distress all hamper immune function. The mechanisms responsible for these changes are not yet fully understood. Scientists do know that stress causes the hypothalamus to promote the release of ACTH from the anterior pituitary. This hormone stimulates the adrenal cortex to release the hormone cortisol, which influences a person's immediate ability to overcome any challenge, even stress itself. However, the abnormally high levels of cortisol that appear during periods of intense stress can actually be harmful. Such levels can:

- inhibit histamine release from damaged tissues, thereby blocking inflammation and the arrival of phagocytic leukocytes.
- reduce phagocytosis in damaged tissues, thus preventing antigen presentation to (and activation of) both killer T cells and helper T cells.
- inhibit interleukin secretion from helper T cells, thus preventing the immune system from mounting a coordinated response to infection.

immunization. The hepatitis B vaccine is produced in this manner.

BOOSTERS In many cases, an active immunity acquired by artificial (or even natural) means does not last a lifetime. Circulating antibodies can decline with time. To help maintain a high titer (level) of antibodies in the blood, repeated inoculations, called *booster shots*, are administered at intervals. The number of booster injections recommended varies with the disease and with an individual's environment or range of exposure. On occasion, epidemics in high schools or colleges may prompt recommendations for specific boosters. Table 17-2 lists the vaccines currently recommended in the United States for childhood immunizations. The number and timing of doses varies with the different vaccines.

PASSport to Success

Nurse practitioners often administer vaccines. Visit *thePoint* or see the Student Resource CD in the back of this book to read about this career, and specifically about pediatric nurse practitioners.

EXAMPLES OF BACTERIAL VACCINES Children are routinely immunized with vaccines against bacteria or their toxins. Because of whooping cough's seriousness in young infants, early inoculation with whooping cough, or **pertussis** (per-TUS-is), vaccine is recommended. A new form of the vaccine containing pertussis toxoid causes fewer adverse reactions than older types that contained heat-killed organisms. This acellular (aP) vaccine usually is given in a mixture with diphtheria toxoid and tetanus tox-

17

Table 17-2	Childhood Immunizations*	
Vaccine	Disease(s)	Schedule
DTaP	Diphtheria, tetanus, pertussis (whooping cough)	2, 4, 6, and 15–18 months; booster at 4–6 years Diphtheria and tetanus toxoid (Td) at 11–12 years
Hib	*Haemophilus influenza* type b (spinal meningitis)	2 and 4 months or 2, 4, and 6 months depending on type used
PCV	Pneumococcus (pneumonia, meningitis)	2, 4, 6, and 12–15 months
MMR	Measles, mumps, rubella	15 months and 4–6 years
HBV	Hepatitis B	Birth, 1–2 months, 6–18 months
Polio vaccine (IPV)	Poliomyelitis	2 and 4 months, 6–18 months, and 4–6 years
Varicella	Chickenpox	12–15 months and 4–6 years
Rotavirus	Rotavirus gastroenteritis	2, 4, and 6 months

*Recommended by the Advisory Committee on Immunization Practices (www.cdc.gov/vaccines/recs/acip), the American Academy of Pediatrics (www.aap.org), and the American Academy of Family Physicians (www.aafp.org). Information is also available through the National Immunization Program website (www.cdc.gov/vaccines).

oid. The combination, referred to as *DTaP*, may be given as early as 2 months of age and should be followed by additional injections at 4, 6, and 15 months and again when the child enters day care, a school, or any other environment in which he or she might be exposed to one of these contagious diseases. Diphtheria and tetanus toxoid (Td) is given again at 11 to 12 years of age. A tetanus booster is given when there is a disease risk and the last booster was administered more than 10 years prior to exposure.

Routine inoculation against *Haemophilus influenzae* type B (Hib) has nearly eliminated the life-threatening meningitis caused by this organism among preschool children. Hib also causes pneumonia and recurrent ear infections in young children. Depending on the type used, the vaccine is given in either two doses or three doses beginning at 2 months of age.

Pneumococcal vaccine (PCV) protects against infection with pneumococcus, an organism that can cause pneumonia and meningitis. Four doses are given between the ages of 2 and 15 months.

EXAMPLES OF VIRAL VACCINES Intensive research on viruses has resulted in the development of vaccines for an increasing number of viral diseases.

- The medical community has achieved spectacular results in eliminating poliomyelitis by the use of vaccines. The first of these was an inactivated polio vaccine (IVP) developed by Dr. Jonas Salk and made with killed poliovirus. A more convenient oral vaccine (OPV), made with live attenuated virus, was then developed by Dr. Albert Sabin. Both vaccine types are presently used in worldwide immunization programs, but IPV is preferred for routine childhood immunizations. A series of three doses is given between 2 and 18 months, and a fourth dose is given before entry into school.

- MMR, made with live attenuated viruses, protects against measles (rubeola), mumps, and rubella (German measles). Rubella is a very mild disease, but it causes birth defects in a developing fetus (see Table 2 in Appendix 5). A first dose of MMR is given at 15 months and a second between 4 and 6 years of age.

- Infants are now routinely immunized against hepatitis B, receiving the first of three shots just after birth and two more before the age of 18 months. The vaccine is also recommended for people at high risk of hepatitis B infection, including healthcare workers, people on kidney dialysis, people receiving blood clotting factors, injecting drug users, and those with multiple sexual partners. A vaccine against hepatitis A virus is recommended for travelers and others at high risk for infection.

- A vaccine against chicken pox (varicella) has been available since 1995. Children who have not had the disease by 1 year of age should be vaccinated. Although chicken pox is usually a mild disease, it can cause encephalitis, and infection in a pregnant woman can cause congenital malformation of the fetus. Because varicella is the same virus that causes shingles, vaccination may prevent this late-life sequel. A live virus shingles vaccine is also now available for people 60 years or older.

- A number of vaccines have been developed against influenza, which is caused by a variety of different viral strains. Laboratories produce a new vaccine each year to combat what they expect will be the most common strains in the population. The elderly, the debilitated, and children, especially those with certain risk factors, including asthma, heart disease, sickle cell disease, HIV infection, and diabetes, should be immunized yearly against influenza.

- Rotavirus causes a highly contagious gastrointestinal infection among babies and toddlers worldwide. The vomiting and diarrhea that result from infection can lead rapidly to life-threatening dehydration. A new vaccine has been approved to prevent this disease and should be administered at 2, 4, and 6 months of age.

- The human papilloma virus (HPV) causes sexually transmitted genital warts in both men and women and is associated with almost all cases of cervical cancer in women. Vaccines against the most prevalent HPV strains are now available and immunization is recommended for girls at age 11 to 12 years and those 13 to 26 years of age who have not yet been vaccinated.

- The rabies vaccine is an exception to the rule that a vaccine should be given before invasion by a disease organism. Rabies is a viral disease transmitted by the bite of wild animals such as raccoons, bats, foxes, and skunks. Mandatory vaccination of domestic animals has practically eliminated this source of rabies in some countries, including the United States, but worldwide, a variety of wild and domestic animals are host to the virus. There is no cure for rabies; it is fatal in nearly all cases. The disease develops so slowly, however, that affected people vaccinated after transmission of the organism still have time to develop an active immunity. The vaccine may be given preventively to people who work with animals.

CHECKPOINT 17-11 ➤ What are some bacterial diseases for which there are vaccines?

CHECKPOINT 17-12 ➤ What are some viral diseases for which there are vaccines?

ARTIFICIAL PASSIVE IMMUNITY It takes several weeks to produce a naturally acquired active immunity and even longer to produce an artificial active immunity through the administration of a vaccine. Therefore, a person who receives a large dose of virulent organisms and has no established immunity to them is in great danger. To prevent illness, the person must quickly receive counteracting antibodies from an outside source. This is accomplished through the administration of an **immune serum**, or **antiserum**. The "ready-made" serum gives short-lived but effective protection against the invaders in the form of an artificially acquired passive immunity. Immune sera are used in emergencies, that is, in situations in which there is no time to wait until an active immunity has developed.

Preparation of Antisera Immune sera often are derived from animals, mainly horses. It has been found that the horse's tissues produce large quantities of antibodies in response to the injection of organisms or their toxins. After repeated injections, the horse is bled according to careful sterile technique; because of the animal's size, it is possible to remove large quantities of blood without causing injury. The blood is allowed to clot, and the serum is removed and packaged in sterile containers.

Injecting humans with serum derived from animals is not without its problems. The foreign proteins in animal sera may cause an often serious sensitivity reaction, called **serum sickness**. To avoid this problem, human antibody in the form of gamma globulin may be used.

CHECKPOINT 17-13 ➤ What is an immune serum and when are immune sera used?

Examples of Antisera Some immune sera contain antibodies, known as **antitoxins**, that neutralize toxins but have no effect on the toxic organisms themselves. Certain antibodies act directly on pathogens, engulfing and destroying them or preventing their continued reproduction. Some antisera are obtained from animal sources, others from human sources. Examples of immune sera are:

- Diphtheria antitoxin is obtained from immunized horses.

- Tetanus immune globulin is effective in preventing lockjaw (tetanus), which is often a complication of neglected wounds. Because tetanus immune globulin is of human origin, it carries less risk of adverse reactions than do sera obtained from horses.

- Immune globulin (human) is given to people exposed to hepatitis A, measles, polio, or chickenpox. It is also given on a regular basis to people with congenital (present at birth) immune deficiencies.

- Hepatitis B immune globulin, used after hepatitis B exposure, is given principally to infants born to mothers who have hepatitis.

- The immune globulin $Rh_o(D)$ (trade name RhoGAM), is a concentrated human antibody given to prevent an Rh-negative mother from forming Rh antibodies. It is given during pregnancy if maternal antibodies develop and after the birth of an Rh-positive infant (or even after a miscarriage of a presumably Rh-positive fetus) (see Chapter 13). It is also given when Rh transfusion incompatibilities occur.

- Anti-snake bite sera, or **antivenins** (an-te-VEN-ins) are used to combat the effects of certain poisonous snake bites.

- Botulism antitoxin, an antiserum from horses, offers the best hope for botulism victims, although only if given early.

- Rabies antiserum, from humans or horses, is used with the vaccine to treat victims of rabid animal bites.

Disorders of the Immune System

Immune system disorders may result from overactivity or underactivity. Allergy and autoimmune diseases fall into the first category; hereditary, infectious, and environmental immune deficiency disease fall into the second.

Allergy

Allergy involves antigens and antibodies, and its chemical processes are much like those of immunity. Allergy—a broader term for which is **hypersensitivity**—can be defined informally as a tendency to react unfavorably to certain substances that are normally harmless to most people.

These reaction-producing substances are called **allergens** (AL-er-jens) and, like most antigens, they are usually proteins. Examples of typical allergens are pollens, house dust, animal dander (*dander* is the term for the minute scales that are found on hairs and feathers), and certain food proteins. Many drugs can induce allergy, particularly aspirin, barbiturates, and antibiotics (especially penicillin).

When a susceptible person's tissues are repeatedly exposed to an allergen—for example, exposure of the nasal mucosa to pollens—those tissues become **sensitized**; that is, antibodies are produced in them. When the next exposure to the allergen occurs, there is an antigen–antibody reaction. Normally, this type of reaction takes place in the blood without harm, as in immunity. In allergy, however, the antigen–antibody reaction takes place within the cells of the sensitized tissues, with results that are disagreeable and sometimes dangerous. In the case of the nasal mucosa that has become sensitized to pollen, the allergic manifestation is **hay fever**, with symptoms much like those of the common cold.

The antigen–antibody reaction in sensitized individuals promotes the release of excessive histamine. Histamine causes dilation and leaking from capillaries as well as contraction of involuntary muscles (e.g., in the bronchi). Antihistamines are drugs that counteract histamine and may be effective in treating the symptoms of certain allergies. Sometimes, it is possible to desensitize an allergic person by repeated intermittent injections of the offending allergen. Unfortunately, this form of protection does not last long.

Serum sickness is an example of an allergic manifestation that may occur in response to various sera. People who are allergic to the proteins in serum from a horse or some other animal show such symptoms as fever, vomit-

17

ing, joint pain, enlargement of the regional lymph nodes, and **urticaria** (ur-tih-KA-re-ah), also called hives. This type of allergic reaction can be severe but is rarely fatal.

ANAPHYLAXIS Anaphylaxis (an-ah-fih-LAK-sis) is a severe, life-threatening allergic response in a sensitized individual. (The term actually means excess "guarding," in this case, immune protection, from the Greek word *phylaxis*.) Any allergen can provoke an anaphylactic response, but common causes are drugs, insect venom, and foods. Symptoms appear within seconds to minutes after contact and include breathing problems, swelling of the throat and tongue, urticaria, edema, and decreased blood pressure with cardiovascular shock. Anaphylaxis is treated with injectable epinephrine, antihistamine, administration of oxygen, and plasma expanders to increase blood volume. People subject to severe allergic reactions must avoid contact with known allergens. They should be sensitivity tested before administration of a new drug and should also carry injectable epinephrine and wear a medical bracelet identifying their allergy.

Autoimmunity

The term **autoimmunity** refers to an abnormal reactivity to one's own tissues. In autoimmunity, the immune system reacts to the body's own antigens, described as "self," as if they were foreign antigens, or "nonself." Normally, the immune system learns before birth to ignore (tolerate) the body's own tissues by eliminating or inactivating those lymphocytes that will attack them. Some factors that might result in autoimmunity include:

- A change in "self" proteins, as a result of disease, for example.
- Loss of immune system control, as through loss of regulatory T cell activity, for example.
- Cross-reaction of antibodies with "self" antigens. This reaction occurs in rheumatic fever, for example, when antibodies to streptococci damage the heart valves.

Autoimmunity is involved in a long list of diseases, including rheumatoid arthritis, multiple sclerosis, lupus erythematosus, psoriasis, inflammatory bowel diseases, Graves disease, glomerulonephritis, and type I diabetes. All of these diseases probably result to varying degrees from the interaction of individual genetic makeup with environmental factors, including infections. Autoimmune diseases are three times more prevalent in women than in men, perhaps related to hormonal differences.

Autoimmunity is treated with drugs that suppress the immune system and with antibodies to lymphocytes. Pure antibodies, such as these, are prepared in the laboratory and are known as *monoclonal antibodies*. A newer approach uses chemotherapy to destroy immune cells followed by their replacement with healthy stem cells from bone marrow.

Immune Deficiency Diseases

An immune deficiency is some type of failure of the immune system. This failure may involve any part of the system, such as T cells, B cells, or the thymus gland, and it may vary in severity. Such disorders may be congenital (present at birth) or may be acquired as a result of malnutrition, infection, or treatment with x-rays or certain drugs.

The disease **AIDS** (acquired immunodeficiency syndrome) is a devastating example of an infection that attacks the immune system. It is caused by **HIV** (human immunodeficiency virus), which destroys the specific helper T cells that have a receptor (CD_4) for the virus. Its first appearance in the United States in the early 1980s was among homosexual men and injecting drug users. It now occurs worldwide in heterosexual populations of all ages. AIDS is considered to be a pandemic, especially in sub-Saharan Africa and in some parts of Asia. It is spread through unprotected sexual activity and the use of contaminated injection needles. It can also be transmitted from a mother to her fetus. The testing of donated blood has virtually eliminated the spread of AIDS through blood transfusions.

HIV belongs to a group of viruses that is unique in its method of reproduction. The group's name, **retroviruses** (RET-ro-vi-rus-es), which means "backward viruses," refers to the way in which the viruses reverse the typical order of genetic action. Retroviruses have RNA instead of DNA as their genetic material. Unlike other RNA viruses, however, they transcribe (copy) the RNA into DNA to reproduce inside the host. To accomplish this unusual feat, the virus has an enzyme called **reverse transcriptase** (tran-SKRIP-tase). The DNA formed using reverse transcriptase enters the host cell's nucleus and becomes part of its genetic material. There, it may direct the formation of more viruses or lie dormant and undetected for long periods, even years, before being triggered to multiply and cause disease. Some retroviruses can transform the host DNA and produce cancer. These viruses have been associated with leukemia in both humans and animals and with other types of tumors in animals.

Diagnosis of HIV infection is based on the presence of HIV antibodies, the virus, or viral components in the blood. The disease is monitored with CD4+ T cell counts and measurement of HIV RNA in the blood.

Patients with AIDS succumb easily to disease, including rare diseases such as a fungal (*Pneumocystis*) pneumonia and an especially malignant skin cancer, **Kaposi** (KAP-o-se) **sarcoma**. Drugs active against HIV stop viral growth at different stages of replication. Some, such as AZT, inhibit reverse transcriptase. These drugs, often used in combination, can slow the progress of HIV replication, but so far, do not prevent infection or cure AIDS. An obstacle to the development of a vaccine against HIV is the tremendous variability of the virus.

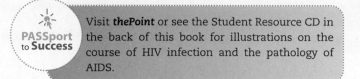

Visit *thePoint* or see the Student Resource CD in the back of this book for illustrations on the course of HIV infection and the pathology of AIDS.

Multiple Myeloma

Multiple myeloma is a cancer of the blood-forming cells in bone marrow, mainly the plasma cells that produce antibodies. These cells produce an excess of a particular antibody, but the antibody is not effective. The disease causes loss of resistance to infection, anemia, bone pain, and bone weakening, owing to production of a factor that accelerates loss of bone tissue. High blood levels of calcium and proteins secreted by the plasma cells often lead to kidney failure. Multiple myeloma is treated with chemotherapy. A new approach is high-dose chemotherapy combined with bone marrow transplants. Blood-forming stem cells in the bone marrow replace cells killed by the chemotherapy. This treatment is expensive, and stem cell transplants in themselves are dangerous, but this combined treatment has improved survival rates.

CHECKPOINT 17-14 ➤ What are some disorders of the immune system?

The Immune System and Cancer

Cancer cells differ slightly from normal body cells and therefore the immune system should recognize them as "nonself." The fact that people with AIDS and other immune deficiencies develop cancer at a higher rate than normal suggests that this is true. Cancer cells probably form continuously in the body but normally are destroyed by NK cells and the immune system, a process called **immune surveillance** (sur-VAY-lans). As a person ages, cell-mediated immunity declines and cancer is more likely to develop.

Medical scientists are attempting to treat cancer by stimulating the patient's immune system, a practice called **immunotherapy**. In one approach, T cells are removed from the patient, activated with interleukin, and then reinjected. This method has given some positive results, especially in treatment of melanoma, a highly malignant form of skin cancer. In the future, a vaccine against cancer may become a reality. Vaccines that target specific proteins produced by cancer cells have already been tested in a few forms of cancer.

Transplantation and the Rejection Syndrome

Transplantation is the grafting to a recipient of an organ or tissue from an animal or other human to replace an injured or incompetent body part. Much experimental work preceded transplantation surgery in humans. Tissues that have been transplanted include: bone marrow, lymphoid tissue, skin, corneas, parathyroid glands, ovaries, kidneys, lungs, heart, and liver.

Every organism's natural tendency to destroy foreign substances, including tissues from another person or any other animal, has been the most formidable obstacle to complete success. This normal antigen–antibody reaction has, in this case, been called the **rejection syndrome**.

In all cases of transplantation or grafting, the tissues of the donor, the person donating the part, should be typed in much the same way that blood is typed when a transfusion is given. Blood type antigens are much fewer in number than tissue antigens; thus, the process of obtaining matching blood is much less involved than is the process of obtaining matching tissues. Laboratories do tissue typing in an effort to obtain donors whose tissues contain relatively few antigens that might cause transplant rejection in a recipient, the person receiving the part. (One exception to the need for careful cross-matching is corneal transplantation in the eye. Corneal proteins don't enter the circulation to stimulate an immune response.)

Because it is impossible to match all of a donor's antigens with those of the recipient, physicians give the recipient drugs that will suppress an immune response to the transplanted tissue. These include drugs that suppress synthesis of nucleic acids; drugs or antibodies that inhibit lymphocytes; and adrenal glucocorticoid hormones, such as cortisol, that suppress immunity. These drugs cause a variety of adverse side effects, such as hypertension, kidney damage, and osteoporosis (glucocorticoids). Most importantly, they reduce a patient's ability to fight infection. Because T cells cause much of the reaction against the foreign material in transplants, scientists are trying to use drugs and antibodies to suppress the action of these lymphocytes without damaging the B cells. B cells produce circulating antibodies and are most important in preventing infections. Success with transplantation will increase when methods are found to selectively suppress the immune attack on transplants without destroying the recipient's ability to combat disease.

CHECKPOINT 17-15 ➤ What is the greatest obstacle to tissue transplantation from one individual to another?

17

Disease in Context revisited

➤ Annual Flu Shots for Maria

Maria has taken precautions against contracting the flu again. Once Dr. Andrews gave her the flu shot, her immune system began to respond to the inactivated viral antigens in the vaccine. Many of the components of Maria's immune system are activated, ending with plasma cells, derived from B cells, producing specific antibodies that will grant immunity to the virus.

Several days later, Maria met Dr. Andrews in the hall. "Thanks for the flu shot," she said. "I guess I'm safe against influenza now for life, or at least for a few years. I remember my mom telling me that if I was good when I had to take my childhood shots, I'd never have to get them again."

"Well, not exactly," the doctor replied. "Your immune system will remember the organisms that were in that vaccine, and protect you against them. But, each year new strains arise in humans or develop in animals and can be transmitted to humans." Maria realized that she'd heard over the years about swine influenza, bird influenza, and different types, such as A and B. She also knew about the Asian flu and the big Spanish flu epidemic of the early 1900s. "The vaccine is made from the three viral strains that are expected to cause the greatest problem each year," Dr. Andrews continued. "But if you get the shot annually, you should be relatively safe."

During this case we learned that vaccination stimulates the immune system to manufacture antibodies against disease organisms. Usually, the immune system protects us from infectious disease, but sometimes the system works to our disadvantage. We saw an example of that in Chapter 9, with Susan's case of multiple sclerosis.

Word Anatomy

Medical terms are built from standardized word parts (prefixes, roots, and suffixes). Learning the meanings of these parts can help you remember words and interpret unfamiliar terms.

WORD PART	MEANING	EXAMPLE
Why Do Infections Occur?		
tox	poison	A *toxin* is a substance that is poisonous.
Disorders of the Immune System		
erg	work	In cases of *allergy*, the immune system overworks.
ana-	excessive	*Anaphylaxis* is a life-threatening condition that results from an excessive immune reaction.
myel/o	marrow	Multiple *myeloma* is a cancer (-oma) of blood-forming cells in bone marrow.

Summary

I. **WHY DO INFECTIONS OCCUR?**
   A. Tissue preference of pathogen
   B. Portal of entry of pathogen
   C. Virulence of pathogen
      1. Invasive power
      2. Production of toxins (poisons)
   D. Dose (number) of pathogens
   E. Predisposition of host

II. **NONSPECIFIC DEFENSES**
   A. Chemical and mechanical barriers
      1. Skin
      2. Mucous membranes
      3. Body secretions
      4. Reflexes—coughing, sneezing, vomiting, diarrhea
   B. Phagocytosis—mainly by neutrophils and macrophages
   C. Natural killer (NK) cells—attack tumor cells and virus-infected cells
   D. Inflammation
   E. Fever
   F. Interferon
      1. Substances released from virus-infected cells
      2. Prevent virus production in nearby cells
      3. Stimulate the immune response nonspecifically

III. **IMMUNITY**—specific defense against disease
   A. Innate immunity
      1. Inborn, inherited with genes
      2. Types: species, individual
   B. Adaptive immunity—acquired after birth
      1. Antigens—stimulate immune response by lymphocytes
      2. T cells (T lymphocytes)
         a. Processed in thymus
         b. Types: cytotoxic, helper, regulatory, memory
         c. Involved in cell-mediated immunity
      3. Macrophages
         a. Derived from monocytes
         b. Present antigen to T cells in combination with MHC ("self") proteins
         c. Stimulate the release of interleukins (IL)
      4. B cells (B lymphocytes)
         a. Mature in lymphoid tissue
         b. Develop into plasma cells
            (1) Produce circulating antibodies
            (2) Antibodies counteract antigens
         c. Also develop into memory cells
         d. Involved in humoral immunity
   C. The antigen–antibody reaction
      1. Shape of antibody matches shape of antigen
      2. Results

      a. Prevention of attachment
      b. Clumping of antigen
      c. Neutralization of toxins
      d. Help in phagocytosis
      e. Activation of complement
      f. Activation of NK cells
   3. Complement
      a. Group of proteins in blood
      b. Actions
         (1) Coats foreign cells
         (2) Damages plasma membranes
         (3) Promotes inflammation
         (4) Attracts phagocytes
   D. Natural adaptive immunity
      1. Active—acquired through contact with the disease
      2. Passive—acquired from antibodies obtained through placenta and mother's milk
   E. Artificial adaptive immunity
      1. Active—immunization with vaccines
         a. Types: live (attenuated), killed, toxoid, recombinant DNA
         b. Boosters—keep antibody titers high
         c. Examples of bacterial vaccines
         d. Examples of viral vaccines
      2. Passive—administration of immune serum (antiserum)

IV. **DISORDERS OF THE IMMUNE SYSTEM**
   A. Allergy—hypersensitivity to normally harmless substances (allergens)
      1. Anaphylaxis—severe, life-threatening allergic response
   B. Autoimmunity—abnormal response to body's own tissues
   C. Immune deficiency diseases—failure in the immune system
      1. Congenital (present at birth)
      2. Acquired (e.g., AIDS)
   D. Multiple myeloma—cancer of blood-forming cells in bone marrow

V. **THE IMMUNE SYSTEM AND CANCER**
   A. Immune surveillance—ability of immune system to find and destroy abnormal cells (e.g., cancer cells)
   B. Immunotherapy—stimulating the immune system to treat cancer

VI. **TRANSPLANTATION AND THE REJECTION SYNDROME**
   A. Grafting of an organ or tissue to replace injured or incompetent part
   B. Requirements
      1. Tissue typing
      2. Suppression of immune system

17

Questions for Study and Review

BUILDING UNDERSTANDING

Fill in the blanks

1. The power of the organism to overcome its host's defenses is called _____.

2. Heat, redness, swelling, and pain are classic signs of _____.

3. Any foreign substance that enters the body and induces an immune response is called a(n)_____.

4. All antibodies are contained in a portion of the blood plasma termed the _____.

5. Substances capable of inducing a hypersensitivity reaction are called _____.

Matching > Match each numbered item with the most closely related lettered item.

___ 6. Destroy foreign cells directly.

___ 7. Release interleukins, which stimulate other cells to join the immune response.

___ 8. Suppress the immune response in order to prevent overactivity.

___ 9. Remember an antigen and start a rapid response if the antigen is contacted again.

___ 10. Manufacture antibodies when activated by antigens.

a. regulatory T cells

b. memory T cells

c. cytotoxic T cells

d. B cells

e. helper T cells

Multiple choice

___ 11. All of the following are part of the first line of defense against invaders *except*

   a. tears
   b. saliva
   c. neutrophils
   d. skin

___ 12. Damaged cells release a vasodilator substance called

   a. interleukin
   b. interferon
   c. histamine
   d. complement

___ 13. Which of the following cells mature in the thymus?

   a. T cell
   b. B cell
   c. plasma cell
   d. natural killer cell

___ 14. Sensitivity to animal-derived immune serum may lead to a serious condition called

   a. serum sickness
   b. hay fever
   c. Kaposi sarcoma
   d. rejection syndrome

___ 15. An abnormal reactivity to one's own tissues is called

   a. allergy
   b. autoimmunity
   c. anaphylaxis
   d. rejection

UNDERSTANDING CONCEPTS

16. Describe four factors that influence the occurrence of infection.

17. What causes the symptoms of inflammation?

18. Differentiate between the terms in each of the following pairs:

    a. interferon and interleukin
    b. antibody and complement
    c. innate immunity and adaptive immunity
    d. cell-mediated immunity and humoral immunity
    e. active immunity and passive immunity
    f. toxin and toxoid

19. Describe the events that must occur for a T cell to react with a foreign antigen. Once activated, what do the T cells do?

20. What role do antibodies play in immunity? How are they produced? How do they work?

21. Compare and contrast the four types of adaptive immunity.

22. What is an immune serum? Give examples. Define antitoxin.

23. Define allergy. How is the process of allergy like that of immunity, and how do they differ?

24. What is meant by rejection syndrome, and what is being done to offset this syndrome?

CONCEPTUAL THINKING

25. While in the garden with his father, Alek, a 4-year-old boy was, in his own words, "kicked by a bee." Shortly afterward, Alek developed hives near the affected area, which he began to scratch. About 10 minutes later, Alek's father noticed that his son was wheezing. What is happening to Alek? Describe the inflammatory events that are occurring in his body. How should Alek's father respond?

26. Why is HIV's attack on helper T cells so devastating to the entire immune system?

27. In Maria's case, she received an injectable influenza vaccine made with killed virus. The nasal spray flu vaccine is made with live attenuated virus. What is the difference between these two types of vaccines? In the future, what other types of influenza vaccines might be developed?

17

UNIT VI

Energy: Supply and Use

The five chapters in this unit show how oxygen and nutrients are processed, taken up by the body fluids, and used by the cells to yield energy. This unit also describes how the stability of body functions (homeostasis) is maintained and how waste products are eliminated.

The Respiratory System

Learning Outcomes

After careful study of this chapter, you should be able to:

1. Define *respiration* and describe the three phases of respiration
2. Name and describe all the structures of the respiratory system
3. Explain the mechanism for pulmonary ventilation
4. List the ways in which oxygen and carbon dioxide are transported in the blood
5. Describe nervous and chemical controls of respiration
6. Give several examples of altered breathing patterns
7. List and define four conditions that result from inadequate breathing
8. Describe several types of respiratory infection
9. Describe some allergic responses that affect the respiratory system
10. Name the diseases involved in chronic obstructive pulmonary disease (COPD)
11. Describe some disorders that involve the pleura
12. Describe equipment used to treat respiratory disorders
13. Show how word parts are used to build words related to respiration (see Word Anatomy at the end of the chapter)

Selected Key Terms

The following terms and other boldface terms in the chapter are defined in the Glossary

alveolus (pl., alveoli)
asthma
bronchiole
bronchus (pl., bronchi)
chemoreceptor
compliance
diaphragm
emphysema
epiglottis
epistaxis
hemoglobin
hilum
hypercapnia
hypoxia
larynx
lung
mediastinum
pharynx
phrenic nerve
pleura
pneumothorax
respiration
surfactant
trachea
ventilation

Disease
in Context

➤ Emily's Case: Advances in Asthma Therapy

"Remind me to mention to Dr. Martinez that Emily still has that nagging cough," Nicole told her husband.

"I've been worried about that," he replied. "You know, I had asthma as a kid—I hope she doesn't. I could hardly do any sports without taking a couple puffs of my inhaler."

Later that week, Dr. Martinez listened carefully to 3-year-old Emily's lungs for any sign of inflammation. He knew that the common symptoms of asthma—coughing, wheezing, and shortness of breath—were due to swelling of the airway tissues and spasm of the smooth muscle wrapped around them. "I don't hear any wheezing, but given the family history, we can't rule out asthma. In addition to the genetic component, asthma can have several environmental triggers such as respiratory infections, allergies, cold air, and exercise."

"Well," replied Nicole, "Emily did have a cold right before the coughing began. I haven't noticed any allergies, but now that I think about it, she did have a persistent cough last winter too. And, she is getting lots of exercise at preschool and dance class. So, if Emily does have asthma, what will that mean for her? I know that it limited my husband's activities when he was a kid."

"Asthma is rarely life-threatening," answered the doctor. "And the drug therapies that we now have to control asthma are much better than when your husband was young. But, first, I think we need to figure out if Emily's cough is really due to asthma. I suggest that you monitor Emily for the next few weeks and see if anything exacerbates it. In the event that she does have asthma, we might be able to treat it with a relatively new medication called an antileukotriene. This medication is taken orally every day and prevents the lungs from producing substances called leukotrienes, which cause the smooth muscle in the airways to constrict. Blocking leukotrienes helps prevent narrowing of the airways, and thus, the symptoms of asthma. With this medication, Emily may not even need an inhaler."

Dr. Martinez su.spects that Emily has asthma, the most common chronic respiratory disease of childhood. In this chapter, we'll examine the respiratory system and the components involved in this disease. Later in the chapter, we'll check in on Emily and learn about other medications used to treat asthma.

Phases of Respiration

Most people think of respiration simply as the process by which air moves into and out of the lungs, that is, *breathing*. By scientific definition, respiration is the process by which oxygen is obtained from the environment and delivered to the cells. Carbon dioxide is transported to the outside in a reverse pathway (Fig. 18-1).

Respiration includes three phases:

- **Pulmonary ventilation,** which is the exchange of air between the atmosphere and the air sacs (alveoli) of the lungs. This is normally accomplished by the inhalation and exhalation of breathing.

- **External exchange of gases,** which occurs in the lungs as oxygen (O_2) diffuses from the air sacs into the blood and carbon dioxide (CO_2) diffuses out of the blood to be eliminated.

- **Internal exchange of gases,** which occurs in the tissues as oxygen diffuses from the blood to the cells, whereas carbon dioxide passes from the cells into the blood.

Gas exchange requires close association of the respiratory system with the circulatory system, as the circulating blood is needed to transport oxygen to the cells and transport carbon dioxide back to the lungs.

The term *respiration* is also used to describe a related process that occurs at the cellular level. In **cellular respiration,** oxygen is taken into a cell and used in the breakdown of nutrients with the release of energy. Carbon dioxide is the waste product of cellular respiration (see Chapter 20's discussion of metabolism).

CHECKPOINT `18-1` ➤ What are the three phases of respiration?

Figure 18-1 **Overview of respiration.** In ventilation, gases are moved into and out of the lungs. In external exchange, gases move between the air sacs (alveoli) of the lungs and the blood. In internal exchange, gases move between the blood and body cells. The circulation transports gases in the blood.

The Respiratory System

The respiratory system is an intricate arrangement of spaces and passageways that conduct air into the lungs (Fig. 18-2). These spaces include the nasal cavities; the pharynx, which is common to the digestive and respiratory systems; the voice box, or larynx; the windpipe, or trachea; and the lungs themselves, with their conducting tubes and air sacs. The entire system might be thought of as a pathway for air between the atmosphere and the blood.

The Nasal Cavities

Air enters the body through the openings in the nose called the **nostrils**, or **nares** (NA-reze) (sing. naris). Immediately inside the nostrils, located between the roof of the mouth and the cranium, are the two spaces known as the **nasal cavities**. These two spaces are separated from each other by a partition, the **nasal septum**. The septum's superior portion is formed by a thin plate of the ethmoid bone that extends downward, and the inferior portion is formed by the vomer (see Fig. 7-5A in Chapter 7). An anterior extension of the septum is made of hyaline cartilage. The sep-

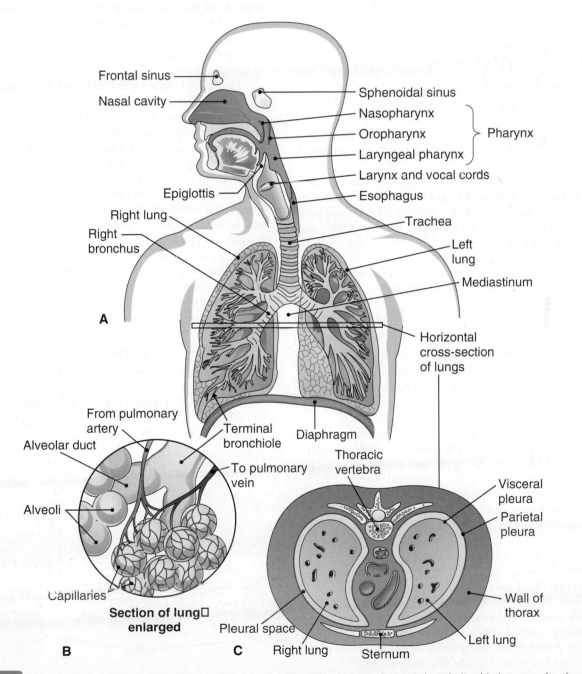

Figure 18-2 **The respiratory system. (A)** Overview. **(B)** Enlarged section of lung tissue showing the relationship between the alveoli (air sacs) of the lungs and the blood capillaries. **(C)** A transverse section through the lungs. [**ZOOMING IN ➤** What organ is located in the medial depression of the left lung?]

tum and the walls of the nasal cavity are covered with mucous membrane, consisting of stratified squamous (flat) epithelium, tissue that is resistant to wear.

On the lateral walls of each nasal cavity are three projections called the **conchae** (KONG-ke) (see Figs. 7-5A and 7-8 in Chapter 7). The shell-like conchae greatly increase the surface area of the mucous membrane over which air travels on its way through the nasal cavities. This membrane contains many blood vessels that deliver heat and moisture. The membrane's cells secrete a large amount of fluid—up to 1 quart each day. The following changes occur as air comes in contact with the nasal lining:

- Foreign bodies, such as dust particles and pathogens, are filtered out by the hairs of the nostrils or caught in the surface mucus.

- Air is warmed by blood in the well-vascularized mucous membrane.

- Air is moistened by the liquid secretion.

To allow for these protective changes to occur, it is preferable to breathe through the nose rather than through the mouth.

The **sinuses** are small cavities lined with mucous membrane in the skull bones. They are resonating chambers for the voice and lessen the skull's weight. The sinuses communicate with the nasal cavities, and they are highly susceptible to infection.

CHECKPOINT 18-2 ➤ What happens to air as it passes over the nasal mucosa?

The Pharynx

The muscular **pharynx** (FAR-inks), or throat, carries air into the respiratory tract and carries foods and liquids into the digestive system (see Fig. 18-2). The superior portion, located immediately behind the nasal cavity, is called the **nasopharynx** (na-zo-FAR-inks); the middle section, located posterior to the mouth, is called the **oropharynx** (o-ro-FAR-inks); and the most inferior portion is called the **laryngeal** (lah-RIN-je-al) **pharynx**. This last section opens into the larynx toward the anterior and into the esophagus toward the posterior.

The Larynx

The **larynx** (LAR-inks), commonly called the *voice box* (Fig. 18-3), is located between the pharynx and the trachea. It has a framework of cartilage, part of which is the thyroid cartilage that protrudes at the anterior of the neck. The projection formed by the thyroid cartilage is commonly called the *Adam's apple* because it is considerably larger in men than in women.

Folds of mucous membrane used in producing speech are located on both sides at the superior portion of the larynx. These are the vocal folds, or **vocal cords** (Fig. 18-4), which vibrate as air flows over them from the lungs. Variations in the length and tension of the vocal cords and the distance between them regulate the pitch of sound. The amount of air forced over them regulates volume. A difference in the size of the larynx and the vocal cords is what accounts for the difference between adult male and female voices. In general, a man's larynx is larger than a woman's. His vocal cords are thicker and longer, so they vibrate more slowly, resulting in a lower range of pitch. Muscles of the pharynx, tongue, lips, and face also are used to form clear pronunciations. The mouth, nasal cavities, paranasal sinuses, and the pharynx all serve as resonating chambers for speech, just as does the cabinet for an audio speaker.

The space between the vocal cords is called the **glottis** (GLOT-is). This is somewhat open during normal breathing but widely open during forced breathing (see Fig. 18-4). The little leaf-shaped cartilage that covers the larynx during swallowing is called the **epiglottis** (ep-ih-GLOT-is). The glottis and epiglottis help keep food and liquids out of the remainder of the respiratory tract. As the larynx moves upward and forward during swallowing, the epiglottis moves downward, covering the opening into the larynx. You can feel the larynx move upward toward the epiglottis during this process by placing the flat ends of your fingers on your larynx as you swallow. Muscles in the larynx assist in keeping foreign materials out of the respiratory tract by closing the glottis during swallowing. Muscles also close the glottis when an individual holds his or her breath and strains, as to defecate or lift a heavy weight.

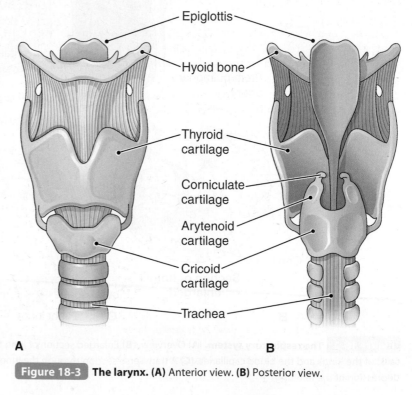

A **B**

Figure 18-3 **The larynx. (A)** Anterior view. **(B)** Posterior view.

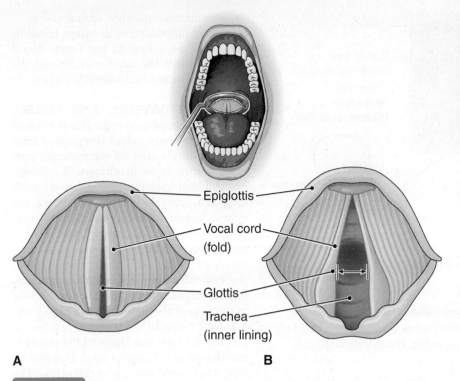

A   **B**

Epiglottis

Vocal cord (fold)

Glottis

Trachea (inner lining)

Figure 18-4 **The vocal cords, superior view. (A)** The glottis in closed position. **(B)** The glottis in open position. **[ZOOMING IN ➤** What cartilage is named for its position above the glottis? **]**

The Trachea

The **trachea** (TRA-ke-ah), commonly called the *windpipe*, is a tube that extends from the inferior edge of the larynx to the upper part of the chest superior to the heart. The trachea's purpose is to conduct air between the larynx and the lungs.

A framework of separate cartilages reinforces the trachea and keeps it open. These cartilages, each shaped somewhat like a tiny horseshoe or the letter **C**, are found along the trachea's entire length. The open sections in the cartilages are lined up at their posterior so that the esophagus can expand into this region during swallowing.

CHECKPOINT 18-3 ➤ What are the scientific names for the throat, voice box, and windpipe?

CHECKPOINT 18-4 ➤ What are the three regions of the pharynx?

The Bronchi

At its inferior end, the trachea divides into two primary, or mainstem, **bronchi** (BRONG-ki), which enter the lungs (see Fig. 18-2). The right bronchus is considerably larger in diameter than the left and extends downward in a more vertical direction. Therefore, if a foreign body is inhaled, it is likely to enter the right lung. Each bronchus enters the lung at a notch or depression called the **hilum** (HI-lum). Blood vessels and

nerves also connect with the lung here and, together with the bronchus, make up a region known as the *root* of the lung.

THE LINING OF THE AIR PAS-SAGEWAYS The trachea, bronchi, and other conducting passageways of the respiratory tract are lined with a special type of epithelium (Fig. 18-5). Basically, it is simple columnar epithelium, but the cells are arranged in such a way that they appear stratified. The tissue is thus described as *pseudostratified*, meaning "falsely stratified." These epithelial cells have cilia to filter out impurities and to create fluid movement within the conducting tubes. The cilia beat to drive impurities toward the throat, where they can be swallowed or eliminated by coughing, sneezing, or blowing the nose.

The Lungs

The **lungs** are the organs in which gas diffusion takes place through the extremely thin and delicate lung tissues (see Fig. 18-2). The two lungs are set side by side in the thoracic (chest) cavity. Between them are the heart, the great blood vessels, and other organs of the **mediastinum** (me-de-as-TI-num), the space between the lungs, including the esophagus, trachea, and lymph nodes. (See Appendix 7 for a dissection photograph showing the lungs in relation to the heart and diaphragm.)

On its medial side, the left lung has an indentation that accommodates the heart. The right lung is subdivided by fissures into three lobes; the left lung is divided into two lobes. Each lobe is then further subdivided into segments and then lobules. These subdivisions correspond to subdivisions of the bronchi as they branch throughout the lungs.

Each primary bronchus enters the lung at the hilum and immediately subdivides. The right bronchus divides into three secondary bronchi, each of which enters one of the right lung's three lobes. The left bronchus gives rise to two secondary bronchi, which enter the left lung's two lobes. Because the bronchial subdivisions resemble the branches of a tree, they have been given the common name *bronchial tree*. The bronchi subdivide again and again, becoming progressively smaller as they branch through lung tissue.

CHECKPOINT 18-5 ➤ The cells that line the respiratory passageways help to keep impurities out of the lungs. What feature of these cells enables them to filter impurities and move fluids?

The smallest of these conducting tubes are called

18

Figure 18-5 **Microscopic view of ciliated epithelium.** Ciliated epithelium lines the respiratory passageways, as shown here in the trachea. (Micrograph reprinted with permission from Cormack DH. *Essential Histology*, 2nd ed. Philadelphia: Lippincott Williams & Wilkins, 2001.)

bronchioles (BRONG-ke-oles). With branching, the histology of the tubes gradually changes. The bronchi contain small bits of cartilage, which give firmness to their walls and hold the passageways open so that air can pass in and out easily. As the bronchi become smaller, however, the cartilage decreases in amount. In the bronchioles, there is no cartilage at all; what remains is mostly smooth muscle, which is under the control of the autonomic (involuntary) nervous system.

THE ALVEOLI At the end of the **terminal bronchioles**, the smallest subdivisions of the bronchial tree, there are clusters of tiny air sacs in which most gas exchange takes place. These sacs are the **alveoli** (al-VE-o-li) (sing. alveolus) (see Fig. 18-2). The wall of each alveolus is made of a single-cell layer of squamous epithelium. This thin wall provides easy passage for the gases entering and leaving the blood as the blood circulates through the millions of tiny capillaries covering the alveoli.

Certain cells in the alveolar wall produce **surfactant** (sur-FAK-tant), a substance that reduces the surface tension ("pull") of the fluids that line the alveoli. This surface action prevents collapse of the alveoli and eases lung expansion.

There are about 300 million alveoli in the human lungs. The resulting surface area in contact with gases approximates 60 square meters (some books say even more). This area is equivalent, as an example, to the floor surface of a classroom that measures about 24 by 24 feet. As with many other body systems, there is great functional reserve; we have about three times as much lung tissue as is minimally necessary to sustain life. Because of the many air spaces, the lung is light in weight; normally, a piece of lung tissue dropped into a glass of water will float. Figure 18-6

shows a microscopic view of lung tissue.

The pulmonary circuit brings blood to and from the lungs. In the lungs, blood passes through the capillaries around the alveoli, where gas exchange takes place.

THE LUNG CAVITIES AND PLEURA

The lungs occupy a considerable portion of the thoracic cavity, which is separated from the abdominal cavity by the muscular partition known as the **diaphragm**. A continuous doubled sac, the **pleura**, covers each lung. The two layers of the pleura are named according to location. The portion of the pleura that is attached to the chest wall is the **parietal pleura**, and the portion that is attached to the lung surface is called the **visceral pleura**. Each closed sac completely surrounds the lung, except at the hilum, where the bronchus and blood vessels enter the lung.

Between the two layers of the pleura is the **pleural space**, containing a thin film of fluid that lubricates the membranes. The effect of this fluid is the same as between two flat pieces of glass joined by a film of water; that is, the surfaces slide easily on each other but strongly resist separation. Thus, the lungs are able to move and enlarge effortlessly in response to changes in the thoracic volume that occur during breathing.

CHECKPOINT 18-6 ➤ In what structures does gas exchange occur in the lung?

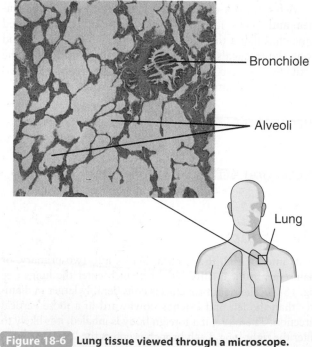

Figure 18-6 **Lung tissue viewed through a microscope.** (Micrograph courtesy of Dana Morse Bittus and BJ Cohen.)

CHECKPOINT 18-7 ➤ What is the name of the membrane that encloses the lung?

The Process of Respiration

Respiration involves ventilation of the lungs, exchange of gases, and their transport in the blood. Respiratory needs are met by central and peripheral controls of breathing.

Pulmonary Ventilation

Ventilation is the movement of air into and out of the lungs, normally accomplished by breathing. There are two phases of ventilation (Fig. 18-7):

- **Inhalation,** or inspiration, is the drawing of air into the lungs.

- **Exhalation,** or expiration, is the expulsion of air from the lungs.

In **inhalation,** the active phase of breathing, respiratory muscles of the thorax and diaphragm contract to en-large the thoracic cavity. During quiet breathing, the diaphragm's movement accounts for most of the increase in thoracic volume. The diaphragm is a strong, dome-shaped muscle attached to the body wall around the base of the rib cage. The diaphragm's contraction and flattening cause a piston-like downward motion that increases the chest's vertical dimension. Other muscles that participate in breathing are the external and internal intercostal muscles. These muscles run at different angles in two layers between the ribs. As the external intercostals contract for inhalation, they lift the rib cage upward and outward. Put the palms of your hands on either side of the rib cage to feel this action as you inhale. During forceful inhalation, the rib cage is moved further up and out by contraction of muscles in the neck and chest wall.

As the thoracic cavity increases in size, gas pressure within the cavity decreases. This phenomenon follows a law in physics stating that when the volume of a given amount of gas increases, the pressure of the gas decreases. Conversely, when the volume decreases, the pressure increases. If you blow air into a tight balloon that does not expand very much, the gas particles are in close contact and will hit the wall of the balloon frequently, creating greater pressure (Fig. 18-8). If you tap this balloon, it will spring back to its original shape. When you blow into a soft balloon that expands easily under pressure, the gas particles spread out into a larger area and will not hit the balloon's wall as often. If you tap the balloon, your finger will make an indentation. Thus, pressure in the chest cavity drops as the thorax expands. When the pressure drops to slightly below the air pressure outside the lungs, air is drawn into the lungs, as by suction.

The ease with which one can expand the lungs and thorax is called **compliance.** Normal elasticity of the lung tissue, aided by surfactant, allows the lungs to expand under pressure and fill adequately with air during inhalation. Compliance is decreased when the lungs resist expansion. Conditions that can decrease compliance include diseases that damage or scar lung tissue, fluid accumulation in the lungs, deficiency of surfactant, and interference with the action of breathing muscles.

Air enters the respiratory passages and flows through the ever-dividing tubes of the bronchial tree. As the air traverses this route, it moves more and more slowly through the great number of bronchial tubes until there is virtually no forward flow as it reaches the alveoli. The incoming air mixes with the residual air remaining in the respiratory passageways, so that the gases

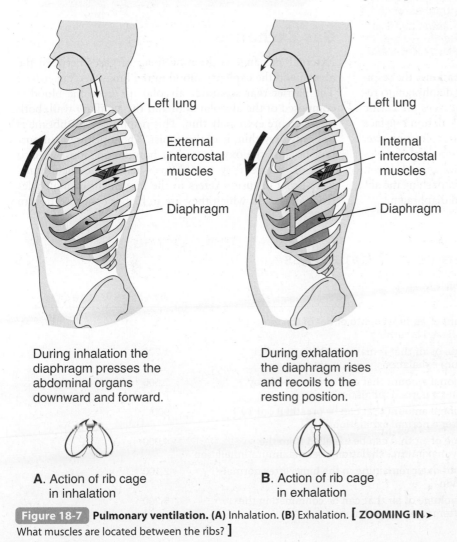

During inhalation the diaphragm presses the abdominal organs downward and forward.

During exhalation the diaphragm rises and recoils to the resting position.

A. Action of rib cage in inhalation

B. Action of rib cage in exhalation

Figure 18-7 **Pulmonary ventilation. (A)** Inhalation. **(B)** Exhalation. **[ZOOMING IN ➤** What muscles are located between the ribs? **]**

18

A　　　　　　　　　　　　　**B**

Figure 18-8 **The relationship of gas pressure to volume. (A)** Inflation of a stiff balloon creates strong air pressure against the wall of the balloon. **(B)** The same amount of air in a soft balloon spreads out into the available space, resulting in lower gas pressure. **[ZOOMING IN ➤** What happens to gas pressure as the volume of its container increases? **]**

soon are evenly distributed. Each breath causes relatively little change in the gas composition of the alveoli, but normal continuous breathing ensures the presence of adequate oxygen and the removal of carbon dioxide.

> **PASSport to Success**
> Visit **thePoint** or see the Student Resource CD in the back of this book for illustrations of the breathing muscles and for the animation *Pulmonary Ventilation.*

In **exhalation,** the passive phase of breathing, the respiratory muscles relax, allowing the ribs and diaphragm to return to their original positions. The lung tissues are elastic and recoil to their original size during exhalation. Surface tension within the alveoli aids in this return to resting size. During forced exhalation, the internal intercostal muscles contract, pulling the bottom of the rib cage in and down. The muscles of the abdominal wall contract, pushing the abdominal viscera upward against the relaxed diaphragm.

Table 18-1 gives the definitions and average values for some of the breathing volumes and capacities that are important in evaluating respiratory function. A lung *capacity* is a sum of volumes. These same values are shown on a graph as they might appear on a tracing made by a **spirometer** (spi-ROM-eh-ter), an instrument for recording lung volumes (Fig. 18-9). The tracing is a **spirogram** (SPI-ro-gram).

CHECKPOINT **18-8** ➤ What are the two phases of breathing? Which is active and which is passive?

> **PASSport to Success**
> Respiratory therapists evaluate and treat breathing disorders. Visit **thePoint** or see the Student Resource CD in the back of this book for a description of this career.

Gas Exchange

External exchange is the movement of gases between the alveoli and the capillary blood in the lungs (see Fig. 18-1). The barrier that separates alveolar air from the blood is composed of the alveolar wall and the capillary wall, both of which are extremely thin. This respiratory membrane is not only very thin, it is also moist. The moisture is important because the oxygen and carbon dioxide must go into solution before they can diffuse across the membrane. Recall that **diffusion** refers to the movement of molecules from an area in which they are in higher concentration to

Table 18-1	**Lung Volumes and Capacities**	
Volume	**Definition**	**Average Value (mL)**
Tidal volume	The amount of air moved into or out of the lungs in quiet, relaxed breathing	500
Residual volume	The volume of air that remains in the lungs after maximum exhalation	1,200
Inspiratory reserve volume	The additional amount that can be breathed in by force after a normal inhalation	2,600
Expiratory reserve volume	The additional amount that can be breathed out by force after a normal exhalation	900
Vital capacity	The volume of air that can be expelled from the lungs by maximum exhalation after maximum inhalation	4,000
Functional residual capacity	The amount of air remaining in the lungs after normal exhalation	2,100
Total lung capacity	The total volume of air that can be contained in the lungs after maximum inhalation	5,200

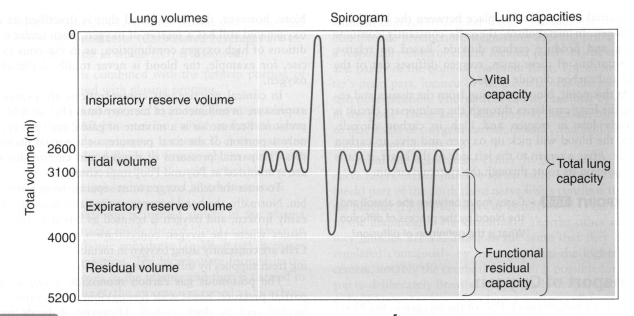

Lung volumes   **Spirogram**   **Lung capacities**

Inspiratory reserve volume

Tidal volume

Expiratory reserve volume

Residual volume

Vital capacity

Total lung capacity

Functional residual capacity

Total volume (ml): 0, 2600, 3100, 4000, 5200

Figure 18-9 **A spirogram.** The tracing of lung volumes is made with a spirometer. [**ZOOMING IN** ➤ What lung volume cannot be measured with a spirometer?]

an area in which they are in lower concentration. Therefore, the relative concentrations of a gas on the two sides of a membrane determine the direction of diffusion. Normally, inspired air contains about 21% oxygen and 0.04% carbon dioxide; expired air has only 16% oxygen and 3.5% carbon dioxide. These values illustrate that a two-way diffusion takes place through the walls of the alveoli and capillaries (Fig. 18-10).

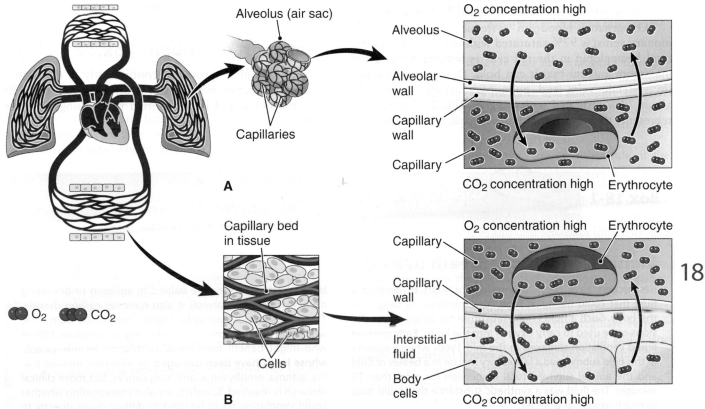

Alveolus (air sac)
Capillaries
O_2 concentration high
Alveolus
Alveolar wall
Capillary wall
Capillary
CO_2 concentration high   Erythrocyte

A

O_2 CO_2

Capillary bed in tissue
O_2 concentration high   Erythrocyte
Capillary
Capillary wall
Interstitial fluid
Body cells
Cells
CO_2 concentration high

B

Figure 18-10 **Gas exchange.** **(A)** External exchange between the alveoli and the blood. Oxygen diffuses into the blood and carbon dioxide diffuses out, based on concentrations of the two gases in the alveoli and in the blood. **(B)** Internal exchange between the blood and the cells. Oxygen diffuses out of the blood and into tissues, while carbon dioxide diffuses from the cells into the blood.

has the most immediate effect in regulating respiration at the level of the central chemoreceptors. When the carbon dioxide level increases, breathing must be increased to blow off the excess gas. Oxygen only becomes a controlling factor when its level falls considerably below normal.

CHECKPOINT 18-14 ➤ What gas is the main chemical controller of respiration?

Abnormal Ventilation

In **hyperventilation** (hi-per-ven-tih-LA-shun), an increased amount of air enters the alveoli. This condition results from deep and rapid respiration that commonly occurs during anxiety attacks, or when a person is experiencing pain or other forms of stress. Hyperventilation causes an increase in the oxygen level and a decrease in the carbon dioxide level of the blood, a condition called **hypocapnia** (hi-po-KAP-ne-ah). The loss of carbon dioxide increases the blood's pH (alkalosis) by removing acidic products, as shown by the equation cited previously. The change in pH results in dizziness and tingling sensations. Breathing may stop because the respiratory control center is not stimulated. Gradually, the carbon dioxide level returns to normal, and a regular breathing pattern is resumed. In extreme cases, a person may faint, and then breathing will involuntarily return to normal. In assisting a person who is hyperventilating, one should speak calmly, reassure him or her that the situation is not dangerous, and encourage even breathing from the diaphragm.

In **hypoventilation**, an insufficient amount of air enters the alveoli. The many possible causes of this condition include respiratory obstruction, lung disease, injury to the respiratory center, depression of the respiratory center, as by drugs, and chest deformity. Hypoventilation results in an increase in the carbon dioxide concentration in the blood, leading to a decrease in the blood's pH (acidosis), again according to the equation previously mentioned.

Breathing Patterns

Normal breathing rates vary from 12 to 20 breaths per minute for adults. In children, rates may vary from 20 to 40 breaths per minute, depending on age and size. In infants, the respiratory rate may be more than 40 breaths per minute. Changes in respiratory rates are important in various disorders and should be recorded carefully. To determine the respiratory rate, the healthcare worker counts the client's breathing for at least 30 seconds, usually by watching the chest rise and fall with each inhalation and exhalation. The count is then multiplied by 2 to obtain the rate in breaths per minute. It is best if the person does not realize that he or she is being observed because awareness of the measurement may cause a change in the breathing rate.

SOME TERMS FOR ALTERED BREATHING The following is a list of terms designating various respiratory abnormalities. These are symptoms, not diseases. Note that the word ending -*pnea* refers to breathing.

- **Hyperpnea** (hi-PERP-ne-ah) refers to an abnormal increase in the depth and rate of breathing.
- **Hypopnea** (hi-POP-ne-ah) is a decrease in the rate and depth of breathing.
- **Tachypnea** (tak-IP-ne-ah) is an excessive rate of breathing that may be normal, as in exercise.
- **Apnea** (AP-ne-ah) is a temporary cessation of breathing. Short periods of apnea occur normally during deep sleep. More severe sleep apnea can result from obstruction of the respiratory passageways or, less commonly, by failure in the central respiratory center.
- **Dyspnea** (disp-NE-ah) is a subjective feeling of difficult or labored breathing.
- **Orthopnea** (or-THOP-ne-ah) refers to a difficulty in breathing that is relieved by sitting in an upright position, either against two pillows in bed or in a chair.
- **Kussmaul** (KOOS-mowl) **respiration** is deep, rapid respiration characteristic of acidosis (overly acidic body fluids) as seen in uncontrolled diabetes.
- **Cheyne-Stokes** (CHANE-stokes) **respiration** is a rhythmic variation in the depth of respiratory movements alternating with periods of apnea. It is caused by depression of the breathing centers and is seen in certain critically ill patients.

RESULTS OF INADEQUATE BREATHING Conditions that may result from decreased respiration include the following:

- **Cyanosis** (si-ah-NO-sis) is a bluish color of the skin and mucous membranes caused by an insufficient amount of oxygen in the blood (see Fig. 6-6).
- **Hypoxia** (hi-POK-se-ah) means a lower than normal oxygen level in the tissues. The term **anoxia** (ah-NOK-se-ah) is sometimes used instead, but is not as accurate because it means a total lack of oxygen.
- **Hypoxemia** (hi-pok-SE-me-ah) refers to a lower than normal oxygen concentration in arterial blood.
- **Suffocation** is the cessation of respiration, often the result of a mechanical blockage of the respiratory passages.

Box 18-2, Adaptations to High Altitudes, offers information on adjusting to high altitudes and other hypoxic conditions.

Disorders of the Respiratory System

Infection is a major cause of respiratory disorders. These may involve any portion of the system. Allergies and environmental factors also affect respiration, and lung cancer is a major cause of cancer deaths in both men and women.

Box 18-2 A Closer Look

Adaptations to High Altitude: Living with Hypoxia

Our bodies work best at low altitudes where oxygen is plentiful. However, people are able to live at high altitudes where oxygen is scarce and can even survive climbing Mount Everest, the tallest peak on our planet, showing that the human body can adapt to hypoxic conditions. This adaptation process compensates for decreased atmospheric oxygen by increasing the efficiency of the respiratory and cardiovascular systems.

The body's immediate response to high altitude is to increase the rate of ventilation (hyperventilation) and raise the heart rate to increase cardiac output. Hyperventilation makes more oxygen available to the cells and increases blood pH (al-

kalosis), which boosts hemoglobin's capacity to bind oxygen. Over time, the body adapts in additional ways. Hypoxia stimulates the kidneys to secrete erythropoietin, prompting red bone marrow to manufacture more erythrocytes and hemoglobin. Also, capillaries proliferate, increasing blood flow to the tissues. Some people are unable to adapt to high altitudes, and for them, hypoxia and alkalosis lead to potentially fatal **altitude sickness**.

Successful adaptation to high altitude illustrates the principle of homeostasis and also helps to explain how the body adjusts to hypoxia associated with disorders such as chronic obstructive pulmonary disease.

Disorders of the Nasal Cavities and Related Structures

The paranasal sinuses are located in the skull bones in the vicinity of the nasal cavities. Infection may easily travel into these sinuses from the mouth, nose, and throat along their mucous membranes. The resulting inflammation is called **sinusitis**. Chronic (long-standing) sinus infection may cause changes in the epithelial cells, resulting in tumor formation. Some of these growths have a grapelike appearance and cause airway obstruction; such tumors are called polyps (POL-ips).

The partition separating the two nasal cavities is called the *nasal septum*. Because of minor structural defects, the nasal septum is rarely exactly in the midline. If it is markedly to one side, it is described as a **deviated septum**. In this condition, one nasal space may be considerably smaller than the other. If an affected person has an attack of hay fever or develops a cold with accompanying swelling of the mucosa, the smaller nasal cavity may be completely closed. Sometimes, the septum is curved in such a way that both nasal cavities are occluded, forcing the person to breathe through his or her mouth. Such an occlusion may also prevent proper drainage from the sinuses and aggravate a case of sinusitis.

The most common cause of nosebleed, also called **epistaxis** (ep-e-STAK-sis) (from a Greek word meaning "to drip"), is injury to the mucous membranes in the nasal cavity. Causes of injury include infection, drying of the membranes, picking the nose, or other forms of trauma. These simple nosebleeds usually stop on their own, but some measures that help are applying pressure to the upper lip under the nose, pinching the nose together, or applying ice to the forehead. Epistaxis may signal more serious problems, such as blood clotting abnormalities, excessively high blood pressure, or tumors.

Serious injuries that lead to nosebleed, or a nosebleed that will not stop, require professional medical care. Treatment may include packing the nose with gauze or other material, administering vasoconstrictors, or cauterizing the wound.

Infection

The respiratory tract mucosa is one of the most important portals of entry for disease-producing organisms. The transfer of disease organisms from one person's respiratory system to another's occurs most rapidly in crowded places, such as schools, theaters, and institutions. Droplets from one sneeze may be loaded with many billions of disease-producing organisms.

Mucous membranes can resist infection to some degree by producing larger quantities of mucus. The runny nose, an unpleasant symptom of the common cold, is the body's attempt to wash away pathogens and protect deeper tissues from further infection. If the membrane's resistance is reduced, however, the membrane may act as a pathway for the spread of disease. The infection may travel by that route into the nasal sinuses, or middle ear, along the respiratory passageways, or into the lung. Each infection is named according to the part involved, such as pharyngitis (commonly called a *sore throat*), laryngitis, or bronchitis.

Among the infections transmitted through the respiratory passageways are the common cold, diphtheria, chickenpox, measles, influenza, pneumonia, and tuberculosis. Any infection that is confined to the nose and throat is called an **upper respiratory infection** (URI). Very often, an upper respiratory infection is the first evidence of infectious disease in children. Such an infection may precede the onset of a serious disease, such as rheumatic fever, which may follow a streptococcal throat infection.

18

Visit *thePoint* or see the Student Resource CD in the back of this book for a summary diagram of respiratory infections.

THE COMMON COLD The common cold is the most widespread of all respiratory diseases—of all communicable diseases, for that matter. More time is lost from school and work because of the common cold than any other disorder. (See Box 5-2 in Chapter 5.) The causative agents are viruses that probably number more than 200 different types. Medical science has yet to establish the effectiveness of any method for preventing the common cold. Because there are so many organisms involved, the production of an effective vaccine against colds seems unlikely.

The symptoms of the common cold are familiar: first the swollen and inflamed mucosa of the nose and the throat, then the copious discharge of watery fluid from the nose, and finally the thick and ropy discharge that occurs when the cold is subsiding. The scientific name for the common cold is **acute coryza** (ko-RI-zah); the word coryza can also mean simply "a nasal discharge."

RESPIRATORY SYNCYTIAL VIRUS (RSV) RSV is the most common cause of lower respiratory tract infections in infants and young children worldwide. The name comes from the fact that the virus induces fusion of cultured cells (formation of a syncytium) when grown in the laboratory. Infection may result in bronchiolitis or pneumonia, but the virus may affect the upper respiratory tract as well. Most susceptible are premature infants, those with congenital heart disease, and those who are immunodeficient. Exposure to cigarette smoke is a definite risk factor.

The virus usually enters through the eyes and nose following contact with contaminated air, nasal secretions, or objects. The incubation period is 3 to 5 days, and an infected person sheds virus particles during the incubation period and up to 2 weeks thereafter. Thorough handwashing helps to reduce spread of the virus. Infection usually resolves in 5 to 7 days, although some cases require hospitalization and antiviral drug treatments.

CROUP Croup usually affects children under 3 years of age and is associated with a number of different infections that result in upper respiratory inflammation. Airway constriction produces a loud, barking cough, wheezing, difficulty in breathing, and hoarseness. If croup is severe, the child may produce a harsh, squeaking noise (stridor) when breathing in through a narrowed trachea. Viral infections, such as those involving parainfluenza, adenovirus, RSV, influenza, or measles, are usually the cause. Although croup may be frightening to parents and children, recovery is complete in most cases within a week. Home treatments include humidifying room air or having the child breathe in steam. Also, cool air may shrink the respiratory tissues enough to bring relief.

INFLUENZA Influenza (in-flu-EN-zah), or "flu," is an acute contagious disease characterized by an inflammatory condition of the upper respiratory tract accompanied by generalized aches and pains. It is caused by a virus and may spread to the sinuses and downward to the lungs. Inflammation of the trachea and the bronchi causes the characteristic cough of influenza, and the general infection causes an extremely weakened condition. The great danger of influenza is its tendency to develop into a particularly severe form of pneumonia. At intervals in history, there have been tremendous epidemics of influenza in which millions of people have died. Vaccines have been effective, although the protection is of short duration.

PNEUMONIA Pneumonia (nu-MO-ne-ah) is an inflammation of the lungs in which the air spaces become filled with fluid. A variety of organisms, including staphylococci, pneumococci, streptococci, *Legionella pneumophila* (cause of Legionnaires disease), chlamydias, and viruses may be responsible. Many of these pathogens may be carried by a healthy person in the upper respiratory mucosa. If the person remains in good health, they may be carried for a long time with no ill effect. If the patient's resistance to infection is lowered, however, the pathogens may invade the tissues and cause disease.

Susceptibility to pneumonia is increased in patients with chronic, debilitating illness or chronic respiratory disease, in smokers, and in people with alcoholism. It is also increased in cases of exposure to toxic gases, suppression of the immune system, or viral respiratory infections.

There are two main kinds of pneumonia as determined by the extent of lung involvement and other factors:

- **Bronchopneumonia**, in which the disease process is scattered throughout the lung. The cause may be infection with a staphylococcus, gram-negative *Proteus* species, colon bacillus (not normally pathogenic), or a virus. Bronchopneumonia most often is secondary to an infection or to some factor that has lowered the patient's resistance to disease. This is the most common form of pneumonia.

- **Lobar pneumonia**, in which an entire lobe of the lung is infected at one time. The causative organism is usually a pneumococcus, although other pathogens may also cause this disease. *Legionella* is the agent of Legionnaires disease, or legionellosis, severe lobar pneumonia that occurs mostly in localized epidemics.

Most types of pneumonia are characterized by the formation of a fluid, or **exudate** (EKS-u-date), in the infected alveoli; this fluid consists chiefly of serum and pus, products of infection. Some red blood cells may be present, as indicated by red streaks in the sputum. Sometimes, so many air sacs become filled with fluid that the victim finds it hard to absorb enough oxygen to maintain life.

Visit *thePoint* or see the Student Resource CD in the back of this book for an illustration of the two types of pneumonia.

Pneumocystis Pneumonia (PCP) PCP occurs mainly in people with weakened immune systems, such as HIV-positive individuals or transplant recipients on immunosuppressant drugs. The infectious agent was originally called P. carinii and classified as a protozoon. It has now been reclassified as an atypical fungus and renamed P. jiroveci. The organism grows in the fluid that lines the alveoli of the lungs. Laboratories diagnose the disease by microscopic identification of the organism in a sputum sample, bronchoscopy specimen, or lung biopsy specimen. PCP is treated with antimicrobial drugs, although these medications may cause serious side effects in immunocompromised patients.

TUBERCULOSIS Tuberculosis (tu-ber-ku-LO-sis) **(TB)** is an infectious disease caused by the bacillus *Mycobacterium tuberculosis*. Although the tubercle bacillus may invade any body tissue, it usually grows in the lung. Tuberculosis remains a leading cause of death from communicable disease, primarily because of the relatively large numbers of cases among recent immigrants, elderly people, and poor people in metropolitan areas. The spread of AIDS has been linked with a rising incidence of TB because this viral disease weakens host defenses.

The name *tuberculosis* comes from the small lesions, or tubercles, that form where the organisms grow. If unchecked, these lesions degenerate and may even liquefy to cause cavities within an organ. In early stages, the disease may lie dormant, only to flare up at a later time. The tuberculosis organism can readily spread into the lymph nodes or into the blood and be carried to other organs. The lymph nodes in the thorax, especially those surrounding the trachea and bronchi, are frequently involved. Infection of the pleura results in tuberculous pleurisy (inflammation of the pleura). In this case, a collection of fluid, known as an effusion (e-FU-zhun), accumulates in the pleural space.

Drugs can be used successfully in many cases of tuberculosis, although strains of the TB organism that are resistant to multiple antibiotics have appeared recently. The best results have been obtained by use of a combination of several drugs, with prompt, intensive, and uninterrupted treatment once a program is begun. Therapy is usually continued for a minimum of 6 to 18 months; therefore, close supervision by the healthcare practitioner is important. Adverse drug reactions are rather common, necessitating changes in the drug combinations. Drug treatment of patients whose infection has not progressed to active disease is particularly effective.

> **PASSport to Success** Visit *thePoint* or see the Student Resource CD in the back of this book for a micrograph of the acid-fast TB organism and a diagram of TB infection.

Hay Fever and Asthma

Hypersensitivity to plant pollens, dust, certain foods, and other allergens may lead to **hay fever** or **asthma** (AZ-mah) or both. Hay fever, known medically as *allergic rhinitis*, is characterized by a watery discharge from the eyes and nose. Hay fever often appears in a seasonal pattern due to pollen allergy. The response may be chronic if the allergen is present year round. The symptoms of asthma are caused by reversible changes, which include inflammation of airway tissues and spasm of the involuntary muscle in bronchial tubes. Spasm constricts the tubes, causing resistance to air flow. The person experiences a sense of suffocation and has labored breathing (dyspnea), often with wheezing. Treatment may include inhaled steroids to prevent inflammation and inhaled bronchodilators to open airways during acute episodes.

Patients vary considerably in their responses, and most cases of asthma involve multiple causes. Respiratory infection, noxious fumes, or drug allergy can initiate episodes, but one of the more common triggers for asthma attacks is exercise. The rapid air movement in sensitive airways causes smooth muscle spasm in the breathing passages.

A great difficulty in the treatment of hay fever or asthma is identification of the particular substance to which the patient is allergic. Allergists usually give a number of skin tests, but in most cases, the results are inconclusive. People with allergies may benefit from a series of injections to reduce their sensitivity to specific substances.

Chronic Obstructive Pulmonary Disease (COPD)

Chronic obstructive pulmonary disease (COPD) is the term used to describe several lung disorders, including **chronic bronchitis** and **emphysema** (em-fih-SE-mah). Most affected patients have symptoms and lung damage characteristic of both diseases. In chronic bronchitis, the airway linings are chronically inflamed and produce excessive secretions. Emphysema is characterized by dilation and finally destruction of the alveoli.

In COPD, respiratory function is impaired by obstruction to normal air flow, reducing exchange of oxygen and carbon dioxide. There is air trapping and over-inflation of parts of the lungs. In the early stages of these diseases, the small airways are involved, and several years may pass before symptoms become evident. Later, the affected person develops dyspnea as a result of difficulty in exhaling air through the obstructed air passages.

In certain smokers, COPD may result in serious disability and death within 10 years of the onset of symptoms. Giving up smoking may reverse progression of the disorder, especially when it is diagnosed early and other respiratory irritants also are eliminated. Sometimes, the word *emphysema* is used to mean COPD.

COPD is also called COLD (chronic obstructive lung disease).

> **PASSport to Success** Visit *thePoint* or see the Student Resource CD in the back of this book for a photograph showing emphysema in lung tissue.

18

Sudden Infant Death Syndrome (SIDS)

SIDS, also called "crib death," is the unexplained death of a seemingly healthy infant under 1 year of age. Death usually occurs during sleep, leaving no signs of its cause. Neither autopsy nor careful investigation of family history and circumstances of death provides any clues. Certain maternal conditions during pregnancy are associated with an increased risk of SIDS, although none is a sure predictor. These include cigarette smoking, age under 20, low weight gain, anemia, illegal drug use, and infections of the reproductive or urinary tracts.

Some guidelines that have reduced the SIDS incidence are:

■ Place the baby supine (on its back) for sleep, unless there is some medical reason not to do so. A reminder for parents and other caregivers is the slogan "Back to sleep." A side position is not as effective, as the baby can roll over, and it should never be put to sleep prone (face down). In the prone position, the baby can rebreathe its own CO_2, building up CO_2 and diminishing blood O_2 levels. The position may also cause obstruction in the upper airways or lead to overheating by reducing loss of body heat.

■ Keep the baby in a smoke-free environment. Maternal smoking during pregnancy, or smoking in the baby's environment after birth, increases the SIDS risk.

■ Use a firm, flat baby mattress, not soft foam, fur, or fiber-filled bedding.

■ Avoid overheating the baby with room air, clothing, or bedding, especially when the baby has a cold or other infection.

CHECKPOINT 18-15 ➤ What does COPD mean and what two diseases are commonly involved in COPD?

Respiratory Distress Syndrome (RDS)

RDS covers a range of inflammatory disorders that result from other medical problems or from direct injury to the lungs. **Acute respiratory distress syndrome** (ARDS), or shock lung, usually appears in adults, in contrast to a form of the syndrome that occurs in premature newborns, as described later. Some causes of ARDS are:

■ Airway obstruction as from mucus, foreign bodies, emboli, or tumors

■ Sepsis (systemic infection)

■ Aspiration (inhalation) of stomach contents

■ Allergy

■ Lung trauma

Inflammation and damage to the alveoli results in pulmonary edema, dyspnea (difficulty in breathing), decreased compliance, hypoxemia, and formation of fibrous scar tissue in the lungs. The incomplete expansion of a lung or portion of a lung, such as results from ARDS, is called **atelectasis** (at-e-LEK-tah-sis), or collapsed lung.

In premature newborns, atelectasis may result from insufficient surfactant production by the immature lungs. **Respiratory distress syndrome of the newborn** is now treated by administration of surfactant that is produced in bacteria by genetic engineering. The syndrome was formerly called *hyaline membrane disease* because of the clear membrane formed from lung exudates in the alveoli.

Cancer

Tumors can arise in all portions of the respiratory tract. Two common sites are described as follows.

LUNG CANCER Cancer of the lungs is the most common cause of cancer-related deaths in both men and women. The incidence rate in women continues to increase, whereas the rate in men has been decreasing recently. By far, the most important cause of lung cancer is cigarette smoking. Smokers suffer from lung cancer 10 times as often as do nonsmokers. The risk of getting lung cancer is increased in people who started smoking early in life, smoke large numbers of cigarettes daily, and inhale deeply. Smokers who are exposed to toxic chemicals or particles in the air have an even higher lung cancer rate. Smoking has also been linked with an increase in COPD and cancers of respiratory passages.

> **PASSport to Success** Visit *thePoint* or see the Student Resource CD in the back of this book for an illustration of the effects of smoking.

A common form of lung cancer is **bronchogenic** (brong-ko-JEN-ik) **carcinoma**, so called because the malignancy originates in a bronchus. The tumor may grow until the bronchus is blocked, cutting off the air supply to that lung. The lung then collapses, and the secretions trapped in the lung spaces become infected, with a resulting pneumonia or lung abscess formation. This type of lung cancer can spread, causing secondary growths in the lymph nodes of the chest and neck and in the brain and other parts of the body. A treatment that offers a possibility of cure before secondary growths have had time to form is complete removal of the lung. This operation is called a **pneumonectomy** (nu-mo-NEK-to-me).

Malignant tumors of the stomach, breast, and other organs may spread to the lungs as secondary growths (metastases).

CANCER OF THE LARYNX Cancer of the larynx usually involves squamous cell carcinoma, and its incidence is definitely linked to cigarette smoking and alcohol consumption. Symptoms include sore throat, hoarseness, ear pain, and enlarged cervical lymph nodes. The cure rate is high for small tumors that have not spread when treated with radiation and (sometimes) surgery. Total or partial removal of the larynx is necessary in cases of advanced cancer that do not respond to radiation or chemotherapy. During and after laryngectomy a patient may need a surgically-created opening, or stoma, in the trachea with a tube (tracheostomy tube) for breathing. Patients have to care for the stoma and the "trach" (trake) tube. If the vocal cords are removed, a patient can learn to speak by using air forced out of the esophagus or by using a mechanical device to generate sound.

Disorders Involving the Pleura

Pleurisy (PLUR-ih-se), or inflammation of the pleura, usually accompanies a lung infection—particularly pneumonia or tuberculosis. This condition can be quite painful because the inflammation produces a sticky exudate that roughens the pleura of both the lung and the chest wall; when the two surfaces rub together during ventilation, the roughness causes acute irritation. The sticking together of two surfaces is called an adhesion (ad-HE-zhun). Infection of the pleura also causes an increase in the amount of pleural fluid. This fluid may accumulate in the pleural space in quantities large enough to compress the lung, resulting in an inability to obtain enough air.

Pneumothorax (nu-mo-THOR-aks) is an accumulation of air in the pleural space (Fig. 18-11). The lung on the affected side collapses, causing the patient to have great difficulty breathing. Pneumothorax may be caused by a wound in the chest wall or by rupture of the lung's air spaces. In pneumothorax caused by a penetrating wound in the chest wall, an airtight cover over the opening prevents further air from entering. The remaining lung can then function to provide adequate oxygen.

Blood in the pleural space, a condition called **hemothorax**, is also caused by penetrating chest wounds. In such cases, the first priority is to stop the bleeding.

The abnormal accumulation of fluid or air in the pleural space from any of the above conditions may call for procedures to promote lung expansion. In **thoracentesis** (thor-ah-sen-TE-sis) a large-bore needle is inserted between ribs into the pleural space to remove fluid (Fig. 18-12). The presence of both air and fluid in the pleural space may require insertion of a chest tube, a large tube with several openings along the internal end. The tube is securely connected to a chest drainage system. These procedures restore negative pressure in the pleural space and allow reexpansion of the lung.

Age and the Respiratory Tract

With age, the tissues of the respiratory tract lose elasticity and become more rigid. Similar rigidity in the chest wall, combined with arthritis and loss of strength in the breathing muscles, results in an overall decrease in compliance and in lung capacity. Reduction in protective mechanisms in the lungs, such as phagocytosis, leads to increased susceptibility to infection. The incidence of lung disease increases with age, hastened by cigarette smoking and by exposure to other environmental irritants. Although there is much individual variation, especially related to one's customary level of activity, these changes gradually lead to reduced capacity for exercise.

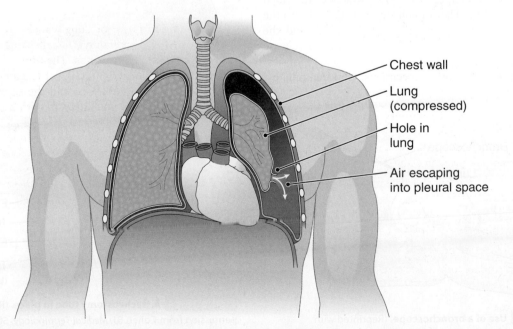

Chest wall

Lung (compressed)

Hole in lung

Air escaping into pleural space

18

Figure 18-11 **Pneumothorax.** Injury to lung tissue allows air to leak into the pleural space and put pressure on the lung. (Reprinted with permission from Cohen BJ. *Medical Terminology*, 5th ed. Philadelphia: Lippincott Williams & Wilkins, 2008.)

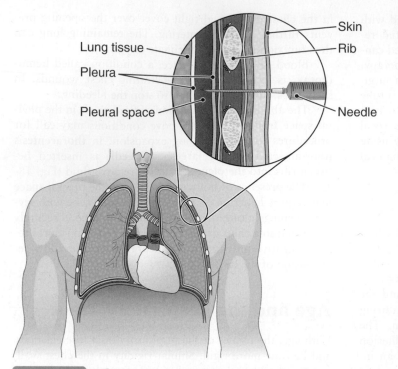

Figure 18-12 **Thoracentesis.** A needle is inserted into the pleural space to withdraw fluid. (Reprinted with permission from Cohen BJ. *Medical Terminology*, 4th ed. Philadelphia: Lippincott Williams & Wilkins, 2004.)

Special Equipment for Respiratory Treatment

The **bronchoscope** (BRONG-ko-skope) is a rigid or flexible fiberoptic tubular instrument used for inspection of the primary bronchi and the larger bronchial tubes (Fig. 18-13). Most bronchoscopes are now attached to video recording equipment. The bronchoscope is passed into the respiratory tract by way of the nose or mouth and the pharynx. Physicians may use a bronchoscope to remove foreign bodies, inspect and take tissue samples (biopsies) from tumors, or collect other specimens. Children inhale a

variety of objects, such as pins, beans, pieces of nuts, and small coins, all of which a physician may remove with the aid of a bronchoscope. If such items are left in the lung, they may cause an abscess or other serious complication and may even lead to death.

Oxygen therapy is used to sustain life when a condition interferes with adequate oxygen supply to the tissues. The oxygen must first have moisture added by bubbling it through water that is at room temperature or heated. Therapists may deliver oxygen to the patient by mask, catheter, or nasal prongs. Because there is danger of fire when oxygen is being administered, smoking in the room is absolutely prohibited.

A **suction apparatus** is used for removing mucus or other substances from the respiratory tract by means of negative pressure. A container to trap secretions is located between the patient and the machine. The tube leading to the patient has an opening to control the suction. When suction is applied, the drainage flows from the patient's respiratory tract into the collection container.

A **tracheostomy** (tra-ke-OS-to-me) **tube** is used if the pharynx or the larynx is obstructed. It is a small metal or plastic tube that is inserted through a cut made in the trachea, and it acts as an artificial airway for ventilation (Fig. 18-14). The procedure

Figure 18-13 **Use of a bronchoscope.** (Reprinted with permission from Cohen BJ. *Medical Terminology*, 4th ed. Philadelphia: Lippincott Williams & Wilkins, 2004.)

Figure 18-14 **A tracheostomy tube in place.** (Reprinted with permission from Cohen BJ. *Medical Terminology*, 5th ed. Philadelphia: Lippincott Williams & Wilkins, 2008.) [**ZOOMING IN ➤** What structure is posterior to the trachea?]

for the insertion of such a tube is a *tracheostomy*. The word **tracheotomy** (tra-ke-OT-o-me) refers to the incision in the trachea.

Artificial respiration is used when a patient has temporarily lost the capacity to perform normal ventilation. Such emergencies include cases of gas or smoke inhalation, electric shock, drowning, poisoning, or paralysis of the breathing muscles. A number of different apparatuses are used for artificial respiration in a clinical setting.

There are also some techniques that can be used in an emergency.

Many public agencies offer classes in the techniques of mouth-to-mouth respiration and cardiac massage to revive people experiencing respiratory or cardiac arrest. This technique is known as **cardiopulmonary resuscitation,** or **CPR.** These classes also include instruction in emergency airway clearance using abdominal thrusts (Heimlich maneuver), chest thrusts, or back blows to open obstructed airways.

Disease in Context revisited

▶ Emily's Asthma

It had been about a month since Emily's appointment with Dr. Martinez. During that time, her parents had monitored her breathing very carefully and had noticed patterns in her coughing bouts. "It does seem that Emily gets out of breath sooner than the other kids when she exercises," Emily's mother reported to Dr. Martinez during her follow-up appointment. "And now that the weather has cooled off, I do notice that she coughs more," continued Nicole.

"Let's take a listen to Emily's lungs," replied the doctor as he placed his stethoscope on the little girl's chest. "Yes," he continued, "I hear wheezing today, which suggests that Emily's airways are narrowed. Based on this finding, your observations, and the family history, I think Emily has asthma."

Although Nicole had expected the doctor's diagnosis, it was still a shock to hear him say it. Seeing her look of alarm, Dr. Martinez continued, "Most kids with asthma lead very normal, active lives. The medications available today target asthma right at its source—inflammation. In fact, with proper treatment, many kids maintain near-normal pulmonary function. Let's start with an oral antileukotriene medication that Emily will take daily to control airway inflammation. If, after a few weeks, we don't see any improvement, we'll supplement her treatment with an anti-inflammatory in the form of a low-dose corticosteroid inhaler. I'm also going to prescribe an inhaler to use if Emily has a severe asthma episode. The inhaler contains a medication that relaxes the smooth muscle of her airways, giving her short-term relief of symptoms."

In this case, we learned that Emily's asthma was caused by airway inflammation. Medications that limit the inflammatory response in the respiratory passages can prevent the symptoms of asthma. For a review of the role of inflammation in normal body defense mechanisms, see Chapter 17.

18

Word Anatomy

Medical terms are built from standardized word parts (prefixes, roots, and suffixes). Learning the meanings of these parts can help you remember words and interpret unfamiliar terms.

WORD PART	MEANING	EXAMPLE
The Respiratory System		
nas/o	nose	The *nasopharynx* is behind the nasal cavity.
or/o	mouth	The *oropharynx* is behind the mouth.
laryng/o	larynx	The *laryngeal* pharynx opens into the larynx.
pleur/o	side, rib	The *pleura* covers the lung and lines the chest wall (rib cage).
The Process of Respiration		
spir/o	breathing	A *spirometer* is an instrument used to record breathing volumes.
capn/o	carbon dioxide	*Hypercapnia* is a rise in the blood level of carbon dioxide.
-pnea	breathing	*Hypopnea* is a decrease in the rate and depth of breathing.
orth/o-	straight	*Orthopnea* can be relieved by sitting in an upright position.
Disorders of the Respiratory System		
pneumon/o	lung	*Pneumonia* is inflammation of the lung.
atel/o	incomplete	*Atelectasis* is incomplete expansion of the lung.
pneum/o	air, gas	*Pneumothorax* is accumulation of air in the pleural space.
–centesis	tapping, perforation	In *thoracentesis* a needle is inserted into the pleural space to remove fluid.

Summary

I. **PHASES OF RESPIRATION**
   A. Pulmonary ventilation
   B. External gas exchange
   C. Internal gas exchange
II. **THE RESPIRATORY SYSTEM**
   A. Nasal cavities—filter, warm, and moisten air
   B. Pharynx (throat)—carries air into respiratory tract and food into digestive tract
   C. Larynx (voice box)—contains vocal cords
      1. Glottis—space between the vocal cords
      2. Epiglottis—covers larynx on swallowing to help prevent food from entering
   D. Trachea (windpipe)
   E. Bronchi—branches of trachea that enter lungs and then subdivide
      1. Bronchioles—smallest subdivisions

F. Lungs
   1. Organs of gas exchange
   2. Lobes—three on right; two on left
   3. Alveoli
      a. Tiny air sacs where gases are exchanged
      b. Surfactant—reduces surface tension in alveoli; eases expansion of lungs
   4. Pleura—membrane that encloses the lung
      a. Visceral pleura—attached to surface of lung
      b. Parietal pleura—attached to chest wall
      c. Pleural space—between layers
   5. Mediastinum—space and organs between lungs
III. **THE PROCESS OF RESPIRATION**
   A. Pulmonary ventilation
      1. Inhalation—drawing of air into lungs

a. Compliance—ease with which lungs and thorax can be expanded
2. Exhalation—expulsion of air from lungs
3. Lung volumes—used to evaluate respiratory function
B. Gas exchange
1. Gases diffuse from area of higher concentration to area of lower concentration
2. In lungs—oxygen enters blood and carbon dioxide leaves (external exchange)
3. In tissues—oxygen leaves blood and carbon dioxide enters (internal exchange)
C. Oxygen transport
1. Almost totally bound to heme portion of hemoglobin in red blood cells
2. Separates from hemoglobin when oxygen concentration is low (in tissues)
a. Carbon monoxide replaces oxygen on hemoglobin
D. Carbon dioxide transport
1. Most carried as bicarbonate ion
2. Regulates pH of blood
E. Regulation of respiration
1. Nervous control—centers in medulla and pons
2. Chemical control
a. Central chemoreceptors respond to CO_2, which decreases pH
b. Peripheral chemorecptors—respond to low levels of O_2
F. Abnormal ventilation
1. Hyperventilation—rapid, deep respiration
2. Hypoventilation—inadequate air in alveoli
G. Breathing patterns
1. Normal—12 to 20 breaths per minute in adult
2. Types of altered breathing
a. Hyperpnea—increase in depth and rate of breathing
b. Tachypnea—excessive rate of breathing

c. Apnea—temporary cessation of breathing
d. Dyspnea—difficulty in breathing
e. Orthopnea—difficulty relieved by upright position
f. Kussmaul—characterizes acidosis
g. Cheyne-Stokes—irregularity found in critically ill
3. Possible results—cyanosis, hypoxia (anoxia), hypoxemia, suffocation
IV. **DISORDERS OF THE RESPIRATORY SYSTEM**
A. Disorders of the nasal cavities and related structures—sinusitis, polyps, deviated septum, nosebleed (epistaxis)
B. Infection—colds, RSV, croup, influenza, pneumonia, tuberculosis
C. Hay fever and asthma—hypersensitivity (allergy)
D. COPD—involves emphysema and bronchitis
E. SIDS—sudden infant death syndrome
F. Respiratory distress syndrome (RDS)
1. Acute (ARDS)—due to other medical problem or direct injury to lung
2. RDS of newborn—due to lack of surfactant
G. Cancer—smoking a major causative factor
H. Disorders involving the pleural space
1. Pleurisy—inflammation of pleura
2. Pneumothorax—air in pleural space
3. Hemothorax—blood in pleural space
V. **AGE AND THE RESPIRATORY TRACT**
VI. **SPECIAL EQUIPMENT FOR RESPIRATORY TREATMENT**
A. Bronchoscope—tube used to examine air passageways and remove foreign bodies
B. Oxygen therapy
C. Suction apparatus—removes mucus and other substances
D. Tracheostomy—artificial airway
a. Tracheotomy—incision into trachea
E. Artificial respiration—cardiopulmonary resuscitation (CPR)

Questions for Study and Review

BUILDING UNDERSTANDING

Fill in the blanks

1. The exchange of air between the atmosphere and the lungs is called _____.
2. The space between the vocal cords is the _____.
3. The ease with which the lungs and thorax can be expanded is termed _____.

4. A lower than normal level of oxygen in the tissues is called _____.
5. Inflammation of the pleura is termed _____.

Matching > Match each numbered item with the most closely related lettered item.

___ **6.** A decrease in the rate and depth of breathing

___ **7.** An increase in the rate and depth of breathing

___ **8.** A temporary cessation of breathing

___ **9.** Difficult or labored breathing

___ **10.** Difficult breathing that is relieved by sitting up

a. dyspnea

b. hyperpnea

c. orthopnea

d. hypopnea

e. apnea

Multiple choice

___ **11.** The bony projections in the nasal cavities that increase surface area are called

    a. nares

    b. septae

    c. conchae

    d. sinuses

___ **12.** Which of the following structures produces speech?

    a. pharynx

    b. larynx

    c. trachea

    d. lungs

___ **13.** The leaf-shaped cartilage that covers the larynx during swallowing is the

    a. epiglottis

    b. glottis

    c. conchae

    d. sinus

___ **14.** Respiration is centrally regulated by the

    a. cerebral cortex

    b. diencephalon

    c. brain stem

    d. cerebellum

___ **15.** Incomplete expansion of a lung or portion of a lung is called

    a. effusion

    b. adhesion

    c. epistaxis

    d. atelectasis

UNDERSTANDING CONCEPTS

16. Differentiate between the terms in each of the following pairs:

    a. internal and external gas exchange

    b. pleura and diaphragm

    c. inhalation and exhalation

    d. spirometer and spirogram

17. Trace the path of air from the nostrils to the lung capillaries.

18. What is the function of the cilia on cells that line the respiratory passageways?

19. Compare and contrast the transport of oxygen and carbon dioxide in the blood.

20. Define hyperventilation and hypoventilation. What is the effect of each on blood CO_2 levels and blood pH?

21. What are chemoreceptors and how do they function to regulate breathing?

22. Describe the structural and functional changes that occur in the respiratory system in chronic obstructive pulmonary disease.

23. Compare and contrast the following disease conditions:

    a. Kussmaul and Cheyne-Stokes respiration

    b. acute coryza and influenza

    c. bronchopneumonia and lobar pneumonia

    d. pneumothorax and hemat[h]orax

CONCEPTUAL THINKING

24. Jake, a sometimes exasperating 4-year-old, threatens his mother that he will hold his breath until "he dies." Should his mother be concerned that he might succeed?

25. Why is it important that airplane interiors are pressurized? If the cabin lost pressure, what physiological adaptations to respiration might occur in the passengers?

26. In Emily's case, an anti-inflammatory medication was used to control her asthma symptoms. Explain how this drug works in the respiratory system.

18

The Digestive System

Learning Outcomes

After careful study of this chapter, you should be able to:

1. Name the three main functions of the digestive system
2. Describe the four layers of the digestive tract wall
3. Differentiate between the two layers of the peritoneum
4. Name and locate the different types of teeth
5. Name and describe the functions of the organs of the digestive tract
6. Name and describe the functions of the accessory organs of digestion
7. Describe how bile functions in digestion
8. Name and locate the ducts that carry bile from the liver into the digestive tract
9. Explain the role of enzymes in digestion and give examples of enzymes
10. Name the digestion products of fats, proteins, and carbohydrates
11. Define *absorption*
12. Define *villi* and state how villi function in absorption
13. Explain the use of feedback in regulating digestion and give several examples
14. List several hormones involved in regulating digestion
15. Describe common disorders of the digestive tract and the accessory organs
16. Show how word parts are used to build words related to digestion (see Word Anatomy at the end of the chapter)

Selected Key Terms

The following terms and other boldface terms in the chapter are defined in the Glossary

absorption
bile
chyle
chyme
defecation
deglutition
digestion
duodenum
emulsify
enzyme
esophagus
gallbladder
hydrolysis
intestine
lacteal
liver
mastication
pancreas
peristalsis
peritoneum
saliva
stomach
ulcer
villi

Disease in Context

► Adam's Case: The Picture of Health

Adam was okay with everything his family doctor had described about his routine physical examination. "We'll draw some blood for testing," Dr. Michaels explained. "You didn't have anything to eat since last night, did you? We'll send your specimen to the lab to get information on your blood cells and blood chemistry, hemoglobin, lipoproteins, and such. You need to leave a urine sample to check for sugar, and then Annette will take your blood pressure and run an ECG. I'll be in to ask you some general questions and do some 'hands-on' examination, including, of course, a check on your prostate. And, Adam, since you are well past your 50th birthday, you need to stop stalling on getting that colonoscopy."

Sending in the stool sample later to test for signs of blood wasn't a problem for Adam, and he could live with the prostate exam, but he wasn't so happy about the colonoscopy! He had heard that the prep to clean out the colon was unpleasant. "You know," Adam protested, "I'm healthy and have no family history of colon cancer or polyps, so why do I need to do this?"

"Actually," replied Dr. Michaels, "most colorectal cancers appear in people with no symptoms and with no family history or genetic predisposition. In that higher risk population, we recommend earlier and more frequent testing. There is a new 'virtual colonoscopy' procedure that uses computerized x-rays instead of an endoscope to generate detailed images of the colon, but for a baseline study, your proctologist might prefer the routine method. Besides, if we have to remove any polyps or other abnormal tissue, we'd have to resort to that anyway. When you're ready to leave the office, ask Jean at the front desk to set up an appointment for you."

As part of Adam's physical, the doctor examined many of Adam's organ systems, including his digestive system. Because of his age, the doctor recommended a closer inspection of Adam's colon. In this chapter, we'll learn about the digestive tract and the accessory organs that contribute to digestion. We'll also visit Adam again and find out how the colonoscopy went!

Function and Design of the Digestive System

Every body cell needs a constant supply of nutrients. The energy contained in these nutrients is used to do cell work. In addition, the cell rearranges the nutrients' chemical building blocks to manufacture cellular materials for metabolism, growth, and repair. Food as we take it in, however, is too large to enter the cells. It must first be broken down into particles small enough to pass through the cells' plasma membrane. This breakdown process is known as **digestion**.

After digestion, the circulation must carry nutrients to the cells in every part of the body. The transfer of nutrients into the circulation is called **absorption**. Finally, undigested waste material must be eliminated. Digestion, absorption, and elimination are the three chief functions of the digestive system.

For our purposes, the digestive system may be divided into two groups of organs:

- The **digestive tract**, a continuous passageway beginning at the mouth, where food is taken in, and terminating at the anus, where the solid waste products of digestion are expelled from the body.

- The **accessory organs**, which are necessary for the digestive process but are not a direct part of the digestive tract. They release substances into the digestive tract through ducts. These organs are the salivary glands, liver, gallbladder, and pancreas.

Before describing the individual organs of the digestive tract, we will pause to discuss the general structure of these organs. We will also describe the large membrane (peritoneum) that lines the abdominopelvic cavity, which contains most of the digestive organs.

CHECKPOINT 19-1 ➤ Why does food have to be digested before cells can use it?

The Wall of the Digestive Tract

Although modified for specific tasks in different organs, the wall of the digestive tract, from the esophagus to the anus, is similar in structure throughout. The general pattern consists of four layers, which are, from innermost to outermost:

1. Mucous membrane
2. Submucosa
3. Smooth muscle
4. Serous membrane

Refer to the diagram of the small intestine in Figure 19-1 as we describe the individual layers of this wall in greater detail.

First is the **mucous membrane**, or **mucosa**, so called because its epithelial layer contains many mucus-secreting cells. From the mouth through the esophagus, and also in the anus, the epithelium consists of multiple layers of squamous (flat) cells, which help to protect deeper tissues.

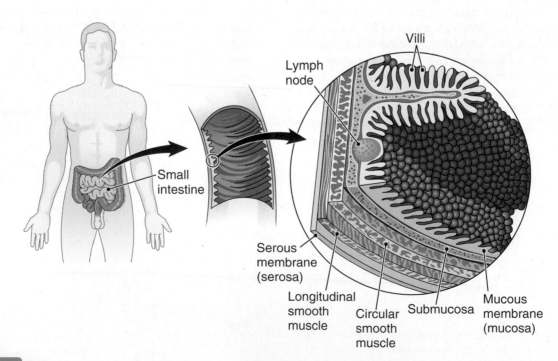

Figure 19-1 **Wall of the digestive tract.** The mucous membrane of the small intestine shown here has numerous projections called villi.

[ZOOMING IN ➤ What type of tissue is between the submucosa and the serous membrane in the digestive tract wall? **]**

Throughout the remainder of the digestive tract, the type of epithelium in the mucosa is simple columnar. Many of the cells that secrete digestive juices are located in the mucosa. Figure 19-2 is a microscopic view of a representative section of the digestive tract taken from the small intestine. Mucus-secreting cells (goblet cells) appear as clear areas between epithelial cells. Note that the small intestine's lining has fingerlike extensions (villi) that aid in the absorption of nutrients, as will be described later.

The layer of connective tissue beneath the mucosa is the **submucosa**, which contains blood vessels and some of the nerves that help regulate digestive activity. In the small intestine, the submucosa has many glands that produce mucus to protect that organ from the highly acidic material it receives from the stomach.

The next layer is composed of **smooth muscle**. Most of the digestive organs have two layers of smooth muscle: an inner layer of circular fibers, and an outer layer of longitudinal fibers. When a section of the circular muscle contracts, the organ's lumen narrows; when the longitudinal muscle contracts, a section of the wall shortens and the lu-

men becomes wider. These alternating muscular contractions create the wavelike movement, called **peristalsis** (per-ih-STAL-sis), that propels food through the digestive tract and mixes it with digestive juices.

The esophagus differs slightly from this pattern in having striated muscle in its upper portion, and the stomach has an additional third layer of smooth muscle in its wall to add strength for churning food.

The digestive organs in the abdominopelvic cavity have an outermost layer of **serous membrane**, or **serosa**, a thin, moist tissue composed of simple squamous epithelium and loose connective tissue. This membrane forms part of the **peritoneum** (per-ih-to-NE-um). The esophagus above the diaphragm has instead an outer layer composed of fibrous connective tissue.

CHECKPOINT **19-2** ➤ The digestive tract has a wall that is basically similar throughout its length and is composed of four layers. What are the typical four layers of this wall?

The Peritoneum

The abdominopelvic cavity is lined with a thin, shiny serous membrane that also folds back to cover most of the organs contained within the cavity (Fig. 19-3). The outer portion of this membrane, the layer that lines the cavity, is called the **parietal** (pah-RI-eh-tal) **peritoneum**; that covering the organs is called the **visceral** (VIS-eh-ral) **peritoneum**. This slippery membrane allows the organs to slide over each other as they function. The peritoneum also carries blood vessels, lymphatic vessels, and nerves. In some places, it supports the organs and binds them to each other. The peritoneal cavity is the potential space between the membrane's two layers and contains serous fluid (peritoneal fluid). The greater peritoneal cavity is the main portion, located in the abdominal cavity and extending into the pelvic cavity (see Fig. 19-3). The lesser peritoneal cavity is formed by a smaller extension of these membranes dorsal to the stomach, extending dorsal to the liver to the posterior attachment of the diaphragm. Subdivisions of the peritoneum around the various organs have special names.

SUBDIVISIONS OF THE PERITONEUM The **mesentery** (MES-en-ter-e) is a double-layered portion of the peritoneum shaped somewhat like a fan. The handle portion is attached to the posterior abdominal wall, and the expanded long edge is attached to the small intestine. Between the two membranous layers of the mesentery are the vessels and nerves that supply the intestine. The section of the peritoneum that extends from the colon to the posterior abdominal wall is the **mesocolon** (mes-o-KO-lon).

19

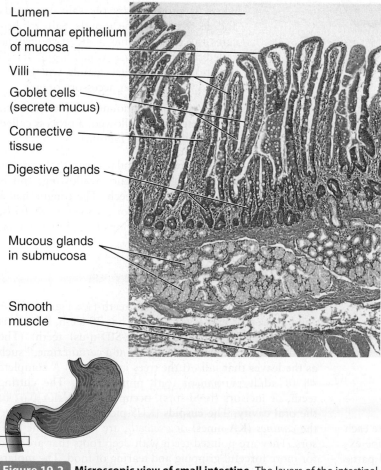

Lumen
Columnar epithelium of mucosa
Villi
Goblet cells (secrete mucus)
Connective tissue
Digestive glands
Mucous glands in submucosa
Smooth muscle

Figure 19-2 **Microscopic view of small intestine.** The layers of the intestinal wall are visible (except for the serous membrane). (Micrograph reprinted with permission from Cormack DH. *Essential Histology*, 2nd ed. Philadelphia: Lippincott Williams & Wilkins, 2001.)

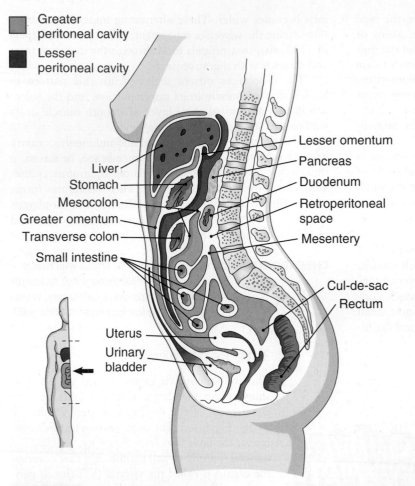

Greater peritoneal cavity

Lesser peritoneal cavity

Liver
Stomach
Mesocolon
Greater omentum
Transverse colon
Small intestine

Lesser omentum
Pancreas
Duodenum
Retroperitoneal space
Mesentery

Cul-de-sac
Rectum

Uterus
Urinary bladder

Figure19-3 **The abdominopelvic cavity.** Subdivisions of the peritoneum fold over, supporting and separating individual organs. [**ZOOMING IN ➤** What part of the peritoneum is around the small intestine?]

A large double layer of the peritoneum containing much fat hangs like an apron over the front of the intestine. This **greater omentum** (o-MEN-tum) extends from the lower border of the stomach into the pelvic cavity and then loops back up to the transverse colon. A smaller membrane, called the **lesser omentum**, extends between the stomach and the liver.

CHECKPOINT **19-3** ➤ What is the name of the large serous membrane that lines the abdominopelvic cavity and covers the organs it contains?

Organs of the Digestive Tract

As we study the organs of the digestive system, locate each in Figure 19-4. The digestive tract is a muscular tube extending through the body. It is composed of several parts: the **mouth, pharynx, esophagus, stomach, small intestine,** and **large intestine.** The digestive tract is sometimes called the alimentary tract, from the word *aliment,* meaning "food." It is more commonly referred to as the **gastroin-**

testinal **(GI)** tract because of the major importance of the stomach and intestine in the digestive process.

The next section describes the structure and function of each digestive organ. These descriptions are followed by an overview of how the organs work together in digestion. See Appendix 7 for a dissection photograph showing the digestive organs in place.

The Mouth

The **mouth,** also called the **oral cavity,** is where a substance begins its travels through the digestive tract (Fig. 19-5). The mouth has the following digestive functions:

- It receives food, a process called **ingestion.**

- It breaks food into small portions. This is done mainly by the teeth in the process of chewing or **mastication** (mas-tih-KA-shun), but the tongue, cheeks, and lips are also used.

- It mixes the food with **saliva** (sah-LI-vah), which is produced by the salivary glands and secreted into the mouth. Saliva lubricates the food and has a digestive enzyme called *salivary amylase,* which begins starch digestion. The salivary glands will be described with the other accessory organs.

- It moves proper amounts of food toward the throat to be swallowed, a process called **deglutition** (deg-lu-TISH-un).

The tongue, a muscular organ that projects into the mouth, aids in chewing and swallowing, and is one of the principal organs of speech. The tongue has a number of special surface receptors, called *taste buds,* which can differentiate taste sensations (e.g., bitter, sweet, sour, or salty) (see Chapter 11).

The Teeth

The oral cavity also contains the teeth (see Fig. 19-5). A child between 2 and 6 years of age has 20 teeth, known as the baby teeth or **deciduous** (de-SID-u-us) teeth. (The word deciduous means "falling off at a certain time," such as the leaves that fall off the trees in autumn.) A complete set of adult permanent teeth numbers 32. The cutting teeth, or **incisors** (in-SI-sors), occupy the anterior part of the oral cavity. The **cuspids** (KUS-pids), commonly called the *canines* (KA-nines) or *eyeteeth,* are lateral to the incisors. They are pointed teeth with deep roots that are used for more forceful gripping and tearing of food. The **molars** (MO-lars), the larger grinding teeth, are posterior. There are two premolars and three molars. In an adult, each quadrant (quarter) of the mouth, moving from anterior to posterior, has two incisors, one cuspid, and five molars.

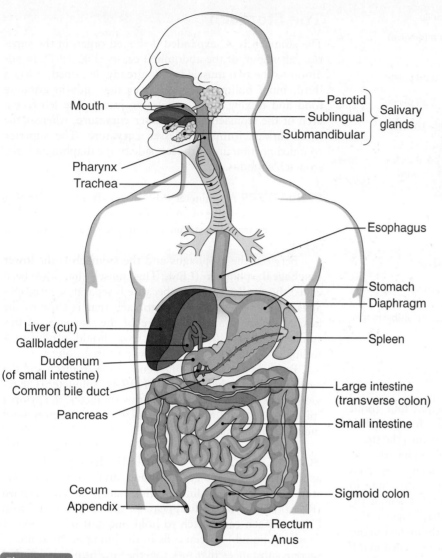

Mouth

Parotid
Sublingual
Submandibular
} Salivary glands

Pharynx

Trachea

Esophagus

Stomach
Diaphragm

Liver (cut)
Gallbladder

Spleen

Duodenum
(of small intestine)

Common bile duct

Large intestine
(transverse colon)

Pancreas

Small intestine

Cecum
Appendix

Sigmoid colon

Rectum
Anus

Figure 19-4 **The digestive system.** The figure also shows nearby structures for orientation. **[ZOOMING IN ➤** What accessory organs of digestion secrete into the mouth? **]**

The first eight deciduous (baby) teeth to appear through the gums are the incisors. Later, the cuspids and molars appear. Usually, the 20 baby teeth all have appeared by the time a child has reached the age of 2 to 3 years. During the first 2 years, the permanent teeth develop within the upper jaw (maxilla) and lower jaw (mandible) from buds that are present at birth. The first permanent teeth to appear are the four 6-year molars, which come in before any baby teeth are lost. Because decay and infection of deciduous molars may spread to new, permanent teeth, deciduous teeth need proper care.

As a child grows, the jawbones grow, making space for additional teeth. After the 6-year molars have appeared, the baby incisors loosen and are replaced by permanent incisors. Next, the baby canines (cuspids) are replaced by permanent canines, and finally, the baby molars are replaced by the permanent bicuspids (premolars).

At this point, the larger jawbones are ready for the appearance of the 12-year, or second, permanent molar teeth. During or after the late teens, the third molars, or so-called *wisdom teeth*, may appear. In some cases, the jaw is not large enough for these teeth, or there are other abnormalities, so that the third molars may not erupt or may have to be removed. Figure 19-6 shows the parts of a molar.

The main substance of the tooth is **dentin**, a calcified substance harder than bone. Within the tooth is a soft pulp containing blood vessels and nerves. The tooth's crown projects above the gum, the **gingiva** (JIN-jih-vah), and is covered with **enamel**, the hardest substance in the body. The roots of the tooth, below the gum line in a bony socket, are covered with a rigid connective tissue (cementum) that helps to hold the tooth in place. Each root has a canal containing extensions of the pulp.

The Pharynx

The **pharynx** (FAR-inks) is commonly referred to as the throat (see Fig. 19-5). The oral part of the pharynx, the oropharynx, is visible when you look into an open mouth and depress the tongue. The palatine tonsils may be seen at either side of the oropharynx. The pharynx also extends upward to the nasal cavity, where it is referred to as the nasopharynx and downward to the larynx, where it is called the laryngeal pharynx. The **soft palate** is tissue that forms the posterior roof of the oral cavity. From it hangs a soft, fleshy, V-shaped mass called the **uvula** (U-vu-lah).

In swallowing, the tongue pushes a **bolus** (BO-lus) of food, a small portion of chewed food mixed with saliva, into the pharynx. Once the food reaches the pharynx, swallowing occurs rapidly by an involuntary reflex action. At the same time, the soft palate and uvula are raised to prevent food and liquid from entering the nasal cavity, and the tongue is raised to seal the back of the oral cavity. The entrance of the trachea is guarded during swallowing by a leaf-shaped cartilage, the **epiglottis**, which covers the opening of the larynx. The swallowed food is then moved into the esophagus.

19

PASSport to Success

Visit *thePoint* or see the Student Resource CD in the back of this book for information on dental hygienists and their role in maintaining the health of the teeth and gums.

CHECKPOINT 19-4 ➤ How many baby teeth are there and what is the scientific name for the baby teeth?

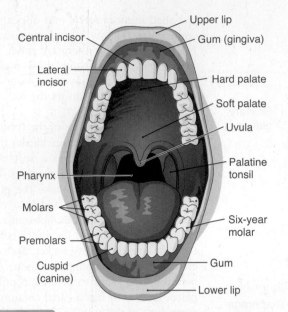

Figure 19-5 **The mouth.** The teeth and tonsils are visible in this view.

The Esophagus

The **esophagus** (eh-SOF-ah-gus) is a muscular tube about 25 cm (10 inches) long. In the esophagus, food is lubricated with mucus and moved by peristalsis into the stomach. No additional digestion occurs in the esophagus.

Before joining the stomach, the esophagus must pass through the diaphragm. It travels through an opening in the diaphragm called the **esophageal hiatus** (eh-sof-ah-JE-al hi-A-tus). If there is a weakness in the diaphragm at this point, a portion of the stomach or other abdominal organ may protrude through the space, a condition called *hiatal hernia*.

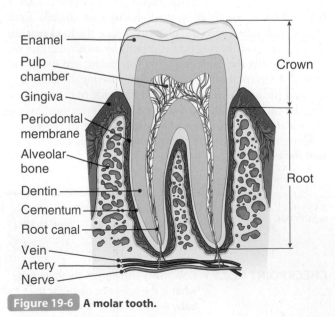

Figure 19-6 **A molar tooth.**

The Stomach

The stomach is an expanded J-shaped organ in the superior left region of the abdominal cavity (Fig. 19-7). In addition to the two muscle layers already described, it has a third, inner oblique (angled) layer that aids in grinding food and mixing it with digestive juices. The left-facing arch of the stomach is the **greater curvature**, whereas the right surface forms the **lesser curvature**. The superior rounded portion under the left side of the diaphragm is the stomach's **fundus**.

SPHINCTERS A sphincter (SFINK-ter) is a muscular ring that regulates the size of an opening. There are two sphincters that separate the stomach from the organs above and below.

Between the esophagus and the stomach is the **lower esophageal sphincter (LES)**. This muscle has also been called the **cardiac sphincter** because it separates the esophagus from the region of the stomach that is close to the heart. We are sometimes aware of the existence of this sphincter when it does not relax as it should, producing a feeling of being unable to swallow past that point.

Between the distal, or far, end of the stomach and the small intestine is the **pyloric** (pi-LOR-ik) **sphincter**. The region of the stomach leading into this sphincter, the **pylorus** (pi-LOR-us), is important in regulating how rapidly food moves into the small intestine.

FUNCTIONS OF THE STOMACH The stomach serves as a storage pouch, digestive organ, and churn. When the stomach is empty, the lining forms many folds called **rugae** (RU-je). These folds disappear as the stomach expands. (The stomach can stretch to hold one half of a gallon of food and liquid.) Special cells in the lining of the stomach secrete substances that mix together to form gastric juice. Some of the cells secrete a great amount of mucus to protect the stomach lining from digestive secretions. Other cells produce the active components of the gastric juice, which are:

- Hydrochloric acid (HCl), a strong acid that helps break down protein and destroys foreign organisms.

- Pepsin, a protein-digesting enzyme produced in an inactive form and activated only when food enters the stomach and HCl is produced.

Chyme (*kime*), from a Greek word meaning "juice," is the highly acidic, semiliquid mixture of gastric juice and food that leaves the stomach to enter the small intestine.

CHECKPOINT 19-5 ➤ What type of food is digested in the stomach?

The Small Intestine

The small intestine is the longest part of the digestive tract (Fig. 19-8). It is known as the small intestine because, although it is longer than the large intestine, it is smaller in di-

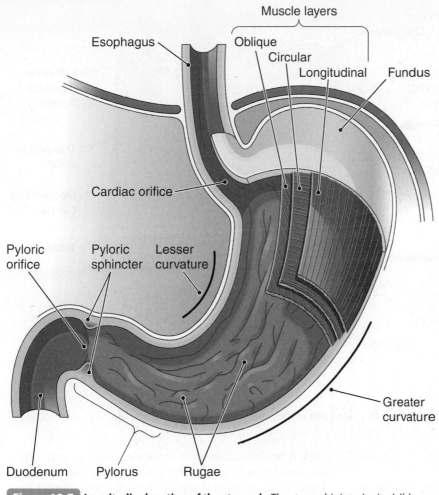

Most absorption of digested food, water, and minerals also occurs through the walls of the small intestine. To increase the organ's surface area for this purpose, the mucosa is formed into millions of tiny, fingerlike projections, called **villi** (VIL-li) (Fig. 19-9), which give the inner surface a velvety appearance (see also Figs. 19-1 and 19-2). The epithelial cells of the villi also have small projecting folds of the plasma membrane known as **microvilli**. These create a remarkable increase in the total surface area available for absorption in the small intestine.

Each villus contains blood vessels through which most digestion products are absorbed into the blood. Each one also contains a specialized lymphatic capillary called a **lacteal** (LAK-tele) through which fats are absorbed into the lymph. Box 19-1, The Folded Intestine, provides more information on the relationship of surface area to absorption.

The Large Intestine

The large intestine is approximately 6.5 cm (2.5 inches) in diameter and approximately 1.5 m (5 feet) long (see Fig. 19-8). It is named for its wide diameter, rather than its length. The outer longitudinal muscle fibers in its wall form three separate surface bands (see Fig. 19-8). These bands, known as **teniae** (TEN-e-e) **coli**, draw up the organ's wall to give it its distinctive puckered appearance. (Spelling is also *taeniae*; the singular is *tenia* or *taenia*).

Visit **thePoint** or see the Student Resource CD in the back of this book for a photomicrograph of a villus showing a lacteal.

CHECKPOINT 19-6 ➤ What are the three divisions of the small intestine?

CHECKPOINT 19-7 ➤ How does the small intestine function in the digestive process?

SUBDIVISIONS OF THE LARGE INTESTINE The large intestine begins in the lower right region of the abdomen. The first part is a small pouch called the **cecum** (SE-kum). Between the ileum of the small intestine and the cecum is a sphincter, the **ileocecal** (il-e-o-SE-kal) **valve**, that prevents food from traveling backward into the small intestine. Attached to the cecum is a small, blind tube containing lymphoid tissue; its full name is **vermiform** (VER-mih-

Figure 19-7 **Longitudinal section of the stomach.** The stomach's interior is visible, along with a portion of the esophagus and the duodenum. [**ZOOMING IN** ➤ What additional muscle layer is in the wall of the stomach that is not found in the rest of the digestive tract?]

ameter, with an average width of approximately 2.5 cm (1 inch). After death, when relaxed to its full length, the small intestine is approximately 6 m (20 feet) long. In life, the small intestine averages 3 m (10 feet) in length. The first 25 cm (10 inches) or so of the small intestine make up the **duodenum** (du-o-DE-num) (named for the Latin word for "twelve," based on its length of twelve finger widths). Beyond the duodenum are two more divisions: the **jejunum** (je-JU-num), which forms the next two-fifths of the small intestine, and the **ileum** (IL-e-um), which constitutes the remaining portion.

FUNCTIONS OF THE SMALL INTESTINE The duodenal mucosa and submucosa contain glands that secrete large amounts of mucus to protect the small intestine from the strongly acidic chyme entering from the stomach. Mucosal cells of the small intestine also secrete enzymes that digest proteins and carbohydrates. In addition, digestive juices from the liver and pancreas enter the small intestine through a small opening in the duodenum. Most digestion takes place in the small intestine under the effects of these juices.

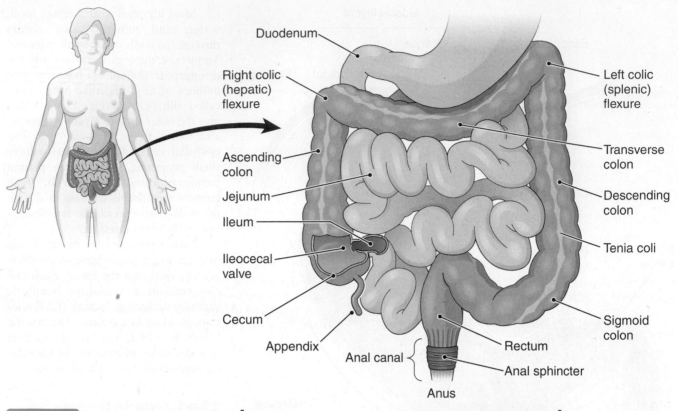

Figure 19-8 labels: Duodenum, Right colic (hepatic) flexure, Ascending colon, Jejunum, Ileum, Ileocecal valve, Cecum, Appendix, Anal canal, Left colic (splenic) flexure, Transverse colon, Descending colon, Tenia coli, Sigmoid colon, Rectum, Anal sphincter, Anus

Figure 19-8 **The small and large intestines.** [**ZOOMING IN** ➤ What part of the small intestine joins the cecum?]

form) **appendix** (*vermiform* means "wormlike"), but usually just "appendix" is used.

The second portion, the **ascending colon**, extends superiorly along the right side of the abdomen toward the

Figure 19-9 labels: Villus, Lacteal, Epithelium, Vein, Capillary, Artery, Small intestine

Figure 19-9 **A villus of the small intestine.** Each villus has blood vessels and a lacteal (lymphatic capillary) for absorption of nutrients.

liver. It bends near the liver at the right colic (hepatic) flexure and extends across the abdomen as the **transverse colon**. It bends again sharply at the left colic (splenic) flexure and extends inferiorly on the left side of the abdomen into the pelvis, forming the **descending colon**. The distal colon bends backward into an **S** shape forming the **sigmoid colon** (named for the Greek letter *sigma*), which continues downward to empty into the **rectum**, a temporary storage area for indigestible or nonabsorbable food residue (see Fig. 19-8). The narrow terminal portion of the large intestine is the **anal canal**, which leads to the outside of the body through an opening called the **anus** (A-nus).

FUNCTIONS OF THE LARGE INTESTINE The large intestine secretes a great quantity of mucus, but no enzymes. Food is not digested in this organ, but some water is reabsorbed, and undigested food is stored, formed into solid waste material, called **feces** (FE-seze) or stool, and then eliminated.

At intervals, usually after meals, the involuntary muscles within the walls of the large intestine propel solid waste toward the rectum. Stretching of the rectum stimulates contraction of smooth muscle in the rectal wall. Aided by voluntary contractions of the diaphragm and the abdominal muscles, the feces are eliminated from the body in a process called **defecation** (def-e-KA-shun). An anal sphincter provides voluntary control over defecation (see Fig. 19-8).

While food residue is stored in the large intestine, bacteria that normally live in the colon act on it to produce

Box 19-1   A Closer Look

The Folded Intestine: More Absorption With Less Length

Whenever materials pass from one system to another, they must travel through a cellular membrane. A major factor in how much transport can occur per unit of time is the total surface area of the membrane; the greater the surface area, the higher the rate of transport. The problem of packing a large amount of surface into a small space is solved in the body by folding the membranes. We do the same thing in everyday life. Imagine trying to store a bed sheet in the closet without folding it!

In the small intestine, where digested food must absorb into the bloodstream, there is folding of membranes down to the level of single cells.

- The 6-meter-long organ is coiled to fit into the abdominal cavity.

- The inner wall of the organ is thrown into circular folds called plicae circulares, which not only increase surface area, but aid in mixing.
- The mucosal villi project into the lumen, providing more surface area than a flat membrane would.
- The individual cells that line the small intestine have microvilli, tiny fingerlike folds of the plasma membrane that increase surface area tremendously.

Together, these structural features of the small intestine result in an absorptive surface area estimated to be about 250 square meters! Folding is present in other parts of the digestive system and in other areas of the body as well. Can you name other systems that show this folding pattern?

---

vitamin K and some of the B-complex vitamins. As mentioned, systemic antibiotic therapy may destroy these symbiotic (helpful) bacteria living in the large intestine, causing undesirable side effects.

CHECKPOINT 19-8 ➤ What are the divisions of the large intestine?

CHECKPOINT 19-9 ➤ What are the functions of the large intestine?

The Accessory Organs

The accessory organs (Fig. 19-10) release secretions through ducts into the digestive tract. The salivary glands deliver their secretions into the mouth. All of the other accessory organs release secretions into the duodenum.

The Salivary Glands

While food is in the mouth, it is mixed with **saliva** (sah-LI-vah), which moistens the food and facilitates mastication (chewing) and deglutition (swallowing). Saliva helps to keep the teeth and mouth clean. It also contains some antibodies and an enzyme (lysozyme) that help reduce bacterial growth.

This watery mixture contains mucus and an enzyme called **salivary amylase** (AM-ih-laze), which begins the

digestive process by converting starch to sugar. Saliva is manufactured by three pairs of glands (see Fig. 19-4):

- The **parotid** (pah-ROT-id) **glands,** the largest of the group, are located inferior and anterior to the ear.

- The **submandibular** (sub-man-DIB-u-lar), or **submaxillary** (sub-MAK-sih-ler-e), **glands** are located near the body of the lower jaw.

- The **sublingual** (sub-LING-gwal) **glands** are under the tongue.

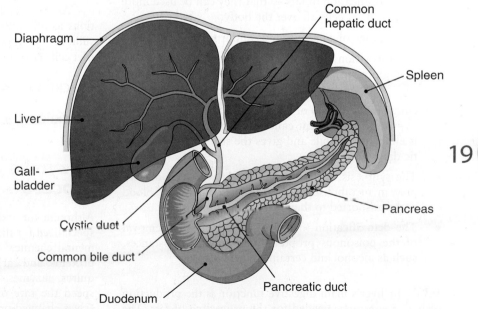

Figure 19-10 **Accessory organs of digestion.** [**ZOOMING IN** ➤ Into what part of the intestine do these accessory organs secrete?]

All these glands empty through ducts into the oral cavity.

The Liver

The **liver** (LIV-er), often referred to by the word root *hepat*, is the body's largest glandular organ (see Fig. 19-10). It is located in the superior right portion of the abdominal cavity under the dome of the diaphragm. The lower edge of a normal-sized liver is level with the lower margin of the ribs. The human liver is the same reddish brown color as animal liver seen in the supermarket. It has a large right lobe and a smaller left lobe; the right lobe includes two inferior smaller lobes. The liver is supplied with blood through two vessels: the portal vein and the hepatic artery (the portal system and blood supply to the liver were described in Chapter 15). These vessels deliver about 1.5 quarts (1.6 L) of blood to the liver every minute. The hepatic artery carries oxygenated blood, whereas the venous portal system carries blood that is rich in digestive end products. This most remarkable organ has many functions that affect digestion, metabolism, blood composition, and elimination of waste. Some of its major activities are:

- The manufacture of **bile**, a substance needed for the digestion of fats.
- The storage of glucose (a simple sugar) in the form of **glycogen**, the animal equivalent of the starch found in plants. When the blood sugar level falls below normal, liver cells convert glycogen to glucose, which is released into the blood to restore the normal blood sugar concentration.
- The modification of fats so that they can be used more efficiently by cells all over the body.
- The storage of some vitamins and iron.
- The formation of blood plasma proteins, such as albumin, globulins, and clotting factors.
- The destruction of old red blood cells and the recycling or elimination of their breakdown products. One byproduct, a pigment called **bilirubin** (BIL-ih-ru-bin), is eliminated in bile and gives the stool its characteristic dark color.
- The synthesis of **urea** (u-RE-ah), a waste product of protein metabolism. Urea is released into the blood and transported to the kidneys for elimination.
- The **detoxification** (de-tok-sih-fih-KA-shun) (removal of the poisonous properties) of harmful substances, such as alcohol and certain drugs.

BILE The liver's main digestive function is the production of bile, a substance needed for the processing of fats. The salts contained in bile act like a detergent to **emulsify** fat, that is, to break up fat into small droplets that can be acted on more effectively by digestive enzymes. Bile also aids in fat absorption from the small intestine.

Bile leaves the lobes of the liver by two ducts that merge to form the **common hepatic duct**. After collecting bile from the gallbladder, this duct, now called the **common bile duct**, delivers bile into the duodenum. These and the other accessory ducts are shown in Figure 19-10.

The Gallbladder

The **gallbladder** (GAWL-blad-er) is a muscular sac on the inferior surface of the liver that stores bile. Although the liver may manufacture bile continuously, the body needs it only a few times a day. Consequently, bile from the liver flows into the hepatic ducts and then up through the **cystic** (SIS-tik) **duct**, connected with the gallbladder (see Fig. 19-10). When chyme enters the duodenum, the gallbladder contracts, squeezing bile through the cystic duct and into the common bile duct, leading to the duodenum.

The Pancreas

The **pancreas** (PAN-kre-as) is a long gland that extends from the duodenum to the spleen (see Fig. 19-10). The pancreas produces enzymes that digest fats, proteins, carbohydrates, and nucleic acids. The protein-digesting enzymes are produced in inactive forms which must be converted to active forms in the small intestine by other enzymes.

The pancreas also releases large amounts of sodium bicarbonate ($NaHCO_3$), an alkaline (basic) fluid that neutralizes the acidic chyme in the small intestine, thus protecting the lining of the digestive tract. These juices collect in a main duct that joins the common bile duct or empties into the duodenum near the common bile duct. Most people have an additional smaller duct that opens into the duodenum.

As described in Chapter 12, the pancreas also functions as an endocrine gland, producing the hormones insulin and glucagon that regulate sugar metabolism. These islet cell secretions are released into the blood.

CHECKPOINT 19-11 ➤ What is the role of the gallbladder?

CHECKPOINT 19-12 ➤ What is the role of bile in digestion?

Enzymes and the Digestive Process

Although the individual organs of the digestive tract are specialized for digesting different types of food, the fundamental chemical process of digestion is the same for fats, proteins, and carbohydrates. In every case, this process requires enzymes. Enzymes are catalysts, substances that speed the rate of chemical reactions, but are not themselves changed or used up in the reaction.

All enzymes are proteins, and they are highly specific in their actions. In digestion, an enzyme acts only in a certain type of reaction involving a certain type of nutrient molecule. For example, the carbohydrate-digesting enzyme amylase only splits starch into the disaccharide (double sugar) maltose. Another enzyme is required to split maltose into two molecules of the monosaccharide (simple sugar) glucose. Other enzymes split fats into their building blocks, glycerol and fatty acids, and still others split proteins into smaller units called *peptides* and into their building blocks, amino acids (see Enzymes in Chapter 2).

The Role of Water

Because water is added to nutrient molecules as they are split by enzymes, the process of digestion is referred to chemically as **hydrolysis** (hi-DROL-ih-sis), which means "splitting by means of water" (see Fig. 2-2). In this chemical process, water's hydroxyl group (OH^-) is added to one fragment and the hydrogen ion (H^+) is added to the other, splitting the molecule. About 7 liters of water are secreted into the digestive tract each day, in addition to the nearly 2 liters taken in with food and drink. You can now understand why so large an amount of water is needed. Water not only is used to produce digestive juices and to dilute food so that it can move more easily through the digestive tract, but also is used in the chemical process of digestion itself.

Digestion, Step-by-Step

Let us see what happens to a mass of food from the time it is taken into the mouth to the moment that it is ready to be absorbed (see Table 19-1).

In the mouth, the food is chewed and mixed with saliva, softening it so that it can be swallowed easily. Salivary amylase initiates the digestive process by changing some of the starches into sugar.

DIGESTION IN THE STOMACH When the food reaches the stomach, it is acted on by gastric juice, with its hydrochloric acid (HCl) and enzymes. The hydrochloric acid has the important function of breaking down proteins and preparing them for digestion. In addition, HCl activates the enzyme pepsin, which is secreted by gastric cells in an inactive form. Once activated by hydrochloric acid, pepsin works to digest protein; this enzyme is the first to digest nearly every type of protein in the diet. The stomach also secretes a fat-digesting enzyme (lipase), but it is of little importance in adults.

The food, gastric juice, and mucus (which is also secreted by cells of the gastric lining) are mixed to form chyme. This semiliquid substance is moved from the stomach to the small intestine for further digestion.

DIGESTION IN THE SMALL INTESTINE In the duodenum, the first part of the small intestine, chyme is mixed with the greenish-yellow bile delivered from the liver and the gallbladder through the common bile duct. Bile does not contain enzymes; instead, it contains salts that emulsify fats to allow the powerful secretions from the pancreas to act on them most efficiently.

Pancreatic juice contains a number of enzymes, including:

- **Lipase**. After bile divides fats into tiny particles, the highly active pancreatic enzyme lipase digests almost all of them. In this process, fats are usually broken down into two simpler compounds, glycerol (glycerin) and fatty acids, which are more readily absorbable. If pancreatic lipase is absent, fats are expelled with the feces in undigested form.

- **Amylase**. This enzyme changes starch to sugar.

Table 19-1	**Summary of Digestion**		
Organ	Activity	Nutrients Digested	Active Secretions
Mouth	Chews food and mixes it with saliva; forms into bolus for swallowing	Starch	Salivary amylase
Esophagus	Moves food by peristalsis into stomach	—	—
Stomach	Stores food, churns food, and mixes it with digestive juices	Proteins	Hydrochloric acid, pepsin
Small intestine	Secretes enzymes, neutralizes acidity, receives secretions from pancreas and liver, absorbs nutrients and water into the blood or lymph	Fats, proteins, carbohydrates, nucleic acids	Intestinal enzymes, pancreatic enzymes, bile from liver
Large intestine	Reabsorbs some water; forms, stores, and eliminates stool	—	—

19

- **Trypsin** (TRIP-sin). This enzyme splits proteins into amino acids, which are small enough to be absorbed through the intestine.
- **Nucleases** (NU-kle-ases). These enzymes digest the nucleic acids DNA and RNA.

It is important to note that most digestion occurs in the small intestine under the action of pancreatic juice, which has the ability to break down all types of foods. When pancreatic juice is absent, serious digestive disturbances always occur.

The small intestine also produces a number of enzymes, including three that act on complex sugars to transform them into simpler, absorbable forms. These enzymes are **maltase**, **sucrase**, and **lactase**, which act on the disaccharides maltose, sucrose, and lactose, respectively.

Table 19-2 summarizes the main substances used in digestion. Note that, except for HCl, sodium bicarbonate, and bile salts, all the substances listed are enzymes.

CHECKPOINT 19-13 ➤ What organ produces the most complete digestive secretions?

Absorption

The means by which digested nutrients reach the blood is known as **absorption**. Most absorption takes place through the villi in the mucosa of the small intestine (see Fig. 19-9). Within each villus is an arteriole and a venule bridged with capillaries. Simple sugars, small proteins (peptides), amino acids, some simple fatty acids, and most of the water in the digestive tract are absorbed into the blood through these capillaries. From here, they pass by way of the portal system to the liver, to be processed, stored, or released as needed.

Absorption of Fats

Most fats have an alternative method of reaching the blood. Instead of entering the blood capillaries, they are absorbed by the villi's more permeable lymphatic capillaries, the lacteals. The absorbed fat droplets give the lymph a milky appearance. The mixture of lymph and fat globules that drains from the small intestine after fat has been digested is called **chyle** (kile). Chyle merges with the lymphatic circulation and eventually enters the blood when the lymph drains into veins near the heart. The absorbed fats then circulate to the liver for further processing.

Absorption of Vitamins and Minerals

Minerals and vitamins ingested with food are also absorbed from the small intestine. The minerals and some of the vitamins dissolve in water and are absorbed directly into the blood. Other vitamins are incorporated in fats and are absorbed along with the fats. Vitamin K and some B vitamins are produced by bacterial action in the colon and are absorbed from the large intestine.

CHECKPOINT 19-14 ➤ What is absorption?

Control of Digestion

As food moves through the digestive tract, its rate of movement and the activity of each organ it passes through must be carefully regulated. If food moves too slowly or digestive secretions are inadequate, the body will not get enough nourishment. If food moves too rapidly or excess secretions are produced, digestion may be incomplete or the digestive tract's lining may be damaged. There are two

Table 19-2	Digestive Juices Produced by Digestive Tract Organs and Accessory Organs	
Organ	**Main Digestive Juices Secreted**	**Action**
Salivary glands	Salivary amylase	Begins starch digestion
Stomach	Hydrochloric acid (HCl)*	Breaks down proteins
	Pepsin	Begins protein digestion
Small intestine	Peptidases	Digests proteins to amino acids
	Lactase, maltase, sucrase	Digests disaccharides to monosaccharides
Pancreas	Sodium bicarbonate*	Neutralizes HCl
	Amylase	Digests starch
	Trypsin	Digests protein to amino acids
	Lipases	Digests fats to fatty acids and glycerol
	Nucleases	Digests nucleic acids
Liver	Bile salts*	Emulsifies fats

*Not enzymes.

types of control over digestion: nervous and hormonal. Both illustrate the principles of feedback control.

The nerves that control digestive activity are located in the submucosa and between the muscle layers of the organ walls. Instructions for action come from the autonomic (visceral) nervous system. In general, parasympathetic stimulation increases activity, and sympathetic stimulation decreases activity. Excess sympathetic stimulation, as in stress, can block food's movement through the digestive tract and inhibit mucus secretion, which is crucial in protecting the lining of the digestive tract.

The digestive organs themselves produce the hormones involved in the regulation of digestion. The following is a discussion of some of these controls (Table 19-3).

The sight, smell, thought, taste, or feel of food in the mouth stimulates, through the nervous system, the secretion of saliva and the release of gastric juice. Once in the stomach, food stimulates the release into the blood of the hormone **gastrin**, which promotes stomach secretions and motility (movement).

When chyme enters the duodenum, nerve impulses inhibit stomach motility, so that food will not move too rapidly into the small intestine. This action is a good example of negative feedback. At the same time, hormones released from the duodenum not only function in digestion, but also feed back to the stomach to reduce its activity. **Gastric-inhibitory peptide (GIP)** is one such hormone. It acts on the stomach to inhibit the release of gastric juice. Its more important action is to stimulate insulin release from the pancreas when glucose enters the duodenum. Another of these hormones, **secretin** (se-KRE-tin) stimulates the pancreas to release water and bicarbonate to dilute and neutralize chyme. **Cholecystokinin** (ko-le-sis-to-KI-nin) **(CCK)**, stimulates the release of enzymes from the pancreas and causes the gallbladder to release bile.

CHECKPOINT `19-15` ➤ What are the two types of control over the digestive process?

Hunger and Appetite

Hunger is the desire for food, which can be satisfied by the ingestion of a filling meal. Hunger is regulated by hypothalamic centers that respond to the levels of nutrients in the blood. When these levels are low, the hypothalamus stimulates a sensation of hunger. Strong, mildly painful contractions of the empty stomach may stimulate a feeling of hunger. Messages received by the hypothalamus reduce hunger as food is chewed and swallowed and begins to fill the stomach. The short-term regulation of food intake works to keep the amount of food eaten within the limits of what the intestine can process. The long-term regulation of food intake maintains appropriate blood levels of nutrients.

Appetite differs from hunger in that, although it is basically a desire for food, it often has no relationship to the need for food. Even after an adequate meal that has relieved hunger, a person may still have an appetite for additional food. A variety of factors, such as emotional state, cultural influences, habit, and memories of past food intake, can affect appetite. The regulation of appetite is not well understood. Despite day-to-day variations in food intake and physical activity, a healthy individual maintains a constant body weight and energy reserves of fat over long periods. With the discovery of the hormone **leptin** (from the Greek word *leptos*, meaning "thin"), researchers have been able to piece together one long-term mechanism for regulating weight. Leptin is produced by adipocytes in adipose tissue. When fat is stored because of excess food intake, the cells release more leptin. Centers in the hypothalamus respond to the hormone by decreasing food intake and increasing energy expenditure, resulting in weight loss. If this feedback mechanism is disrupted, obesity will result. Early hopes of using leptin to treat human obesity have dimmed, however, because obese people do not have a leptin deficiency. This system's failure in humans appears to be caused by the hypothalamus' inability to respond to leptin rather than our inability to make the hormone.

Table 19-3	Hormones Active in Digestion	
Hormone	**Source**	**Action**
Gastrin	Stomach	Stimulates release of gastric juice
Gastric-inhibitory peptide (GIP)	Duodenum	Stimulates insulin release from pancreas when glucose enters duodenum; inhibits release of gastric juice
Secretin	Duodenum	Stimulates release of water and bicarbonate from pancreas, stimulates release of bile from liver; inhibits the stomach
Cholecystokinin (CCK)	Duodenum	Stimulates release of digestive enzymes from pancreas, stimulates release of bile from gallbladder; inhibits the stomach

19

CHECKPOINT **19-16** ➤ What is the difference between hunger and appetite?

Eating Disorders

A chronic loss of appetite, called **anorexia** (an-o-REK-se-ah), may be caused by a great variety of physical and mental disorders. Because the hypothalamus and the higher brain centers are involved in the regulation of hunger, it is possible that emotional and social factors contribute to the development of anorexia.

Anorexia nervosa is a psychological disorder that predominantly afflicts young women. In a desire to be excessively thin, affected people literally starve themselves, sometimes to the point of death. A related disorder, **bulimia** (bu-LIM-e-ah), is also called the *binge-purge syndrome*. Affected individuals eat huge quantities of food at one time, and then induce vomiting or take large doses of laxatives to prevent absorption of the food.

These disorders stress all body systems. In women, a lack of estrogen production may cause menstrual periods to cease. Loss of bone mass may lead to osteoporosis. Degeneration of the myocardium can result in heart failure. Mental function is impaired. The reflux of acidic substances in bulimia causes erosion of the esophagus and destruction of tooth enamel.

Disorders of the Digestive System

Infections, ulcers, cancer, and structural abnormalities all affect the digestive system at almost any level. Stones may form in the accessory organs or their ducts. Mechanical, nervous, chemical, and hormonal factors may be at the source of digestive problems.

Peritonitis

Inflammation of the peritoneum, termed **peritonitis** (per-ih-to-NI-tis), is a serious complication that may follow infection of an organ covered by the peritoneum—often, the appendix. The frequency and severity of peritonitis have been greatly reduced by the use of antibiotics. The disorder still occurs, however, and can be dangerous. If the infection is kept in one area, it is said to be *localized peritonitis*. A *generalized peritonitis*, as may be caused by a ruptured appendix, a perforated ulcer, or a penetrating wound, may lead to the growth of so many disease organisms and the release of so much bacterial toxin as to be fatal. Immediate surgery to repair the rupture and medical care are needed.

Diseases of the Mouth and Teeth

Tooth decay is also termed dental **caries** (KA-reze) (from Latin meaning "rottenness"). It has a number of causes, including diet, heredity, mechanical problems, and endocrine disorders. People who ingest a lot of sugar are particularly prone to this disease. Because a baby's teeth begin to develop before birth, a mother's diet during pregnancy is important in ensuring the formation of healthy teeth in her baby.

Any infection of the gum is called **gingivitis** (jin-jih-VI-tis). If such an infection continues untreated, it may lead to a more serious condition, **periodontitis** (per-e-o-don-TI-tis), which involves not only the gum tissue but also the teeth's supporting bone. Tooth loosening and bone destruction follow unless periodontitis is halted by proper treatment and improved dental hygiene. Periodontitis is responsible for nearly 80% of tooth loss in people older than 45 years of age.

Vincent disease, a kind of gingivitis caused by a spirochete or a bacillus, is most prevalent in teenagers and young adults. Characterized by inflammation, ulceration, and infection of the oral mucous membranes, this disorder is highly contagious, particularly by oral contact. Patients on antibiotic therapy are more likely than normal to develop fungal infections of the mouth and tongue because these drugs may destroy the normal bacterial flora and allow other organisms to grow.

Leukoplakia (lu-ko-PLA-ke-ah) is characterized by thickened white patches on the mucous membranes of the mouth. It is common in smokers and is considered precancerous.

CHECKPOINT **19-17** ➤ What are some common diseases of the mouth and teeth?

Disorders of the Esophagus and Stomach

The distal portion of the esophagus is a common site for ulcer development due to acid reflux (backflow) from the stomach. In cases of liver disease, the esophagus is prone to develop varicose veins, which are subject to severe bleeding.

As noted, a weakness in the diaphragm at the point where the esophagus joins the stomach may allow the stomach to protrude upward as a **hiatal** (hi-A-tal) **hernia**. Minor irregularities in this area are common and may cause no problem, but the incidence and severity of hiatal hernia increase with age. A hiatal hernia may cause discomfort after meals, gastritis, or ulceration, and serious cases may need surgical repair.

> **PASSport to Success**
> Visit **thePoint** or see the Student Resource CD in the back of this book for an illustration of hiatal hernia.

Weakness in the lower esophageal sphincter (LES) may allow the acidic stomach contents to flow back into the distal esophagus. The result is a burning sensation below or behind the sternum that is described as *heartburn*. The symptom does not involve the heart in any way, but is felt in the vicinity of the heart. Often it is mistaken for a heart attack. More dangerously, a heart attack can be mistaken for heartburn, and people may fail to seek medical attention thinking they have a minor disturbance. Chronic reflux is referred to as **gastroesophageal reflux disease (GERD)**. Overfilling of the stomach and meals high in fat contribute to reflux and GERD by initiating nervous responses that relax the LES. Acid reflux irritates the esophageal mucous membrane, leading to esophagitis. Eventually there may be edema and scar tissue formation that narrows the esophagus and interferes with digestion. GERD also increases the risk of esophageal cancer.

> **PASSport to Success**
> Visit *thePoint* or see the Student Resource CD in the back of this book for an illustration of the causes and effects of GERD.

Acid reflux and GERD are treated with antacids and drugs that inhibit the production of HCl. People with this problem should avoid certain foods and beverages, including fats, caffeine, chocolate, and alcohol, and should not smoke. Other measures that may help are eating in an upright position, not bending down for long periods, not lying down for several hours after eating, and sleeping with the head elevated. Weight loss may also help in cases of obesity.

Nausea is an unpleasant sensation that may follow distention or irritation of the distal esophagus or the stomach as a result of various nervous and mechanical factors. It may be a symptom of interference with normal peristalsis in the stomach and intestine, and thus may be followed by vomiting.

Vomiting, also called **emesis** (EM-eh-sis), is the expulsion of gastric (and sometimes intestinal) contents through the mouth by reverse peristalsis. The contraction of muscles in the abdominal wall forcibly empties the stomach. Vomiting is frequently caused by overeating or by inflammation of the stomach lining, a condition called **gastritis** (gas-TRI-tis). Gastritis results from irritation of the mucosa by certain drugs, food, or drinks. For example, the long-term use of aspirin, highly spiced foods, or alcohol can lead to gastritis. The nicotine in cigarettes can also cause gastritis.

Flatus (FLA-tus) usually refers to excessive amounts of air (gas) in the stomach or intestine. The resulting condition is referred to as **flatulence** (FLAT-u-lens). In some cases, a physician may need to insert a tube into the stomach or rectum to aid the patient in expelling flatus.

STOMACH CANCER Although stomach cancer has become rare in the United States, it is common in many parts of the world, and it is a serious disorder because of its high death rate. Men are more susceptible than women to stomach cancer. The tumor nearly always develops from the stomach's epithelial or mucosal lining, and is often of the type called **adenocarcinoma** (ad-en-o-kar-sih-NO-mah). Sometimes, the victim has suffered from long-standing indigestion (discomfort after meals) but has failed to consult a physician until the cancer has metastasized (spread) to other organs, such as the liver or lymph nodes. Persistent indigestion is one of the important warning signs of stomach cancer.

PEPTIC ULCER An ulcer is an area of the skin or mucous membrane in which the tissues are gradually destroyed. **Peptic ulcers** (named for the enzyme pepsin) occur in the mucous membrane of the esophagus, stomach, or duodenum (the first part of the small intestine) and are most common in people between the ages of 30 and 45 years. Peptic ulcers in the stomach are termed *gastric ulcers*; those in the duodenum are *duodenal* (du-o-DE-nal) *ulcers*.

Smoking cigarettes and taking aspirin or other anti-inflammatory drugs are major causative factors. It also has been found that infection with a bacterium, *Helicobacter pylori*, is a factor in causing peptic ulcers. The organism is associated with inflammation of the stomach and duodenum, and most people with ulcers who have an *H. pylori* infection are cured when the organism is eliminated with antibiotics. Drugs that inhibit the secretion of stomach acids are often effective in treating peptic ulcers.

> **PASSport to Success**
> Visit *thePoint* or see the Student Resource CD in the back of this book for common ulcer types and sites.

PYLORIC STENOSIS Normally, the stomach contents are moved through the pyloric sphincter within approximately 2 to 6 hours after eating. Some infants, however, most often boys, are born with an obstruction of the pyloric sphincter, a condition called **pyloric stenosis** (steh-NO-sis). Usually, surgery is required in these cases to modify the muscle, so that food can pass from the stomach into the duodenum.

> **PASSport to Success**
> Visit *thePoint* or see the Student Resource CD in the back of this book for an illustration of pyloric stenosis.

Intestinal Disorders

Many intestinal disorders involve inflammation. **Appendicitis** (ah-pen-dih-SI-tis) is inflammation of the appendix, which may result from infection or obstruction. The cause of obstruction is usually a **fecalith** (FE-cah-lith), a hardened piece of fecal material. The first sign of acute appendicitis is usually abdominal pain, with loss of appetite and sometimes nausea or vomiting. Pain eventually localizes in the right lower quadrant of the abdomen. Laboratory blood tests show elevated leukocytes. Surgery (appendectomy) is required to remove an inflamed appendix. Untreated, it can rupture to spread infection into the peritoneal cavity.

Two similar diseases are included under the heading of **inflammatory bowel disease (IBD)**: **Crohn** (krone) **disease** and **ulcerative colitis**. Both occur mainly in adolescents and young adults and cause similar symptoms of pain, diarrhea, weight loss, and rectal bleeding. Crohn disease usually involves inflammation of the distal small intestine. It is an autoimmune disease, which may in part be hereditary. Ulcerative colitis involves inflammation and ulceration of the colon, and usually the rectum.

PASSport to Success

Visit **thePoint** or see the Student Resource CD in the back of this book for information on the complications of ulcerative colitis.

Irritable bowel syndrome (IBS) is a common gastrointestinal disorder seen typically in young to middle-aged women. Symptoms include pain and constipation or diarrhea, or sometimes both conditions in alternation. In IBS, the intestine is overly sensitive to stimulation, often brought on by stress. Although the condition is chronic and causes much pain, frustration, and anxiety, it is not life-threatening and does not develop into more serious bowel diseases.

Difficulties with digestion or absorption may be due to **enteritis** (en-ter-I-tis), an intestinal inflammation. When both the stomach and the small intestine are involved, the disorder is called **gastroenteritis** (gas-tro-en-ter-I-tis). The symptoms of gastroenteritis include nausea, vomiting, and diarrhea as well as acute abdominal pain (colic). The disorder may be caused by a variety of pathogenic organisms, including viruses, bacteria, and protozoa. Chemical irritants, such as alcohol, certain drugs (e.g., aspirin), and other toxins, have been known to cause this disorder as well.

Diverticula (di-ver-TIK-u-lah) are small pouches in the wall of the intestine, most commonly in the colon. A diet low in fiber contributes to the formation of large numbers of diverticula, a condition called **diverticulosis** (di-ver-tik-u-LO-sis). Collection of waste and bacteria in these sacs leads to **diverticulitis** (di-ver-tik-u-LI-tis), which is accompanied by pain and sometimes bleeding. There is no cure for diverticulitis; it is treated with diet, stool softeners, and drugs to reduce intestinal motility.

PASSport to Success

Visit **thePoint** or see the Student Resource CD in the back of this book for an illustration of diverticulitis.

CHECKPOINT 19-18 ▸ What two diseases fall into the category of inflammatory bowel disease?

DIARRHEA Diarrhea is a symptom characterized by abnormally frequent watery bowel movements. The danger of diarrhea is dehydration and loss of salts, especially in infants. Diarrhea may result from excess activity of the colon, faulty absorption, or infection. Infections resulting in diarrhea include cholera, dysentery, and food poisoning. Tables 1 and 5 in Appendix 5 list some of the organisms causing these diseases. Such infections are often spread by poor sanitation and contaminated food, milk, or water. A stool examination may be required to establish the cause of diarrhea; examination may reveal the presence of pathogenic organisms, worm eggs, or blood.

CONSTIPATION Millions of dollars are spent each year in an effort to remedy a condition called **constipation**. What is constipation? Many people erroneously think they are constipated if they go a day or more without having a bowel movement. Actually, what is normal varies greatly; one person may normally have a bowel movement only once every 2 or 3 days, whereas another may normally have more than one movement daily. The term *constipation* is also used to refer to hard stools or difficulty with defecation.

On the basis of its onset, constipation may be classified as acute or chronic. Acute constipation occurs suddenly and may be due to an intestinal obstruction, such as a tumor or diverticulitis. Extreme constipation is termed **obstipation** (ob-stih-PA-shun). Chronic constipation, in contrast, has a more gradual onset and may be divided into two groups:

■ **Spastic constipation**, in which the intestinal musculature is overstimulated so that the canal becomes narrowed and the lumen (space) inside the intestine is not large enough to permit the passage of fecal material.

■ **Flaccid** (FLAK-sid) **constipation**, which is characterized by a lazy, or **atonic** (ah-TON-ik), intestinal muscle. Elderly people and those on bed rest are particularly susceptible to this condition. Often, it results from repeated denial of the urge to defecate. Regular bowel habits, moderate exercise, eating more vegetables and other bulky foods, and an increase in fluid may help people who have sluggish intestinal muscles.

People should avoid the chronic use of laxatives and enemas, which interfere with the natural defecation reflex. They may also alter electrolyte balance and result in fluid loss. The streams of fluid used in enemas may injure the intestinal lining by removing the normal protective mucus. In addition, enemas aggravate hemorrhoids. Enemas should be done only on a physician's order, and sparingly.

INTESTINAL OBSTRUCTION Intussusception (in-tuh-suh-SEP-shun) is the slipping of a part of the intestine into an adjacent part (Fig. 19-11). It occurs mainly in male infants in the ileocecal region. **Volvulus** (VOL-vu-lus) is a twisting of the intestine, usually the sigmoid colon. It may be a congenital malformation or the result of a foreign body. Both intussusception and volvulus can be fatal if not treated quickly. **Ileus** (IL-e-us) is an intestinal obstruction caused by lack of peristalsis or by muscle contraction. A physician can insert a tube to release intestinal material. **Hemorrhoids** (HEM-o-roydz) are varicose veins in the rectum. These enlarged veins may cause pain and bleeding and may eventually extend out through the rectum.

CANCER OF THE COLON AND RECTUM Tumors of the colon and rectum are among the six most common types of cancer in the United States. These tumors are usually adenocarcinomas that arise from the mucosal lining.

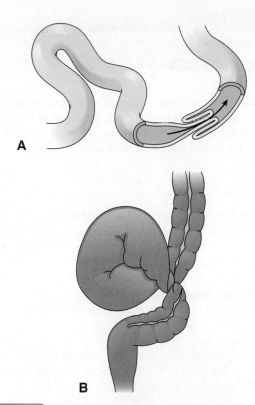

A

B

Figure 19-11 **Intestinal obstructions. (A)** Intussusception. A part of the intestine slips into an adjacent part. **(B)** Volvulus. A twisting of the intestine. (Modified with permission from Cohen BJ. *Medical Terminology*, 5th ed. Philadelphia: Lippincott Williams & Wilkins, 2008.)

The occurrence of colon cancer is evenly divided between the sexes, but malignant tumors of the rectum are more common in men than in women.

Tumors may be detected by direct examination of the rectum and lower colon with an instrument called a **sigmoidoscope** (sig-MOY-do-skope) (named for the sigmoid colon). A **colonoscope** (ko-LON-o-skope) is used to examine deeper regions of the colon (see Box 19-2, Endoscopy). The presence of blood in the stool may indicate cancer of the bowel or some other gastrointestinal disturbance. A simple chemical test can detect extremely small quantities of blood in the stool, referred to as *occult* ("hidden") *blood*. Early detection and treatment are the keys to increasing survival rates.

> **PASSport to Success** Visit **thePoint** or see the Student Resource CD in the back of this book for illustrations of colonoscopy and a colonoscopic image.

Infection of the Salivary Glands

The contagious disease commonly called *mumps* is a viral infection of the parotid salivary glands. This type of **parotitis** (par-o-TI-tis), or inflammation of the parotid glands, may lead to inflammation of the testicles by the same virus. Males affected after puberty are at risk for permanent damage to these sex organs, resulting in sterility. Another complication of mumps that occurs in about 10% of cases is meningitis. Mumps now can be prevented by childhood immunization with a vaccine (MMR).

Cirrhosis and Other Liver Diseases

Cirrhosis (sih-RO-sis) of the liver is a chronic disease in which active liver cells are replaced by inactive connective (scar) tissue. The most common type of cirrhosis is alcoholic

---

Box 19-2　🩺　**Clinical Perspectives**

Endoscopy: A View From Within

Modern medicine has made great strides toward looking into the body without resorting to invasive surgery. An instrument that has made this possible in many cases is the **endoscope**, which is inserted into the body through an orifice or small incision and used to examine passageways, hollow organs, and body cavities. The first endoscopes were rigid lighted telescopes that could be inserted only a short distance into the body. Today, physicians are able to navigate the twists and turns of the digestive tract using long **fiberoptic endoscopes** composed of flexible bundles of glass or plastic that transmit light.

In the gastrointestinal tract, endoscopy can detect structural abnormalities, bleeding ulcers, inflammation, and tumors. In addition, endoscopes can be used to remove fluid samples or tissue biopsy specimens. Some surgery can even be done with an endoscope, such as polyp removal from the colon or expansion of a sphincter. Endoscopy can also be used to examine and operate on joints (arthroscopy), the bladder (cystoscopy), respiratory passages (bronchoscopy), and the abdominal cavity (laparoscopy).

Capsular endoscopy, a recent technological advance, has made examination of the gastrointestinal tract even easier. It uses a pill-sized camera that can be swallowed! As the camera moves through the digestive tract, it transmits video images to a data recorder worn on the patient's belt.

19

(portal) cirrhosis. Alcohol has a direct damaging effect on liver cells that is compounded by malnutrition. Hepatic cell destruction hampers the portal circulation, causing blood to accumulate in the spleen and gastrointestinal tract and causing fluid (ascites) to accumulate in the peritoneal cavity.

PASSport to Success — Visit *thePoint* or see the Student Resource CD in the back of this book for a photograph of a cirrhotic liver.

JAUNDICE Damage to the liver or blockage in any of the bile ducts may cause bile pigment to accumulate in the blood. As a result, the stool may become pale in color and the skin and sclera of the eyes may become yellowish; this symptom is called **jaundice** (JAWN-dis) (from French *jaune* for "yellow") (see Fig. 6-6B). Jaundice may also be caused by excess destruction of red blood cells. In addition, it is often seen in newborns, in whom the liver is immature and not yet functioning efficiently.

HEPATITIS Inflammation of the liver, called **hepatitis** (hep-ah-TI-tis), may be caused by drugs, alcohol, or infection (see Table 2 in Appendix 5). The known viruses that cause hepatitis are named A through E. These vary in route (pathway) of infection, severity, and complications. All types of hepatitis are marked by hepatic cell destruction and such symptoms as loss of appetite, jaundice, and liver enlargement. In most patients, the liver cells regenerate with little residual damage. The types of hepatitis virus and their primary routes of transmission are as follows:

Hepatitis A (HAV): commonly transmitted in fecal matter and contaminated food and water. There is a vaccine for hepatitis A, which is recommended for people traveling to areas where this disease is a threat.

Hepatitis B (HBV): transmitted by exposure to the virus in blood or body fluids, although it also can be spread by fecal contamination. This is the most prevalent form of hepatitis. HBV and other blood-borne types of hepatitis virus (C and D) have been linked to long-term development of liver cancer. Also, people with these forms of hepatitis may develop into carriers, able to transmit the disease but not showing any symptoms. HBV is usually transmitted by use of improperly sterilized needles. A vaccine is available that is now recommended for childhood immunization and for people working in healthcare and childcare.

Hepatitis C (HCV): transmitted primarily by exposure to infected blood. There is some evidence of limited sexual transmission. Clinical symptoms of hepatitis C may develop many years after exposure to the virus.

Hepatitis D (HDV): transmitted by direct exchange of blood. It occurs only in those with hepatitis B infection.

Hepatitis E (HEV): transmitted by fecal contamination of water. Most cases have been linked to epidemics in Asia, Africa, and Central America.

An additional related virus has been designated hepatitis G. It is similar in structure to HCV and is found in blood, but does not appear to cause hepatitis.

There is no specific treatment for hepatitis.

CHECKPOINT 19-19 ➤ What is hepatitis?

CANCER The metastasis (spread) of cancer to the liver is common in cases that begin as cancer in one of the abdominal organs; the tumor cells are carried in the blood through the portal system to the liver.

Gallstones

The most common disease of the gallbladder is the formation of stones, or **cholelithiasis** (ko-le-lih-THI-ah-sis). Stones are formed from the substances contained in bile, mainly cholesterol. They may remain in the gallbladder or may lodge in the bile ducts, causing extreme pain. Cholelithiasis is usually associated with inflammation of the gallbladder, or **cholecystitis** (ko-le-sis-TI-tis).

PASSport to Success — Visit *thePoint* or see the Student Resource CD in the back of this book for an illustration of gallstones.

Pancreatitis

Because they are usually confined to proper channels, pancreatic enzymes do not damage body tissues. If the bile ducts become blocked, however, pancreatic enzymes back up into the pancreas. Also, in some cases of gastric inflammation from excess alcohol consumption or in gallbladder disease, irritation may extend to the pancreas and cause abnormal activation of the pancreatic enzymes. In either circumstance, the pancreas suffers destruction by its own juice, and the outcome can be fatal; this condition is known as **acute pancreatitis**.

Aging and the Digestive System

With age, receptors for taste and smell deteriorate, leading to a loss of appetite and decreased enjoyment of food. A decrease in saliva and poor gag reflex make swallowing more difficult. Tooth loss or poorly fitting dentures may make chewing food more difficult.

Activity of the digestive organs decreases. These changes can be seen in poor absorption of certain vitamins and poor protein digestion. Slowing of peristalsis in the large intestine and increased consumption of easily chewed, refined foods contribute to the common occurrence of constipation.

The tissues of the digestive system require constant replacement. Slowing of this process contributes to a variety of digestive disorders, including gastritis, ulcers, and diverticulosis. As with many body systems, tumors and cancer occur more frequently with age.

Disease in Context revisited

Adam's Colonoscopy

At his scheduled time, Adam reported to the hospital as an outpatient for his colonoscopy. He had stayed on a clear liquid diet for a day and done the required laxative prep to clear his colon. He met with Dr. Clarkson who described the procedure. "We'll give you light sedation, and then use a flexible lighted endoscope with a camera to examine the entire colon. The procedure should take only about half an hour and has a very low risk. You have made arrangements for someone to go home with you, haven't you?" Adam said his brother was coming. After the test Dr. Clarkson reported that everything looked fine and that he would send the results to Dr. Michaels. "The good news, Adam, is that you have 10 years before you have to do this again.

Maybe next time we'll be able to get our pictures with a small camera in a pill that you can swallow. That's already being tested. With the excellent medical care you're getting, you'll probably be alive to see the screening done by genetic study of cells sloughed off in the stool—and that won't require a prep."

Adam's case shows the importance of anatomic studies in the diagnosis and treatment of disease. Box 1-2 has general information on medical imaging, and various methods are mentioned in chapters and cases throughout this book. We'll visit Adam again in Chapter 22 when he finds out that his prostate gland is affecting his urinary system.

Word Anatomy

Medical terms are built from standardized word parts (prefixes, roots, and suffixes). Learning the meanings of these parts can help you remember words and interpret unfamiliar terms.

WORD PART	MEANING	EXAMPLE
Function and Design of the Digestive System		
ab-	away from	In *absorption*, digested materials are taken from the digestive tract into the circulation.
enter/o	intestine	The *mesentery* is the portion of the peritoneum around the intestine.
mes/o-	middle	The *mesocolon*, like the mesentery, comes from the middle layer of cells in the embryo, the mesoderm.
Organs of the Digestive Tract		
gastr/o	stomach	The *gastrointestinal* tract consists mainly of the stomach and intestine.
The Accessory Organs		
amyl/o	starch	The starch-digesting enzyme in saliva is salivary *amylase*.
lingu/o	tongue	The *sublingual* salivary glands are under the tongue.
hepat/o	liver	The *hepatic* portal system carries blood to the liver.
bil/i	bile	*Bilirubin* is a pigment found in bile.
cyst/o	bladder, sac	The *cystic* duct carries bile into and out of the gallbladder.

19

WORD PART	MEANING	EXAMPLE
Control of Digestion		
chole	bile, gall	*Cholecystokinin* is a hormone that activates the gallbladder (cholecyst/o).
Disorders of the Digestive System		
odont/o	tooth	*Periodontitis* is a disease of the gums and the tissue around a tooth.
-lith	stone	A *fecalith* is a hardened piece of fecal material.
-rhea (the r is doubled when added to a word)	flow, discharge	*Diarrhea* is flow of watery bowel movements through (dia-) the digestive tract.

Summary

I. **FUNCTION AND DESIGN OF THE DIGESTIVE SYSTEM**
   A. Functions—digestion, absorption, elimination
   B. Two groups of organs—digestive tract and accessory organs
   C. The wall of the digestive tract—mucous membrane (mucosa), submucosa, smooth muscle, serous membrane (serosa)
   D. The peritoneum
      1. Serous membrane that lines the abdominal cavity and folds over organs
      2. Divisions—mesentery, mesocolon, greater omentum, lesser omentum

II. **ORGANS OF THE DIGESTIVE TRACT**
   A. Mouth
      1. Functions
         a. Ingest food
         b. Begin digestion of starch with salivary amylase
         c. Mastication (chewing)
         d. Deglutition (swallowing)
      2. Tongue—aids mastication and deglutition; has taste buds
   B. Teeth
      1. Deciduous (baby) teeth—20 (incisors, canines, molars)
      2. Permanent teeth—32 (incisors, canines, premolars, molars)
   C. Pharynx (throat)—moves bolus (portion) of food into esophagus by reflex swallowing
   D. Esophagus—long muscular tube that carries food to stomach by peristalsis
   E. Stomach
      1. Functions
         a. Storage of food
         b. Breakdown of food by churning to form chyme
         c. Breakdown of protein with hydrochloric acid (HCl)
         d. Digestion of protein with enzyme pepsin
   F. Small intestine
      1. Functions
         a. Digestion of food
         b. Absorption of nutrients and water through villi (small projections of intestinal lining)
      2. Divisions—duodenum, jejunum, ileum
   G. Large intestine
      1. Functions
         a. Storage and elimination of waste (defecation)
         b. Reabsorption of water
      2. Divisions—cecum; ascending, transverse, descending, and sigmoid colons; rectum; anus

III. **ACCESSORY ORGANS**
   A. Salivary glands—secrete saliva
      1. Functions of saliva
         a. Moistening food—aids chewing and swallowing
         b. Cleaning of mouth and teeth
         c. Digestion of starch with amylase
      2. Three pairs—parotid, submandibular, sublingual
   B. Liver
      1. Functions
         a. Manufacture of bile—emulsifies fats
         b. Storage of glucose
         c. Modification of fats
         d. Storage of vitamins and iron
         e. Formation of blood plasma proteins
         f. Destruction of old red blood cells
         g. Synthesis of urea—waste product of proteins
         h. Detoxification of harmful substances

C. Gallbladder
   1. Stores bile until needed for digestion
D. Pancreas
   1. Secretes powerful digestive juice
   2. Secretes sodium bicarbonate ($NaHCO_3$), an alkali (base) to neutralize chyme
IV. **ENZYMES AND THE DIGESTIVE PROCESS**
   A. Enzymes—catalysts that speed reactions
      1. Products of digestion
         a. Simple sugars (monosaccharides) from carbohydrates
         b. Peptides and amino acids from proteins
         c. Glycerol and fatty acids from fats
   B. The role of water
      1. Used to split foods (hydrolysis)
      2. Lubricates and dilutes food
   C. Digestion, step-by-step
      1. Mouth—starch
      2. Stomach—protein
      3. Small intestine—remainder of food
V. **ABSORPTION**
   A. Movement of nutrients into the circulation
   B. Absorption of fats—most enter lymphatic system
   C. Absorption of vitamins and minerals
VI. **CONTROL OF DIGESTION**
   A. Nervous control
      1. Parasympathetic system—generally increases activity
      2. Sympathetic system—generally decreases activity
   B. Hormonal control
      1. Stimulation of digestive activity
      2. Feedback to inhibit stomach activity
      3. Examples—gastrin, GIP, secretin, CCK
   C. Hunger and appetite

D. Eating disorders—e.g., anorexia, bulimia
VII. **DISORDERS OF THE DIGESTIVE SYSTEM**
   A. Peritonitis
   B. Diseases of the mouth and teeth—caries, gingivitis, periodontitis, Vincent disease, leukoplakia
   C. Disorders involving the esophagus and stomach
      1. Hiatal hernia—protrusion of organ through diaphragm
      2. Gastroesophageal reflux disease (GERD)
      3. Nausea, vomiting (emesis)
      4. Cancer
      5. Ulcer—peptic ulcer in esophagus, stomach, or duodenum
      6. Pyloric stenosis
   D. Intestinal disorders
      1. Inflammatory diseases—appendicitis, Crohn disease, ulcerative colitis, irritable bowel syndrome (IBS), diverticulitis
      2. Diarrhea
      3. Constipation
      4. Obstruction—intussuception, volvulus, ileus, hemorrhoids
      5. Cancer
   E. Infection of the salivary glands
      1. Mumps—viral infection of parotid salivary gland
   F. Cirrhosis and other diseases of the liver
      1. Jaundice—yellow color due to bile pigments in blood
      2. Hepatitis—viruses A to E
      3. Cancer
   G. Gallstones—cholelithiasis
   H. Pancreatitis
VIII. **AGING AND THE DIGESTIVE SYSTEM**

Questions for Study and Review

BUILDING UNDERSTANDING

Fill in the blanks

1. The wave-like movement of the digestive tract wall is called _____.
2. The small intestine is connected to the posterior abdominal wall by _____.
3. The liver can store glucose in the form of _____.
4. The parotid glands secrete ____ ,
5. Inflammation of the gallbladder is termed _____.

Matching > Match each numbered item with the most closely related lettered item.

___ **6.** Digests starch

___ **7.** Begins protein digestion

___ **8.** Digests fats

___ **9.** Digests protein to amino acids

___ **10.** Emulsify fats

a. lipase

b. amylase

c. trypsin

d. pepsin

e. bile salts

Multiple choice

___ **11.** The teeth break up food into small parts by a process called

   a. absorption
   b. deglutition
   c. ingestion
   d. mastication

___ **12.** Hydrochloric acid and pepsin are secreted by the

   a. salivary glands
   b. stomach
   c. pancreas
   d. liver

___ **13.** The double layer of peritoneum that extends from the lower border of the stomach and hangs over the intestine is the

   a. greater omentum
   b. lesser omentum
   c. mesentery
   d. mesocolon

___ **14.** The soft, fleshy V-shaped mass of tissue that hangs from the soft palate is the

   a. epiglottis
   b. esophageal hiatus
   c. uvula
   d. gingiva

___ **15.** Thickened white patches on the oral mucous membranes characterizes the disorder called

   a. periodontitis
   b. cholelithiasis
   c. pancreatitis
   d. leukoplakia

UNDERSTANDING CONCEPTS

16. Differentiate between the terms in each of the following pairs:

   a. digestion and absorption
   b. parietal and visceral peritoneum
   c. gastrin and gastric-inhibitory peptide
   d. secretin and cholecystokinin

17. Name the four layers of the digestive tract. What tissue makes up each layer? What is the function of each layer?

18. Trace the path of a bolus of food through the digestive system.

19. Describe the structure and function of the liver, pancreas, and gallbladder. How are the products of these organs delivered to the digestive tract?

20. Where does absorption occur in the digestive tract, and what structures are needed for absorption? What types of nutrients are absorbed into the blood? Into the lymph?

21. Name several hormones that regulate digestion.

22. Compare and contrast the following disorders:

   a. anorexia and bulimia
   b. inflammatory bowel disease and irritable bowel syndrome
   c. intussusception and volvulus

23. What are the causes and effects of hepatitis?

CONCEPTUAL THINKING

24. Why should a person who suffers from peptic ulcers avoid the use of aspirin (acetylsalicylic acid)?

25. Cholelithiasis can cause pancreatitis. Why?

26. In Adam's case, the proctologist described a future test in which pathologists would look for genetic changes in sloughed off colon cells. What kind of changes might they look for?

27. Colorectal cancer often develops from polyps in the intestinal lining. What is a polyp and why might a polyp become cancerous?

19

CHAPTER 20

Metabolism, Nutrition, and Body Temperature

Learning Outcomes

After careful study of this chapter, you should be able to:

1. Differentiate between catabolism and anabolism
2. Differentiate between the anaerobic and aerobic phases of cellular respiration and give the end products and the relative amount of energy released by each
3. Define *metabolic rate* and name several factors that affect the metabolic rate
4. Explain the roles of glucose and glycogen in metabolism
5. Compare the energy contents of fats, proteins, and carbohydrates
6. Define *essential amino acid*
7. Explain the roles of minerals and vitamins in nutrition and give examples of each
8. List the recommended percentages of carbohydrate, fat, and protein in the diet
9. Distinguish between simple and complex carbohydrates, giving examples of each
10. Compare saturated and unsaturated fats
11. List some adverse effects of alcohol consumption
12. Describe some nutritional disorders
13. Explain how heat is produced and lost in the body
14. Describe the role of the hypothalamus in regulating body temperature
15. Explain the role of fever in disease
16. Describe some adverse effects of excessive heat and cold
17. Show how word parts are used to build words related to metabolism, nutrition, and body temperature (see Word Anatomy at the end of the chapter)

Selected Key Terms

The following terms and other boldface terms in the chapter are defined in the Glossary

anabolism
catabolism
fever
glucose
glycogen
hypothalamus
hypothermia
kilocalorie
malnutrition
metabolic rate
mineral
oxidation
pyrogen
vitamin

Disease in Context

➤ Becky's Second Case: Managing Her Metabolism

"Becky, are you sure you packed everything? Glucose monitor, insulin, needles..." asked Becky's mom as she loaded her daughter's knapsack and sleeping bag into the car. Becky rolled her eyes and said, "Yeah mom, I've got everything. Don't worry; I'll only be at camp for a week!"

Becky's mom sighed. She knew her daughter was right. Besides, *this* summer camp was for children with diabetes mellitus. Not only would she get to do all the fun things that kids normally do at camp, she would also be safe. After all, there was experienced medical staff on site and many of the camp counselors were diabetic themselves. Becky's mom knew that this was a great opportunity for her daughter to learn more about managing her condition and meet other kids with diabetes.

At camp, Becky was having a great time. Her cabin leader, Wanda, was really cool. Today, Wanda was going to teach them how to paddle a canoe! "OK girls," said Wanda, "before we head out to the dock, we need to check our blood glucose levels. Does anyone remember why?"

"Paddling a canoe takes a lot of effort and we have to make sure that we have energy for our muscles to do the work," answered Becky's bunkmate.

"That's right!" replied Wanda. She went on to explain that blood glucose is the main energy source for the body. The pancreas releases the hormone insulin, which signals body cells to absorb glucose from the blood stream. Then, the cells run a series of chemical reactions (called cellular respiration) that convert glucose into carbon dioxide and water. During these catabolic reactions, the cells manufacture adenosine triphosphate (ATP), which they use to run their cellular activities. People with diabetes mellitus don't make enough insulin, so their cells aren't able to absorb glucose from the bloodstream and use it to make ATP. To ensure a constant supply of cellular ATP, diabetics must monitor their blood glucose levels and inject themselves with insulin.

Diabetes mellitus is a disorder that affects glucose metabolism. In this chapter, we'll learn more about metabolism as well as nutrition and body temperature regulation. Later in the chapter, we'll revisit Becky and see what else she's learned at camp.

Metabolism

Nutrients absorbed from the digestive tract are used for all the body's cellular activities, which together make up **metabolism**. These activities fall into two categories:

- **Catabolism**, the breakdown of complex compounds into simpler compounds. Catabolism includes the digestion of food into small molecules and the release of energy from these molecules within the cell.

- **Anabolism**, the building of simple compounds into substances needed for cellular activities and for the growth and repair of tissues.

Through the steps of catabolism and anabolism, there is a constant turnover of body materials as energy is consumed, cells function and grow, and waste products are generated.

CHECKPOINT 20-1 ➤ What are the two phases of metabolism?

Cellular Respiration

Energy is released from nutrients in a series of reactions called **cellular respiration** (Table 20-1 and Fig. 20-1). Early studies on cellular respiration were done with **glucose** as the starting compound. Glucose is a simple sugar that is the body's main energy source.

THE ANAEROBIC PHASE The first steps in the breakdown of glucose do not require oxygen; that is, they are **anaerobic**. This phase of catabolism, known as **glycolysis** (gli-KOL-ih-sis), occurs in the cell's cytoplasm. It yields a small amount of energy, which is used to make ATP (adenosine triphosphate), the cell's energy compound. Each glucose molecule yields enough energy by this process to produce two molecules of ATP.

The anaerobic breakdown of glucose is incomplete and ends with formation of an organic product called **pyruvic** (pi-RU-vik) **acid**. This organic acid is further metabolized in the next phase of cellular respiration, which requires oxygen. In muscle cells operating briefly under anaerobic conditions, pyruvic acid is converted to lactic acid, which accumulates as the cells build up an oxygen debt (described in Chapter 8). Lactic acid induces muscle fatigue, so the body is forced to rest and recover. During the recovery phase immediately after exercise, breathing

ANAEROBIC

AEROBIC

Figure 20-1 **Cellular respiration.** This diagram shows the catabolism of glucose without oxygen (anaerobic) and with oxygen (aerobic). (c, carbon atoms in one molecule of a substance.) In cellular respiration, glucose first yields two molecules of pyruvic acid, which will convert to lactic acid under anaerobic conditions, as during intense exercise. (Lactic acid must eventually be converted back to pyruvic acid.) Typically, however, pyruvic acid is broken down aerobically (using oxygen) to CO_2 and H_2O. **[ZOOMING IN ➤** What does pyruvic acid produce in cellular respiration under anaerobic conditions? Under aerobic conditions? **]**

restores the oxygen needed to convert lactic acid back to pyruvic acid, which is then metabolized further. During this recovery phase, reserves stored in muscles are also replenished. These compounds are myoglobin, which stores oxygen; glycogen, which can be broken down into glucose; and creatine phosphate, which stores energy.

THE AEROBIC PHASE To generate enough energy for survival, the body's cells must break pyruvic acid down more completely in the second phase of cellular respiration, which requires oxygen. These **aerobic** reactions occur within the cell's mitochondria. They result in transfer of most of the energy remaining in the nutrients to ATP. On

Table 20-1	Summary of Cellular Respiration of Glucose		
Phase	**Location in Cell**	**End Product(s)**	**Energy Yield/Glucose**
Anaerobic (glycolysis)	Cytoplasm	Pyruvic acid	2 ATP
Aerobic	Mitochondria	Carbon dioxide and water	30 ATP

average, cells are able to form about 30 molecules of ATP aerobically per glucose molecule. Statements on energy yields may differ slightly, because cells in different tissues vary in their metabolic pathways and in the amount of energy they use to power cellular respiration. In any case, this additional yield is quite an increase over anaerobic metabolism alone, resulting in a total of 32 molecules of ATP per glucose as compared to two.

During the aerobic steps of cellular respiration, the cells form carbon dioxide, which then must be transported to the lungs for elimination. In addition, water is formed by the combination of oxygen with the hydrogen that is removed from nutrient molecules. Because of the type of chemical reactions involved, and because oxygen is used in the final steps, cellular respiration is described as an **oxidation** of nutrients. Note that enzymes are required as catalysts in all these metabolic reactions. Many of the vitamins and minerals described later in this chapter are parts of these enzymes.

Although the oxidation of food is often compared to the burning of fuel, this comparison is inaccurate. Burning fuel results in a sudden and often wasteful release of energy in the form of heat and light. In contrast, metabolic oxidation occurs in small steps, and much of the energy released is stored as ATP for later use by the cells; some of

the energy is released as heat, which is used to maintain body temperature, as discussed later in this chapter.

For those who know how to read chemical equations, the net balanced equation for cellular respiration, starting with glucose, is as follows:

$$C_6H_{12}O_6 + 6O_2 \rightarrow 6CO_2 + 6H_2O$$

glucose   oxygen   carbon dioxide   water

CHECKPOINT 20-2 ➤ What name is given to the series of cellular reactions that releases energy from nutrients?

METABOLIC RATE **Metabolic rate** refers to the rate at which energy is released from nutrients in the cells. It is affected by a person's size, body fat, sex, age, activity, and hormones, especially thyroid hormone (thyroxine). Metabolic rate is high in children and adolescents and decreases with age. **Basal metabolism** is the amount of energy needed to maintain life functions while the body is at rest.

The unit used to measure energy is the kilocalorie (kcal), which is the amount of heat needed to raise 1 kilogram of water 1°C. To estimate the daily calories needed taking activity level into account, see Box 20-1, Calorie Counting.

Box 20-1   A Closer Look

Calorie Counting: Estimating Daily Energy Needs

Basal energy requirements for a day can be estimated with a simple formula. An average woman requires 0.9 kcal/kg/hour, and a man, 1.0 kcal/kg/hour. Multiplying 0.9 by body weight in kilograms* by 24 for a woman, or 1.0 by body weight in kilograms by 24 for a man, yields the daily basal energy requirement. For example, if a woman weighed 132 pounds, the equation would be as follows:

132 pounds ÷ 2.2 pounds/kg = 60 kg

0.9 kcal/kg/hour × 60 kg = 54 kcal/hour

54 kcal/hour × 24 hours/day = 1,296 kcal/day

To estimate total energy needs for a day, a percentage based on activity level ("couch potato" to serious athlete) must also be added to the basal requirement. These percentages are shown in the table that follows.

The equation to calculate total energy needs for a day is:

Basal energy requirement + (basal energy requirement × activity level)

Using our previous example, and assuming light activity levels, the following equations apply:

At 40% activity:

1,296 kcal/day + (1,296 kcal/day × 40%) = 1,814.4 kcal/day

At 60% activity:

1,296 kcal/day + (1,296 kcal/day × 60%) = 2,073.6 kcal/day

Therefore, the woman in our example would require between 1,814 and 2,073 kcal/day.

Activity Level	Male	Female
Little activity ("couch potato")	25%–40%	25%–35%
Light activity (e.g., walking to and from class, but little or no intentional exercise)	50%–75%	40%–60%
Moderate activity (e.g., aerobics several times a week)	65%–80%	50%–70%
Heavy activity (serious athlete)	90%–120%	80%–100%

*To convert pounds to kilograms, divide weight in pounds by 2.2.

The Use of Nutrients for Energy

As noted, glucose is the body's main energy source. Most of the carbohydrates in the diet are converted to glucose in the course of metabolism. Reserves of glucose are stored in liver and muscle cells as **glycogen** (GLI-ko-jen), a compound built from glucose molecules. When glucose is needed for energy, glycogen is broken down to yield glucose. Glycerol and fatty acids (from fat digestion) and amino acids (from protein digestion) can also be used for energy, but they enter the breakdown process at different points.

Fat in the diet yields more than twice as much energy as do protein and carbohydrate (e.g., it is more "fattening"); fat yields 9 kcal of energy per gram, whereas protein and carbohydrate each yield 4 kcal per gram. Calories that are ingested in excess of need are converted to fat and stored in adipose tissue.

Before they are oxidized for energy, amino acids must have their nitrogen (amine) groups removed. This removal, called **deamination** (de-am-ih-NA-shun), occurs in the liver, where the nitrogen groups are then formed into urea by combination with carbon dioxide. The blood transports urea to the kidneys to be eliminated.

There are no specialized storage forms of proteins, as there are for carbohydrates (glycogen) and fats (adipose tissue). Therefore, when one needs more proteins than are supplied in the diet, they must be obtained from body substance, such as muscle tissue or plasma proteins. Drawing on these resources becomes dangerous when needs are extreme. Fats and carbohydrates are described as "protein sparing," because they are used for energy before proteins are and thus spare proteins for the synthesis of necessary body components.

CHECKPOINT 20-3 ➤ What is the main energy source for the cells?

Anabolism

Nutrient molecules are built into body materials by anabolic steps, all of which are catalyzed by enzymes.

ESSENTIAL AMINO ACIDS Eleven of the 20 amino acids needed to build proteins can be synthesized internally by metabolic reactions. These 11 amino acids are described as *nonessential* because they need not be taken in as food (Table 20-2). The remaining 9 amino acids cannot be made metabolically and therefore must be taken in as part of the diet; these are the **essential amino acids**. Note that some nonessential amino acids may become essential under certain conditions, as during extreme physical stress, or in certain hereditary metabolic diseases.

ESSENTIAL FATTY ACIDS There are also two essential fatty acids, **linoleic** (lin-o-LE-ik) **acid** and **linolenic** (lin-o-LEN-ik) **acid**, that must be taken in as food. These are easily obtained through a healthful, balanced diet.

CHECKPOINT 20-4 ➤ What is meant when an amino acid or a fatty acid is described as essential?

Minerals and Vitamins

In addition to needing fats, proteins, and carbohydrates, the body requires minerals and vitamins.

Table 20-2	**Amino acids**

Nonessential Amino Acids*		Essential Amino Acids**	
Name	**Pronunciation**	**Name*****	**Pronunciation**
Alanine	AL-ah-nene	Histidine	HIS-tih-dene
Arginine	AR-jih-nene	Isoleucine	i-so-LU-sene
Asparagine	ah-SPAR-ah-jene	Leucine	LU-sene
Aspartic acid	ah-SPAR-tik AH-sid	Lysine	LI-sene
Cysteine	SIS-teh-ene	Methionine	meh-THI-o-nene
Glutamic acid	glu-TAM-ik AH-sid	Phenylalanine	fen-il-AL-ah-nene
Glutamine	GLU-tah-mene	Threonine	THRE-o-nene
Glycine	GLY-sene	Tryptophan	TRIP-to-fane
Proline	PRO-lene	Valine	VA-lene
Serine	SERE-ene		
Tyrosine	TI-ro-sene		

*Nonessential amino acids can be synthesized by the body.

**Essential amino acids cannot be synthesized by the body; they must be taken in as part of the diet.

***If you are ever called upon to memorize the essential amino acids, the mnemonic (memory device) Pvt. T. M. Hill gives the first letter of each name.

Minerals are chemical elements needed for body structure, fluid balance, and such activities as muscle contraction, nerve impulse conduction, and blood clotting. Some minerals are components of vitamins. A list of the main minerals needed in a proper diet is given in Table 20-3. Some additional minerals not listed are also required for good health. Minerals needed in extremely small amounts are referred to as **trace elements**.

Vitamins are complex organic substances needed in very small quantities. Vitamins are parts of enzymes or other substances essential for metabolism, and vitamin deficiencies lead to a variety of nutritional diseases.

The water-soluble vitamins are the B vitamins and vitamin C. These are not stored and must be taken in regularly with food. The fat-soluble vitamins are A, D, E, and K. These vitamins are kept in reserve in fatty tissue. Excess intake of the fat-soluble vitamins can lead to toxicity. A list of vitamins is given in Table 20-4.

Certain substances are valuable in the diet as **antioxidants**. They defend against the harmful effects of **free radicals**, highly reactive and unstable molecules produced from oxygen in the normal course of metabolism (and also from UV radiation, air pollution, and tobacco smoke). Free radicals contribute to aging and disease. Antioxidants react with free radicals to stabilize them and minimize their harmful effects on cells. Vitamins C and E and beta-carotene, an orange pigment found in plants that is converted to vitamin A, are antioxidants. There are also many compounds found in plants (e.g., soybeans and tomatoes) that are antioxidants.

CHECKPOINT 20-5 ➤ Both vitamins and minerals are needed in metabolism. What is the difference between vitamins and minerals?

Table 20-3	**Minerals**		
Mineral	**Functions**	**Sources**	**Results of Deficiency**
Calcium (Ca)	Formation of bones and teeth, blood clotting, nerve conduction, muscle contraction	Dairy products, eggs, green vegetables, legumes (peas and beans)	Rickets, tetany, osteoporosis
Phosphorus (P)	Formation of bones and teeth; found in ATP, nucleic acids	Meat, fish, poultry, egg yolk, dairy products	Osteoporosis, abnormal metabolism
Sodium (Na)	Fluid balance; nerve impulse conduction, muscle contraction	Most foods, especially processed foods, table salt	Weakness, cramps, diarrhea, dehydration
Potassium (K)	Fluid balance, nerve and muscle activity	Fruits, meats, seafood, milk, vegetables, grains	Muscular and neurologic disorders
Chloride (Cl)	Fluid balance, hydrochloric acid in stomach	Meat, milk, eggs, processed foods, table salt	Rarely occurs
Iron (Fe)	Oxygen carrier (hemoglobin, myoglobin)	Meat, eggs, fortified cereals, legumes, dried fruit	Anemia, dry skin, indigestion
Iodine (I)	Thyroid hormones	Seafood, iodized salt	Hypothyroidism, goiter
Magnesium (Mg)	Catalyst for enzyme reactions, carbohydrate metabolism	Green vegetables, grains, nuts, legumes	Spasticity, arrhythmia, vasodilation
Manganese (Mn)	Catalyst in actions of calcium and phosphorus; facilitator of many cellular processes	Many foods	Possible reproductive disorders
Copper (Cu)	Necessary for absorption and use of iron in formation of hemoglobin; part of some enzymes	Meat, water	Anemia
Chromium (Cr)	Works with insulin to regulate blood glucose levels	Meat, unrefined food, fats and oils	Inability to use glucose
Cobalt (Co)	Part of vitamin B_{12}	Animal products	Pernicious anemia
Zinc (Zn)	Promotes carbon dioxide transport and energy metabolism; found in enzymes	Meat, fish, poultry, grains, vegetables	Alopecia (baldness); possibly related to diabetes
Fluoride (F)	Prevents tooth decay	Fluoridated water, tea, seafood	Dental caries

20

Table 20-4	Vitamins		
Vitamins	**Functions**	**Sources**	**Results of Deficiency**
A (retinol)	Required for healthy epithelial tissue and for eye pigments; involved in reproduction and immunity	Orange fruits and vegetables, liver, eggs, dairy products, dark green vegetables	Night blindness; dry, scaly skin; decreased immunity
B_1 (thiamin)	Required for enzymes involved in oxidation of nutrients; nerve function	Pork, cereal, grains, meats, legumes, nuts	Beriberi, a disease of nerves
B_2 (riboflavin)	In enzymes required for oxidation of nutrients	Milk, eggs, liver, green leafy vegetables, grains	Skin and tongue disorders
B_3 (niacin, nicotinic acid)	Involved in oxidation of nutrients	Yeast, meat, liver, grains, legumes, nuts	Pellagra with dermatitis, diarrhea, mental disorders
B_6 (pyridoxine)	Amino acid and fatty acid metabolism; formation of niacin; manufacture of red blood cells	Meat, fish, poultry, fruit, grains, legumes, vegetables	Anemia, irritability, convulsions, muscle twitching, skin disorders
Pantothenic acid	Essential for normal growth; energy metabolism	Yeast, liver, eggs, and many other foods	Sleep disturbances, digestive upset
B_{12} (cyanocobalamin)	Production of cells; maintenance of nerve cells; fatty acid and amino acid metabolism	Animal products	Pernicious anemia
Biotin (a B vitamin)	Involved in fat and glycogen formation, amino acid metabolism	Peanuts, liver, tomatoes, eggs, oatmeal, soy, and many other foods	Lack of coordination, dermatitis, fatigue
Folate (folic acid, a B vitamin)	Required for amino acid metabolism, DNA synthesis, maturation of red blood cells	Vegetables, liver, legumes, seeds	Anemia, digestive disorders, neural tube defects in the embryo
C (ascorbic acid)	Maintains healthy skin and mucous membranes; involved in synthesis of collagen; antioxidant	Citrus fruits, green vegetables, potatoes, orange fruits	Scurvy, poor wound healing, anemia, weak bones
D (calciferol)	Aids in absorption of calcium and phosphorus from intestinal tract	Fatty fish, liver, eggs, fortified milk	Rickets, bone deformities
E (tocopherol)	Protects cell membranes; antioxidant	Seeds, green vegetables, nuts, grains, oils	Anemia, muscle and liver degeneration, pain
K	Synthesis of blood clotting factors, bone formation	Bacteria in digestive tract, liver, cabbage, and leafy green vegetables	Hemorrhage

Nutritional Guidelines

The relative amounts of carbohydrates, fats, and proteins that should be in the daily diet vary somewhat with the individual. Typical recommendations for the number of calories derived each day from the three types of food are as follows:

- Carbohydrate: 55% to 60%.
- Fat: 30% or less.
- Protein: 15% to 20%.

It is important to realize that the type as well as the amount of each nutrient is a factor in good health. A weight loss diet should follow the same proportions as given above, but with a reduction in portion sizes.

Carbohydrates

Carbohydrates in the diet should be mainly complex, naturally occurring carbohydrates, and one should keep simple sugars to a minimum. Simple sugars are monosaccharides, such as glucose and fructose (fruit sugar), and disaccharides, such as sucrose (table sugar) and lactose (milk sugar). Simple sugars are a source of fast energy because they are metabolized rapidly. However, they boost pancreatic insulin output, and as a result, they cause blood glucose levels to rise and fall rapidly. It is healthier to maintain steady glucose levels, which normally range from approximately 85 to 125 mg/dL throughout the day.

The **glycemic effect** is a measure of how rapidly a particular food raises the blood glucose level and stimulates the release of insulin. The effect is generally low for whole grains, fruit, and dairy products and high for sweets and refined ("white") grains. Note, however, that the glycemic effect of a food also depends on when it is eaten during the day, and if or how it is combined with other foods.

Complex carbohydrates are polysaccharides. Examples are:

- Starches, found in grains, legumes, and potatoes
- Fibers, such as cellulose, pectins, and gums, which are the structural materials of plants

Fiber adds bulk to the stool and promotes elimination of toxins and waste. It also slows the digestion and absorption of carbohydrates, thus regulating the release of glucose. It helps in weight control by providing a sense of fullness and limiting caloric intake. Adequate fiber in the diet lowers cholesterol and helps to prevent diabetes, colon cancer, hemorrhoids, appendicitis, and diverticulitis. Foods high in fiber, such as whole grains, fruits, and vegetables, are also rich in vitamins and minerals (see Box 20-2).

CHECKPOINT 20-6 ➤ What is the normal range of blood glucose?

Fats

Fats are subdivided into saturated and unsaturated forms based on their chemical structure. The fatty acids in **saturated fats** have more hydrogen atoms in their molecules and fewer double bonds between carbons atoms than do those of unsaturated fats (Fig. 20-2). Most saturated fats are from animal sources and are solid at room temperature, such as butter and lard. Also included in this group are the so-called "tropical oils": coconut oil and palm oil. **Unsaturated fats** are derived from plants. They are liquid at room temperature and are generally referred to as oils, such as corn, peanut, olive, and canola oils.

Saturated fats should make up less than one third of the fat in the diet (less than 10% of total calories). Diets high in saturated fats are associated with a higher than normal incidence of cancer, heart disease, and cardiovascular problems, although the relation between these factors is not fully understood.

Many commercial products contain fats that are artificially saturated to prevent rancidity and provide a more solid consistency. These are listed on food labels as partially hydrogenated (HI-dro-jen-a-ted) vegetable oils and are found in baked goods, processed peanut butter, vegetable shortening, and solid margarine. Evidence shows that components of hydrogenated fats, known as *trans-fatty acids*, may be just as harmful, if not more so, than natural saturated fats and should be avoided.

Proteins

Because proteins, unlike carbohydrates and fats, are not stored in special reserves, protein foods should be taken in on a regular basis, with attention to obtaining the essential amino acids. Most animal proteins supply all of the essential amino acids and are described as complete proteins. Most vegetables are lacking in one or more of the essential amino acids. People on strict vegetarian diets must learn to combine foods, such as legumes (e.g., beans and peas) with

---

Box 20-2 **Health Maintenance**

Dietary Fiber: Bulking Up

Dietary fiber is best known for its ability to improve bowel habits and ease weight loss. But fiber may also help to prevent diabetes, heart disease, and certain digestive disorders such as diverticulitis and gallstones.

Dietary fiber is an indigestible type of carbohydrate found in fruit, vegetables, and whole grains. The amount of fiber recommended for a 2,000-calorie diet is 25 grams per day, but most people in the United States tend to get only half this amount. One should eat fiber-rich foods throughout the day to meet the requirement. It is best to increase fiber in the diet gradually to avoid unpleasant symptoms, such as intestinal bloating and flatulence. If your diet lacks fiber, try adding the following foods over a period of several weeks:

- Whole grain breads, cereals, pasta, and brown rice. These add 1 to 3 more grams of fiber per serving than the "white" product.
- Legumes, which include beans, peas, and lentils. These add 4 to 12 grams of fiber per serving.
- Fruits and vegetables. Whole, raw, unpeeled versions contain the most fiber, and juices, the least. Apple juice has no fiber, whereas a whole apple has 3 grams.
- Unprocessed bran. This can be sprinkled over almost any food: cereal, soups, and casseroles. One tablespoon adds 2 grams of fiber. Be sure to take adequate fluids with bran.

20

Saturated
fatty acid
(stearic acid)

Unsaturated
fatty acid
(linoleic acid)

A   **B**

Figure 20-2 **Saturated and unsaturated fats. (A)** Saturated fatty acids contain the maximum numbers of hydrogen atoms attached to carbons and no double bonds between carbon atoms. **(B)** Unsaturated fatty acids have less than the maximum number of hydrogen atoms attached to carbons and one or more double bonds between carbon atoms (highlighted).

grains (e.g., rice, corn, or wheat), to obtain all the essential amino acids each day. Table 20-5 demonstrates the principles of combining two foods, legumes and grains, to supply essential amino acids that might be missing in one food or the other. Legumes are rich in isoleucine and lysine but poor in methionine and tryptophan, while grains are just the opposite. For illustration purposes, the table includes only the four missing essential amino acids (there are nine total). Traditional ethnic diets reflect these healthy combinations, for example, beans with corn or rice in Mexican dishes or chickpeas and lentils with wheat in Middle Eastern fare.

Vitamin and Mineral Supplements

The need for mineral and vitamin supplements to the diet is a subject of controversy. Some researchers maintain that adequate amounts of these substances can be obtained from a varied, healthful diet. Many commercial foods, including milk, cereal, and bread, are already fortified with minerals and vitamins. Others hold that pollution, depletion of the soils, and the storage, refining, and processing of foods make additional supplementation beneficial. Most agree, however, that children, elderly people, pregnant and lactating women, and teenagers, who often do not get enough of the proper foods, would profit from additional minerals and vitamins.

When required, supplements should be selected by a physician or nutritionist to fit an individual's particular needs. Megavitamin dosages may cause unpleasant reactions and in some cases are hazardous. Vitamins A and D have both been found to cause serious toxic effects when taken in excess.

U.S. Dietary Guidelines

The United States Department of Agriculture (USDA) has published dietary guidelines at regular intervals since 1916. The newest version, incorporating updated nutritional information, is the 2005 guide, MyPyramid (Fig. 20-3). The colored bands in the pyramid show five different categories of foods in widths that indicate relative amounts that should be chosen from each group daily. The narrow yellow band

Table 20-5 Combining Foods for Essential Amino Acids

	Essential Amino Acids*			
	Isoleucine	Lysine	Methionine	Tryptophan
Legumes	+	+		
Grains			+	+
Legumes and grains combined	+	+	+	+

*There are 9 essential amino acids; the table includes 4 for the purposes of illustration.

GRAINS | VEGETABLES | FRUITS | MILK | MEAT & BEANS

Figure 20-3 **U.S. Dietary Guidelines.** (MyPyramid, U.S. Department of Agriculture/Center for Nutrition Policy and Promotion.)

between the fruits (red) and milk (blue) represents oils, which should be consumed in moderation.

The pyramid and accompanying guidelines stress:

- Variety in the diet. Foods in all the groups are needed each day for good health.

- Moderation. A single serving or portion is smaller than most people think.

- Eating fruits and vegetables. Most people need more of these in their diets.

- Choice of "nutrient dense" foods that are rich in nutrients compared to their calorie content. This recommendation also includes eating unrefined foods, such as whole grains, and unprocessed foods.

- The importance of exercise, as represented by the climbing figure on the side of the pyramid.

The pyramid graphic does not include sugar, solid fats, or alcohol. The USDA guidelines explain that these are considered "discretionary calories," that is, "extras" that you can eat within your recommended daily energy limit after nutrient needs are met. Of course, you could also select additional foods from among the recommended nutrient-rich groups to satisfy energy needs.

The new guidelines also stress individual variation. On the Internet at http://www.mypyramid.gov/ you can get a personalized estimate of what and how much you should eat based on your height, weight, age, sex, and level of physical activity. You can also access your diet online with MyPyramid Tracker. Most people will need to make gradual shifts in their diets to reach their healthier eating goals, as suggested by the steps on the side of the pyramid.

Alcohol

Alcohol yields energy in the amount of 7 kcal per gram, but it is not considered a nutrient because it does not yield

useful end products. In fact, alcohol interferes with metabolism and contributes to a variety of disorders.

The body can metabolize about one-half ounce of pure alcohol (ethanol) per hour. This amount translates into one glass of wine, one can of beer, or one shot of hard liquor. Consumed at a more rapid rate, alcohol enters the bloodstream and affects many cells, notably in the brain.

Alcohol is rapidly absorbed through the stomach and small intestine and is detoxified by the liver. When delivered in excess to the liver, alcohol can lead to the accumulation of fat as well as inflammation and scarring of liver tissue. It can eventually cause cirrhosis (*sih-RO-sis*), which involves irreversible changes in liver structure. Alcohol metabolism ties up enzymes needed for oxidation of nutrients and also results in byproducts that acidify body fluids. Other effects of alcoholism include obesity, malnutrition, cancer, ulcers, and fetal alcohol syndrome. Health professionals advise pregnant women not to drink any alcohol. In addition, alcohol impairs judgment and leads to increased involvement in accidents.

Although alcohol consumption is compatible with good health and may even have a beneficial effect on the cardiovascular system, alcohol should be consumed only in moderation.

PASSport to Success

Visit **thePoint** or see the Student Resource CD in the back of this book for a summary of the effects of alcohol abuse and photographs of its effects on liver and brain tissue.

CHECKPOINT **20-7** ➤ What are typical recommendations for the relative amounts of carbohydrates, fats, and proteins in the diet?

Nutritional Disorders

Diet-related problems may originate from an excess or shortage of necessary nutrients. Another issue in the news today is weight control. Food allergies may also affect some people.

Food Allergies

Some people develop clear allergic (hypersensitive) symptoms if they eat certain foods. Common food allergens are wheat, nuts, milk, shellfish, and eggs, but almost any food might cause an allergic reaction in a given individual. People may also have allergic reactions to food additives, such as flavorings, colorings, or preservatives. Signs of allergic reactions usually involve the skin, respiratory tract, or gastrointestinal tract. Food allergies may provoke potentially fatal anaphylactic shock in extremely sensitive individuals.

20

Malnutrition

If any vital nutrient is missing from the diet, the body will suffer from malnutrition. One commonly thinks of a malnourished person as someone who does not have enough to eat, but malnutrition can also occur from eating too much of the wrong foods. Factors that contribute to malnutrition are poverty, old age, chronic illness, anorexia, poor dental health, and drug or alcohol addiction.

In poor and underdeveloped countries, many children suffer from protein and energy malnutrition (PEM). **Marasmus** (mah-RAZ-mus) is a term used for severe malnutrition in infancy (from Greek meaning "dying away").

Kwashiorkor (kwash-e-OR-kor) typically affects older children when they are weaned because another child is born (and the name means just that). A low protein level in the blood plasma interferes with fluid return to the capillaries, resulting in edema. Often excess fluid accumulates in the abdomen as ascites (ah-SI-teze) fluid, causing the stomach to bulge.

Visit **thePoint** or see the Student Resource CD in the back of this book for the effects of kwashiorkor.

Overweight and Obesity

The causes of obesity are complex, involving social, economic, genetic, psychological, and metabolic factors. It is common knowledge that overweight and obesity have increased in the past several decades in many countries. In the US, 35% of adults are overweight and an additional 30% are obese (see "Body Mass Index" below.) Obesity shortens the life span and is associated with cardiovascular disease, diabetes, some cancers, and other diseases. The incidence of type 2 diabetes, once considered to have an adult onset, has increased greatly among children. Some researchers hold that obesity has a closer correlation to chronic disease than poverty, smoking, or drinking alcohol.

Visit **thePoint** or see the Student Resource CD in the back of this book for a summary of the long-term complications of diabetes.

Scientists are studying the nervous and hormonal controls over weight, but so far they have not found any effective and safe drugs for weight control. For most people, a varied diet eaten in moderation and regular exercise are the surest ways to avoid obesity. At least 30 minutes of moderate to vigorous exercise every day is recommended for health and weight control.

BODY MASS INDEX Body mass index (BMI) is a measurement used to evaluate body size. It is based on the ratio of weight to height (Fig. 20-4). BMI is calculated by

Calculation of body mass index (BMI)

Formula:

$$BMI = \frac{Weight\ (kg)}{Height\ (m)^2}$$

Conversion:

Kilograms = pounds ÷ 2.2

Meters = inches ÷ 39.4

Example:

A woman who is 5′4″ tall and weighs 134 pounds has a BMI of 23.5.

Weight: 134 pounds ÷ 2.2 = 61 kg

Height: 64 inches ÷ 39.4 = 1.6 m; $(1.6)^2 = 2.6$

$$BMI = \frac{61\ kg}{2.6\ m} = 23.5$$

Figure 20-4 **Calculation of body mass index (BMI).**
[ZOOMING IN ➤ What is the BMI of a male 5′10″ in height who weighs 170 pounds? (Round off to one decimal place.) **]**

dividing weight in kilograms by height in meters squared. (For those not accustomed to using the metric system, an alternate method is to divide weight in pounds by the square of height in inches and multiply by 703.) A healthy range for this measurement is 19 to 24. Overweight is defined as a BMI of 25 to 30, and obesity as a BMI greater than 30. However, BMI does not take into account the relative amount of muscle and fat in the body. For example, a bodybuilder might be healthy with a higher than typical BMI because muscle has a higher density than fat.

Underweight

People who are underweight have as much difficulty gaining weight as others have losing it. The problem of underweight may result from rapid growth, eating disorders, allergies, illness, or psychological factors. It is associated with low reserves of energy, reproductive disturbances, and nutritional deficiencies. A BMI of less than 18.5 is defined as underweight. To gain weight, people have to increase their intake of calories, but they should also exercise to add muscle tissue and not just fat.

Nutrition and Aging

With age, a person may find it difficult to maintain a balanced diet. Often, the elderly lose interest in buying and preparing food or are unable to do so. Because metabolism generally slows, and less food is required to meet energy needs, nutritional deficiencies may develop. Medications may interfere with appetite and with the absorption and use of specific nutrients.

It is important for older people to seek out foods that are "nutrient dense," that is, foods that have a high proportion of nutrients in comparison with the number of calories they provide. Exercise helps to boost appetite and maintains muscle tissue, which is more active metabolically.

Body Temperature

Heat is an important byproduct of the many chemical activities constantly occurring in body tissues. At the same time, heat is always being lost through a variety of outlets. Under normal conditions, a number of regulatory devices keep body temperature constant within quite narrow limits. Maintenance of a constant temperature despite both internal and external influences is one phase of homeostasis, the tendency of all body processes to maintain a normal state despite forces that tend to alter them.

Heat Production

Heat is a byproduct of the cellular oxidations that generate energy. The amount of heat produced by a given organ varies with the kind of tissue and its activity. While at rest, muscles may produce as little as 25% of total body heat, but when muscles contract, heat production is greatly multiplied, owing to their increased metabolic rate. Under basal conditions (at rest), the liver and other abdominal organs produce about 50% of total body heat. The brain produces only 15% of body heat at rest, and an increase in nervous tissue activity produces little increase in heat production. High heat-generating tissues do not become much warmer than others because the circulating blood distributes the heat fairly evenly.

FACTORS AFFECTING HEAT PRODUCTION The rate at which heat is produced is affected by a number of factors, including exercise, hormone production, food intake, and age. Hormones, such as thyroxine from the thyroid gland and epinephrine (adrenaline) from the adrenal medulla, increase heat production.

The intake of food is also accompanied by increased heat production. The nutrients that enter the blood after digestion are available for increased cellular metabolism. In addition, the glands and muscles of the digestive system generate heat as they set to work. These responses do not account for all the increase, however, nor do they account for the much greater increase in metabolism after a meal containing a large amount of protein.

CHECKPOINT 20-8 ➤ What are some factors that affect heat production in the body?

Heat Loss

Although 15% to 20% of heat loss occurs through the respiratory system and with urine and feces, more than 80% of heat loss occurs through the skin. Networks of blood vessels in the skin's dermis (deeper part) can bring considerable quantities of blood near the surface, so that heat can be dissipated to the outside. This release can occur in several ways.

- Heat can be transferred directly to the surrounding air by means of **conduction**.

- Heat also travels from its source as heat waves or rays, a process termed **radiation**.

- If the air is moving, so that the layer of heated air next to the body is constantly being carried away and replaced with cooler air (as by an electric fan), the process is known as **convection**.

- Finally, heat may be lost by **evaporation**, the process by which liquid changes to the vapor state.

To illustrate evaporation, rub some alcohol on your skin; it evaporates rapidly, using so much heat that your skin feels cold. Perspiration does the same thing, although not as quickly. The rate of heat loss through evaporation depends on the humidity of the surrounding air. When humidity exceeds 60% or so, perspiration does not evaporate so readily, making one feel very uncomfortable unless some other means of heat loss is available, such as convection caused by a fan.

PREVENTION OF HEAT LOSS Factors that play a part in heat loss through the skin include the volume of tissue compared with the amount of skin surface. A child loses heat more rapidly than does an adult. Such parts as fingers and toes are affected most by exposure to cold because they have a great amount of skin compared with total tissue volume.

If the surrounding air temperature is lower than that of the body, excessive heat loss is prevented by both natural and artificial means. Clothing checks heat loss by trapping insulating air in both its material and its layers. An effective natural insulation against cold is the layer of fat under the skin. The degree of insulation depends on the thickness of the subcutaneous layer. Even when skin temperature is low, this fatty tissue prevents the deeper tissues from losing much heat. On the average, this layer is slightly thicker in females than in males.

Temperature Regulation

Body temperature remains almost constant despite wide variations in the rate of heat production or loss, because of internal temperature-regulating mechanisms.

THE ROLE OF THE HYPOTHALAMUS Many body areas take part in heat regulation, but the most important center is the hypothalamus, the area of the brain located just above the pituitary gland. One group of hypothalamic cells controls heat production in body tissues, whereas another group controls heat loss. Regulation is based on the temperature of the blood circulating through the brain and also on input from temperature receptors in the skin.

If these two factors indicate that too much heat is being lost, impulses are sent quickly from the hypothalamus to the autonomic (involuntary) nervous system, which in turn causes constriction of the skin's blood vessels to reduce heat loss. Other impulses are sent to the muscles to

20

cause shivering, a rhythmic contraction that result in increased heat production. Furthermore, epinephrine output may be increased if necessary. Epinephrine increases cellular metabolism for a short period, and this in turn increases heat production.

If there is danger of overheating, the hypothalamus stimulates the sweat glands to increase their activity. Impulses from the hypothalamus also cause cutaneous blood vessels to dilate, so that increased blood flow will promote heat loss. The hypothalamus may also induce muscle relaxation to minimize heat production.

Muscles are especially important in temperature regulation because variations in the activity of these large tissue masses can readily increase or decrease heat generation. Because muscles form roughly one-third of the body, either an involuntary or an intentional increase in their activity can form enough heat to offset a considerable decrease in the temperature of the environment.

CHECKPOINT 20-9 ➤ What part of the brain is responsible for regulating body temperature?

AGE FACTORS Very young and very old people are limited in their ability to regulate body temperature when exposed to environmental extremes. A newborn infant's body temperature decreases if the infant is exposed to a cool environment for a long period. Elderly people also are not able to produce enough heat to maintain body temperature in a cool environment.

With regard to overheating in these age groups, heat loss mechanisms are not fully developed in the newborn. The elderly do not lose as much heat from their skin as do younger people. Both groups should be protected from extreme temperatures.

NORMAL BODY TEMPERATURE The normal temperature range obtained by either a mercury or an electronic thermometer may extend from 36.2°C to 37.6°C (97°F to 100°F). Body temperature varies with the time of day. Usually, it is lowest in the early morning because the muscles have been relaxed and no food has been taken in for several hours. Temperature tends to be higher in the late afternoon and evening because of physical activity and food consumption.

Normal temperature also varies in different parts of the body. Skin temperature obtained in the axilla (armpit) is lower than mouth temperature, and mouth temperature is a degree or so lower than rectal temperature. It is believed that, if it were possible to place a thermometer inside the liver, it would register a degree or more higher than rectal temperature. The temperature within a muscle might be even higher during activity.

Although the Fahrenheit scale is used in the United States, in most parts of the world, temperature is measured with the **Celsius** (SEL-se-us) thermometer. On this scale, the ice point is at 0° and the normal boiling point of water is at 100°, the interval between these two points being divided into 100 equal units. The Celsius scale is also called

the **centigrade scale** (think of 100 cents in a dollar). See Appendix 2 for a comparison of the Celsius and Fahrenheit scales and formulas for converting from one to the other.

CHECKPOINT 20-10 ➤ What is normal body temperature?

Fever

Fever is a condition in which the body temperature is higher than normal. An individual with a fever is described as **febrile** (FEB-ril). Usually, the presence of fever is due to an infection, but there can be many other causes, such as malignancies, brain injuries, toxic reactions, reactions to vaccines, and diseases involving the central nervous system (CNS). Sometimes, emotional upsets can bring on a fever. Whatever the cause, the effect is to reset the body's thermostat in the hypothalamus.

Curiously enough, fever usually is preceded by a chill—that is, a violent attack of shivering and a sensation of cold that blankets and heating pads seem unable to relieve. As a result of these reactions, heat is generated and stored and, when the chill subsides, the body temperature is elevated.

The old adage that a fever should be starved is completely wrong. During a fever, there is an increase in metabolism that is usually proportional to the fever's intensity. The body uses available sugars and fats, and there is an increase in the use of protein. During the first week or so of a fever, there is definite evidence of protein destruction, so a high-calorie diet with plenty of protein is recommended.

When a fever ends, sometimes the drop in temperature to normal occurs very rapidly. This sudden fall in temperature is called the **crisis**, and it is usually accompanied by symptoms indicating rapid heat loss: profuse perspiration, muscular relaxation, and dilation of blood vessels in the skin. A gradual drop in temperature, in contrast, is known as **lysis**. A drug that reduces fever is described as **antipyretic** (an-ti-pi-RET-ik).

The mechanism of fever production is not completely understood, but we might think of the hypothalamus as a thermostat that during fever is set higher than normal. This change in the heat-regulating mechanism often follows the introduction of a foreign protein or the entrance into the bloodstream of bacteria or their toxins. Substances that produce fever are called **pyrogens** (PI-ro-jens).

Up to a point, fever may be beneficial because it steps up phagocytosis (the process by which white blood cells destroy bacteria and other foreign material), inhibits the growth of certain organisms, and increases cellular metabolism, which may help recovery from disease.

Responses to Excessive Heat

The body's heat-regulating devices are efficient, but there is a limit to what they can accomplish. High outside temperature may overcome the body's heat loss mechanisms, in which case body temperature rises and cellular metabolism with accompanying heat production increases. When body temperature rises, the affected person is apt to suffer from a series of disorders: heat cramps are followed by heat exhaustion, which, if untreated, is followed by heat stroke.

In **heat cramps**, there is localized muscle cramping of the extremities and occasionally of the abdomen. The condition abates with rest in a cool environment and adequate fluids.

With further heat retention and more fluid loss, **heat exhaustion** occurs. Symptoms of this disorder include headache, tiredness, vomiting, and a rapid pulse. The victim feels hot, but the skin is cool due to evaporation of sweat. There may be a decrease in circulating blood volume and lowered blood pressure. Heat exhaustion is also treated by rest and fluid replacement.

Heat stroke (also called sunstroke) is a medical emergency. Heat stroke can be recognized by a body temperature of up to 41°C (105°F); hot, dry skin; and CNS symptoms, including confusion, dizziness, and loss of consciousness. The body has responded to the loss of circulating fluid by reducing blood flow to the skin and sweat glands.

It is important to lower the heatstroke victim's body temperature immediately by removing the individual's clothing, placing him or her in a cool environment, and cooling the body with cold water or ice. The patient should be treated with appropriate fluids containing necessary electrolytes, including sodium, potassium, calcium, and chloride. Supportive medical care is also needed to avoid fatal complications.

CHECKPOINT **20-11** ➤ What are some conditions brought on by excessive heat?

Responses to Excessive Cold

The body is no more capable of coping with prolonged exposure to cold than with prolonged exposure to heat. If, for example, the body is immersed in cold water for a time, the water (a better heat conductor than air) removes more heat from the body than can be replaced, and temperature falls. Cold air can produce the same result, particularly when clothing is inadequate. The main effects of an excessively low body temperature, termed **hypothermia** (hi-po-THER-me-ah), are uncontrolled shivering, lack of coordination, and decreased heart and respiratory rates. Speech becomes slurred, and there is overpowering sleepiness, which may lead to coma and death. Outdoor activities in cool, not necessarily cold, weather cause many unrecognized cases of hypothermia. Wind, fatigue, and depletion of water and energy stores all play a part.

When the body is cooled below a certain point, cellular metabolism slows, and heat production is inadequate to maintain a normal temperature. The person must then be warmed gradually by heat from an outside source. The best first aid measure is to remove the person's clothing and put him or her in a warmed sleeping bag with an unclothed companion until shivering stops. Administration of warm, sweetened fluids also helps.

Exposure to cold, particularly to moist cold, may result in **frostbite**, which can cause permanent local tissue damage. The areas most likely to be affected by frostbite are the face, ears, and extremities. Formation of ice crystals and reduction of blood supply to an area leads to necrosis (death) of tissue and possible gangrene. The very young, the very old, and those who suffer from circulatory disorders are particularly susceptible to cold injuries.

A frostbitten area should never be rubbed; rather, it should be thawed by application of warm towels or immersion in circulating lukewarm (not hot) water for 20 to 30 minutes. The affected area should be treated gently; a person with frostbitten feet should not be permitted to walk. People with cold-damaged extremities frequently have some lowering of body temperature. The whole body should be warmed at the same time that the affected part is warmed.

Hypothermia is employed in certain types of surgery. In these circumstances, drugs are used to depress the hypothalamus and reduce the body temperature to as low as 25°C (77°F) before the surgeon begins the operation. In heart surgery, the blood is cooled further to 20°C (68°F) as it goes through the heart-lung machine. This method has been successful even in infants.

CHECKPOINT **20-12** ➤ What is the term for excessively low body temperature?

Disease in Context revisited

▶ Becky Learns to Manage Her Diabetes

"Hi Mom!" Becky shouted into the camp phone. "No, everything's fine... Actually, I'm calling because I knew you were probably worried! I'm having an awesome time. I've gone canoeing, hiking, and swimming every day. At night, we've been sitting around the campfire telling ghost stories... Yeah, I've made some new friends too—everyone's really great. Wanda, my cabin leader, is so cool. She has diabetes too and she knows a lot about it. We did this neat experiment the other day where we tested our blood glucose levels before and after going on a hike. Did you know that glucose levels drop after exercise because the body uses glucose to make ATP? ... And at lunch today we learned that foods are made up of car-bohydrates, fats, and proteins. Did you know that glucose is a carbohydrate? And that some foods can raise your blood sugar really fast. Wanda called it the 'glycemic effect' or some-thing like that. Anyways, that's why it's better to eat brown bread and fruit instead of white bread and candy. We also learned about saturated and unsaturated fats. Tell Dad that when I get home he and I need to talk. If he keeps eating all those fatty foods he likes, he's going to get heart dis-ease!"

In this case, we saw that diabetes mellitus is an endocrine disorder that prevents cells from metabolizing glucose. To review the topic of dia-betes mellitus, refer back to Chapter 12.

Word Anatomy

Medical terms are built from standardized word parts (prefixes, roots, and suffixes). Learning the meanings of these parts can help you remember words and interpret unfamiliar terms.

WORD PART	MEANING	EXAMPLE
Metabolism		
glyc/o	sugar, sweet	*Glycogen* yields glucose molecules when it breaks down.
-lysis	separating, dissolving	*Glycolysis* is the breakdown of glucose for energy.
Body Temperature		
pyr/o	fire, fever	An *antipyretic* drug reduces fever.
therm/o	heat	*Hypothermia* is an excessively low body temperature.

Summary

I. **METABOLISM**
   A. Phases
      1. Catabolism—breakdown of complex com-pounds into simpler compounds
      2. Anabolism—building of simple compounds into substances needed for cellular activities, growth, and repair

   B. Cellular respiration—a series of reactions in which food is oxidized for energy
      1. Anaerobic phase—does not require oxygen
         a. Location—cytoplasm
         b. Yield—2 ATP per glucose
         c. End product—organic (i.e., pyruvic acid)

2. Aerobic phase—requires oxygen
   a. Location—mitochondria
   b. Yield—30 ATP per glucose on average
   c. End products—carbon dioxide and water
3. Metabolic rate—rate at which energy is released from food in the cells
   a. Basal metabolism—amount of energy needed to maintain life functions while at rest
C. Use of nutrients for energy
   1. Glucose—main energy source
   2. Fats—highest energy yield
   3. Proteins—can be used for energy after removal of nitrogen (deamination)
D. Anabolism
   1. Essential amino acids and fatty acids must be taken in as part of diet
E. Minerals and vitamins
   1. Minerals—elements needed for body structure and cell activities
      a. Trace elements—elements needed in extremely small amounts
   2. Vitamins—organic substances needed in small amounts
      a. Antioxidants (e.g., vitamins C and E) protect against free radicals

II. **NUTRITIONAL GUIDELINES**
A. Carbohydrates
   1. 55% to 60% of calories
   2. Should be complex (unrefined) not simple (sugars)
      a. Glycemic effect—how quickly a food raises blood glucose and insulin
      b. Plant fiber important
B. Fats
   1. 30% or less of calories
   2. Unsaturated healthier than saturated
      a. Hydrogenated fats artificially saturated
C. Proteins
   1. 15% to 20% of calories
   2. Complete—all essential amino acids
      a. Need to combine plant foods
D. Vitamin and mineral supplements
E. U.S. dietary guidelines—USDA MyPyramid
F. Alcohol—metabolized in liver

III. **NUTRITIONAL DISORDERS**
A. Food allergies
B. Malnutrition

C. Overweight and obesity
   1. Body mass index (BMI)—weight (kg) ÷ (height [m])^2
D. Underweight

IV. **NUTRITION AND AGING**
V. **BODY TEMPERATURE**
A. Heat production
   1. Most heat produced in muscles and glands
   2. Distributed by the circulation
   3. Affected by exercise, hormones, food, age
B. Heat loss
   1. Avenues—skin, urine, feces, respiratory system
   2. Mechanisms—conduction, radiation, convection, evaporation
   3. Prevention of heat loss—clothing, subcutaneous fat
C. Temperature regulation
   1. Hypothalamus—main temperature-regulating center
      a. Responds to temperature of blood in brain and temperature receptors in skin
   2. Conservation of heat
      a. Constriction of blood vessels in skin
      b. Shivering
      c. Increased release of epinephrine
   3. Release of heat
      a. Dilation of skin vessels
      b. Sweating
      c. Relaxation of muscles
   4. Age factors
   5. Normal body temperature—ranges from 36.2°C to 37.6°C; varies with time of day and location measured
D. Fever—higher than normal body temperature resulting from infection, injury, toxin, damage to CNS, etc.
   1. Pyrogen—substance that produces fever
   2. Antipyretic—drug that reduces fever
E. Response to excessive heat—heat cramps, heat exhaustion, heat stroke
F. Response to excessive cold
   1. Hypothermia—low body temperature
      a. Results—coma and death
      b. Uses—surgery
   2. Frostbite—reduction of blood supply to areas such as face, ears, toes, fingers
      a. Results—necrosis and gangrene

20

Questions for Study and Review

BUILDING UNDERSTANDING

Fill in the blanks

1. Building glycogen from glucose is an example of _____.

2. The amount of energy needed to maintain life functions while at rest is _____.

3. Reserves of glucose are stored in liver and muscle as _____.

4. The most important area of the brain for temperature regulation is the _____.

5. A drug that reduces fever is described as _____.

Matching > Match each numbered item with the most closely related lettered item.

___ **6.** Main energy source for the body

___ **7.** Chemical element required for normal body function

___ **8.** Complex organic substance required for normal body function

___ **9.** Energy storage molecule with only single bonds between carbon atoms

___ **10.** Energy storage molecule with one or more double bonds between carbon atoms

a. saturated fat

b. vitamin

c. mineral

d. unsaturated fat

e. glucose

Multiple choice

___ **11.** During amino acid catabolism, nitrogen is removed by
   a. oxidation
   b. the glycemic effect
   c. lysis
   d. deamination

___ **12.** Which of the following would have the lowest glycemic effect?
   a. glucose
   b. sucrose
   c. lactose
   d. starch

___ **13.** Alcohol is catabolized by the
   a. small intestine
   b. liver
   c. pancreas
   d. spleen

___ **14.** Amino acids that cannot be made by metabolism are said to be
   a. essential
   b. nonessential
   c. antioxidants
   d. free radicals

UNDERSTANDING CONCEPTS

15. In what part of the cell does anaerobic respiration occur and what are its end products? In what part of the cell does aerobic respiration occur? What are its end products?

16. About how many kilocalories are released from a tablespoon of butter (14 grams)? a tablespoon of sugar (12 grams)? a tablespoon of egg white (15 grams)?

17. If you eat 2,000 kcal a day, how many kilocalories should come from carbohydrates? from fats? from protein?

18. How is heat produced in the body? What structures produce the most heat during increased activity?

19. Emily's body temperature increased from 36.2°C to 36.5°C and then decreased to 36.2°C. Describe the feedback mechanism regulating Emily's body temperature.

20. Define *fever*. Name some aspects of the course of fever, and list some of its beneficial and harmful effects.

21. What is hypothermia? Under what circumstances does it usually occur? List some of its effects.

22. Differentiate between the terms in the following pairs:
   a. conduction and convection
   b. radiation and evaporation
   c. marasmus and kwashiorkor
   d. lysis and crisis
   e. heat exhaustion and heat stroke

CONCEPTUAL THINKING

23. The oxidation of glucose to form ATP is often compared to the burning of fuel. Why is this analogy inaccurate?

24. In the case story, Becky learned about the glycemic effect. In order to prevent hyperglycemia, which foods should Becky avoid or eat in moderation?

25. Richard M, a self-described couch potato, is 6 feet tall and weighs 240 pounds. Calculate Richard's body mass index. Is Richard overweight or obese? List some diseases associated with obesity.

20

CHAPTER 21

Body Fluids

Learning Outcomes

After careful study of this chapter, you should be able to:

1. Compare intracellular and extracellular fluids
2. List four types of extracellular fluids
3. Name the systems that are involved in water balance
4. Explain how thirst is regulated
5. Define *electrolytes* and describe some of their functions
6. Describe the role of hormones in electrolyte balance
7. Describe three methods for regulating the pH of body fluids
8. Compare acidosis and alkalosis, including possible causes
9. Describe three disorders involving body fluids
10. Specify some fluids used in therapy
11. Show how word parts are used to build words related to bodily fluids (see Word Anatomy at the end of the chapter)

Selected Key Terms

The following terms and other boldface terms in the chapter are defined in the Glossary

acidosis
alkalosis
ascites
buffer
dehydration
edema
effusion
electrolyte
extracellular
interstitial
intracellular
pH

PASSport to Success

Visit **thePoint** or see the Student Resource CD in the back of this book for definitions and pronunciations of key terms as well as a pretest for this chapter.

Disease
in Context

▶ Margaret's Second Case: A Fluid Balancing Act

Angela, a nurse in the intensive care unit (ICU), sat down at her station to review her patient's chart. During last week's heat wave, Margaret Ringland, 78-years-old, was admitted to the hospital with dehydration (severe water loss). This was evident by her low urine output and high urine concentration. While in emergency, she received intravenous fluids to replace the water she had lost. In the ICU, Margaret was encouraged to drink plenty of fluids so that she would remain hydrated. Over the past several days, the ICU team had kept a 24-hour intake–output record of all the liquid Margaret had ingested and excreted. Today, she was going home. But before Margaret could be discharged, Angela needed to provide her with some information to help prevent this condition from happening again.

Given the current heat wave, Angela wasn't surprised with Margaret's diagnosis. Elderly patients like Margaret are particularly susceptible to dehydration because they often have less water stored in their body fluid compartments than younger adults. In addition, their kidneys tend to be less efficient at reabsorbing water. Margaret also presented with hypernatremia (excess sodium ions in the body fluids). Angela knew this was directly related to Margaret's water loss—as her total body fluid volume dropped, the concentration of

sodium in that fluid increased. Sodium is essential for body functions such as nerve impulse transmission. However, too much sodium can cause problems, including hypertension, edema, convulsions, and even coma. Now that Margaret was rehydrated, her sodium ion concentration had dropped to normal levels as well.

While reviewing Margaret's chart, Angela noted that Margaret was also deficient in two other essential electrolytes—potassium and calcium. Like sodium, potassium is required for proper nerve impulse conduction. Calcium is required for bone formation and blood clotting. Margaret's hypokalemia was probably due to the diuretic medication her doctor had prescribed to lower her blood pressure, which caused her to lose potassium as a side effect. Her hypocalcemia was probably associated with her age-related osteoporosis. Angela reminded herself that she would have to give Margaret a list of foods rich in potassium and calcium.

For Margaret, abnormal body water volume and ion concentrations had serious health consequences. In this chapter we'll learn more about body fluid and electrolyte balance. Later, we'll check in on Margaret as Angela prepares her for discharge.

The Importance of Water

Water is important to living cells as a solvent, a transport medium, and a participant in metabolic reactions. The normal proportion of body water varies from 50% to 70% of a person's weight. It is highest in the young and in thin, muscular individuals. As the amount of fat increases, the percentage of water in the body decreases, because adipose tissue holds very little water compared with muscle tissue. In infants, water makes up 75% of the total body mass. That's why infants are in greater danger from dehydration than adults.

Various electrolytes (salts), nutrients, gases, waste, and special substances, such as enzymes and hormones, are dissolved or suspended in body water. The composition of body fluids is an important factor in homeostasis. Whenever the volume or chemical makeup of these fluids deviates even slightly from normal, disease results. (See Appendix 4, Table 3, for normal values.) The constancy of body fluids is maintained in the following ways:

■ The thirst mechanism maintains the volume of water at a constant level

■ Kidney activity regulates the volume and composition of body fluids (see Chapter 22)

■ Hormones serve to regulate fluid volume and electrolytes (see section on electrolytes later in the chapter)

■ Regulators of pH (acidity and alkalinity), including buffers, respiration, and kidney function

The maintenance of proper fluid balance involves many of the principles discussed in earlier chapters, such as pH and buffers, the effects of respiration on pH, tonicity of solutions, and forces influencing capillary exchange. Some of these chapters will be referenced in the following sections. Additional information follows in Chapter 22 on the urinary system.

Fluid Compartments

Although body fluids have much in common no matter where they are located, there are some important differences between fluid inside and outside cells. Accordingly, fluids are grouped into two main compartments (Fig. 21-1):

■ **Intracellular fluid** (ICF) is contained within the cells. About two-thirds to three-fourths of all body fluids are in this category.

■ **Extracellular fluid** (ECF) includes all body fluids outside of cells. In this group are included the following:

> **Interstitial** (in-ter-STISH-al) **fluid,** or more simply, tissue fluid. This fluid is located in the spaces between the cells in tissues all over the body. It is estimated that tissue fluid constitutes about 15% of body weight.

> **Blood plasma,** which constitutes about 4% of a person's body weight.

> **Lymph,** the fluid that drains from the tissues into the lymphatic system. This is about 1% of body weight.

> **Fluid in special compartments,** such as cerebrospinal fluid, the aqueous and vitreous humors of the eye, serous fluid, and synovial fluid. Together, these make up about 1% to 3% of total body fluids.

Fluids are not locked into one compartment. There is a constant interchange between compartments as fluids are transferred across semipermeable plasma membranes by diffusion and osmosis (see Fig. 21-1). Also, fluids are lost and replaced on a daily basis.

Figure 21-1   **Main fluid compartments showing relative percentage by weight of body fluid.** Fluid percentages vary but total about 60% of body weight. Fluids are constantly exchanged among compartments, and each day fluids are lost and replaced. **[ZOOMING IN ➤** What are some avenues through which water is lost? **]**

Water Balance

In a healthy person, the quantity of water gained in a day is approximately equal to the quantity lost (output) (Fig. 21-2). The quantity of water consumed in a day (intake) varies considerably. The average adult in a comfortable environment takes in about 2,300 mL of water (about 2 1/2 quarts) daily. About two-thirds of this quantity comes from drinking water and other beverages; about one-third comes from foods—fruits, vegetables, and soups. About 200 mL of water is produced each day as a by-product of cellular respiration. This water, described as *metabolic water*, brings the total average gain to 2,500 mL each day.

The same volume of water is constantly being lost from the body by the following routes:

- The **kidneys** excrete the largest quantity of water lost each day. About 1 to 1.5 liters of water are eliminated daily in the urine. (Note that beverages containing alcohol or caffeine act as diuretics and increase water loss through the kidneys.)
- The **skin**. Although sebum and keratin help prevent dehydration, water is constantly evaporating from the skin's surface. Larger amounts of water are lost from the skin as sweat when it is necessary to cool the body.

- The **lungs** expel water along with carbon dioxide.
- The **intestinal tract** eliminates water along with the feces.

In many disorders, it is important for the healthcare team to know whether a patient's intake and output are equal; in such a case, a 24-hour intake–output record is kept. The intake record includes *all* the liquid the patient has taken in. This means fluids administered intravenously as well as those consumed by mouth. The healthcare worker must account for water, other beverages, and liquid foods, such as soup and ice cream. The output record includes the quantity of urine excreted in the same 24-hour period as well as an estimation of fluid losses due to fever, vomiting, diarrhea, bleeding, wound discharge, or other causes.

Sense of Thirst

The control center for the sense of thirst is located in the brain's hypothalamus. This center plays a major role in the regulation of total fluid volume. A decrease in fluid volume or an increase in the concentration of body fluids stimulates the thirst center, causing a person to drink water or other fluids containing large amounts of water. Dryness of the mouth also causes a sensation of thirst. Excessive thirst, such as that caused by excessive urine loss in cases of diabetes, is called **polydipsia** (pol-e-DIP-se-ah).

The thirst center should stimulate enough drinking to balance fluids, but this is not always the case. During vigorous exercise, especially in hot weather, the body can dehydrate rapidly. People may not drink enough to replace needed fluids. In addition, if plain water is consumed, the dilution of body fluids may depress the thirst center. Athletes who are exercising very strenuously may need to drink beverages with some carbohydrates for energy and also some electrolytes to keep fluids in balance. (See Box 21-1, Osmoreceptors: Thinking About Thirst, for more about thirst regulation.)

Electrolytes and Their Functions

Electrolytes are important constituents of body fluids. These compounds separate into positively and negatively charged ions in solution. Positively charged ions are called *cations*; negatively charged ions are called *anions*. Electrolytes are so-named because they conduct an electrical current in solution. A few of the most important ions are reviewed next:

- Positive ions (cations):
    - > **Sodium** is chiefly responsible for maintaining osmotic balance and body fluid volume. It is the main positive ion in extracellular fluids. Sodium is

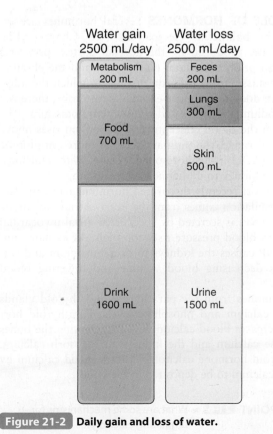

Water gain 2500 mL/day	Water loss 2500 mL/day
Metabolism 200 mL	Feces 200 mL
Food 700 mL	Lungs 300 mL
	Skin 500 mL
Drink 1600 mL	Urine 1500 mL

Figure 21-2 **Daily gain and loss of water.**

Box 21-1   A Closer Look

Osmoreceptors: Thinking About Thirst

Osmoreceptors are specialized neurons that help to maintain water balances by detecting changes in the concentration of extracellular fluid (ECF). They are located in the hypothalamus of the brain in an area adjacent to the third ventricle, where they monitor the osmotic pressure (concentration) of the circulating blood plasma.

Osmoreceptors respond primarily to small increases in sodium, the most common cation in ECF. As the blood becomes more concentrated, sodium draws water out of the cells, initiating nerve impulses. Traveling to different regions of the hypothalamus, these impulses may have two different but related effects:

■ They stimulate the hypothalamus to produce antidiuretic hormone (ADH), which is then released from the posterior pituitary. ADH travels to the kidneys and causes these organs to conserve water.

■ They stimulate the thirst center of the hypothalamus, causing increased consumption of water. Almost as soon as water consumption begins, however, the sensation of thirst disappears. Receptors in the throat and stomach send inhibitory signals to the thirst center, preventing overconsumption of water and allowing time for ADH to affect the kidneys.

Both of these mechanisms serve to dilute the blood and other body fluids. Either mechanism alone can maintain water balance. If both fail, a person soon becomes dehydrated.

---

required for nerve impulse conduction and is important in maintaining acid–base balance.

> **Potassium** is also important in the transmission of nerve impulses and is the major positive ion in intracellular fluids. Potassium is involved in enzymatic activities, and it helps regulate the chemical reactions by which carbohydrate is converted to energy and amino acids are converted to protein.

> **Calcium** is required for bone formation, muscle contraction, nerve impulse transmission, and blood clotting.

■ Negative ions (anions):

> **Phosphate** is essential in carbohydrate metabolism, bone formation, and acid–base balance. Phosphates are found in plasma membranes, nucleic acids (DNA and RNA), and ATP.

> **Chloride** is essential for the formation of hydrochloric acid in the stomach. It also helps to regulate fluid balance and pH. It is the most abundant anion in extracellular fluids.

CHECKPOINT 21-4 ➤ What is the main cation in extracellular fluid? In intracellular fluid?

CHECKPOINT 21-5 ➤ What is the main anion in extracellular fluid?

Electrolyte Balance

The body must keep electrolytes in the proper concentration in both intracellular and extracellular fluids (see Box 21-2, Sodium and Potassium). The maintenance of water and electrolyte balance is one of the most difficult problems for health workers in caring for patients. Although some electrolytes are lost in the feces and through the skin as sweat, the job of balancing electrolytes is left mainly to the kidneys, as described in Chapter 22 on the urinary system.

THE ROLE OF HORMONES Several hormones are involved in balancing electrolytes (see Chapter 12). Aldosterone, produced by the adrenal cortex, promotes the reabsorption of sodium (and water) and the elimination of potassium. In Addison disease, in which the adrenal cortex does not produce enough aldosterone, there is a loss of sodium and water and an excess of potassium.

When the blood concentration of sodium rises above the normal range, the pituitary secretes more antidiuretic hormone (ADH). This hormone increases water reabsorption in the kidney to dilute the excess sodium.

The most recently discovered hormone active in electrolyte regulation comes from the heart. Atrial natriuretic peptide (ANP) is secreted by specialized atrial myocardial cells when blood pressure rises too high. As its name implies, ANP causes the kidneys to excrete sodium and water, thus decreasing blood volume and lowering blood pressure.

Hormones from the parathyroid and thyroid glands regulate calcium and phosphate levels. Parathyroid hormone increases blood calcium levels by causing the bones to release calcium and the kidneys to reabsorb calcium. The thyroid hormone calcitonin lowers blood calcium by causing calcium to be deposited in the bones.

CHECKPOINT 21-6 ➤ What are some mechanisms for regulating electrolytes in body fluids?

Sodium and Potassium: Causes and Consequences of Imbalance

The concentrations of sodium and potassium in body fluids are important measures of water and electrolyte balance. An excess of sodium in body fluids is termed **hypernatremia**, taken from the Latin name for sodium, *natrium*. This condition accompanies dehydration and severe vomiting and may cause hypertension, edema, convulsions, and coma. **Hyponatremia**, a deficiency of sodium in body fluids, can come from water intoxication, heart failure, kidney failure, cirrhosis of the liver, pH imbalance, or endocrine disorders. It can cause muscle weakness, hypotension, confusion, shock, convulsions, and coma.

The term **hyperkalemia** is taken from the Latin name for potassium, *kalium*. It refers to excess potassium in body fluids, which may result from kidney failure, dehydration, and other causes. Its signs and symptoms include nausea, vomiting, muscular weakness, and severe cardiac arrhythmias. **Hypokalemia**, or low potassium in body fluids, may result from taking diuretics, which cause potassium to be lost along with water. It may also result from pH imbalance or secretion of too much aldosterone from the adrenal cortex, and it causes muscle fatigue, paralysis, confusion, hypoventilation, and cardiac arrhythmias.

PASSport to Success

Visit **thePoint** or see the Student Resource CD in the back of this book for a summary chart of hormones and electrolyte balance.

Acid–Base Balance

The pH scale is a measure of how acidic or basic (alkaline) a solution is. As described in Chapter 2, the pH scale measures the hydrogen ion (H^+) concentration in a solution. Body fluids are slightly alkaline, with a pH range of 7.35 to 7.45. These fluids must be kept within a narrow pH range, or damage, even death, will result. A shift in either direction by three tenths of a point on the pH scale, to 7.0 or 7.7, is fatal.

Regulation of pH

The body constantly produces acids in the course of metabolism. Catabolism of fats yields fatty acids and other acidic byproducts; cellular respiration yields pyruvic acid and, under anaerobic conditions, lactic acid; carbon dioxide dissolves in the blood and yields carbonic acid (see Chapter 18). Conversely, a few abnormal conditions may cause alkaline shifts in pH. Several systems act together to counteract these changes and maintain acid–base balance:

- **Buffer systems.** Buffers are substances that prevent sharp changes in hydrogen ion (H^+) concentration and thus maintain a relatively constant pH. Buffers work by accepting or releasing these ions as needed to keep the pH steady. The main buffer systems in the body are bicarbonate buffers, phosphate buffers, and proteins, such as hemoglobin in red blood cells and plasma proteins.

- **Respiration.** The role of respiration in controlling pH was described in Chapter 18. Recall that carbon dioxide release from the lungs makes the blood more alkaline by reducing the amount of carbonic acid formed. In contrast, carbon dioxide retention makes the blood more acidic. Respiratory rate can adjust pH for short-term regulation.

- **Kidney function.** The kidneys regulate pH by reabsorbing or eliminating hydrogen ions as needed. The kidneys are responsible for long-term pH regulation. The activity of the kidneys is described in Chapter 22.

CHECKPOINT 21-7 ➤ What are three mechanisms for maintaining the acid–base balance of body fluids?

Abnormal pH

If shifts in pH cannot be controlled, either acidosis or alkalosis results (Table 21-1). **Acidosis** (as-ih-DO-sis) is a condition produced by a drop in the pH of body fluids to less than pH 7.35. This condition depresses the nervous system, leading to mental confusion and ultimately coma. Acidosis may result from a respiratory obstruction or any lung disease which prevents the release of CO_2. It may also arise from kidney failure or prolonged diarrhea, which drains the alkaline contents of the intestine. Long-term excessive exercise under anaerobic conditions can produce lactic acidosis.

Acidosis may also result from inadequate carbohydrate metabolism, as occurs in diabetes mellitus, ingestion of a low-carbohydrate diet, or starvation. In these cases, the body metabolizes too much fat and protein from food or body materials, leading to the production of excess acid. When acidosis results from the accumulation of

21

Table 21-1	Causes of Acidosis and Alkalosis	
	Acidosis	**Alkalosis**
Metabolic	Kidney failure; anaerobic metabolism; lack of carbohydrate metabolism, as in diabetes, starvation; prolonged diarrhea	Overuse of antacids; prolonged vomiting
Respiratory	Respiratory obstruction, lung disease such as asthma or emphysema, apnea or decreased ventilation	Hyperventilation (overbreathing due to anxiety or oxygen deficiency)

ketone bodies, as in the case of diabetes, the condition is more accurately described as ketoacidosis.

Alkalosis (al-kah-LO-sis) results from an increase in pH to greater than 7.45. This abnormality excites the nervous system to produce tingling sensations, muscle twitches, and eventually paralysis. The possible causes of alkalosis include hyperventilation (the release of too much carbon dioxide), ingestion of too much antacid, and prolonged vomiting with loss of stomach acids.

It is convenient to categorize acidosis and alkalosis as having either respiratory or metabolic origins. Respiratory acidosis or alkalosis results from either an increase or a decrease in blood CO_2. Metabolic acidosis or alkalosis results from unregulated increases or decreases in any other acids (see Table 21-1).

CHECKPOINT 21-8 ➤ What are the conditions that arise from abnormally low or high pH of body fluids?

Disorders of Body Fluids

Edema is the accumulation of excessive fluid in the intercellular spaces (Fig. 21-3).

Some causes of edema are as follows:

■ Interference with normal fluid return to the heart, as caused by congestive heart failure or blockage in the venous or lymphatic systems (see Chapters 14 and 15). A backup of fluid in the lungs, **pulmonary edema**, is a serious potential consequence of congestive heart failure.

■ Lack of protein in the blood. This deficiency may result from protein loss or ingestion of too little dietary protein for an extended period. It may also result from failure of the liver to manufacture adequate amounts of the protein albumin, as frequently occurs in liver disease. The decrease in protein lowers the blood's osmotic pressure and reduces fluid return to the circulation. Diminished fluid return results in accumulation of fluid in the tissues.

■ Kidney failure, a common clinical cause of edema, resulting from the inability of the kidneys to eliminate adequate amounts of urine.

■ Increased loss of fluid through the capillaries, as caused by injury, allergic reaction, or certain infections.

Water intoxication involves dilution of body fluids in both the intracellular and extracellular compartments. Transport of water into the cells results in swelling. In the brain, cellular swelling may lead to convulsions, coma, and finally death. Causes of water intoxication include an excess of ADH and intake of excess fluids by mouth or by intravenous injection.

Effusion (e-FU-zhun) is the escape of fluid into a cavity or a space. An example is pleural effusion, fluid within the pleural space; in this condition fluid compresses the lung, so that normal breathing is not possible. Tuberculosis, cancer, and some infections may give rise to effusion. Effusion into the pericardial sac, which encloses the heart, may occur in autoimmune disorders, such as lupus erythematosus and rheumatoid arthritis. Infection is

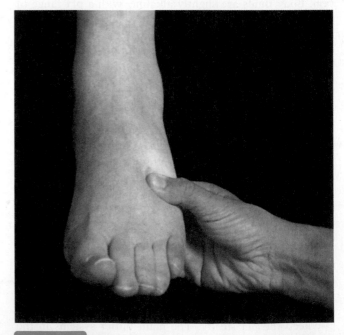

Figure 21-3 Edema of the foot. (Reprinted with permission from Bickley LS. *Bates' Guide to Physical Examination and History Taking*, 8th ed. Philadelphia: Lippincott Williams & Wilkins, 2003.)

Disease in Context revisited

➤ Margaret Learns to Avoid Dehydration

"Hello, Margaret. Are you ready to go home today?" Angela asked her patient.

"Oh yes," answered Margaret. "You've made me feel so comfortable, but I'm looking forward to sleeping in my own bed tonight!"

"Well," continued Angela, "before you leave, can we talk a bit about taking care of yourself at home?" With Margaret's permission, Angela explained that Margaret needed to match her fluid intake with her fluid loss to ensure water balance and prevent dehydration. "I know that 2½ quarts of water per day seems like a lot, but don't forget that drinks aren't your only source. You can also get water from foods like fruits, vegetables, and soups," she recommended.

Angela advised Margaret to think about her electrolytes as well. She encouraged Margaret to eat foods low in sodium—not only would it help

her stay hydrated, but it would also help her avoid high blood pressure. Since Margaret's potassium levels were a little low (due to a blood pressure medication she was taking), Angela suggested that she eat potassium-rich foods like cantaloupe, apricots, raisins, and tomatoes. Margaret's calcium levels were also a little low, so Angela suggested that Margaret eat calcium-rich foods like dairy products, fish, and leafy green vegetables such as spinach and broccoli.

During this case, we saw the importance of fluid and electrolyte balance to maintain health. Many of the mechanisms that the body uses to regulate fluid volume and ion concentration occur in the kidneys. In Chapter 22, The Urinary System, we'll examine some of these homeostatic mechanisms.

another cause of pericardial effusion. The fluid may interfere with normal heart contractions and can cause death.

Ascites (ah-SI-teze) is effusion with accumulation of fluid within the abdominal cavity. It may occur in disorders of the liver, kidneys, and heart, as well as in cancers, infection, or malnutrition.

Dehydration (de-hi-DRA-shun), a severe deficit of body fluids, will result in death if it is prolonged. The causes include vomiting, diarrhea, drainage from burns or wounds, excessive perspiration, and inadequate fluid intake, as in cases of damage to the thirst mechanism. In such cases, it may be necessary to administer intravenous fluids to correct fluid and electrolyte imbalances.

CHECKPOINT 21-9 ➤ What is edema?

Fluid Therapy

Chapter 3 discussed the rules concerning movement of water into and out of cells when they are placed in different solutions. Recall that an isotonic solution has the same concentration as the cellular fluids and will not cause a net loss or gain of water. A hypertonic solution is more concentrated than cellular fluid and will draw water out of the cells. A hypotonic solution is less concentrated than the cellular fluids and a cell will take in water when placed in this type of solution. These rules must be considered when fluid is administered.

Fluids are administered into a vein under a wide variety of conditions to help maintain normal body functions when natural intake is not possible. Fluids are also administered to correct specific fluid and electrolyte imbalances in cases of losses due to disease or injury.

 PASSport to Success Visit **thePoint** or see the Student Resource CD in the back of this book for information on emergency medical technicians who often must administer fluids in providing health care.

The first fluid administered intravenously in emergencies is normal saline, which contains 0.9% sodium chloride, a concentration equal to that of plasma. Because it is isotonic, this type of solution does not change the ion distribution in the body fluid compartments.

Frequently, a patient receives 5% dextrose (glucose) in 0.45% (1/2 normal) saline. This solution is hypertonic when infused, but becomes hypotonic after the sugar is metabolized. Another common fluid is 5% dextrose in water. This solution is slightly hypotonic when infused. The amount of sugar contained in a liter of this fluid is equal to 170 calories. The sugar is soon used up, resulting in a fluid that is effectively pure water. Use of these hypotonic fluids is not advisable for long-term therapy because of the common occurrence of water intoxication. Both these dextrose solutions increase the

21

plasma fluid volume. Small amounts of potassium chloride are often added to replace electrolytes lost by vomiting or diarrhea.

Ringer lactate solution contains sodium, potassium, calcium, chloride, and lactate. In this formulation, the electrolyte concentrations are equal to normal plasma values. The lactate is metabolized to bicarbonate, which acts as a buffer. This fluid is given when the need is for additional plasma volume with the electrolyte concentration equal to that of the blood.

In 25% serum albumin, the concentration of the plasma protein albumin is five times normal. This hypertonic solution draws fluid from the interstitial spaces into the circulation.

Fluids containing varied concentrations of dextrose, sodium chloride, potassium, and other electrolytes and substances are manufactured. These fluids are used to correct specific imbalances. Nutritional solutions containing concentrated sugar, protein, and fat are available for administration when oral intake is not possible for an extended period.

Word Anatomy

Medical terms are built from standardized word parts (prefixes, roots, and suffixes). Learning the meanings of these parts can help you remember words and interpret unfamiliar terms.

WORD PART	MEANING	EXAMPLE
Fluid Compartments		
intra-	within	*Intracellular* fluid is within a cell.
extra-	outside of, beyond	*Extracellular* fluid is outside the cells.
semi-	partial, half	A *semipermeable* membrane is partially permeable.
Water Balance		
poly-	many	*Polydipsia* is excessive thirst.
osmo-	osmosis	*Osmoreceptors* detect changes in osmotic concentration of fluids.
Acid–Base Balance		
-o/sis	condition, process	*Acidosis* is a condition produced by a drop in the pH of body fluids.
Disorders of Body Fluids		
tox/o	poison	Water *intoxication* is dilution of body fluids by excess water.
hydr/o	water	*Dehydration* is a severe deficit of body fluids.

Summary

I. **THE IMPORTANCE OF WATER**
  A. Functions
    1. Solvent
    2. Transport medium
    3. Participant in metabolic reactions
  B. 50% to 70% of body weight
  C. Contains electrolytes, nutrients, gases, wastes, hormones, and other substances
  D. Important in homeostasis

II. **FLUID COMPARTMENTS**
  A. Intracellular fluid—contained within the cells
  B. Extracellular fluid—outside the cells
    1. Blood plasma
    2. Interstitial (tissue) fluid
    3. Lymph
    4. Fluid in special compartments

III. **WATER BALANCE**
  A. Loss—through kidneys, skin, lungs, intestinal tract

B. Gain—through beverages, food, metabolic water
C. Sense of thirst
  1. Control center in hypothalamus
  2. Responds to fluid volume and concentration of body fluids
IV. **ELECTROLYTES AND THEIR FUNCTIONS**
  A. Electrolytes release ions in solution
   1. Positive ions (cations)—e.g., sodium, potassium, calcium
   2. Negative ions (anions)—e.g., phosphate, chloride
  B. Electrolyte balance
   1. Kidneys—main regulators
   2. Role of hormones
    a. Aldosterone (from adrenal cortex)
     (1) Promotes reabsorption of sodium
     (2) Promotes excretion of potassium
    b. ADH (from pituitary)
     (1) Causes kidney to retain water
    c. ANP (from heart)
     (1) Causes kidney to excrete sodium and water
    d. Parathyroid hormone (from parathyroid glands)
     (1) Increases blood calcium level
    e. Calcitonin (from thyroid)
     (1) Decreases blood calcium level
V. **ACID–BASE BALANCE**
  A. Normal pH range is 7.35 to 7.45
  B. Regulation of pH
   1. Buffers—maintain constant pH
   2. Respiration—release of carbon dioxide increases alkalinity; retention of carbon dioxide increases acidity

  3. Kidney—regulates amount of hydrogen ion excreted
  C. Abnormal pH
   1. Acidosis—decrease in pH; causes: respiratory obstruction, lung disease, kidney failure, diarrhea, diabetes mellitus, starvation
   2. Alkalosis—increase in pH; causes: hyperventilation, ingestion of antacids, prolonged vomiting
VI. **DISORDERS OF BODY FLUIDS**
  A. Edema—accumulation of fluid in tissues
   1. Causes
    a. Interference with fluid return to heart
    b. Lack of proteins in blood
    c. Kidney failure
    d. Fluid loss from capillaries
  B. Water intoxication—dilution of body fluids
  C. Effusion—escape of fluid into a cavity or space
  D. Ascites—accumulation of fluid in abdominal cavity
  E. Dehydration—deficiency of fluid
VII. **FLUID THERAPY**
  A. Purpose
   1. Correct fluid balance
   2. Correct electrolyte balance
   3. Provide nourishment
  B. Commonly used solutions
   1. Normal saline
   2. 5% dextrose (glucose) in 0.45% (1/2 normal) saline
   3. 5% dextrose in water
   4. Ringer lactate
   5. 25% serum albumin

Questions for Study and Review

BUILDING UNDERSTANDING

Fill in the blanks

1. Excessive thirst is termed_____.
2. Loss of sodium and an excess of potassium are classic signs of _____ disease.
3. Substances in the blood that prevent sharp changes in hydrogen ion concentration are called_____.
4. Effusion with accumulation of fluid within the abdominal cavity is termed _____.
5. A severe deficit in body fluid is called _____.

21

Matching > Match each numbered item with the most closely related lettered item.

___ **6.** Essential for maintaining osmotic balance and body fluid volume; this cation is abundant in extracellular fluid

___ **7.** Important in the transmission of nerve impulses and enzyme activities; this cation is abundant in intracellular fluid

___ **8.** Required for bone formation, muscle contraction, and blood clotting

___ **9.** Essential in bone formation and acid–base balance; this anion is found in plasma membranes, ATP, and nucleic acids

___ **10.** Important for gastric acid formation; this anion is abundant in extracellular fluid

a. sodium
b. potassium
c. calcium
d. phosphate
e. chloride

Multiple choice

___ **11.** Body water content is greatest in

a. infants
b. children
c. young adults
d. elderly adults

___ **12.** Fluid located in the spaces between the cells is called

a. cytoplasm
b. plasma
c. interstitial fluid
d. lymph

___ **13.** The organ(s) responsible for water loss through evaporation is (are) the

a. kidneys
b. skin
c. lungs
d. intestinal tract

___ **14.** Which of the following is responsible for long-term regulation of pH?

a. buffer system
b. digestive system
c. respiratory system
d. urinary system

___ **15.** Increased blood CO_2 causes

a. respiratory acidosis
b. respiratory alkalosis
c. metabolic acidosis
d. metabolic alkalosis

UNDERSTANDING CONCEPTS

16. Compare the terms in each of the following pairs:

a. intracellular and extracellular fluid
b. aldosterone and antidiuretic hormone
c. calcitonin and parathyroid hormone

17. In a healthy person, what is the ratio of fluid intake to output?

18. Explain the role of the hypothalamus in water balance.

19. How do the respiratory and urinary systems regulate pH?

20. Compare and contrast the following disorders:

a. acidosis and alkalosis
b. edema and effusion
c. water intoxication and dehydration

21. List some causes of edema.

22. List three purposes for administering intravenous fluids.

23. Compare and contrast the following types of intravenous fluids:

a. normal saline and 5% dextrose saline
b. Ringer solution and serum albumin

CONCEPTUAL THINKING

24. Patty Grant, 55-years-old, reports severe headaches and excessive thirst and urination. What is the probable cause of Patty's symptoms?

25. Why is emphysema associated with decreased urine pH?

26. In Margaret's case, her dehydration was treated with an isotonic IV solution. What would happen to her intracellular fluid volume if she received a hypertonic IV solution?

21

CHAPTER 22

The Urinary System

Learning Outcomes

After careful study of this chapter, you should be able to:

1. List the systems that eliminate waste and name the substances eliminated by each
2. Describe the parts of the urinary system and give the functions of each
3. List the activities of the kidneys in maintaining homeostasis
4. Trace the path of a drop of blood as it flows through the kidney
5. Describe a nephron
6. Name the four processes involved in urine formation and describe the action of each
7. Identify the role of antidiuretic hormone (ADH) in urine formation
8. Describe the components and functions of the juxtaglomerular (JG) apparatus
9. Describe the process of micturition
10. Name three normal and six abnormal constituents of urine
11. List the common disorders of the urinary system
12. List six signs of chronic renal failure
13. Explain the principle and the purpose of kidney dialysis
14. Show how word parts are used to build words related to the urinary system (see Word Anatomy at the end of the chapter)

Disease in Context

➤ Adam's Second Case: Urinary Blockade

Adam rolled out of bed and glanced at the clock as he rushed to the bathroom. *Jeez, it's only been a couple of hours since the last time I had to pee*, he thought. *Hopefully this time it won't take as long.* Sure enough, Adam had difficulty voiding. Even once he was able to get started, he only managed to produce a small volume of urine. Lately, this was happening more and more frequently. At first, he chalked it up to getting older, but now he wondered if he had some sort of bladder or kidney infection. As he climbed back into bed, Adam decided that he would make an appointment with his family doctor.

"So let me get this straight," said Dr. Singh. "Over the last several weeks, you've experienced increased frequency and urgency of urination, even at night (nocturia). While urinating, you've had hesitation in starting, decreased volume, and diminished force of the stream. And even after urination, you still feel that your urinary bladder is not completely empty." Based on Adam's symptoms, Dr. Singh suspected that Adam's prostate gland (a male reproductive organ) was causing problems for his urinary system. The prostate gland lies immediately inferior to the urinary bladder, where it surrounds the first part of the urethra. If the gland becomes enlarged, it can obstruct the urethra and prevent the urinary bladder from emptying completely. At 55 years old, Adam was in the right age range for this condition.

Dr. Singh's suspicions were confirmed by the digital rectal exam. Adam's prostate was large and rubbery. The doctor carefully palpated the prostate's surface with his finger—he could not detect any nodules on its smooth surface. "Adam, my initial diagnosis is that you have benign prostatic hypertrophy—your prostate has grown larger and is preventing urine from passing out of your urinary bladder. Your prostate's surface is smooth though, which suggests that the growth is not cancerous, but we'll have to get that ruled out. I'm going to order some blood tests and urinalyses, as well as refer you to a urologist."

Adam's prostate is causing problems for his urinary system. In this chapter, we'll examine the anatomy and physiology of the urinary system. Later, we'll learn how Adam's disorder is resolved.

Excretion

The urinary system is also called the *excretory system* because one of its main functions is **excretion**, removal and elimination of metabolic waste products from the blood. It has many other functions as well, including regulation of the volume, acid–base balance (pH), and electrolyte composition of body fluids.

Although the focus of this chapter is the urinary system, certain aspects of other systems are also discussed, because body systems work interdependently to maintain homeostasis (internal balance). The systems active in excretion and some of the substances they eliminate are the following:

- The **urinary system** excretes water, nitrogen-containing waste products, and salts. These are all constituents of the urine.

- The **digestive system** eliminates water, some salts, and bile, in addition to digestive residue, all of which are contained in the feces. The liver is important in eliminating the products of red blood cell destruction and in breaking down certain drugs and toxins.

- The **respiratory system** eliminates carbon dioxide and water. The latter appears as vapor, as can be demonstrated by breathing on a windowpane or a mirror, where the water condenses.

- The skin, or **integumentary system**, excretes water, salts, and very small quantities of nitrogenous wastes. These all appear in perspiration, although water also evaporates continuously from the skin without our being conscious of it.

CHECKPOINT 22-1 ➤ The main function of the urinary system is to eliminate waste. What are some other systems that eliminate waste?

Organs of the Urinary System

The main parts of the urinary system, shown in Figure 22-1, are as follows:

- Two **kidneys**. These organs extract wastes from the blood, balance body fluids, and form urine.

- Two **ureters** (U-re-ters). These tubes conduct urine from the kidneys to the urinary bladder.

- A single **urinary bladder**. This reservoir receives and stores the urine brought to it by the two ureters.

- A single **urethra** (u-RE-thrah). This tube conducts urine from the bladder to the outside of the body for elimination.

CHECKPOINT 22-2 ➤ What are the organs of the urinary system?

The Kidneys

The kidneys interact with other systems as prime regulators of homeostasis. After a brief overview of the kidney's many activities, we'll describe its structure and specific roles in urine formation and regulation of blood pressure.

Kidney Activities

The kidneys are involved in the following processes:

- Excretion of unwanted substances, such as cellular metabolic waste, excess salts, and toxins. One product of amino acid metabolism is nitrogen-containing waste material, chiefly **urea** (u-RE-ah). After synthesis in the liver, urea is transported in the blood to the kidneys for elimination. The kidneys have a specialized mechanism for the elimination of urea and other nitrogenous (ni-TROJ-en-us) wastes.

- Water balance. Although the amount of water gained and lost in a day can vary tremendously, the kidneys can adapt to these variations, so that the volume of body water remains remarkably stable from day to day.

- Acid–base balance of body fluids. Acids are constantly being produced by cellular metabolism. Certain foods can yield acids or bases, and people may also ingest antacids, such as bicarbonate. However, if the body is to function normally, the pH of body fluids must remain in the range of 7.35 to 7.45 (see Chapter 21).

- Blood pressure regulation. The kidneys depend on blood pressure to filter the blood. If blood pressure falls too low for effective filtration, specialized kidney cells release renin. This enzyme activates a blood protein, angiotensin, that causes blood vessels to constrict, thus raising blood pressure. Angiotensin has additional effects as described later in the chapter.

- Regulation of red blood cell production. When the kidneys do not get enough oxygen, they produce the hormone **erythropoietin** (eh-rith-ro-POY-eh-tin) (**EPO**), which stimulates red cell production in the bone marrow. EPO made by genetic engineering is now available to treat severe anemia, such as occurs in the end stage of kidney failure.

Kidney Structure

The kidneys lie against the back muscles in the upper abdomen at about the level of the last thoracic and first three lumbar vertebrae. The right kidney is slightly lower than the left to accommodate the liver. Each kidney is firmly enclosed in a membranous **renal capsule** made of fibrous connective tissue. In addition, there is a protective layer of fat called the **adipose capsule** around the organ. An outermost layer of fascia (connective tissue) anchors the kidney to the peritoneum and abdominal wall. The kidneys, as well as the ureters, lie posterior to

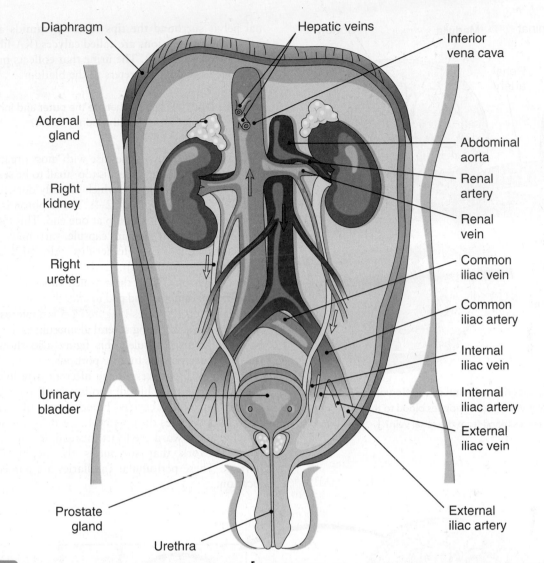

Diaphragm

Hepatic veins

Inferior vena cava

Adrenal gland

Abdominal aorta

Renal artery

Right kidney

Renal vein

Common iliac vein

Right ureter

Common iliac artery

Internal iliac vein

Urinary bladder

Internal iliac artery

External iliac vein

Prostate gland

External iliac artery

Urethra

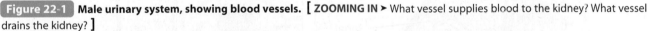

Figure 22-1 **Male urinary system, showing blood vessels.** [ZOOMING IN ➤ What vessel supplies blood to the kidney? What vessel drains the kidney?]

the peritoneum. Thus, they are not in the peritoneal cavity but rather in an area known as the **retroperitoneal** (ret-ro-per-ih-to-NE-al) **space.** See Appendix 7 for a dissection photograph showing the kidneys and renal vessels in place.

CHECKPOINT **22-3** ➤ The kidneys are located in the retroperitoneal space. Where is this space?

BLOOD SUPPLY The kidney's blood supply is illustrated in Figure 22-2. Blood is brought to the kidney by a short branch of the abdominal aorta called the **renal artery.**

After entering the kidney, the renal artery subdivides into smaller and smaller branches, which eventually make contact with the kidney's functional units, the **nephrons** (NEF-ronz). Blood leaves the kidney by vessels that finally merge to form the **renal vein,** which carries blood into the inferior vena cava for return to the heart.

CHECKPOINT **22-4** ➤ What vessel supplies blood to the kidney and what vessel drains blood from the kidney?

ORGANIZATION The kidney is a somewhat flattened organ approximately 10 cm (4 inches) long, 5 cm (2 inches) wide, and 2.5 cm (1 inch) thick (Fig. 22-3). On the medial border there is a notch called the **hilum,** where the renal artery, the renal vein, and the ureter connect with the kidney. The lateral border is convex (curved outward), giving the entire organ a bean-shaped appearance.

The kidney is divided into two regions: the renal cortex and the renal medulla (Fig. 22-3). The **renal cortex** is the kidney's outer portion. The internal **renal medulla** contains tubes in which urine is formed and collected. These tubes form a number of cone-shaped structures called **renal pyramids.** The tips of the pyramids point toward the **renal pelvis,** a funnel-shaped basin that forms the upper end of the ureter. Cuplike extensions of the re-

22

Abdominal aorta
Medulla
Cortex
Renal artery
Inferior vena cava
Renal vein
Ureter

Figure 22-2 **Blood supply and circulation of the kidney.**
[**ZOOMING IN** ➤ What vessel supplies blood to the renal artery? What vessel receives blood from the renal vein?]

nal pelvis surround the tips of the pyramids and collect urine; these extensions are called **calyces** (KA-lih-seze; singular, **calyx**, KA-liks). The urine that collects in the pelvis then passes down the ureters to the bladder.

CHECKPOINT 22-5 ➤ What are the outer and inner regions of the kidney called?

THE NEPHRON As is the case with most organs, the kidney's most fascinating aspect is too small to be seen with the naked eye. This basic unit, which actually does the kidney's work, is the **nephron** (Fig. 22-4). The nephron is essentially a tiny coiled tube with a bulb at one end. This bulb, known as the **glomerular (Bowman) capsule**, surrounds a cluster of capillaries called the **glomerulus** (glo-MER-u-lus) (pl., glomeruli [glo-MER-u-li]). Each kidney contains about 1 million nephrons; if all these coiled tubes were separated, straightened out, and laid end to end, they would span some 120 kilometers (75 miles)! Figure 22-5 is a microscopic view of kidney tissue showing several glomeruli, each surrounded by a glomerular capsule. This figure also shows sections through the nephron's tubular portions.

A small blood vessel, the **afferent arteriole**, supplies the glomerulus with blood; another small vessel, called the **efferent arteriole**, carries blood from the glomerulus. When blood leaves the glomerulus, it does not head immediately back toward the heart. Instead, it flows into a capillary network that surrounds the nephron's tubular portion. These **peritubular capillaries** are named for their location.

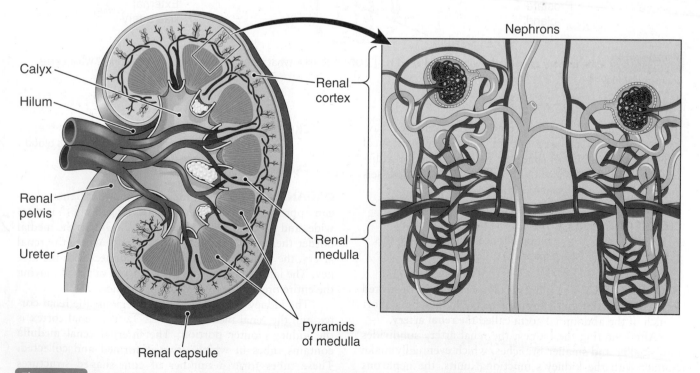

Nephrons
Calyx
Hilum
Renal cortex
Renal pelvis
Renal medulla
Ureter
Pyramids of medulla
Renal capsule

Figure 22-3 **Longitudinal section through the kidney.** Its internal structure is shown (left), along with an enlarged diagram of nephrons (right). Each kidney contains more than 1 million nephrons. [**ZOOMING IN** ➤ What is the outer region of the kidney called? What is the inner region of the kidney called?]

Afferent arteriole Efferent arteriole Glomerulus Glomerular (Bowman) capsule

Distal convoluted tubule

Proximal convoluted tubule

From renal artery →

To renal vein ←

Peritubular capillaries

Loop of Henle
{ Ascending limb
  Descending limb }

Collecting duct

Calyx

Figure 22-4 **A nephron and its blood supply.** The nephron regulates the proportions of water, waste, and other materials according to the body's constantly changing needs. Materials that enter the nephron can be returned to the blood through the surrounding capillaries. [**ZOOMING IN ➤** Which of the two convoluted tubules is closer to the glomerular capsule? Which convoluted tubule is farther away?]

Glomerulus

Renal tubules

Glomerular capsule

Figure 22-5 **Microscopic view of the kidney.** (Courtesy of Dana Morse Bittus and BJ Cohen.)

The nephron's tubular portion consists of several parts. The coiled part leading from the glomerular capsule is called the **proximal convoluted** (KON-vo-lu-ted) **tubule** (**PCT**, or just proximal tubule). The tubule then uncoils to form a hairpin-shaped segment called the **nephron loop**, or loop of Henle. The first part of the loop, which carries fluid toward the medulla, is the **descending limb** (see Fig. 22-4). The part that continues from the loop's turn and carries fluid away from the medulla, is the **ascending limb**. Continuing from the ascending limb, the tubule coils once again into the **distal convoluted tubule** (**DCT**, or just distal tubule), so called because it is farther along the tubule from the glomerular capsule than is the PCT. Each tubule empties into a collecting duct, which then continues through the medulla toward the renal pelvis.

The glomerulus, glomerular capsule, and the proximal and distal convoluted tubules of the nephron are within the renal cortex. The nephron loop and collecting duct extend into the medulla (see Fig. 22-3).

CHECKPOINT 22-6 ➤ What is the functional unit of the kidney called?

CHECKPOINT 22-7 ➤ What name is given to the coil of capillaries in the glomerular (Bowman) capsule?

Formation of Urine

The following explanation of urine formation describes a complex process, involving many back-and-forth exchanges between the bloodstream and the kidney tubules. As fluid filtered from the blood travels slowly through the nephron's twists and turns, there is ample time for exchanges to take place. These processes together allow the kidney to "fine tune" body fluids as they adjust the composition of the urine.

22

Visit *thePoint* or see the Student Resource CD in the back of this book for the animation Renal Function, which shows the process of urine formation in action.

GLOMERULAR FILTRATION The process of urine formation begins with the glomerulus in the glomerular capsule. The walls of the glomerular capillaries are sievelike and permit the free flow of water and soluble materials through them. Like other capillary walls, however, they are impermeable (im-PER-me-abl) to blood cells and large protein molecules, and these components remain in the blood (Fig. 22-6).

Because the diameter of the afferent arteriole is slightly larger than that of the efferent arteriole (see Fig. 22-6), blood can enter the glomerulus more easily than it can leave. Thus, blood pressure in the glomerulus is about three to four times higher than it is in other capillaries. To understand this effect, think of placing your thumb over the end of a garden hose as water comes through. As you make the diameter of the opening smaller, water is forced out under higher pressure. As a result of increased fluid (hydrostatic) pressure in the glomerulus, materials are constantly being pushed out of the blood and into the nephron's glomerular capsule. As described in Chapter 3, movement of water and dissolved materials through a membrane under pressure is called *filtration*. This movement of materials under pressure from the blood into the capsule is therefore known as **glomerular filtration**.

The fluid that enters the glomerular capsule, called the **glomerular filtrate**, begins its journey along the nephron's tubular system. In addition to water and the normal soluble substances in the blood, other substances, such as vitamins and drugs, also may be filtered and become part of the glomerular filtrate.

CHECKPOINT 22-8 ➤ The first step in urine formation is glomerular filtration. What is glomerular filtration?

TUBULAR REABSORPTION The kidneys form about 160 to 180 liters of filtrate each day. However, only 1 to 1.5 liters of urine are eliminated daily. Clearly, most of the water that enters the nephron is not excreted with the urine, but rather, is returned to the circulation. In addition to water, many other substances the body needs, such as nutrients and ions, pass into the nephron as part of the filtrate, and these also must be returned. Therefore, the process of filtration that occurs in the glomerular capsule is followed by a process of **tubular reabsorption**. As the filtrate travels through the nephron's tubular system, water and other needed substances leave the tubule and enter the surrounding tissue fluid, the interstitial fluid (IF). They move by several processes previously described in Chapter 3, including:

- Diffusion. The movement of substances from an area of higher concentration to an area of lower concentration (following the concentration gradient).

- Osmosis. Diffusion of water through a semipermeable membrane.

- Active transport. Movement of materials through the plasma membrane against the concentration gradient using energy and transporters.

Several hormones noted in Chapter 21, including aldosterone and ANP (atrial natriuretic peptide) affect these changes (Table 22-1).

The substances that leave the nephron and enter the interstitial fluid then enter the peritubular capillaries and return to the circulation. In contrast, most of the urea and other nitrogenous waste materials are kept within the tubule to be eliminated with the urine. Box 22-1, Transport Maximum, presents additional information on tubular reabsorption in the nephron.

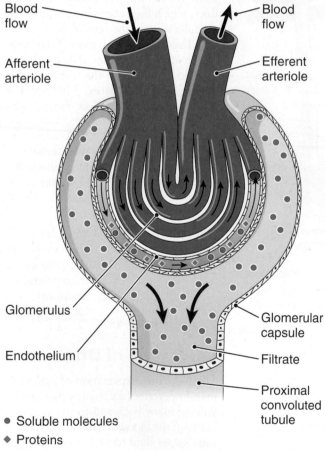

Blood flow

Afferent arteriole

Blood flow

Efferent arteriole

Glomerulus

Endothelium

Glomerular capsule

Filtrate

Proximal convoluted tubule

- Soluble molecules
- Proteins
- Blood cells

Figure 22-6 **Filtration process in the formation of urine.** Blood pressure inside the glomerulus forces water and dissolved substances into the glomerular (Bowman) capsule. Blood cells and proteins remain behind in the blood. The smaller diameter of the efferent arteriole as compared with that of the afferent arteriole maintains the hydrostatic (fluid) pressure. **[ZOOMING IN ➤** Which arteriole associated with the glomerulus has the wider diameter? **]**

Table 22-1	Substances that Affect Renal Function		
Substance	**Source**	**Action**	
Aldosterone (al-DOS-ter-one)	Hormone released from the adrenal cortex under effects of angiotensin	Promotes reabsorption of sodium and water in the kidney to conserve water and increase blood pressure	
Atrial natriuretic peptide (na-tre-u-RET-ik) (ANP)	Atrial myocardial cells; released when blood pressure is too high	Causes kidney to excrete sodium and water to decrease blood volume and blood pressure	
Antidiuretic hormone (an-te-di-u-RET-ik) (ADH)	Made in the hypothalamus and released from the posterior pituitary; released when blood becomes too concentrated	Promotes reabsorption of water from the distal convoluted tubule and collecting duct to concentrate the urine and conserve water	
Renin (RE-nin)	Enzyme produced by renal cells when blood pressure falls too low for effective filtration	Activates angiotensin in the blood	
Angiotensin (an-je-o-TEN-sin)	Protein in the blood that is activated by renin	Causes constriction of blood vessels to raise blood pressure; also stimulates release of aldosterone from the adrenal cortex and ADH from the posterior pituitary	

TUBULAR SECRETION Before the filtrate leaves the body as urine, the kidney makes final adjustments in composition by means of **tubular secretion**. In this process, some substances are actively moved from the blood into the nephron. Potassium ions are moved into the urine in this manner. Importantly, the kidneys regulate the acid–base (pH) balance of body fluids by the active secretion of hydrogen ions. Some drugs, such as penicillin, also are actively secreted into the nephron for elimination.

CONCENTRATION OF THE URINE The amount of water that is eliminated with the urine is regulated by a complex mechanism within the nephron that is influenced by **antidiuretic hormone (ADH)**, a hormone released from the posterior pituitary gland (see Table 22-1). The process is

called the **countercurrent mechanism** because it involves fluid traveling in opposite directions within the ascending and descending limbs of the nephron loop. The countercurrent mechanism is illustrated in Figure 22-7. Its essentials are as follows.

As the filtrate passes through the nephron loop, electrolytes, especially sodium, are actively pumped out by the nephron's cells, resulting in an increased concentration of the interstitial fluid. Because the ascending limb of the loop is not very permeable to water, the filtrate at this point becomes increasingly dilute (see Fig. 22-7). As the filtrate then passes through the more permeable DCT and collecting duct, the concentrated fluids around the nephron draw water out to be returned to the blood. (Remember, according to the laws of osmosis, water fol-

Box 22-1   Clinical Perspectives

Transport Maximum

The kidneys work efficiently to return valuable substances to the blood after glomerular filtration. However, the carriers that are needed for active transport of these substances can become overloaded. Thus, there is a limit to the amount of each substance that can be reabsorbed in a given time period. The limit of this reabsorption rate is called the **transport maximum (Tm)**, or tubular maximum, and it is measured in milligrams (mg) per minute. For example, the Tm for glucose is approximately 375 mg/minute.

If a substance is present in excess in the blood, it may exceed its transport maximum and then, because it cannot be

totally reabsorbed, some will be excreted in the urine. Thus, the transport maximum determines the **renal threshold**—the plasma concentration at which a substance will begin to be excreted in the urine, which is measured in mg per deciliter (dL). For example, if the concentration of glucose in the blood exceeds its renal threshold (180 mg/dL), glucose will begin to appear in the urine, a condition called **glycosuria**. The most common cause of glycosuria is uncontrolled diabetes mellitus.

22

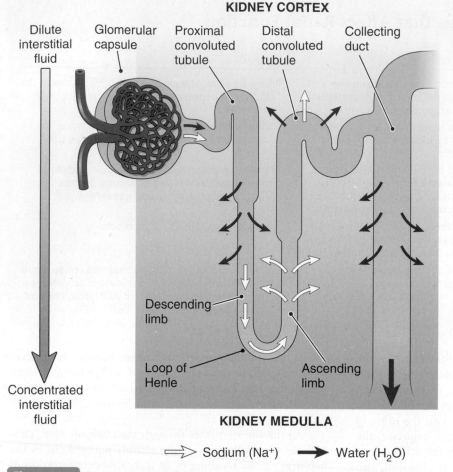

KIDNEY CORTEX

Dilute interstitial fluid — Glomerular capsule — Proximal convoluted tubule — Distal convoluted tubule — Collecting duct

Concentrated interstitial fluid

Descending limb

Loop of Henle — Ascending limb

KIDNEY MEDULLA

⟹ Sodium (Na$^+$)   ⟶ Water (H$_2$O)

Figure 22-7 **Countercurrent mechanism for concentration of urine.** Concentration is regulated by means of intricate exchanges of water and electrolytes, mainly sodium, in the nephron loop, distal convoluted tubule, and collecting duct. The intensity of color shows changing concentrations of the interstitial fluid and filtrate.

lows salt.) In this manner, the urine becomes more concentrated as it leaves the nephron and its volume is reduced.

The hormone ADH makes the walls of the DCT and collecting duct more permeable to water, so that more water will be reabsorbed and less will be excreted with the urine. The release of ADH from the posterior pituitary is regulated by a feedback system. As the blood becomes more concentrated, the hypothalamus triggers more ADH release from the posterior pituitary; as the blood becomes more dilute, less ADH is released. In the disease diabetes insipidus, there is inadequate secretion of ADH from the hypothalamus, which results in the elimination of large amounts of dilute urine accompanied by excessive thirst.

SUMMARY OF URINE FORMATION The processes involved in urine formation are summarized below and illustrated in Figure 22-8.

1. Glomerular filtration allows diffusible materials to pass from the blood into the nephron.

2. Tubular reabsorption moves useful substances back into the blood while keeping waste products in the nephron to be eliminated in the urine.

3. Tubular secretion moves additional substances from the blood into the nephron for elimination. Movement of hydrogen ions is one means by which the pH of body fluids is balanced.

4. The countercurrent mechanism concentrates the urine and reduces the volume excreted. The pituitary hormone ADH allows more water to be reabsorbed from the nephron.

❶ Filtration from blood into nephron

Glomerular capsule

Filtrate

ADH

Afferent arteriole

Efferent arteriole

Urine (excreted)

Blood with reabsorbed substances

Peritubular capillaries

❷ Reabsorption from filtrate into blood

❸ Tubular secretion from blood into filtrate

❹ Reabsorption of water under effects of ADH

Figure 22-8   **Summary of urine formation in a nephron.**

CHECKPOINT 22-9 ➤ What are the four processes involved in the formation of urine?

Control of Blood Pressure

The kidneys have an internal mechanism for maintaining adequate filtration pressure. A specialized portion of the nephron, the **juxtaglomerular (JG) apparatus**, is involved in this control. The JG apparatus includes cells in the DCT, which carries urine from the nephron into the collecting duct, and cells in the afferent arteriole, which carries blood into the glomerulus. As seen in Figure 22-9, the first portion of the DCT curves backward toward the glomerulus to pass between the afferent and efferent arterioles (*juxtaglomerular* means "near the glomerulus"). At the point where the DCT makes contact with the afferent arteriole, there are specialized cells in each that together make up the JG apparatus.

When receptors in the DCT detect low volume or low sodium content in the filtrate leaving the nephron, they trigger cells in the afferent arteriole to secrete the enzyme **renin** (RE-nin) (see Table 22-1). This enzyme initiates the process that activates angiotensin, a protein that elevates blood pressure by several mechanisms. It promotes the release of aldosterone and ADH and stimulates thirst, raising blood pressure by increasing blood volume. It also causes vasoconstriction and stimulates heart activity through the sympathetic nervous system. Box 22-2, The Renin-Angiotensin Pathway, has more details on these events and their clinical applications.

PASSport to Success — Visit *thePoint* or see the Student Resource CD in the back of this book for a flow chart summarizing kidney regulation of blood pressure.

CHECKPOINT 22-10 ➤ What substance is produced by the JG apparatus and under what conditions is it produced?

The Ureters

Each of the two ureters is a long, slender, muscular tube that extends from the kidney down to and through the inferior portion of the urinary bladder (see Fig. 22-1). The ureters, which are located posterior to the peritoneum and distally below the peritoneum, are entirely extraperitoneal. Their length naturally varies with the size of the individual, and they may be anywhere from 25 cm to 32 cm (10 to 13 inches) long. Nearly 2.5 cm (1 inch) of the terminal distal ureter enters the bladder by passing obliquely (at an angle) through the inferior bladder wall. Because of this oblique path through the wall, a full bladder compresses the ureter and prevents the backflow of urine.

The ureteral wall includes a lining of epithelial cells, a relatively thick layer of involuntary muscle, and finally, an outer coat of fibrous connective tissue. The epithelium is the transitional type, which flattens from a cuboidal shape as the tube stretches. This same type of epithelium lines the renal pelvis, the bladder, and the proximal portion of the urethra. The ureteral muscles are capable of the same rhythmic contraction (peristalsis) that occurs in the digestive

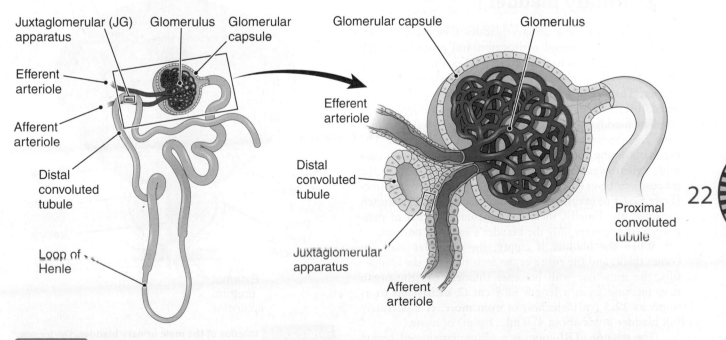

Figure 22-9 Structure of the juxtaglomerular (JG) apparatus. Note how the distal convoluted tubule contacts the afferent arteriole *(right)*. Cells in these two structures make up the JG apparatus. [**ZOOMING IN ➤** The JG apparatus is made up of cells from which two structures?]

The Renin-Angiotensin Pathway: The Renal Route to Blood Pressure Control

In addition to forming urine, the kidneys play an integral role in regulating blood pressure. When blood pressure drops, cells of the juxtaglomerular (JG) apparatus secrete the enzyme renin into the blood. Renin acts on another blood protein, **angiotensinogen**, which is manufactured by the liver. Renin converts angiotensinogen into **angiotensin I** by cleaving off some amino acids from the end of the protein. Angiotensin I is then converted into **angiotensin II** by yet another enzyme called angiotensin-converting enzyme (ACE), which is manufactured by capillary endothelium, especially in the lungs. Angiotensin II increases blood pressure in four ways:

1. It increases cardiac output and stimulates vasoconstriction.

2. It stimulates the release of aldosterone, a hormone that acts on the nephron's distal convoluted tubule to increase sodium reabsorption, and secondarily, water reabsorption.

3. It stimulates the release of antidiuretic hormone (ADH), which acts directly on the distal convoluted tubules to increase water reabsorption.

4. It stimulates thirst centers in the hypothalamus, resulting in increased fluid consumption.

The combined effects of angiotensin II produce a dramatic increase in blood pressure. In fact, angiotensin II is estimated to be four to eight times more powerful than norepinephrine, another potent stimulator of hypertension, and thus is a good target for blood pressure-controlling drugs. One class of drugs used to treat hypertension is the **ACE inhibitors** (angiotensin-converting enzyme inhibitors), which control blood pressure by blocking the production of angiotensin II.

---

system. Urine is moved along the ureter from the kidneys to the bladder by gravity and by peristalsis at frequent intervals.

The Urinary Bladder

When it is empty, the urinary bladder (Fig. 22-10) is located below the parietal peritoneum and posterior to the pubic symphysis. When filled, it pushes the peritoneum upward and may extend well into the abdominal cavity proper. The urinary bladder is a temporary reservoir for urine, just as the gallbladder is a storage sac for bile.

The bladder wall has many layers. It is lined with mucous membrane containing transitional epithelium. The bladder's lining, like that of the stomach, is thrown into folds called *rugae* when the organ is empty. Beneath the mucosa is a layer of connective tissue, followed by a three-layered coat of involuntary smooth muscle that can stretch considerably. Finally, there is an incomplete coat of peritoneum that covers only the bladder's superior portion.

When the bladder is empty, the muscular wall becomes thick, and the entire organ feels firm. As the bladder fills, the muscular wall becomes thinner, and the organ may increase from a length of 5 cm (2 inches) up to as much as 12.5 cm (5 inches) or even more. A moderately full bladder holds about 470 mL (1 pint) of urine.

The **trigone** (TRI-gone) is a triangular-shaped region in the floor of the bladder. It is marked by the openings of the two ureters and the urethra (see Fig. 22-10). As the bladder fills with urine, it expands upward, leaving the

Figure 22-10 **Interior of the male urinary bladder.** The trigone is a triangular region in the floor of the bladder marked by the openings of the ureters and the urethra. [**ZOOMING IN** ➤ What gland does the urethra pass through in the male?]

trigone at the base stationary. This stability prevents stretching of the ureteral openings and the possible backflow of urine into the ureters.

The Urethra

The **urethra** is the tube that extends from the bladder to the outside (see Fig. 22-1) and is the means by which the bladder is emptied. The urethra differs in males and females; in the male, it is part of both the reproductive system and the urinary system, and it is much longer than is the female urethra.

The male urethra is approximately 20 cm (8 inches) in length. Proximally, it passes through the prostate gland, where it is joined by two ducts carrying male germ cells (spermatozoa) from the testes and glandular secretions. From here, it leads to the outside through the **penis** (PE-nis), the male organ of copulation. The male urethra serves the dual purpose of conveying semen with the germ cells and draining the bladder.

The urethra in the female is a thin-walled tube about 4 cm (1.5 inches) long. It is posterior to the pubic symphysis and is embedded in the muscle of the anterior vaginal wall. The external opening, called the **urinary meatus** (me-A-tus), is located just anterior to the vaginal opening between the labia minora. The female urethra drains the bladder only and is entirely separate from the reproductive system.

Urination

The process of expelling (voiding) urine from the bladder is called **urination** or **micturition** (mik-tu-RISH-un). This process is controlled both voluntarily and involuntarily with the aid of two rings of muscle (sphincters) that surround the urethra (see Fig. 22-10). Near the bladder's outlet is an involuntary **internal urethral sphincter** formed by a continuation of the bladder's smooth muscle. Below this muscle is a voluntary **external urethral** sphincter formed by the muscles of the pelvic floor. By learning to control the voluntary sphincter, one can gain control over the bladder's emptying.

As the bladder fills with urine, stretch receptors in its wall send impulses to a center in the lower part of the spinal cord. Motor impulses from this center stimulate contraction of the bladder wall, forcing urine outward as both the internal and external sphincters are made to relax. In the infant, this emptying occurs automatically as a simple reflex. Early in life, a person learns to control urination from higher centers in the brain until an appropriate time, a process known as *toilet training*. The impulse to urinate will override conscious controls if the bladder becomes too full.

The bladder can be emptied voluntarily by relaxing the muscles of the pelvic floor and increasing the pressure in the abdomen. The resulting increased pressure in the bladder triggers the spinal reflex that leads to urination.

CHECKPOINT 22-11 ➤ What is the name of the tube that carries urine from the kidney to the bladder?

CHECKPOINT 22-12 ➤ What is the name of the tube that carries urine from the bladder to the outside?

The Urine

Urine is a yellowish liquid that is approximately 95% water and 5% dissolved solids and gases. The pH of freshly collected urine averages 6.0, with a range of 4.5 to 8.0. Diet may cause considerable variation in pH.

The amount of dissolved substances in urine is indicated by its **specific gravity**. The specific gravity of pure water, used as a standard, is 1.000. Because of the dissolved materials it contains, urine has a specific gravity that normally varies from 1.002 (very dilute urine) to 1.040 (very concentrated urine). When the kidneys are diseased, they lose the ability to concentrate urine, and the specific gravity no longer varies as it does when the kidneys function normally.

Normal Constituents

Some of the dissolved substances normally found in the urine are the following:

- **Nitrogenous waste products**, including urea, uric acid, and **creatinine** (kre-AT-ih-nin).
- **Electrolytes**, including sodium chloride (as in common table salt) and different kinds of sulfates and phosphates. Electrolytes are excreted in appropriate amounts to keep their blood concentration constant.
- **Pigment**, mainly yellow pigment derived from certain bile compounds. Pigments from foods and drugs also may appear in the urine.

Abnormal Constituents

Examination of urine, called a **urinalysis** (u-rin-AL-ih-sis) **(UA)**, is one of the most important parts of a medical evaluation. A routine urinalysis includes observation of color and turbidity (cloudiness) as well as measurement of pH and specific gravity. Laboratories also test for a variety of abnormal components, including:

- **Glucose** is usually an important indicator of diabetes mellitus, in which the cells do not adequately metabolize blood sugar. The excess glucose, which cannot be reabsorbed, is excreted in the urine. The presence of glucose in the urine is known as glycosuria (gli-ko-SU-re-ah) or glucosuria.
- **Albumin**. The presence of this protein, which is normally retained in the blood, may indicate a kidney disorder, such as glomerulonephritis. Albumin in the urine is known as **albuminuria** (al-bu-mih-NU-re-ah).
- **Blood** in the urine is usually an important indicator of urinary system disease, including nephritis. Blood in the urine is known as **hematuria** (hem-ah-TU-re-ah).

- **Ketones** (KE-tones) are produced when fats are incompletely oxidized; ketones in the urine are seen in diabetes mellitus and starvation.

- **White blood cells** (pus) are evidence of infection; they can be seen by microscopic examination of a centrifuged specimen. Pus in the urine is known as **pyuria** (pi-U-re-ah).

- **Casts** are solid materials molded within the microscopic kidney tubules. They consist of cells or proteins and, when present in large number, they usually indicate disease of the nephrons.

More extensive tests on urine may include analysis for drugs, enzymes, hormones, and other metabolites, as well as cultures for microorganisms. Normal values for common urine tests are given in Appendix 4, Table 1.

Disorders of the Urinary System

The kidney is more prone to disorders than any other portion of the urinary system.

Kidney Disorders

Kidney disorders may be acute or chronic. Acute conditions usually arise suddenly, most frequently as the result of infection with inflammation of the nephrons. These diseases commonly run a course of a few weeks and are followed by complete recovery. Chronic conditions arise slowly and are often progressive, with gradual loss of kidney function.

Acute glomerulonephritis (glo-mer-u-lo-nef-RI-tis), also known as *acute poststreptococcal glomerulonephritis*, is the most common renal disease. This condition usually occurs in children about 1 to 4 weeks after a streptococcal throat infection. Antibodies formed in response to the streptococci attach to the glomerular membrane and cause injury. These damaged glomeruli allow protein, especially albumin, to filter into the glomerular capsule and ultimately to appear in the urine (albuminuria). They also allow red blood cells to filter into the urine (hematuria). Usually, the patient recovers without permanent kidney damage. In adult patients, the disease is more likely to become chronic, with a gradual decrease in the number of functioning nephrons, leading to chronic renal failure.

Pyelonephritis (pi-el-o-nef-RI-tis), an inflammation of the renal pelvis and the kidney tissue, may be either acute or chronic. In acute pyelonephritis, the inflammation results from a bacterial infection. Bacteria most commonly reach the kidney by ascending along the lining membrane from a distal urinary tract infection (see Fig. 23-14 in Chapter 23). More rarely, the blood carries bacteria to the kidney.

Acute pyelonephritis is often seen in people with partial obstruction of urine flow with stagnation (urinary stasis). It is most likely to occur in pregnant women and in men with an enlarged prostate, because the prostate surrounds the first portion of the urethra in males. Other causes of stasis include neurogenic bladder, which is bladder dysfunction resulting from neurologic lesions, as seen in diabetes mellitus, and structural defects in the area where the ureters enter the bladder. Pyelonephritis usually responds to antibiotic treatment, fluid replacement, rest, and fever control.

Chronic pyelonephritis, a more serious disease, is frequently seen in patients with urinary tract stasis or backflow. It may be caused by persistent or repeated bacterial infections. Progressive kidney damage is evidenced by high blood pressure, continual loss of protein in the urine, and dilute urine.

Hydronephrosis (hi-dro-nef-RO-sis) is the distention of the renal pelvis and calyces with accumulated fluid as a result of urinary tract obstruction. The most common causes of obstruction, in addition to pregnancy or an enlarged prostate, are a kidney stone that has formed in the pelvis and dropped into the ureter, a tumor that presses on a ureter, and scars due to inflammation. Prompt removal of the obstruction may result in complete recovery. If the obstruction is not removed, the kidney will be permanently damaged.

A **polycystic** (pol-e-SIS-tik) **kidney** is one in which many fluid-containing sacs develop in the active tissue and gradually destroy it by pressure. This disorder may run in families, and treatment has not proved very satisfactory, except for the use of dialysis machines or kidney transplantation.

Tumors of the kidneys usually grow rather slowly, but rapidly invading types are occasionally found. Blood in the urine and dull pain in the kidney region are warnings that should be heeded at once. Surgical removal of the kidney offers the best chance of cure because most renal cancers do not respond to chemotherapy or radiation.

> **PASSport to Success**
>
> Visit **thePoint** or see the Student Resource CD in the back of this book for illustrations of the kidney disorders discussed here.

KIDNEY STONES Kidney stones, or **calculi** (KAL-ku-li), are made of substances, such as calcium salts or uric acid, that precipitate out of the urine instead of remaining in solution. They usually form in the renal pelvis, but may also form in the bladder.

The causes of stone formation include dehydration, urinary stasis (stagnation), and urinary tract infection. The stones may vary in size from tiny grains resembling bits of gravel up to large masses that fill the renal pelvis and extend into the calyces. The latter are described as **staghorn calculi**.

There is no way of dissolving these stones because substances that could do so would also destroy renal tissue. Sometimes, instruments can be used to crush small stones and thus allow them to be expelled with the urine, but more often, surgical removal is required. A **litho-triptor** (LITH-o-trip-tor), literally a "stone-cracker," is a device that employs external shock waves to shatter kidney stones. The procedure is called **lithotripsy** (LITH-o-trip-se).

Visit **thePoint** or see the Student Resource CD in the back of this book for illustrations of kidney stones.

RENAL FAILURE Acute renal failure may result from a medical or surgical emergency or from toxins that damage the tubules. This condition is characterized by a sudden, serious decrease in kidney function accompanied by electrolyte and acid–base imbalances. Acute renal failure occurs as a serious complication of other severe illness and may be fatal.

Chronic renal failure results from a gradual loss of nephrons. As more and more nephrons are destroyed, the kidneys slowly lose the ability to perform their normal functions. As the disease progresses, nitrogenous waste products accumulate to high levels in the blood, causing a condition known as **uremia** (u-RE-me-ah). In many cases, there is a lesser decrease in renal function, known as **renal insufficiency**, that produces fewer symptoms.

A few of the characteristic signs and symptoms of chronic renal failure are the following:

- **Dehydration** (de-hi-DRA-shun). Excessive loss of body fluid may occur early in renal failure, when the kidneys cannot concentrate the urine and large amounts of water are eliminated.

- **Edema** (eh-DE-mah). Accumulation of fluid in the tissue spaces may occur late in chronic renal disease, when the kidneys cannot eliminate water in adequate amounts.

- **Electrolyte imbalance**, including retention of sodium and accumulation of potassium.

- **Hypertension** may occur as the result of fluid overload and increased renin production (see Box 22-2).

- **Anemia** occurs when the kidneys cannot produce the hormone erythropoietin to activate red blood cell production in bone marrow.

- **Uremia** (u-RE-me-ah), an excess of nitrogenous waste products in the blood. When these levels are very high, urea can be changed into ammonia in the stomach and intestine and cause ulcerations and bleeding.

CHECKPOINT 22-13 ➤ What is the difference between acute and chronic kidney disorders?

RENAL DIALYSIS AND KIDNEY TRANSPLANTATION Dialysis (di-AL-ih-sis) means "the separation of dissolved molecules based on their ability to pass through a semipermeable membrane" (Fig. 22-11A). Molecules that can pass through the membrane move from an area of greater concentration to one of lesser concentration. In patients who have defective renal function, the accumulation

Figure 22-11 **A hemodialysis system and a peritoneal dialysis system. (A)** In hemodialysis, a cellophane membrane separates the blood compartment and dialysis fluid compartment. This membrane is porous enough to allow all of the constituents except the plasma proteins (PRO) and blood cells (WBC, RBC) to diffuse between the two compartments. **(B)** In peritoneal dialysis, a semipermeable membrane richly supplied with blood vessels lines the peritoneal cavity. With dialysate dwelling in the peritoneal cavity, waste products diffuse from the network of blood vessels into the dialysate. (A, Reprinted with permission from Porth CM. *Pathophysiology*, 7th ed. Philadelphia: Lippincott Williams & Wilkins, 2004; B, reprinted with permission from Cohen BJ. *Medical Terminology*, 5th ed. Philadelphia: Lippincott Williams & Wilkins, 2008.)

of urea and other nitrogenous waste products can be reduced by passage of the patient's blood through a dialysis machine. The principle of "molecules leaving the area of greater concentration" thus operates to remove wastes from the blood. The fluid in the dialysis machine, the dialysate, can be adjusted to regulate the flow of substances out of the blood.

There are two methods of dialysis in use: hemodialysis (blood dialysis) and peritoneal dialysis (dialysis in the abdominal cavity). In hemodialysis, the dialysis membrane is made of cellophane or other synthetic material. In peritoneal dialysis, the surface area of the peritoneum acts as the membrane (see Fig. 22-11B). Dialysis fluid is introduced into the peritoneal cavity and then periodically removed along with waste products. This procedure may be done at intervals through the day or during the night.

A 1973 amendment to the Social Security Act provides federal financial assistance for people who have chronic renal disease and require dialysis. Most hemodialysis is performed in freestanding clinics. Treatment time has been reduced; a typical schedule involves 2 to 3 hours, three times a week. Access to the bloodstream has been made safer and easier through surgical establishment of a permanent exchange site (shunt). Peritoneal dialysis also has been improved and simplified, enabling patients to manage treatment at home.

Visit *thePoint* or see the Student Resource CD in the back of this book for a description of the career of hemodialysis technician.

The final option for treatment of renal failure is kidney transplantation. Surgeons have successfully performed many of these procedures. Kidneys have so much extra functioning tissue that the loss of one kidney normally poses no problem to the donor. Records show that transplantation success is greatest when surgeons use a kidney from a living donor who is closely related to the patient. Organs from deceased donors have also proved satisfactory in many cases. The problem of tissue rejection (the rejection syndrome) is discussed in Chapter 17.

Disorders of the Ureters

Abnormalities in structure of the ureter include subdivision at the renal pelvis and constricted or abnormally narrow parts, called **strictures** (STRICK-tures). Abnormal pressure from tumors or other outside masses may cause ureteral narrowing. Obstruction also may be caused by stones from the kidneys, or kinking of the tube because of a dropped kidney, a condition known as **renal ptosis** (TO-

Disease in Context revisited

▶ Adam Has Prostate Surgery to Prevent Kidney Damage

The urologist inserted the cystoscope into Adam's urethra, carefully guiding it toward the urinary bladder. When he examined the bladder's mucous membrane lining, he did not see any urinary stones or tumors of the rugae. He did note that the neck of Adam's urinary bladder was occluded by his enlarged prostate. This observation fit with the results of the pyelogram (a special radiograph of the urinary system) he had ordered for Adam a week earlier. The x-ray images indicated a blockage in the neck of the urinary bladder, which prevented urine from exiting. The back-pressure of the urine was causing distention of the ureters (hydroureter) and kidneys (hydronephrosis). The doctor removed the cystoscope and reported his findings to his patient. "Adam, Dr. Singh's diagnosis was correct. The blockage in your urinary system is due to enlargement of your prostate gland. If we don't treat this now, your kidneys are at risk of severe

damage and renal failure. I suggest we do a procedure called a *transurethral prostatectomy* to remove the prostatic overgrowth and reestablish urine flow."

A few days later, Adam was back at the hospital for his surgery. The urologist inserted an instrument called a resectoscope into Adam's urethra. With the electrical loop at the end of the instrument, he removed pieces of the prostate and cauterized blood vessels to control bleeding. By the end of the surgery, the urologist had resected enough of the prostate to restore normal urine flow. It would take Adam a few weeks to recover, but soon he would be back to normal.

During this case, we saw that enlargement of the prostate gland can seriously affect urinary system function. To learn more about the prostate gland and other organs of the male reproductive system, see Chapter 23.

sis). In cases of **ureterocele** (u-RE-ter-o-sele), the end of the ureter bulges into the bladder (Fig. 22-12). The result is urinary obstruction that leads to distention of the ureter (hydroureter) and renal pelvis (hydronephrosis). The usual cause of ureterocele is a congenital (present at birth) narrowing of the ureteral opening.

URETERAL STONES The passage of a small stone along the ureter causes excruciating pain, called *renal colic.* Relief of this pain usually requires morphine or an equally powerful drug. The first "barber surgeons," operating without benefit of anesthesia, were permitted by their patients to cut through the skin and the muscles of the back to remove stones from the ureters. "Cutting for stone" in this way was relatively successful, despite the lack of sterile technique, because the approach through the back avoided the peritoneal cavity and the serious risk of peritonitis.

Modern surgery employs a variety of instruments for removal of stones from the ureter, including endoscopes similar to those described in Chapter 19. The transurethral route through the urethra and urinary bladder and then into the ureter, as well as entrance through the skin and muscles of the back, may be used to remove calculi from the kidney pelvis or from the ureter.

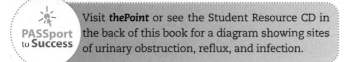

PASSport to Success Visit **thePoint** or see the Student Resource CD in the back of this book for a diagram showing sites of urinary obstruction, reflux, and infection.

CHECKPOINT 22-14 ➤ What is the scientific name for stones, as may occur in the urinary tract?

Bladder Disorders

A full (distended) bladder lies in an unprotected position in the lower abdomen, and a blow may rupture it, necessitating immediate surgical repair. Blood in the urine is a rather common symptom of infection or tumors, which may involve the bladder.

CYSTITIS Inflammation of the bladder, called **cystitis** (sis-TI-tis), is 10 times as common in women as in men. This may be due, at least in part, to the very short urethra of the female compared with that of the male. The usual path of infection is that bacteria ascend from the outside through the urethra into the bladder (see Fig. 23-14 in Chapter 23). The common contaminants are colon bacteria, such as *E. coli*, carried to the urethra from the anus. Urinary stasis and catheterization to remove urine from the bladder are other possible sources of infection. Pain, urgency to urinate, and urinary frequency are common symptoms of cystitis.

Another type of cystitis, called **interstitial cystitis**, may cause pelvic pain with discomfort before and after urination. The tissues below the mucosa are involved. The dis-

Figure 22-12 Ureterocele. The ureter bulges into the bladder. The resulting obstruction causes urine to back up into the ureter and renal pelvis. (Reprinted with permission from Cohen BJ. *Medical Terminology*, 5th ed. Philadelphia: Lippincott Williams & Wilkins, 2008.)

ease can be diagnosed only with the use of a **cystoscope**, a type of endoscope used to examine the bladder (Fig. 22-13). Because no bacteria are involved, antibiotics are not effective treatment and may even be harmful.

Obstruction by an enlarged prostate gland in a male or from pregnancy may lead to urinary stasis and cystitis. Reduction of a person's general resistance to infection, as in diabetes, may also lead to cystitis. The danger of cystitis is that the infection may ascend to other parts of the urinary tract.

TUMORS Bladder tumors, which are most prevalent in men older than 50 years of age, include benign papillomas and various kinds of cancer. About 90% of these tumors arise from the bladder's epithelial lining. Possible causes include toxins (particularly certain aniline dyes), chronic infestations (e.g., schistosomiasis), heavy cigarette smoking, and the presence of urinary stones, which may develop and increase in size within the bladder.

Blood in the urine (hematuria) and frequent urination, in the absence of pain or fever, are early signs of a bladder tumor. A cystoscopic examination (see Fig. 22-13) and biopsy should be performed as soon as these signs are detected. Treatment includes removal of the tumor, which may be done cystoscopically, and localized chemotherapy. More serious cases may require irradiation. Removal before the tumor invades the muscle wall gives the best prognosis.

If it is necessary to remove the bladder in a **cystectomy** (sis-TEK-to-me), the ureters must be vented elsewhere. They may be diverted to the body surface through a segment of the ileum, a procedure known as an **ileal conduit** (Fig. 22-14), or diverted to some other portion of the intestine. Alternatively, surgeons may create a bladder from a section of the colon.

URINARY INCONTINENCE Urinary incontinence (in-KON-tin-ens) refers to an involuntary loss of urine. The

Light cord

Urinary bladder

Tube for fluid

Prostate

Scrotum

Figure 22-13 **Cystoscopy.** A lighted cystoscope is introduced through the urethra into the bladder of a male subject. Sterile fluid is used to inflate the bladder. The cystoscope is used to examine the bladder, remove specimens for biopsy, and remove tumors. (Reprinted with permission from Cohen BJ. *Medical Terminology*, 5th ed. Philadelphia: Lippincott Williams & Wilkins, 2008.)

condition may originate with a neurologic disorder, trauma to the spinal cord, weakness of the pelvic muscles, impaired bladder function, or medications. Different forms of urinary incontinence have specific names:

- Stress incontinence results from urethral incompetence that allows small amounts of urine to be released when an activity increases pressure in the abdomen. These activities include coughing, sneezing, laughing, lifting, or exercising.

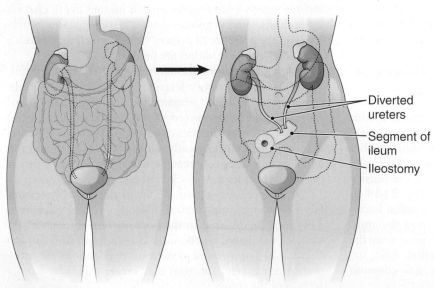

Diverted ureters

Segment of ileum

Ileostomy

Figure 22-14 **Ileal conduit.** The ureters are vented through a segment of the ileum to open at the body surface through an ileostomy. (Reprinted with permission from Cohen BJ. *Medical Terminology*, 5th ed. Philadelphia: Lippincott Williams & Wilkins, 2008.)

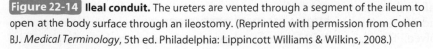

- Urge incontinence, also called *overactive bladder*, results from an inability to control bladder contractions once the sensation of bladder fullness is perceived.

- Overflow incontinence arises from neurologic damage or urinary obstruction that causes the bladder to overfill. Excess pressure in the bladder results in involuntary loss of urine.

- **Enuresis** (en-u-RE-sis) is involuntary urination, usually during the night (bed-wetting).

Some treatment approaches to incontinence include muscle exercises, dietary changes, biofeedback, medication, surgery or, in serious cases, self-catheterization.

CHECKPOINT 22-15 ➤ What is the term for inflammation of the bladder?

Disorders of the Urethra

Congenital anomalies may involve the urethra as well as other parts of the urinary tract. The opening of the urethra to the outside may be too small, or the urethra itself may be narrowed. Occasionally, an abnormal valve-like structure is found at the point where the urethra enters the bladder. If it is not removed surgically, it can cause back pressure of the urine, with serious consequences. There is also a condition in the male in which the urethra opens on the undersurface of the penis instead of at the end. This is called **hypospadias** (hi-po-SPA-de-as) (Fig. 22-15).

Urethritis, which is characterized by inflammation of the mucous membrane and the glands of the urethra, is much more common in men than in women. It is often caused by infection with gonococci or chlamydias, although many other bacteria may be involved.

"Straddle" injuries to the urethra are common in men. This type of injury occurs when, for example, a man walking along a raised beam slips and lands with the beam between his legs. Such an accident may catch the urethra between the hard surfaces of the beam and the pubic arch and rupture the urethra. In accidents in which the bones of the pelvis are fractured, rupture of the urethra is fairly common.

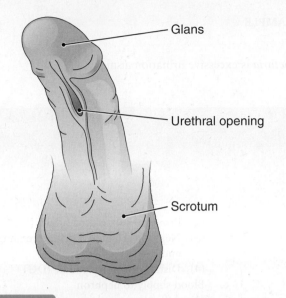

— Glans

— Urethral opening

— Scrotum

Figure 22-15 Hypospadias. A ventral view of the penis is shown here. (Reprinted with permission from Cohen BJ. *Medical Terminology,* 5th ed. Philadelphia: Lippincott Williams & Wilkins, 2008.)

The Effects of Aging

Even without renal disease, aging causes the kidneys to lose some of their ability to concentrate urine. With aging, progressively more water is needed to excrete the same amount of waste. Older people find it necessary to drink more water than young people, and they eliminate larger amounts of urine (polyuria), even at night (nocturia).

Beginning at about 40 years of age, there is a decrease in the number and size of the nephrons. Often, more than half of them are lost before the age of 80 years. There may be an increase in blood urea nitrogen (BUN) without serious symptoms. Elderly people are more susceptible than young people to urinary system infections. Childbearing may cause damage to the musculature of the pelvic floor, resulting in urinary tract problems in later years.

Enlargement of the prostate, common in older men, may cause obstruction and back pressure in the ureters and kidneys. If this condition is untreated, it will cause permanent damage to the kidneys. Changes with age, including decreased bladder capacity and decreased muscle tone in the bladder and urinary sphincters, may predispose to incontinence. However, most elderly people (60% in nursing homes, and up to 85% living independently) have no incontinence.

Word Anatomy

Medical terms are built from standardized word parts (prefixes, roots, and suffixes). Learning the meanings of these parts can help you remember words and interpret unfamiliar terms.

WORD PART	MEANING	EXAMPLE
The Kidneys		
retro-	backward, behind	The *retroperitoneal* space is posterior to the peritoneal cavity.
ren/o	kidney	The *renal* artery carries blood to the kidney.
nephr/o	kidney	The *nephron* is the functional unit of the kidney.
juxta-	next to	The *juxtaglomerular* apparatus is next to the glomerulus.
The Ureters		
extra-	beyond, outside of	The ureters are *extraperitoneal*.
Disorders of the Urinary System		
pyel/o	renal pelvis	*Pyelonephritis* is inflammation of the nephrons and renal pelvis.
cyst/o	sac, bladder	A *polycystic* kidney develops many fluid-containing sacs.
dia-	through	*Dialysis* is the separation (-lysis) of molecules based on their ability to pass through a semipermeable membrane.
-cele	swelling, enlarged space	A *uterocele* is formed as the end of the ureter bulges into the bladder.
trans-	across, through	A *transurethral* route is through the urethra.

22

WORD PART	MEANING	EXAMPLE

The Effects of Aging

| noct/i | night | *Nocturia* is excessive urination at night. |

Summary

I. **EXCRETION**
   A. Removal and elimination of metabolic waste
   B. Systems that eliminate waste
      1. Urinary—removes waste from blood
         a. Other functions—regulates blood volume, pH, and electrolytes
      2. Digestive system—eliminates water, salts, bile with digestive residue
      3. Respiratory system—eliminates carbon dioxide, water
      4. Skin—eliminates water, salts, nitrogenous waste

II. **ORGANS OF THE URINARY SYSTEM**
   A. Kidneys (2)
   B. Ureters (2)
   C. Urinary bladder (1)
   D. Urethra (1)

III. **KIDNEYS**
   A. Kidney activities
      1. Excretion of waste, excess salts, toxins
      2. Water balance
      3. Acid–base balance (pH)
      4. Blood pressure regulation
      5. Erythropoietin (EPO) secretion—hormone stimulates red blood cell production
   B. Kidney structure
      1. Location
         a. In upper abdomen against the back
         b. In retroperitoneal space (posterior to the peritoneum)
      2. Blood supply
         a. Renal artery—carries blood to kidney from aorta
         b. Renal vein—carries blood from kidney to inferior vena cava
      3. Organization
         a. Cortex—outer portion
         b. Medulla—inner portion
         c. Pelvis
            (1) Upper end of ureter
            (2) Calyces—cuplike extensions that receive urine
      4. Nephron
         a. Functional unit of kidney
         b. Parts
            (1) Glomerular (Bowman) capsule—around glomerulus
            (2) Proximal convoluted tubule (PCT)
            (3) Nephron (Henle) loop—descending and ascending limbs
            (4) Distal convoluted tubule (DCT)
         c. Blood supply to nephron
            (1) Afferent arteriole—enters glomerular capsule
            (2) Glomerulus—coil of capillaries in glomerular capsule
            (3) Efferent arteriole—leaves glomerular capsule
            (4) Peritubular capillaries—surround nephron
   C. Formation of urine
      1. Glomerular filtration—driven by blood pressure in glomerulus
         a. Water and soluble substances forced out of blood and into glomerular capsule
         b. Blood cells and proteins remain in blood
         c. Glomerular filtrate—material that leaves blood and enters the nephron
      2. Tubular reabsorption
         a. Most of filtrate leaves nephron by diffusion, osmosis, and active transport
         b. Influenced by hormones (e.g. aldosterone, ANP)
         c. Returns to blood through peritubular capillaries
      3. Tubular secretion—materials moved from blood into nephron for excretion
      4. Concentration of urine
         a. Countercurrent mechanism—method for concentrating urine based on movement of ions and permeability of tubule
         b. ADH
            (1) Hormone from posterior pituitary
            (2) Promotes reabsorption of water
   D. Regulation of blood pressure
      1. Kidneys need adequate blood pressure to filter blood
      2. Juxtaglomerular apparatus
         a. Consists of cells in afferent arteriole and distal convoluted tubule
         b. Releases renin when blood pressure low

c. Renin activates angiotensin to raise blood pressure
   (1) Stimulates release of aldosterone
   (2) Stimulates release of ADH
   (3) Promotes vasoconstriction
   (4) Stimulates thirst
   (5) Stimulates sympathetic nervous system

IV. **URETERS**
   A. Carry urine from the kidneys to the bladder

V. **URINARY BLADDER**
   A. Stores urine until it is eliminated
   B. Trigone—triangular region in base of bladder; remains stable as bladder fills

VI. **URETHRA**
   A. Carries urine out of body
   B. Male urethra—20 cm long; carries both urine and semen
   C. Female urethra—4 cm long; opening anterior to vagina
   D. Urination (micturition)
      1. Both voluntary and involuntary
      2. Sphincters
         a. Internal urethral sphincter—involuntary (smooth muscle)
         b. External urethral sphincter—voluntary (skeletal muscle)
      3. Stretch receptors in bladder wall signal reflex emptying
      4. Can be controlled through higher brain centers

VII. **URINE**
   A. pH averages 6.0
   B. Specific gravity—measures dissolved substances
   C. Normal constituents—water, nitrogenous waste, electrolytes, pigments
   D. Abnormal constituents—glucose, albumin, blood, ketones, white blood cells, casts

VIII. **DISORDERS OF THE URINARY SYSTEM**
   A. Kidney disorders
      1. Examples
         a. Acute glomerulonephritis—damages glomeruli
         b. Pyelonephritis—inflammation of kidney and renal pelvis
         c. Hydronephrosis—distention with obstructed fluids
         d. Polycystic kidney—fluid-containing sacs develop
         e. Tumors
      2. Kidney stones—calculi
      3. Renal failure
         a. Types
            (1) Acute—results from medical emergency or toxins
            (2) Chronic—signs include dehydration, electrolyte imbalance, edema, hypertension, anemia, uremia
      4. Treatment
         a. Renal dialysis—removes unwanted substances from blood when kidneys fail
            (1) Hemodialysis—exchange through synthetic membrane
            (2) Peritoneal dialysis—peritoneum is exchange membrane
         b. Kidney transplantation
   B. Disorders of the ureters
      1. Stricture (narrowing)
      2. Stones (calculi)
   C. Disorders of the bladder
      1. Cystitis—inflammation; most common in females
      2. Tumors
      3. Urinary incontinence
   D. Disorders of the urethra
      1. Hypospadias—urethra opens on underside of penis
      2. Urethritis—inflammation

IX. **EFFECTS OF AGING**
   A. Polyuria—increased elimination of urine
   B. Nocturia—urination at night
   C. Incontinence
   D. Increased blood urea nitrogen (BUN)
   E. Prostate enlargement

Questions for Study and Review

22

BUILDING UNDERSTANDING

Fill in the blanks

1. Each kidney is located outside the abdominal cavity in the _____ space.

2. The renal artery, renal vein, and ureter connect to the kidney at the _____.

3. The part of the bladder marked by the openings of the ureters and urethra is called the _____.

4. The amount of dissolved substances in urine is indicated by its _____.

5. The presence of glucose in the urine is known as _____.

Matching > Match each numbered item with the most closely related lettered item.

___ **6.** Produced by the kidney in response to low blood pressure

___ **7.** Stimulates vasoconstriction

___ **8.** Produced by the kidney in response to hypoxia

___ **9.** Stimulates kidneys to produce concentrated urine

___ **10.** Produced by the liver during protein catabolism

a. urea

b. erythropoietin

c. antidiuretic hormone

d. renin

e. angiotensin

Multiple choice

___ **11.** The functional unit of the renal system is the
  a. renal capsule
  b. kidney
  c. nephron
  d. juxtaglomerular apparatus

___ **12.** The nephron loop is located in the renal
  a. cortex
  b. medulla
  c. pelvis
  d. calyx

___ **13.** Fluid moves out of the glomerulus by
  a. filtration
  b. diffusion
  c. osmosis
  d. active transport

___ **14.** One's ability to delay urination is due to voluntary control of the
  a. trigone
  b. internal urethral sphincter
  c. external urethral sphincter
  d. urinary meatus

___ **15.** Pus in the urine is termed
  a. pyuria
  b. uremia
  c. anemia
  d. enuresis

UNDERSTANDING CONCEPTS

16. List four organ systems active in excretion. What are the products eliminated by each?

17. Compare and contrast the following terms:
  a. glomerular capsule and glomerulus
  b. afferent and efferent arteriole
  c. proximal and distal convoluted tubule
  d. ureter and urethra

18. Trace the pathway of a urea molecule from the afferent arteriole to the urinary meatus.

19. Describe the four processes involved in the formation of urine.

20. Compare the male urethra and female urethra in structure and function. Why is cystitis more common in women than in men?

21. List some of the dissolved substances normally found in the urine.

22. Differentiate between the following disorders:
  a. albuminuria and hematuria
  b. glomerulonephritis and pyelonephritis
  c. hydronephrosis and polycystic kidney
  d. renal ptosis and ureterocele

23. What is meant by the word *dialysis* and how is this principle used for patients with kidney failure? What kinds of membranes are used for hemodialysis? for peritoneal dialysis?

CONCEPTUAL THINKING

24. Christie is 14 years old and suffers from anorexia nervosa. Her parents take her to the hospital after she reports sharp pain in the lumbar region of her back. While there, she is diagnosed with hydronephrosis. What is the relationship between her eating disorder and her renal disorder?

25. A class of antihypertensive drugs called loop diuretics prevents sodium reabsorption in the nephron loop. How could a drug like this lower blood pressure?

26. In Adam's second case, enlargement of the prostate gland led to hydronephrosis. What effect might this have on glomerular filtration?

The final unit includes three chapters on the structures and functions related to reproduction and heredity. The reproductive system is not necessary for the continuation of the life of the individual but rather is needed for the continuation of the human species. The reproductive cells and their genes have been studied intensively during recent years as part of the rapidly advancing science of genetics.

CHAPTER 23

The Male and Female Reproductive Systems

Learning Outcomes

After careful study of this chapter, you should be able to:

1. Name the male and female gonads and describe the function of each
2. State the purpose of meiosis
3. List the accessory organs of the male and female reproductive tracts and cite the function of each
4. Describe the composition and function of semen
5. Draw and label a spermatozoon
6. List in the correct order the hormones produced during the menstrual cycle and cite the source of each
7. Describe the functions of the main male and female sex hormones
8. Explain how negative feedback regulates reproductive function in both males and females
9. Describe the changes that occur during and after menopause
10. Cite the main methods of birth control in use
11. Briefly describe the major disorders of the male and female reproductive tracts
12. Show how word parts are used to build words related to the reproductive systems (see Word Anatomy at the end of the chapter)

Selected Key Terms

The following terms and other boldface terms in the chapter are defined in the Glossary

contraception
corpus luteum
endometrium
estrogen
follicle
follicle-stimulating hormone (FSH)
gamete
infertility
luteinizing hormone (LH)
menopause
menses
menstruation
ovary
ovulation
ovum (pl., ova)
progesterone
semen
spermatozoon (pl., spermatozoa)
testis (pl., testes)
testosterone
uterus

PASSport to Success

Visit *thePoint* or see the Student Resource CD in the back of this book for definitions and pronunciations of key terms as well as a pretest for this chapter.

Disease
in Context

> ## Sylvie's Case: Removal of a Benign Uterine Tumor

"Ooh," Sylvie complained to her husband as she came into the house from gardening. "I know it's unusually hot this summer, but I'm having a hard time gardening this year for some reason. I feel a pull in my hip and groin and some discomfort in my belly. Maybe I've pulled a muscle; I should make an appointment for a massage and maybe talk to the trainers at the gym about getting some exercises to stretch out my hip muscles." "Maybe you should make an extra visit to your gynecologist," Jon suggested. "Remember he said something about a tumor last time you went?" "Right," Sylvie replied, "he said something about a small, benign tumor in my uterus. A fibroid, I think he called it. He didn't think it would cause problems, at least for a while, but maybe I should check it out. I've noticed some irregular bleeding, but chalked that up to my approaching menopause."

When Sylvie later consulted with her gynecologist, Dr. Bernard, she had already had a pelvic ultrasound to check on her uterus. After looking over her results, the doctor told her, "I don't know if this fibroid is the cause of your symptoms, but it has increased in size since your last visit. The ultrasound shows that the myoma, or fibroid, is about 3.5 cm, just about the size of a golf ball. I'm surprised that it has changed so rapidly, but that may be related to hormonal changes. I think because of its interior location we can remove it and repair the uterus through the vagina. We'll schedule you for outpatient surgery at Lincoln Hospital. If all goes well, you should have a very brief recovery period."

Sylvie's case uses some of the terms related to the female reproductive tract. Later, we'll revisit Sylvie to find out the results of her surgery.

Reproduction

The chapters in this unit deal with what is certainly one of the most interesting and mysterious attributes of life: the ability to reproduce. The simplest forms of life, one-celled organisms, usually need no partner to reproduce; they simply divide by themselves. This form of reproduction is known as **asexual** (nonsexual) reproduction.

In most animals, however, reproduction is **sexual**, meaning that there are two kinds of individuals, males and females, each of which has specialized cells designed specifically for the perpetuation of the species. These specialized sex cells are known as **germ cells** or **gametes** (GAM-etes). In the male, they are called **spermatozoa** (sper-mah-to-ZO-ah, sing., **spermatozoon**) or simply sperm cells; in the female, they are called **ova** (O-vah; sing., **ovum**), or egg cells.

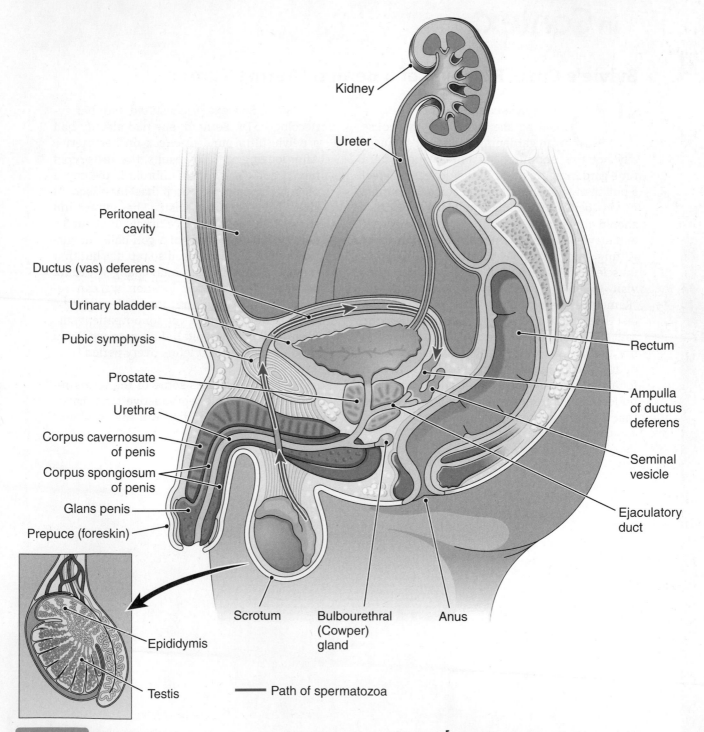

Figure 23-1   **Male reproductive system.** Organs of the urinary system are also shown. **[ZOOMING IN ➤** What four glands empty secretions into the urethra? **]**

Meiosis

Gametes are characterized by having half as many chromosomes as are found in any other body cell. During their formation, they go through a special process of cell division, called **meiosis** (mi-O-sis), which halves the number of chromosomes. In humans, meiosis reduces the chromosome number in a cell from 46 to 23. The role of meiosis in reproduction is explained in more detail in Chapter 25.

CHECKPOINT 23-1 ➤ What is the process of cell division that halves the chromosome number in a cell to produce a gamete?

The Male Reproductive System

The male reproductive system, like that of the female, may be divided into two groups of organs: primary and accessory (see Fig. 23-1).

- The primary organs are the **gonads** (GO-nads), or sex glands; they produce the germ cells and manufacture hormones. The male gonad is the testis. (In comparison, the female gonad is the ovary, as explained below.)

- The **accessory organs** include a series of ducts that transport the germ cells as well as various exocrine glands.

See Appendix 7 for a dissection photograph of the male reproductive system.

The Testes

The male gonads, the paired **testes** (TES-teze) (sing. **testis**), are located outside of the body proper, suspended between the thighs in a sac called the **scrotum** (SKRO-tum). The testes are oval organs measuring approximately 4.0 cm (1.5 inches) in length and approximately 2.5 cm (1 inch) in each of the other two dimensions. During embryonic life, each testis develops from tissue near the kidney.

A month or two before birth, the testis normally descends (moves downward) through the **inguinal** (ING-gwih-nal) **canal** in the abdominal wall into the scrotum. The testis then remains suspended by a **spermatic cord** (Fig. 23-2) that extends through the inguinal canal. This cord contains blood vessels, lymphatic vessels, nerves, and the tube (ductus deferens) that transports spermatozoa away from the testis. The gland must descend completely if it is to function normally; to produce spermatozoa, the testis must be kept at the temperature of the scrotum, which is several degrees lower than that of the abdominal cavity.

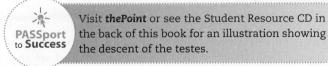

Visit **thePoint** or see the Student Resource CD in the back of this book for an illustration showing the descent of the testes.

INTERNAL STRUCTURE Most of the specialized tissue of the testis consists of tiny coiled **seminiferous** (seh-mih-

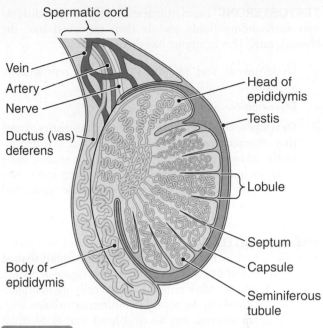

Figure 23-2 **Structure of the testis.** The epididymis and spermatic cord are also shown. [ZOOMING IN ➤ What duct receives secretions from the epididymis?]

NIF-er-us) **tubules.** Primitive cells in the walls of these tubules develop into mature spermatozoa, aided by neighboring cells called **sustentacular** (sus-ten-TAK-u-lar) **(Sertoli) cells.** These so-called "nurse" cells nourish and protect the developing spermatozoa. They also secrete a protein that binds testosterone in the seminiferous tubules.

Specialized **interstitial** (in-ter-STISH-al) **cells** that secrete the male sex hormone **testosterone** (tes-TOS-teh-rone) are located between the seminiferous tubules. Figure 23-3 is a microscopic view of the testis in cross-section, showing the seminiferous tubules, interstitial cells, and developing spermatozoa.

Figure 23-3 **Microscopic view of the testis.** (Courtesy of Dana Morse Bittus and BJ Cohen.)

TESTOSTERONE From the testis, testosterone diffuses into surrounding fluids and is then absorbed into the bloodstream. This hormone has three functions:

■ Development and maintenance of the reproductive structures.

■ Development of spermatozoa.

■ Development of **secondary sex characteristics**, traits that characterize males and females but are not directly concerned with reproduction. In males, these traits include a deeper voice, broader shoulders, narrower hips, a greater percentage of muscle tissue, and more body hair than are found in females.

THE SPERMATOZOA Spermatozoa are tiny individual cells illustrated in Figure 23-4. They are so small that at least 200 million are contained in the average ejaculation (release of semen). After puberty, sperm cells are manufactured continuously in the testes' seminiferous tubules.

The spermatozoon has an oval head that is mostly a nucleus containing chromosomes. The **acrosome** (AK-ro-some), which covers the head like a cap, contains enzymes that help the sperm cell to penetrate the ovum.

Whiplike movements of the tail (flagellum) propel the sperm through the female reproductive system to the ovum. The cell's middle region (midpiece) contains many mitochondria that provide energy for movement.

CHECKPOINT 23-2 ➤ What is the male gonad? What is the main male sex hormone?

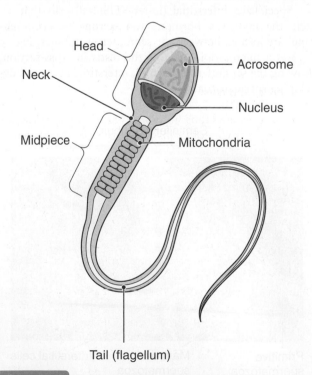

Tail (flagellum)

Figure 23-4   Diagram of a human spermatozoon. Major structural features are shown. [**ZOOMING IN** ➤ What organelles provide energy for sperm cell motility?]

CHECKPOINT 23-3 ➤ What is the male sex cell (gamete) called?

CHECKPOINT 23-4 ➤ What are the main subdivisions of a spermatozoon?

Accessory Organs

The system of ducts that transports the spermatozoa begins with tubules inside the testis itself. From these tubules, the cells collect in a greatly coiled tube called the **epididymis** (ep-ih-DID-ih-mis), which is 6 meters (20 feet) long and is located on the surface of the testis inside the scrotal sac (see Fig. 23-2). While they are temporarily stored in the epididymis, the sperm cells mature and become motile, able to move or "swim" by themselves.

The epididymis finally extends upward at the **ductus deferens** (DEF-er-enz), also called the **vas deferens**. This tube, contained in the spermatic cord, continues through the inguinal canal into the abdominal cavity. Here, it separates from the remainder of the spermatic cord and curves behind the urinary bladder. The ductus deferens then joins with the duct of the **seminal vesicle** (VES-ih-kl) on the same side to form the **ejaculatory** (e-JAK-u-lah-to-re) **duct**. The right and left ejaculatory ducts travel through the body of the prostate gland and then empty into the urethra.

CHECKPOINT 23-5 ➤ What is the order in which sperm cells travel through the ducts of the male reproductive system?

Semen

Semen (SE-men) (meaning "seed") is the mixture of sperm cells and various secretions that is expelled from the body. It is a sticky fluid with a milky appearance. The pH is in the alkaline range of 7.2 to 7.8. The secretions in semen serve several functions:

■ Nourish the spermatozoa

■ Transport the spermatozoa

■ Neutralize the acidity of the male urethra and the female vaginal tract

■ Lubricate the reproductive tract during sexual intercourse

■ Prevent infection with antibacterial enzymes and antibodies

The glands discussed next contribute secretions to the semen (see Fig. 23-1).

THE SEMINAL VESICLES The seminal vesicles are twisted muscular tubes with many small outpouchings. They are approximately 7.5 cm (3 inches) long and are attached to the connective tissue at the posterior of the urinary bladder. The glandular lining produces a thick, yellow, alkaline secretion containing large quantities of simple sugar and other substances that provide nourishment for the sperm. The seminal fluid makes up a large part of the semen's volume.

THE PROSTATE GLAND The **prostate gland** lies immediately inferior to the urinary bladder, where it surrounds the first part of the urethra. Ducts from the prostate carry its secretions into the urethra. The thin, alkaline prostatic secretion helps neutralize the acidity of the vaginal tract and enhance the spermatozoa's motility. The prostate gland is also supplied with muscular tissue, which, upon signals from the nervous system, contracts to aid in the expulsion of the semen from the body.

BULBOURETHRAL GLANDS The **bulbourethral** (bul-bo-u-RE-thral) **glands**, also called **Cowper glands**, are a pair of pea-sized organs located in the pelvic floor just inferior to the prostate gland. They secrete mucus to lubricate the urethra and tip of the penis during sexual stimulation. The ducts of these glands extend approximately 2.5 cm (1 inch) from each side and empty into the urethra before it extends into the penis.

Other very small glands secrete mucus into the urethra as it passes through the penis.

CHECKPOINT 23-6 ➤ What glands, aside from the testis, contribute secretions to semen?

The Urethra and Penis

The male urethra, as discussed in Chapter 22, serves the dual purpose of conveying urine from the bladder and carrying the reproductive cells with their accompanying secretions to the outside. The ejection of semen is made possible by **erection**, the stiffening and enlargement of the penis, through which the longest part of the urethra extends. The penis is made of spongy tissue containing many blood spaces that are relatively empty when the organ is flaccid but that fill with blood and distend when the penis is erect. This tissue is subdivided into three segments, each called a **corpus** (body) (Fig. 23-5). A single, ventrally located **corpus spongiosum** contains the urethra. On either side is a larger **corpus cavernosum** (pl., corpora cavernosa). At the distal end of the penis, the corpus spongiosum enlarges to form the **glans penis**, which is covered with a loose fold of skin, the **prepuce** (PRE-puse), commonly called the *foreskin*. It is the end of the foreskin that is removed in a **circumcision** (sir-kum-SIZH-un), a surgery frequently performed on male babies for religious or cultural reasons. Experts disagree on the medical value of circumcision with regard to improved cleanliness and disease prevention.

The penis and scrotum together make up the male **external genitalia** (jen-ih-TA-le-ah).

EJACULATION Ejaculation (e-jak-u-LA-shun) is the forceful expulsion of semen through the urethra to the outside. The process is initiated by reflex centers in the spinal cord that stimulate smooth muscle contraction in the prostate.

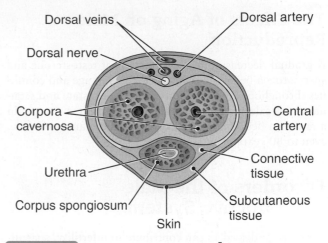

Figure 23-5 **Cross-section of the penis.** [ZOOMING IN ➤ What subdivision of the penis contains the urethra?]

This is followed by contraction of skeletal muscle in the pelvic floor, which provides the force needed for expulsion. During ejaculation, the involuntary sphincter at the base of the bladder closes to prevent the release of urine.

A male typically ejaculates 2 to 5 mL of semen containing 50 to 150 million sperm cells per mL. Out of the millions of spermatozoa in an ejaculation, only one, if any, can fertilize an ovum. The remainder of the cells live from only a few hours up to a maximum of 3 days.

Hormonal Control of Male Reproduction

The activities of the testes are under the control of two hormones produced by the anterior pituitary. These hormones are named for their activity in female reproduction (described later), although they are chemically the same in both males and females.

- **Follicle-stimulating hormone (FSH)** stimulates the sustentacular (Sertoli) cells and promotes the formation of spermatozoa.

- **Luteinizing hormone (LH)** stimulates the interstitial cells between the seminiferous tubules to produce testosterone, which is also needed for sperm cell development.

Starting at puberty, the hypothalamus begins to secrete hormones that trigger the release of FSH and LH. These hormones are secreted continuously in the male. The activity of the hypothalamus is in turn regulated by a negative feedback mechanism involving testosterone. As the blood level of testosterone increases, the hypothalamus secretes less releasing hormone; as the level of testosterone decreases, the hypothalamus secretes more releasing hormone (see Fig. 12-3 in Chapter 12).

CHECKPOINT 23-7 ➤ What two pituitary hormones regulate both male and female reproduction?

23

The Effects of Aging on Male Reproduction

A gradual decrease in the production of testosterone and spermatozoa begins as early as 20 years of age and continues throughout life. Secretions from the prostate and seminal vesicles decrease in amount and become less viscous. In a few men (less than 10%), sperm cells remain late in life, even to 80 years of age.

Disorders of the Male Reproductive System

A variety of disorders can contribute to **infertility**, a significantly lower than normal ability to reproduce. If the inability is complete, the condition is termed **sterility**. The proportion of infertility in couples that can be attributed to defects involving the male has been estimated from 40% to 50%. (See also Box 23-1, Treating Erectile Dysfunction.)

The tubules of the testes are sensitive to x-rays, infections, toxins, and malnutrition, all of which bring about degenerative changes. Such damage may cause a decrease in the numbers of spermatozoa produced, leading to a condition called **oligospermia** (ol-ih-go-SPER-me-ah). Adequate numbers of sperm are required to disperse the coating around the ovum so that one sperm can fertilize it. Absence of or an inadequate number of sperm cells is a significant cause of infertility.

A male may be intentionally sterilized by an operation called a **vasectomy** (vah-SEK-to-me). In this procedure, a portion of the ductus deferens on each side is removed, and the cut end is closed to keep spermatozoa from reaching the urethra. The tiny sperm cells are simply reabsorbed. A man who has had a vasectomy retains the ability to produce hormones and all other seminal secretions as well as the ability to perform the sex act, but no fertilization can occur.

Structural Disorders

Cryptorchidism (kript-OR-kid-izm) is a failure of the testis to descend into the scrotum. Unless corrected in childhood, this condition results in sterility. Undescended testes are also particularly subject to tumor formation. Most testes that are undescended at birth descend spontaneously by 1 year of age. Surgical correction is the usual remedy in the remaining cases.

Torsion of the testis is a twisting of the spermatic cord that results from rotation of the testis (Fig. 23-6). This turning may occur during descent of the testis or later in life, most commonly between the ages of 8 to 18 years. The condition is accompanied by acute pain, swelling, and shortening of the spermatic cord. It requires emergency surgery to correct the defect, and may involve removal of the testis (orchiectomy). Torsion of the testis is a developmental disorder that often affects both glands, so the other testis must be examined to determine whether or not preventive surgery is needed.

Hernia (HER-ne-ah), or rupture, refers to the abnormal protrusion of an organ or organ part through the wall of the cavity in which it is normally contained (Fig. 23-7).

Box 23-1 **Clinical Perspectives**

Treating Erectile Dysfunction: When NO Means Yes

Approximately 25 million American men and their partners are affected by **erectile dysfunction** (ED), the inability to achieve an erection. Although ED is more common in men over the age of 65, it can occur at any age and can have many causes. Until recently, ED was believed to be caused by psychological factors, such as stress or depression. It is now known that many cases of ED are caused by physical factors, including cardiovascular disease, diabetes, spinal cord injury, and damage to penile nerves during prostate surgery. Antidepressant and antihypertensive medications also can produce erectile dysfunction.

Erection results from interaction between the autonomic nervous system and penile blood vessels. Sexual arousal stimulates parasympathetic nerves in the penis to release a compound called nitric oxide (NO), which activates the vascular smooth muscle enzyme guanylyl cyclase. This enzyme catalyzes production of cyclic GMP (cGMP), a potent vasodilator that in-

creases blood flow into the penis to cause erection. Physical factors that cause ED prevent these physiologic occurrences.

Until recently, treatment options for ED, such as penile injections, vacuum pumps, and insertion of medications into the penile urethra, were inadequate, inconvenient, and painful. Today, drugs that target the physiologic mechanisms that underlie erection are giving men who suffer from ED new hope. The best known of these is sildenafil (Viagra), which works by inhibiting the enzyme that breaks down cGMP, thus prolonging the effects of NO.

Although effective in about 80% of all ED cases, Viagra can cause some relatively minor side effects, including headache, nasal congestion, stomach upset, and blue-tinged vision. Viagra should never be used by men who are taking nitrate drugs to treat angina. Because nitrate drugs elevate NO levels, taking them with Viagra, a drug that prolongs the effects of NO, can cause life-threatening hypotension.

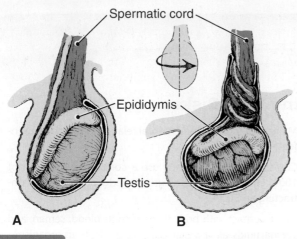

Figure 23-6 Torsion of the testis. (A) Normal. **(B)** Torsion. The testis rotates, twisting the spermatic cord. (Reprinted with permission from LifeART Pediatrics 1 [CD-ROM]. Baltimore: Lippincott Williams & Wilkins, 2000.)

Hernias most often occur where there is a weak area in the abdominal wall, at the inguinal canal for example. In this region, during development, the testis pushes its way through the muscles and connective tissues of the abdominal wall, carrying with it the blood vessels and other structures that form the spermatic cord.

Normally, in the adult, the inguinal area is fairly well reinforced with connective tissue, and there is no direct connection between the abdominal cavity and the scrotal sac. As in other regions where an opening permits a structure's passage through the abdominal wall, however, this area constitutes a weak place where a hernia may occur.

Phimosis (fi-MO-sis) is a tightness of the foreskin (prepuce), so that it cannot be drawn back. Phimosis may

Figure 23-7 Inguinal hernia. (A) Normal. **(B)** Hernia. The intestine protrudes through a weakness in the abdominal wall at the inguinal canal. (Reprinted with permission from Cohen BJ. *Medical Terminology*, 4th ed. Philadelphia: Lippincott Williams & Wilkins, 2004.)

be remedied by circumcision, in which part or all of the foreskin is surgically removed.

Infections

Sexually transmitted infections (STI), formerly known as *sexually transmitted diseases* (STD) or *venereal diseases* (VD), are spread through sexual contact in both males and females. They most commonly involve chlamydial infections and gonococcal infections (gonorrhea). In males, these diseases are manifested by a discharge from the urethra, which may be accompanied by burning and pain, especially during urination. The infection may travel along the mucous membrane into the prostate gland and the epididymis; if both sides are affected and enough scar tissue is formed to destroy the tubules, sterility may result.

Another common STI is a persistent infection called **genital herpes**. Caused by a virus, this disorder is characterized by fluid-filled vesicles (blisters) on and around the genital organs.

The sexually transmitted disease **syphilis** is caused by a spirochete (*Treponema pallidum*). Because syphilis spreads quickly in the bloodstream, it is regarded as a systemic disorder (see Appendix 5, Table 1). The genital ulcers caused by syphilis increase the chances of infection with the AIDS virus. HIV itself is considered an STI because of its most common route of spread. (See Box 23-2, Sexually Transmitted Infections.)

EPIDIDYMITIS Organisms from an STI or urinary tract infection (UTI) may travel through the ducts of the reproductive system to the epididymis. A congenital malformation in the urinary tract can predispose to **epididymitis** (ep-ih-did-ih-MI-tis), and infection may also be carried to the organ systemically by blood or lymph. Treatment includes an antibiotic along with bed rest and support of the scrotum to promote lymphatic drainage.

PROSTATITIS The usual cause of prostatic inflammation is bacterial infection secondary to an ascending urinary tract infection. A variety of intestinal organisms and bacteria from other sources may be involved, but *E. coli* is the most common. Treatment with antibiotics usually clears the infection, but tests to diagnose the source of infection may be needed if the condition persists. Other possible causes of **prostatitis** (pros-tah-TI-tis) are bladder-neck obstruction that forces urine into the prostate and autoimmunity.

ORCHITIS Orchitis (or-KI-tis) is inflammation of the testis, which also may follow from infection of the urinary or reproductive tract. Mumps, a viral infection of the parotid salivary gland, may also involve the testes. A mumps infection during or after puberty may result in testicular inflammation, which could lead to sterility.

CHECKPOINT 23-8 ➤ What are some infectious diseases of the reproductive tract?

23

Box 23-2 **Health Maintenance**

Sexually Transmitted Infections: Lowering Your Risks

Sexually transmitted infections (STIs) such as chlamydia, gonorrhea, genital herpes, HIV, and syphilis are some of the most common infectious diseases in the United States, affecting more than 13 million men and women each year. These diseases are associated with complications such as pelvic inflammatory disease, epididymitis, infertility, liver failure, neurological disorders, cancer, and AIDS. Women are more likely to contract STIs than are men. The same mechanisms that transport sperm cells through the female reproductive tract also move infectious organisms. The surest way to prevent STIs is to avoid sexual contact with others. If you are sexually active, the following techniques can lower your risks:

- Maintain a monogamous sexual relationship with an uninfected partner.

- Correctly and consistently use a condom. Although not 100% effective, condoms greatly reduce the risk of contracting an STI.

- Avoid contact with body fluids such as blood, semen, and vaginal fluids, all of which may harbor infectious organisms.

- Urinate and wash the genitals after sex. This may help remove infectious organisms before they cause disease.

- Have regular checkups for STIs. Most of the time STIs cause no symptoms, particularly in women.

Tumors

Tumors of the prostate may be benign or malignant. Both types cause such pressure on the urethra that urination becomes difficult. Back pressure may destroy kidney tissue and may lead to stasis of urine in the bladder with a resulting susceptibility to infection. Men with benign prostate enlargement, known as benign prostatic hyperplasia (BPH), may respond to medication to shrink the prostate. An herbal remedy that may help to slow progress of BPH is an extract of berries of the saw palmetto, a low-growing palm tree. If urinary function is threatened, however, surgery is needed to reduce the obstruction. Traditionally, this surgery has been performed through the urethra, in a transurethral prostatectomy (TURP). Newer methods include use of laser and ultrasound to destroy excess tissue or placement of a stent to widen the urethra.

Prostatic cancer is the most common cancer of males in the United States, especially among men older than 50 years of age. Other risk factors, in addition to age, are race, family history, and certain environmental agents. A high-fat diet may increase risk by promoting production of male sex hormones. Prostatic cancer is frequently detected as a nodule during rectal examination. Early detection has improved with annual blood tests for prostate-specific antigen (PSA). This protein increases in cases of prostate cancer, although it may increase in other prostatic disorders as well. Depending on the age of the patient and the nature of the cancer, the course of treatment may include surveillance, radiation therapy, surgery, or hormone treatments.

PASSport to Success   Visit *thePoint* or see the Student Resource CD in the back of this book for illustrations of prostate surgery procedures.

Testicular cancer affects young to middle-aged adults. Almost all testicular cancers arise in the germ cells, and a tumor can metastasize through the lymphatic system at an early stage of development. Early detection with regular testicular self-examination (TSE), however, improves the chances for effective treatment. The 5-year survival rate for this form of cancer is now greater than 95%. Often fertility can be preserved, although sperm banking is an option for men about to undergo treatment for testicular cancer.

The Female Reproductive System

The female gonads are the paired **ovaries** (O-vah-reze), where the female sex cells, or ova, are formed (Fig. 23-8). The remainder of the female reproductive tract consists of an organ (uterus) to hold and nourish a developing infant, various passageways, and the external genital organs. See Appendix 7 for a dissection photograph of the female reproductive system.

CHECKPOINT **23-9** ➤ What is the female gonad called?

CHECKPOINT **23-10** ➤ What is the female gamete called?

The Ovaries

The ovary is a small, somewhat flattened oval body measuring approximately 4 cm (1.6 inches) in length, 2 cm (0.8 inch) in width, and 1 cm (0.4 inch) in depth. Like the testes, the ovaries descend, but only as far as the pelvic cavity. Here, they are held in place by ligaments, including the broad ligament, the ovarian ligament, and others, that attach them to the uterus and the body wall.

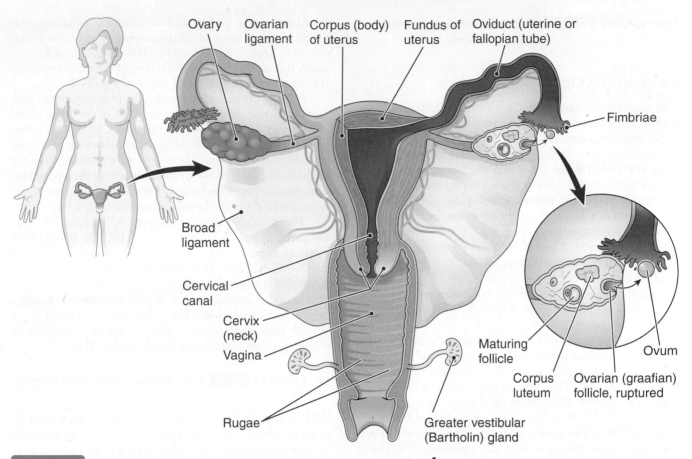

Ovary
Ovarian ligament
Corpus (body) of uterus
Fundus of uterus
Oviduct (uterine or fallopian tube)
Fimbriae
Broad ligament
Cervical canal
Cervix (neck)
Vagina
Rugae
Greater vestibular (Bartholin) gland
Maturing follicle
Corpus luteum
Ovarian (graafian) follicle, ruptured
Ovum

Figure 23-8 **Female reproductive system.** The enlargement (*right*) shows ovulation. [**ZOOMING IN** ➤ What is the deepest part of the uterus called?]

The Ova and Ovulation

The outer layer of the ovary is made of a single layer of epithelium. Beneath this layer, the female gametes, the ova, are produced. The ovaries of a newborn female contain a large number of potential ova. Each month during the reproductive years, several ripen, but usually only one is released.

The complicated process of maturation, or "ripening," of an ovum takes place in a small fluid-filled cluster of cells called the **ovarian follicle** (o-VA-re-an FOL-ih-kl) or **graafian** (GRAF-e-an) **follicle** (Fig. 23-9). As the follicle develops, cells in its wall secrete the hormone estrogen (ES-tro-jen), which stimulates growth of the uterine lining. When an ovum has ripened, the ovarian follicle may rupture and discharge the egg cell from the ovary's surface. The rupture of a follicle allowing an ovum's escape into the pelvic cavity is called **ovulation** (ov-u-LA-shun). Any developing ova that are not released simply degenerate.

After it is released, the egg cell is swept into the nearest **oviduct** (O-vih-dukt), a tube that arches over the ovary and leads to the uterus (see Fig. 23-8).

CHECKPOINT 23-11 ➤ What is the structure that surrounds the egg as it ripens?

CHECKPOINT 23-12 ➤ What is the process of releasing an egg cell from the ovary called?

THE CORPUS LUTEUM After the ovum has been expelled, the remaining follicle is transformed into a solid glandular mass called the **corpus luteum** (LU-te-um). This structure secretes estrogen and also progesterone (pro-JES-ter-one), another hormone needed in the reproductive cycle. Commonly, the corpus luteum shrinks and is replaced by scar tissue. When a pregnancy occurs, however, this structure remains active for a while. Sometimes, as a result of normal ovulation, the corpus luteum persists and forms a small ovarian cyst (fluid-filled sac). This condition usually resolves without treatment.

Ovum
Ovarian (graafian) follicle

Figure 23-9 **Microscopic view of the ovary.** The photomicrograph shows egg cells (ova) developing within ovarian (graafian) follicles. (Courtesy of Dana Morse Bittus and BJ Cohen.)

23

CHECKPOINT **23-13** ➤ What does the follicle become after its egg is released?

Accessory Organs

The accessory organs in the female are the oviducts, the uterus, the vagina, the greater vestibular glands, and the vulva and perineum.

THE OVIDUCTS The tubes that transport the ova in the female reproductive system, the oviducts, are also known as **uterine** (U-ter-in) **tubes**, or **fallopian** (fah-LO-pe-an) **tubes**. Each is a small, muscular structure, nearly 12.5 cm (5 inches) long, extending from a point near the ovary to the uterus (womb). There is no direct connection between the ovary and this tube. The ovum is swept into the oviduct by a current in the peritoneal fluid produced by the small, fringelike extensions called **fimbriae** (FIM-bre-e) that are located at the edge of the tube's opening into the pelvic cavity (see Fig. 23-8).

Unlike the sperm cell, the ovum cannot move by itself. Its progress through the oviduct toward the uterus depends on the sweeping action of cilia in the tube's lining and on peristalsis of the tube. It takes about 5 days for an ovum to reach the uterus from the ovary.

THE UTERUS The oviducts lead to the **uterus** (U-ter-us), the organ in which a fetus develops to maturity. The uterus is a pear-shaped, muscular organ approximately 7.5 cm (3 inches) long, 5 cm (2 inches) wide, and 2.5 cm (1 inch) deep. (The organ is typically larger in women who have borne children and smaller in postmenopausal women.) The superior portion rests on the upper surface of the urinary bladder; the inferior portion is embedded in the pelvic

floor between the bladder and the rectum. The wider upper region of the uterus is called the **corpus**, or body; the lower, narrower region is the **cervix** (SER-viks), or neck. The small, rounded region above the level of the tubal entrances is known as the **fundus** (FUN-dus) (see Fig. 23-8).

Folds of the peritoneum called the *broad ligaments* support the uterus, extending from each side of the organ to the lateral body wall. Along with the uterus, these two membranes form a partition dividing the female pelvis into anterior and posterior areas. The ovaries are suspended from the broad ligaments, and the oviducts lie within the upper borders. Blood vessels that supply these organs are found between the layers of the broad ligament (see Fig. 23-8).

The muscular wall of the uterus is called the **myometrium** (mi-o-ME-tre-um) (Fig. 23-10). The lining of the uterus is a specialized epithelium known as **endometrium** (en-do-ME-tre-um). This inner layer changes during the menstrual cycle, first preparing to nourish a fertilized egg, then breaking down if no fertilization occurs to be released as the menstrual flow. The cavity inside the uterus is shaped somewhat like a capital T, but it is capable of changing shape and dilating as a fetus develops.

CHECKPOINT **23-14** ➤ In what organ does a fetus develop?

THE VAGINA The cervix leads to the **vagina** (vah-JI-nah), the distal part of the birth canal, which opens to the outside of the body. The vagina is a muscular tube approximately 7.5 cm (3 inches) long. The cervix dips into the superior portion of the vagina forming a circular recess known as the **fornix** (FOR-niks). The deepest area of the fornix, located behind the cervix, is the **posterior fornix** (Fig. 23-11). This recess in the posterior vagina lies adjacent to the most inferior portion of the peritoneal cavity, a

Figure 23-10 **The uterus as seen under the microscope.** The photomicrographs show the myometrium and endometrium and illustrate the changes that occur in the endometrium during the menstrual cycle. **(A)** Proliferative phase (first part of cycle). **(B)** Secretory phase (second part of cycle). (Reprinted with permission from Cormack DH. *Essential Histology*, 2nd ed. Philadelphia: Lippincott Williams & Wilkins, 2001.) **[ZOOMING IN ➤** In which part of the menstrual cycle is the endometrium most highly developed? **]**

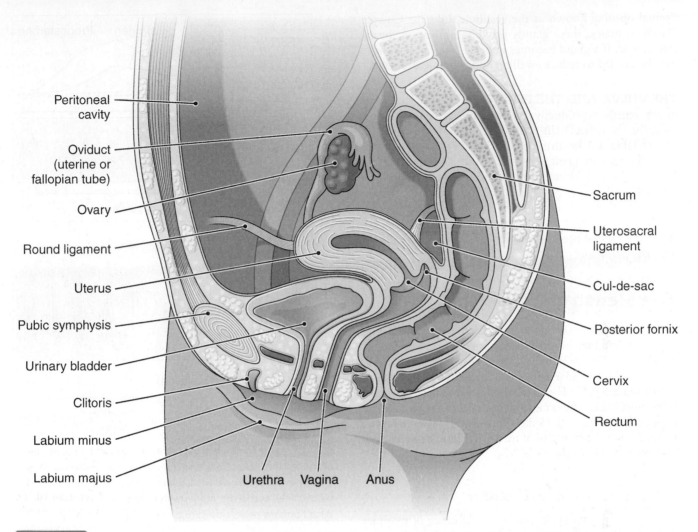

Figure 23-11 **Female reproductive system (sagittal section).** This view shows the relationship of the reproductive organs to each other and to other structures in the pelvic cavity. **[ZOOMING IN ➤** Which has the more anterior opening, the vagina or the urethra? **]**

narrow passage between the uterus and the rectum named the **cul-de-sac** (from the French meaning "bottom of the sack"). This area is also known as the *rectouterine pouch* or the *pouch of Douglas*. A rather thin layer of tissue separates the posterior fornix from this region, so that abscesses or tumors in the peritoneal cavity can sometimes be detected by vaginal examination.

The lining of the vagina is a wrinkled mucous membrane similar to that found in the stomach. The folds (rugae) permit enlargement so that childbirth usually does not tear the lining. In addition to being a part of the birth canal, the vagina is the organ that receives the penis during sexual intercourse. A fold of membrane called the **hymen** (HI-men) may sometimes be found at or near the vaginal (VAJ-ih-nal) canal opening (Fig. 23-12).

THE GREATER VESTIBULAR GLANDS Just superior and lateral to the vaginal opening are the two mucus-producing **greater vestibular** (ves-TIB-u-lar) (**Bartholin**) **glands** (see Fig. 23-8). These glands secrete into an area near the

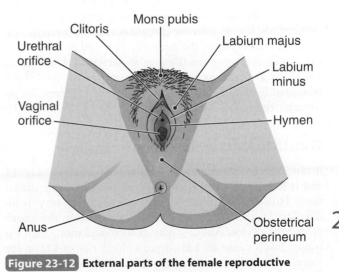

Figure 23-12 **External parts of the female reproductive system.** Nearby structures are also shown.

23

vaginal opening known as the **vestibule**. Like the Cowper glands in males, these glands provide lubrication during intercourse. If a gland becomes infected, a surgical incision may be needed to reduce swelling and promote drainage.

THE VULVA AND THE PERINEUM The external parts of the female reproductive system, or external genitalia, comprise the **vulva** (VUL-vah), which includes two pairs of lips, or **labia** (LA-be-ah); the **clitoris** (KLIT-o-ris), which is a small organ of great sensitivity; and related structures (see Fig. 23-12). Although the entire pelvic floor in both the male and female (see Fig. 8-15 in Chapter 8) is properly called the **perineum** (per-ih-NE-um), those who care for pregnant women usually refer to the limited area between the vaginal opening and the anus as the *perineum* or *obstetric perineum*.

The Menstrual Cycle

In the female, as in the male, reproductive function is controlled by pituitary hormones that are regulated by the hypothalamus. Female activity differs, however, in that it is cyclic; it shows regular patterns of increases and decreases in hormone levels. These changes are regulated by hormonal feedback. The typical length of the menstrual cycle varies between 22 and 45 days, but 28 days is taken as an average, with the first day of menstrual flow being considered the first day of the cycle (Fig. 23-13).

Beginning of the Cycle

At the start of each cycle, under the influence of pituitary FSH, several follicles, each containing an ovum, begin to develop in the ovary. Usually, only one of these follicles will ultimately release an ovum from the ovary in a single month. The follicle produces increasing amounts of **estrogen** as it matures (see Fig. 23-13). (*Estrogen* is the term used for a group of related hormones, the most active of which is estradiol.) The estrogen is carried in the bloodstream to the uterus, where it starts preparing the endometrium for a possible pregnancy. This preparation includes thickening of the endometrium and elongation of the glands that produce the uterine secretion. Estrogen in the blood also acts as a feedback messenger to inhibit the release of FSH and stimulate the release of LH from the pituitary (see Fig. 12-3 in Chapter 12).

Ovulation

In an average 28-day cycle, ovulation occurs on day 14 and is followed 2 weeks later by the start of the menstrual flow. However, an ovum can be released any time from day 7 to 21, thus accounting for the variation in the length of normal cycles. About 1 day before ovulation, high estrogen levels cause an **LH surge**, a sharp rise of LH in the blood. (Note that there is also a small rise in FSH at this time—shown in Figure 23-13—caused by the increase in

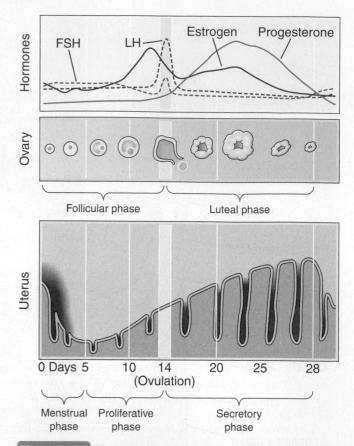

Figure 23-13 **The menstrual cycle.** Changes in hormones, the ovary, and the uterus are shown during a typical 28-day menstrual cycle with ovulation on day 14. (Pituitary hormones are shown with dashed lines, ovarian hormones with solid lines.) **[ZOOMING IN ➤** What hormone peaks closest to ovulation? **]**

gonadotropin-releasing hormone [Gn-RH] from the hypothalamus that promotes the rise in LH.) It is LH that causes ovulation and transforms the ruptured follicle into the corpus luteum, which produces some estrogen and large amounts of **progesterone**. Under the influence of these hormones, the endometrium continues to thicken, and the glands and blood vessels increase in size. The rising levels of estrogen and progesterone feed back to inhibit the release of FSH and LH from the pituitary. During this time, the ovum makes its journey to the uterus by way of the oviduct. If the ovum is not fertilized while passing through the uterine tube, it dies within 2 to 3 days and then disintegrates.

During each menstrual cycle, changes occur in both the ovary and the uterus (see Fig. 23-13). The time before ovulation is described as the follicular phase in the ovary, because it encompasses development of the ovarian follicle. The uterus during this same time is in a proliferative phase, marked by growth of the endometrium. After ovulation, the ovary is in a luteal phase, with conversion of the follicle to the corpus luteum, and the uterus is described as being in a secretory phase, based on activity of the endometrial glands.

CHECKPOINT **23-15** ➤ What are the two hormones produced in the ovaries?

Visit ***thePoint*** or see the Student Resource CD in the back of this book for a summary chart on reproductive hormones and the animation *Ovulation and Fertilization.*

PASSport to **Success**

The Menstrual Phase

If fertilization does not occur, the corpus luteum degenerates, and the levels of estrogen and progesterone decrease. Without the hormones to support growth, the endometrium degenerates. Small hemorrhages appear in this tissue, producing the bloody discharge known as **menstrual flow**, or **menses** (MEN-seze). Bits of endometrium break away and accompany the blood flow during this period of **menstruation** (men-stru-A-shun). The average duration of menstruation is 2 to 6 days.

Even before the menstrual flow ceases, the endometrium begins to repair itself through the growth of new cells. The low levels of estrogen and progesterone allow the release of FSH from the anterior pituitary. FSH causes new follicles to begin to ripen within the ovaries, and the cycle begins anew.

The activity of ovarian hormones as negative feedback messengers is the basis of hormonal methods of contraception (birth control). Estrogen and progesterone inhibit the release of FSH and LH from the pituitary, preventing ovulation. The menstrual period that follows withdrawal of estrogen and progesterone supplementation is anovulatory, that is, it is not preceded by ovulation.

Menopause

Menopause (MEN-o-pawz) is the period during which menstruation ceases altogether. It ordinarily occurs gradually between the ages of 45 and 55 years and is caused by a normal decline in ovarian function. The ovary becomes chiefly scar tissue and no longer produces ripe follicles or appreciable amounts of estrogen. Eventually, the uterus, oviducts, vagina, and vulva all become somewhat atrophied and the vaginal mucosa becomes thinner, dryer, and more sensitive.

Menopause is an entirely normal condition, but its onset sometimes brings about effects that are temporarily disturbing. The decrease in estrogen levels can cause nervous symptoms, such as anxiety and insomnia. Because estrogen also helps maintain the vascular dilation that promotes heat loss, low levels may result in "hot flashes."

Hormone Replacement Therapy

Physicians may prescribe hormone replacement therapy (HRT) to relieve the discomforts associated with menopause. This medication is usually a combination of estrogen with a synthetic progesterone (progestin), which is included to prevent overgrowth of the endometrium and the risk of endometrial cancer. Early assumptions about the role of estrogen in preventing heart attacks have been disproved by carefully controlled studies, at least with regard to the most commonly prescribed form of HRT. The hormone therapy did lower the incidence of colorectal cancer and hip fractures, a sign of osteoporosis. Studies are continuing with estrogen alone, generally prescribed for women who have undergone a hysterectomy and do not have a uterus.

In addition to an increased risk of breast cancer, HRT also carries a risk of thrombosis and embolism, which is highest among women who smoke. All HRT risks increase with the duration of therapy. Therefore, treatment should be given for a short time and at the lowest effective dose. Women with a history or family history of breast cancer or circulatory problems should not take HRT.

CHECKPOINT **23-16** ➤ What is the definition of menopause?

Birth Control

Birth control is most commonly achieved by **contraception**, which is the use of artificial methods to prevent fertilization of the ovum. Birth control measures that prevent implantation of the fertilized ovum are also considered contraceptives, although technically they do not prevent conception and are more accurately called **abortifacients** (ah-bor-tih-FA-shents) (agents that cause abortion). Some of the birth control methods act by both mechanisms. Table 23-1 presents a brief description of the main contraceptive methods currently in use along with some advantages and disadvantages of each. The list is given in rough order of decreasing effectiveness. Unless specifically mentioned as doing so, a given method does *not* prevent the transmission of STIs.

Visit ***thePoint*** or see the Student Resource CD in the back of this book for an illustration of surgical sterilization.

PASSport to **Success**

The various hormonal methods of birth control basically differ in how they administer the hormones. The emergency contraceptive pill (ECP) is a synthetic progesterone (progestin) taken within 72 hours after intercourse, usually in two doses 12 hours apart. It reduces the risk of pregnancy following unprotected intercourse. This so-called "morning after pill" is intended for emergency use and not as a regular birth control method. Birth control hormones can also be implanted as capsules under the skin of the upper arm. This method is highly effective and lasts for 3 to 5 years, but the capsules must be implanted and removed by a health professional, and they have been difficult to remove in some cases.

Researchers have done trials with a male contraceptive pill, but none is on the market as yet. The male version

23

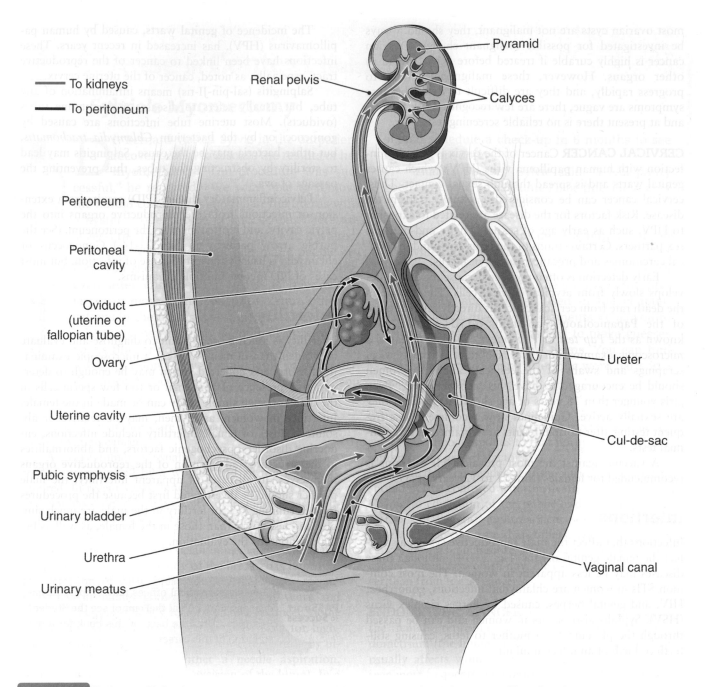

Legend:
- To kidneys
- To peritoneum

Labels (left side):
- Peritoneum
- Peritoneal cavity
- Oviduct (uterine or fallopian tube)
- Ovary
- Uterine cavity
- Pubic symphysis
- Urinary bladder
- Urethra
- Urinary meatus

Labels (right side):
- Pyramid
- Renal pelvis
- Calyces
- Ureter
- Cul-de-sac
- Vaginal canal

Figure 23-14 **Pathway of infection.** Disease organisms can travel from outside to the peritoneum and into the urinary system.

Word Anatomy

Medical terms are built from standardized word parts (prefixes, roots, and suffixes). Learning the meanings of these parts can help you remember words and interpret unfamiliar terms.

WORD PART	MEANING	EXAMPLE
The Male Reproductive System		
semin/o	semen, seed	Sperm cells are produced in the *seminiferous* tubules.
test/o	testis	The hormone *testosterone* is produced in the testis.
acr/o	extremity, end	The *acrosome* covers the head of a sperm cell.
fer	to carry	The ductus *deferens* carries spermatozoa away from (de-) the testis.
circum-	around	A cut is made around the glans to remove part of the foreskin in a *circumcision*.
Disorders of the Male Reproductive System		
oligo/o-	few, deficiency	*Oligospermia* is a deficiency in the numbers of spermatozoa produced.
crypto/o-	hidden	*Cryptorchidism* refers to an undescended testis (orchid/o).
orchid/o, orchi/o	testis	*Orchiectomy* is removal of the testis.
The Female Reproductive System		
ov/o, ov/i	egg	An *ovum* is an egg cell.
ovar, ovari/o	ovary	The *ovarian* follicle encloses a maturing ovum.
metr/o	uterus	The *myometrium* is the muscular (my/o) layer of the uterus.
rect/o	rectum	The *rectouterine* pouch is between the uterus and rectum.
Disorders of the Female Reproductive System		
men/o	uterine bleeding; menses	*Amenorrhea* is absence of menstrual flow.
hyster/o	uterus	*Hysterectomy* is surgical removal of the uterus.
mamm/o	breast, mammary gland	A *mammogram* is radiographic study of the breast.
mast/o	breast	A *mastectomy* is surgical removal of the breast.
salping/o	tube	*Salpingitis* is inflammation of a tube, such as the oviduct.

Summary

I. **REPRODUCTION**
  A. Meiosis—reduces chromosome number from 46 to 23
    1. Gametes (sex cells)
      a. Spermatozoa (sperm cells)—male
      b. Ova (egg cells)—female
II. **MALE REPRODUCTIVE SYSTEM**
  A. Primary organs—gonads
  B. Accessory organs—ducts and exocrine glands

  C. Testes
    1. Scrotum—sac that holds the testes
    2. Inguinal canal—channel through which testis descends
    3. Internal structure
      a. Seminiferous tubules—tubes in which sperm cells are produced
        (1) Sustentacular (Sertoli) cells—aid in development of spermatozoa

23

b. Interstitial cells (between tubules)—secrete hormones

4. Testosterone—main male hormone
   a. Maintains reproductive structures
   b. Aids development of secondary sex characteristics

5. Spermatozoa
   a. Head—contains chromosomes
   b. Acrosome—covers head; has enzymes to help penetration of ovum
   c. Midpiece—contains mitochondria
   d. Tail (flagellum)—propels sperm

D. Accessory organs
   1. Epididymis—stores spermatozoa until ejaculation
   2. Ductus (vas) deferens—conducts sperm cells through spermatic cord
   3. Ejaculatory duct—empties into urethra

E. Semen
   1. Functions
      a. Nourish spermatozoa
      b. Transport spermatozoa
      c. Neutralize male urethra and vaginal tract
      d. Lubricate reproductive tract during intercourse
      e. Prevent infection
   2. Glands
      a. Seminal vesicles
      b. Prostate—around first portion of urethra
      c. Bulbourethral (Cowper) glands

F. Urethra and penis
   1. Urethra
      a. Conveys urine and semen through penis
   2. Penis
      a. Structure
         (1) Corpus spongiosum—central; contains urethra
         (2) Corpora cavernosa—lateral
         (3) Glands—distal enlargement of corpus spongiosum
         (4) Prepuce—foreskin
      b. Erection—stiffening and enlargement of penis
   3. Ejaculation—forceful expulsion of semen

III. **HORMONAL CONTROL OF MALE REPRODUCTION**
A. Pituitary hormones
   1. FSH (follicle stimulating hormone)
      a. Stimulates Sertoli cells
      b. Promotes formation of spermatozoa
   2. LH (luteinizing hormone)
      a. Stimulates interstitial cells to produce testosterone
B. Effects of aging on male reproduction
   1. Decline in testosterone, spermatozoa, and semen

IV. **DISORDERS OF THE MALE REPRODUCTIVE SYSTEM**
A. Infertility—lower than normal ability to reproduce
B. Structural disorders
   1. Cryptorchidism—failure of testis to descend

2. Torsion of the testis—twisting of spermatic cord
3. Inguinal hernia
4. Phimosis—tightness of the foreskin

C. Infections
   1. Sexually transmitted infections (STI)
   2. Epididymitis—inflammation of the epididymis
   3. Prostatitis—inflammation of the prostate
   4. Orchitis—inflammation of the testis

D. Tumors
   1. Tumors of the prostate
      a. Benign prostatic hyperplasia (BPH)
   2. Cancer of the testis

V. **FEMALE REPRODUCTIVE SYSTEM**
A. Ovaries—gonads in which ova form
B. Ova and ovulation
   1. Egg ripens in graafian follicle
   2. Ovulation—release of ovum from ovary
   3. Corpus luteum
      a. Remainder of follicle in ovary
      b. Continues to function if egg fertilized
      c. Disintegrates if egg not fertilized

C. Accessory organs
   1. Oviducts (uterine tubes, fallopian tubes)
      a. Fimbriae—fringelike extensions that sweep egg into oviduct
   2. Uterus
      a. Holds developing fetus
      b. Supported by broad ligament
      c. Endometrium—lining of uterus
      d. Myometrium—muscle layer
      e. Cervix—narrow, lower part
   3. Vagina
      a. Tube connecting uterus to outside
      b. Hymen—fold of membrane over vaginal opening
      c. Greater vestibular (Bartholin) glands—secrete mucus
   4. Vulva and perineum
      a. Vulva—external genitalia
         (1) Labia—two sets of folds (majora, minora)
         (2) Clitoris—organ of great sensitivity
      b. Perineum—pelvic floor
         (1) In obstetrics—area between vagina and anus

VI. **MENSTRUAL CYCLE**
A. Average 28 days
B. Beginning of the cycle
   1. FSH stimulates follicle—follicular phase
   2. Follicle secretes estrogen
   3. Estrogen thickens lining of uterus—proliferative phase
C. Ovulation
   1. LH surge 1 day before
   2. Corpus luteum produces progesterone—luteal phase

3. Progesterone continues growth of endometrium—secretory phase
4. Ovum disintegrates if not fertilized
D. Menstrual phase (menstruation)
  1. If egg not fertilized, corpus luteum degenerates
  2. Lining of uterus breaks down releasing menses
VII. **MENOPAUSE**
A. Period during which menstuation stops
B. Hormone replacement therapy (HRT)
  1. Reduces adverse symptoms of menopause
  2. Risks of HRT—cardiovascular disorders, breast cancer
VIII. **BIRTH CONTROL**
A. Contraception—use of artificial methods to prevent fertilization or implantation of fertilized egg
B. Methods—surgery, hormonal, barrier, IUD, spermicides, fertility awareness
IX. **DISORDERS OF THE FEMALE REPRODUCTIVE SYSTEM**
A. Menstrual disorders
  1. Amenorrhea—absence of menstrual flow
  2. Dysmenorrhea—painful or difficult menstruation

3. Abnormal uterine bleeding
4. Premenstrual syndrome
B. Benign and malignant tumors
  1. Fibroids (myomas)—common tumors of uterus
  2. Breast cancer
    a. Mammogram—radiographic study of the breast
    b. Mastectomy—removal of breast or breast tissue
  3. Endometrial cancer—cancer of uterine lining
  4. Ovarian cancer
  5. Cervical cancer—due to human papilloma virus (HPV) infection
    a. Pap test (smear) for cervical cancer
D. Infections
  1. Sexually transmitted infections
  2. Genital warts—caused by HPV
  3. Salpingitis—inflammation of uterine tubes
  4. Pelvic inflammatory disease (PID)
E. Infertility

Review

BUILDING UNDERSTANDING

Fill in the blanks

1. Gametes go through a special process of cell division called _____.

2. Spermatozoa begin their development in tiny coiled _____.

3. An ovum matures in a small fluid-filled cluster of cells called the _____.

4. Failure of the testis to descend into the scrotum results in the disorder _____.

5. Surgical removal of the uterus is called a(n) _____.

Matching > Match each numbered item with the most closely related lettered item.

___ **6.** A hormone released by the pituitary that promotes follicular development in the ovary

___ **7.** A hormone released by developing follicles that promotes thickening of the endometrium

___ **8.** A hormone released by the pituitary that stimulates ovulation

___ **9.** A hormone released by the corpus luteum that promotes thickening of the endometrium

a. follicle stimulating hormone

b. estrogen

c. luteinizing hormone

d. progesterone

Multiple choice

___ **10.** A month or two before birth, the testis travels from the abdominal cavity to the scrotum through the
   a. spermatic cord
   b. inguinal canal
   c. seminiferous tubule
   d. vas deferens

___ **11.** Enzymes that help the sperm cell to penetrate the ovum are found in the
   a. acrosome
   b. head
   c. midpiece
   d. flagellum

___ **12.** Inflammation of the testis is called
   a. phimosis
   b. epididymitis
   c. prostatitis
   d. orchitis

___ **13.** The uterus and ovaries are supported by the
   a. uterine tubes
   b. broad ligaments
   c. fimbriae
   d. fornix

___ **14.** The area between the vaginal opening and the anus is referred to as the
   a. vestibule
   b. vulva
   c. hymen
   d. perineum

___ **15.** The most common site of cancer in the female reproductive tract is the
   a. endometrium
   b. myometrium
   c. ovaries
   d. cervix

UNDERSTANDING CONCEPTS

16. Compare and contrast the following terms:
   a. asexual reproduction and sexual reproduction
   b. spermatozoa and ova
   c. sustentacular cell and interstitial cell
   d. ovarian follicle and corpus luteum
   e. myometrium and endometrium

17. Trace the pathway of sperm from the site of production to the urethra.

18. Describe the components of semen, their sites of production, and their functions.

19. List the hormones that control male reproduction and state their functions.

20. Trace the pathway of an ovum from the site of production to the site of implantation.

21. Beginning with the first day of the menstrual flow, describe the events of one complete cycle, including the role of the hormones involved.

22. Define *contraception*. Describe methods of contraception that involve (1) barriers; (2) chemicals; (3) hormones; (4) prevention of implantation.

23. Compare and contrast the following disorders:
   a. epididymitis and prostatitis
   b. benign prostatic hyperplasia and prostatic cancer
   c. amenorrhea and dysmenorrhea
   d. fibroids and endometrial cancer
   e. ovarian cancer and cervical cancer

CONCEPTUAL THINKING

24. Theoretically, it is possible for a brain-dead man to ejaculate. What anatomical and physiological feature makes this possible?

25. Nicole, a middle-aged mother of three, is considering a tubal ligation, a contraceptive procedure that involves cutting the uterine tubes. Nicole is worried that this might cause her to enter early menopause. Should she be worried?

26. Sylvie's case involves a myoma. Define a myoma. Identify the two word parts in the term *myoma* and give the meaning of each. Identify and define the word parts in other terms used in the case history and the remainder of the chapter, including fibroid, myomectomy, hysteroscope, and laparoscope.

23

CHAPTER 24

Development and Birth

Learning Outcomes

After careful study of this chapter, you should be able to:

1. Describe fertilization and the early development of the fertilized egg
2. Describe the structure and function of the placenta
3. Describe how fetal circulation differs from adult circulation
4. Briefly describe changes that occur in the fetus and the mother during pregnancy
5. Briefly describe the four stages of labor
6. Compare fraternal and identical twins
7. Cite the advantages of breastfeeding
8. Describe several disorders associated with pregnancy, childbirth, and lactation
9. Show how word parts are used to build words related to development and birth (see Word Anatomy at the end of the chapter)

PASSport to Success

Visit *thePoint* or see the Student Resource CD in the back of this book for definitions and pronunciations of key terms as well as a pretest for this chapter.

Disease in Context

Sue's Third Case: Emma's Arrival

"Your reflexes are fine," said Sue's neurologist. "Have you had any unusual symptoms since your last appointment?"

"No," replied Sue. "I feel really good. My MS hasn't been a problem lately."

"That's excellent," replied the neurologist. "I'll write a refill for your medications—is there anything else for you today?"

"Actually, there is," replied Sue. She told her doctor that she and her husband were thinking about starting a family, but were concerned about the potential negative effects of multiple sclerosis on fetal development. Sue also worried that pregnancy might aggravate the neurological disorder.

"There's no evidence that multiple sclerosis negatively affects pregnancy, labor, or delivery, nor does it pose significant risks to the fetus," replied the neurologist. "Pregnancy doesn't seem to have a negative effect on MS either. In fact, many women with MS find that their symptoms actually lessen during pregnancy, especially in the second and third trimesters. We think this is because a pregnant woman's ovaries produce hormones, like progesterone, that act as natural immunosuppressants, preventing her body from rejecting her fetus. Most women do report an in increase in the frequency and severity of their MS symptoms in the first 6 months postpartum. And as you already know, future flare-ups may cause increased fatigue, and pose physical limitations. It will be important for you and your husband to look ahead and make sure you have the resources and people you can rely on for support."

"When you and your husband feel ready to conceive," the doctor continued, "You'll need to come and see me so we can adjust your medications. Unfortunately, corticosteroids and interferon can cross the placenta and have adverse effects on fetal development. Like any other woman in childbearing years, you should also start taking a folic acid supplement. This has been shown to lower the risk of embryonic neural tube defects like spina bifida."

Sue is relieved that her MS will not impact on her desire to start a family. In this chapter, you will learn about pregnancy, labor, and delivery. Later, we will return to Sue as she prepares to deliver her baby.

Pregnancy

Pregnancy begins with fertilization of an ovum and ends with delivery of the fetus and afterbirth. During this approximately 38-week period of development, known as **gestation** (jes-TA-shun), all fetal tissues differentiate from a single fertilized egg. Along the way, many changes occur in both the mother and the developing infant.

Fertilization and the Start of Pregnancy

When semen is deposited in the vagina, the many spermatozoa immediately wriggle about in all directions, some traveling into the uterus and oviducts (Fig. 24-1). If an egg cell is present in the oviduct, many spermatozoa cluster around it. Using enzymes, they dissolve the coating around the ovum, so that eventually one sperm cell can penetrate its plasma membrane. The nuclei of the sperm and egg then combine. (See Box 24-1, Assisted Reproductive Technology.)

The result of this union is a single cell, called a **zygote** (ZI-gote), with the full human chromosome number of 46. The zygote divides rapidly into two cells and then four

cells and soon forms a ball of cells. During this time, the cell cluster is traveling toward the uterine cavity, pushed along by cilia lining the oviduct and by peristalsis (contractions) of the tube. After reaching the uterus, the little ball of cells burrows into the greatly thickened uterine lining and is soon implanted and completely covered. After **implantation** in the uterus, a group of cells within the dividing cluster becomes an **embryo** (EM-bre-o), the term used for the growing offspring in the early stage of gestation. The other cells within the cluster will differentiate into tissue that will support the developing offspring throughout gestation.

CHECKPOINT 24-1 ➤ What structure is formed by the union of an ovum and a spermatozoon?

The Placenta

For a few days after implantation, the embryo gets nourishment from the endometrium. By the end of the second week, however, the outer cells of the embryonic cluster form villi (projections) that invade the uterine wall and maternal blood channels (venous sinuses). Gradually, tissue in the outer embryonic layer and in the uterine lining

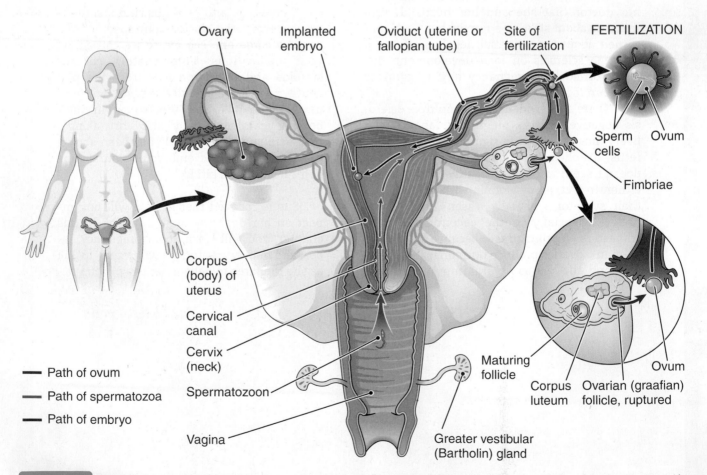

Path of ovum
Path of spermatozoa
Path of embryo

Ovary · Implanted embryo · Oviduct (uterine or fallopian tube) · Site of fertilization · FERTILIZATION · Sperm cells · Ovum · Fimbriae · Corpus (body) of uterus · Cervical canal · Cervix (neck) · Spermatozoon · Vagina · Greater vestibular (Bartholin) gland · Maturing follicle · Corpus luteum · Ovarian (graafian) follicle, ruptured · Ovum

Figure 24-1 **The female reproductive system.** Arrows show the pathway of the spermatozoa and ovum and also of the fertilization and implantation of the fertilized ovum. [**ZOOMING IN ➤** Where is the ovum fertilized?]

Assisted Reproductive Technology: The "Art" of Conception

At least one in ten American couples is affected by infertility. Assisted reproductive technologies such as in vitro fertilization (IVF), gamete intrafallopian transfer (GIFT), and zygote intrafallopian transfer (ZIFT) can help these couples become pregnant.

In vitro fertilization refers to fertilization of an ovum outside the mother's body in a laboratory dish. It is often used when a woman's oviducts are blocked or when a man has a low sperm count. The woman participating in IVF is given hormones to cause ovulation of several ova. These are then withdrawn with a needle and fertilized with the father's sperm. After a few divisions, some of the fertilized ova are placed in the uterus, thus bypassing the oviducts. Additional fertilized ova can be frozen to repeat the procedure in case of failure or for later pregnancies.

GIFT can be used when the woman has at least one normal oviduct and the man has an adequate sperm count. As in

IVF, the woman is given hormones to cause ovulation of several ova, which are collected. Then, the ova and the father's sperm are placed into the oviduct using a catheter. Thus, in GIFT, fertilization occurs inside the woman, not in a laboratory dish.

ZIFT is a combination of both IVF and GIFT. Fertilization takes place in a laboratory dish, and then the zygote is placed into the oviduct.

Because of a lack of guidelines or restrictions in the United States in the field of assisted reproductive technology, some problems have arisen. These issues concern the use of stored embryos and gametes, use of embryos without consent, and improper screening for disease among donors. In addition, the implantation of more than one fertilized ovum has resulted in a high incidence of multiple births, even up to seven or eight offspring in a single pregnancy, a situation that imperils the survival and health of the babies.

together form the **placenta** (plah-SEN-tah), a flat, circular organ that consists of a spongy network of blood-filled channels and capillary-containing villi (Fig. 24-2). (*Placenta* is from a Latin word meaning "pancake.") The placenta is the organ of nutrition, respiration, and excretion for the developing offspring throughout gestation. Although the blood of the mother and her offspring do not mix—each has its own blood and cardiovascular system—exchanges take place through the capillaries of the placental villi. In this manner, gases (CO_2 and O_2) are exchanged, nutrients are provided to the developing infant, and waste products are released into the maternal blood to be eliminated.

THE UMBILICAL CORD The embryo is connected to the developing placenta by a stalk of tissue that eventually becomes the **umbilical** (um-BIL-ih-kal) **cord.** This structure carries blood to and from the embryo, later called the **fetus** (FE-tus). The cord encloses two arteries that carry deoxygenated blood from the fetus to the placenta, and one vein that carries oxygenated blood from the placenta to the fetus (see Fig. 24-2). (Note that, like the pulmonary vessels, these arteries carry blood low in oxygen and this vein carries blood high in oxygen.)

FETAL CIRCULATION The fetus has special circulatory adaptations to carry blood to and from the umbilical cord and to bypass the non-functional lungs. A small amount of the oxygenated blood traveling toward the fetus in the **umbilical vein** is delivered directly to the liver. However, most of the blood is added to the deoxygenated blood in the inferior vena cava through a small vessel, the **ductus venosus.**

Although mixed, this blood still contains enough oxygen to nourish fetal tissues. Once in the right atrium, some of the blood flows directly into the left atrium through a small hole in the atrial septum, the **foramen ovale** (o-VA-le). This blood bypasses the right ventricle and the pulmonary circuit. Blood that does enter the right ventricle is pumped into the pulmonary artery. Although a small amount of this blood goes to the lungs, most of it shunts directly into the systemic circuit through a small vessel, the **ductus arteriosus,** which connects the pulmonary artery to the descending aorta (see Fig. 24-2). Blood returns to the placenta to be oxygenated through the two **umbilical arteries.** See Appendix 7 for a dissection photograph showing fetal circulation.

After birth, when the baby's lungs are functioning, these adaptations begin to close. The foramen ovale gradually seals and the various vessels constrict into fibrous cords, usually within minutes after birth (only the proximal parts of the umbilical arteries persist as arteries to the urinary bladder). Failure to close results in congenital heart defects, as shown in Figure 14-13B and C.

PASSport to Success Visit thePoint or see the Student Resource CD in the back of this book to view the animation *Fetal Circulation.*

PLACENTAL HORMONES In addition to maintaining the fetus, the placenta is an endocrine organ. Beginning soon after implantation, some embryonic cells produce the hormone **human chorionic gonadotropin** (ko-re-ON-ik gon-ah-do-TRO-pin) (**hCG**). This hormone stimulates the

Fetal circulation

Oxygen-rich blood
Oxygen-poor blood
Mixed blood

Venous sinus
Uterine arteriole
Uterine venule
Placental capillaries
Placental villi
Uterine wall
Placenta

Umbilical vein (from placenta)
Liver
Portal vein
Umbilical cord
Umbilical arteries (to placenta)

Aortic arch
Ductus arteriosus
Foramen ovale
Left pulmonary artery
Heart
Ductus venosus
Descending aorta
Inferior vena cava

Figure 24-2 **Fetal circulation and section of placenta.** Colors show relative oxygen content of blood. [**ZOOMING IN** ➤ What is signified by the purple color in this illustration?]

ovarian corpus luteum, prolonging its life-span to 11 or 12 weeks and causing it to secrete increasing amounts of progesterone and estrogen. It is hCG that is used in tests as an indicator of pregnancy.

Progesterone is essential for the maintenance of pregnancy. It promotes endometrial secretion to nourish the embryo, maintains the endometrium, and decreases the uterine muscle's ability to contract, thus preventing the embryo from being expelled from the body. During pregnancy, progesterone also helps prepare the breasts for milk secretion. Estrogen promotes enlargement of the uterus and breasts. By the 11th or 12th week of pregnancy, the corpus luteum is no longer needed; by this time, the placenta itself can secrete adequate amounts of progesterone and estrogen, and the corpus luteum disintegrates. Miscarriages (loss of an embryo or fetus) are most likely to occur during this critical time when hormone secretion is shifting from the corpus luteum to the placenta.

Human placental lactogen (hPL) is a hormone secreted by the placenta during pregnancy, reaching a peak at term, the normal conclusion of pregnancy. hPL stimulates growth of the breasts to prepare the mother for production of milk, or **lactation** (lak-TA-shun). More importantly, it regulates the levels of nutrients in the mother's blood to keep them available for the fetus. This second function leads to an alternate name for this hormone: human chorionic somatomammotropin.

Relaxin is a placental hormone that softens the cervix and relaxes the sacral joints and the pubic symphysis. These changes help to widen the birth canal and aid in delivery.

PASSport to Success — Visit *thePoint* or see the Student Resource CD in the back of this book for a summary chart on placental hormones.

CHECKPOINT 24-2 ➤ What organ nourishes the developing fetus?

CHECKPOINT 24-3 ➤ What is the function of the umbilical cord?

CHECKPOINT 24-4 ➤ Fetal circulation is adapted to bypass what organs?

Development of the Embryo

The developing offspring is referred to as an embryo for the first 8 weeks of life (Fig. 24-3), and the study of growth during this period is called **embryology** (em-bre-OL-o-je). The beginnings of all body systems are established during this time. The heart and the brain are among

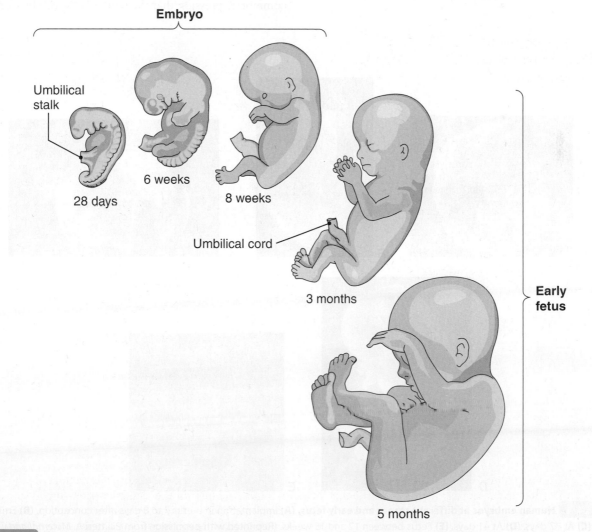

Embryo

Umbilical stalk

28 days

6 weeks

8 weeks

Umbilical cord

3 months

Early fetus

5 months

Figure 24-3 **Development of an embryo and early fetus.**

the first organs to develop. A primitive nervous system begins to form in the third week. The heart and blood vessels originate during the second week, and the first heartbeat appears during week 4, at the same time that other muscles begin to develop.

By the end of the first month, the embryo is approximately 0.62 cm (0.25 inches) long, with four small swellings at the sides called **limb buds**, which will develop into the four extremities. At this time, the heart produces a prominent bulge at the anterior of the embryo.

By the end of the second month, the embryo takes on an appearance that is recognizably human. In male embryos, the primitive testes have formed and have begun to secrete testosterone, which will direct formation of the male reproductive organs as gestation continues. Figure 24-4 shows photographs of embryonic and early fetal development.

CHECKPOINT 24-5 ➤ All body systems originate during the early development of the embryo. At about what time in gestation does the heartbeat first appear?

The Fetus

The term *fetus* is used for the developing offspring from the beginning of the third month until birth. During this period, the organ systems continue to grow and mature. The ovaries form in the female early in this fetal period, and at this stage they contain all the primitive cells (oocytes) that can later develop into mature ova (egg cells).

For study, the entire gestation period may be divided into three equal segments or **trimesters**. The fetus's most rapid growth occurs during the second trimester (months 4 to 6). By the end of the fourth month, the fetus is almost 15 cm (6 inches) long, and its external genitalia are sufficiently developed to reveal its sex. By the seventh month, the fetus is usually approximately 35 cm (14 inches) long and weighs approximately 1.1 kg (2.4 pounds). At the end of pregnancy, the normal length of the fetus is 45 to 56 cm (18 to 22.5 inches), and the weight varies from 2.7 to 4.5 kg (6 to 10 pounds).

The **amniotic** (am-ne-OT-ik) **sac**, which is filled with a clear liquid known as **amniotic fluid**, surrounds the fetus and serves as a protective cushion for it (Fig. 24-5). The amniotic sac ruptures at birth, an event marked by the common expression that the mother's "water broke."

Figure 24-4 **Human embryos at different stages and early fetus. (A)** Implantation in uterus 7 to 8 days after conception. **(B)** Embryo at 32 days. **(C)** At 37 days. **(D)** At 41 days. **(E)** Fetus between 12 and 15 weeks. (Reprinted with permission from Pillitteri A. *Maternal and Child Health Nursing*, 4th ed. Philadelphia: Lippincott Williams & Wilkins, 2003.)

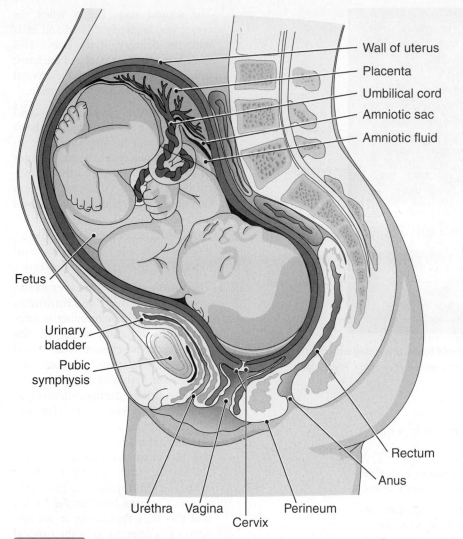

Fetus

Urinary
bladder

Pubic
symphysis

Urethra   Vagina   Perineum
              Cervix

Wall of uterus
Placenta
Umbilical cord
Amniotic sac
Amniotic fluid

Rectum

Anus

Figure 24-5 **Midsagittal section of a pregnant uterus with intact fetus.** [ZOOMING IN ➤ What structure connects the fetus to the placenta?]

- The lungs provide more oxygen by increasing the rate and depth of respiration.

- The kidneys excrete nitrogenous wastes from both the fetus and the mother.

- The digestive system supplies additional nutrients for the growth of maternal organs (uterus and breasts) and fetal growth, as well as for subsequent labor and milk secretion.

Nausea and vomiting are common discomforts in early pregnancy. These most often occur upon arising or during periods of fatigue, and are more common in women who smoke cigarettes. The specific cause of these symptoms is not known, but they may be a result of the great changes in hormone levels that occur at this time. The nausea and vomiting usually last for only a few weeks to several months.

Urinary frequency and constipation are often present during the early stages of pregnancy and then usually disappear. They may reappear late in pregnancy as the head of the fetus drops from the abdominal region down into the pelvis, pressing on the rectum and the urinary bladder.

THE USE OF ULTRASOUND IN OBSTETRICS Ultrasonography (ul-trah-son-OG-rah-fe) is a safe, painless, and noninvasive method for studying soft tissue. It has proved extremely valuable for monitoring pregnancies and deliveries.

An ultrasound image, called a *sonogram*, is made by sending high-frequency sound waves into the body (Fig. 24-6). Each time a wave meets an interface between two tissues of different densities, an echo is produced. An instrument called a *transducer* converts the reflected sound waves into electrical energy, and a computer is used to generate an image on a viewing screen.

Ultrasound scans can be used in obstetrics to diagnose pregnancy, judge fetal age, and determine the location of the placenta. The technique can also show the presence of excess amniotic fluid and fetal abnormalities.

CHECKPOINT **24-7** ➤ What is the approximate duration of pregnancy in days?

During development, the fetal skin is protected by a layer of cheeselike material called the **vernix caseosa** (VER-niks ka-se-O-sah) (literally, "cheesy varnish").

CHECKPOINT **24-6** ➤ What is the name of the fluid-filled sac that holds the fetus?

The Mother

The total period of pregnancy, from fertilization of the ovum to birth, is approximately 266 days, also given as 280 days or 40 weeks from the last menstrual period (LMP). During this time, the mother must supply all the food and oxygen for the fetus and eliminate its waste materials. To support the additional demands of the growing fetus, the mother's metabolism changes markedly, and several organ systems increase their output:

- The heart pumps more blood to supply the needs of the uterus and the fetus.

Childbirth

The exact mechanisms that trigger the beginning of uterine contractions for childbirth are still not completely known.

24

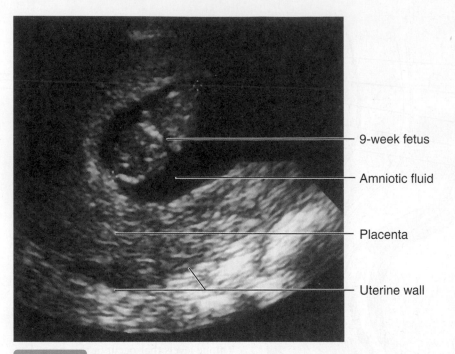

9-week fetus

Amniotic fluid

Placenta

Uterine wall

Figure 24-6 **Sonogram showing a 9-week-old fetus.** (Reprinted with permission from Erkonen WE. *Radiology 101: Basics and Fundamentals of Imaging.* Philadelphia: Lippincott Williams & Wilkins, 1998.)

Some fetal and maternal factors that probably work in combination to start labor are:

- Stretching of the uterine muscle stimulates production of prostaglandin, which promotes uterine contractions.

- Pressure on the cervix from the baby stimulates release of **oxytocin** (ok-se-TO-sin) from the posterior pituitary. The uterine muscle becomes increasingly sensitive to this hormone late in pregnancy.

- Changes in the placenta that occur with time may contribute to the start of labor.

- Cortisol from the fetal adrenal cortex inhibits the mother's progesterone. Increase in the relative amount of estrogen as compared to progesterone stimulates uterine contractions.

After labor begins, stimuli from the cervix and vagina produce reflex secretion of oxytocin, which in turn increases the uterine contractions (an example of positive feedback).

The Four Stages of Labor

The process by which the fetus is expelled from the uterus is known as **labor** and **delivery**; it also may be called **parturition** (par-tu-RISH-un). It is divided into four stages:

1. The **first stage** begins with the onset of regular uterine contractions. With each contraction, the cervix becomes thinner and the opening larger. Rupture of the amniotic sac may occur at any time, with a gush of fluid from the vagina.

2. The **second stage** begins when the cervix is completely dilated and ends with the delivery of the baby. This stage involves the passage of the fetus, usually head first, through the cervical canal and the vagina to the outside.

3. The **third stage** begins after the child is born and ends with the expulsion of the afterbirth. The afterbirth includes the placenta, the membranes of the amniotic sac, and the umbilical cord, except for a small portion remaining attached to the baby's umbilicus (um-BIL-ih-kus), or navel. (Box 24-2, Umbilical Cord Blood, discusses the medical uses of cord blood.)

4. The **fourth stage** begins after expulsion of the afterbirth and constitutes a period in which bleeding is controlled. Contraction of the uterine muscle acts to close off the blood vessels leading to the placental site. To prevent tissues of the pelvic floor from being torn during childbirth, as often happens, the obstetrician may cut the mother's perineum just before her infant is born and then repair this clean cut immediately after childbirth; such an operation is called an **episiotomy** (eh-piz-e-OT-o-me). The area between the vagina and the anus that is cut in an episiotomy is referred to as the surgical or obstetrical perineum (see Fig. 23-12 in Chapter 23).

CHECKPOINT 24-8 ➤ What is parturition?

Cesarean Section

A **cesarean** (se-ZAR-re-an) **section** (C section) is an incision made in the abdominal wall and uterine wall for delivery of a fetus. A cesarean section may be required for a variety of reasons, including placental abnormalities, abnormal fetal position, disproportion between the head of the fetus and the mother's pelvis that makes vaginal delivery difficult or dangerous, and other problems that may arise during pregnancy and delivery.

CHECKPOINT 24-9 ➤ What is a cesarean section?

Multiple Births

Until recently, statistics indicated that twins occurred in about 1 of every 80 to 90 births, varying somewhat in different countries. Triplets occurred much less frequently, usually once in several thousand births, whereas quadru-

Disease in Context revisited

› Sue Experiences the Four Stages of Labor

"Ooh, I think it's time," gasped Sue as another wave of uterine contractions began.

"I'll call Dr. Philips and let her know we're on our way," replied Sue's husband, and went to get Sue's overnight bag.

"Hurry, Shawn! I think my water just broke!"

Dr. Philips examined Sue in the labor and delivery room. Sue's cervix was dilating, signaling that she was in the first stage of labor. At Sue's request, the anesthetist gave her an epidural block to help control pain. He inserted a needle between Sue's lumbar vertebrae into the epidural space. Through the needle, he threaded a catheter, which would remain in Sue's back for her entire labor. He removed the needle and administered the pain medication via the catheter.

About an hour later, Sue's labor progressed into the second stage. Her cervix was completely dilated and she was encouraged to push with each contraction. After the baby's head was de-

livered, the obstetrician cleared its airway and checked to make sure that the umbilical cord was free. Shortly after, Sue gave a final push and her baby girl, Emma, was born. The nurse wrapped her in a warm blanket and placed her on Sue's chest. While Sue and Shawn admired their new daughter, Dr. Philips delivered Sue's placenta. This marked the end of the third stage of labor. A couple of hours later, Sue and Emma were in their hospital room resting comfortably. As Sue breastfed Emma, her uterus contracted and began to shrink to its original size. Although Sue was too enamored with her baby daughter to notice, she had just completed the fourth stage of labor.

In this case, Sue learned that multiple sclerosis would not affect her ability to have a baby. Following a normal pregnancy, she successfully delivered a healthy baby girl. To review some of the reproductive anatomy discussed in this case, see Chapter 23.

Box 24-2   Hot Topics

Umbilical Cord Blood: Giving Life After Birth

Following childbirth, the umbilical cord and placenta are usually discarded. However, research suggests that blood harvested from these structures could save lives. Like bone marrow, umbilical cord blood contains stem cells capable of differentiating into all blood cell types. Cancer patients whose bone marrow is destroyed by chemotherapy often require stem cell transplants, as do those with leukemia, anemia, or certain immune disorders.

Stem cells obtained from umbilical cord blood offer some important advantages over those acquired from bone marrow. These advantages include:

■ Greater ease of collection and storage. Whereas bone marrow collection is a surgical procedure, cord blood can be collected immediately after the umbilical cord is cut. The blood can then be stored frozen in a blood bank.

■ No risk to the donor. Because cord blood is collected after the cord is cut, the procedure is not dangerous to the donor.

■ Lower risk to the recipient. Since cord blood is immature, it does not have to match the recipient's tissues as closely as bone marrow does, so there is less chance of transplant rejection and graft-versus-host disease than with bone marrow. In addition, umbilical cord blood is less likely to contain infectious organisms than is bone marrow.

■ Higher chance of finding a donor. Since umbilical cord blood need not closely match a recipient's tissues, the likelihood of finding a match between donor and recipient is higher.

Although umbilical cord blood is a promising stem cell source, only enough cells to treat a child or small adult can be harvested from a single donor. Scientists hope that improved collection techniques and advances in cell culture will increase the number of stem cells available from a single donor, enabling all patients in need to benefit from this treatment.

24

plets occurred very rarely. The birth of quintuplets represented a historic event unless the mother had taken fertility drugs. Now these fertility drugs, usually gonadotropins, are given more commonly, and the number of multiple births has increased significantly. Multiple fetuses tend to be born prematurely and therefore have a high death rate. However, better care of infants and newer treatments have resulted in more living multiple births than ever.

Twins originate in two different ways, and on this basis are divided into two types:

- **Fraternal twins** result from the fertilization of two different ova by two spermatozoa. Two completely different individuals, as distinct from each other as brothers and sisters of different ages, are produced. Each fetus has its own placenta and surrounding sac.

- **Identical twins** develop from a single zygote formed from a single ovum fertilized by a single spermatozoon. Sometime during the early stages of development, the embryonic cells separate into two units. Usually, there is a single placenta, although there must be a separate umbilical cord for each fetus. Identical twins are always the same sex and carry the same inherited traits.

Other multiple births may be fraternal, identical, or combinations of these. The tendency to multiple births seems to be hereditary.

Termination of Pregnancy

A pregnancy may end before its full term has been completed. The term **live birth** is used if the baby breathes or shows any evidence of life such as heartbeat, pulsation of the umbilical cord, or movement of voluntary muscles. An **immature** or **premature** infant is one born before the organ systems are mature. Infants born before the 37th week of gestation or weighing less than 2,500 grams (5.5 pounds) are considered **preterm**.

Loss of the fetus is classified according to the duration of the pregnancy:

- The term **abortion** refers to loss of the embryo or fetus before the 20th week or weight of about 500 grams (1.1 pound). This loss can be either spontaneous or induced.

  > **Spontaneous abortion** occurs naturally with no interference. The most common causes are related to an abnormality of the embryo or fetus. Other causes include abnormality of the mother's reproductive organs, infections, or chronic disorders, such as kidney disease or hypertension. **Miscarriage** is the lay term for spontaneous abortion.

  > **Induced abortion** occurs as a result of artificial or mechanical interruption of pregnancy. A **therapeutic abortion** is an abortion performed by a physician as a treatment for a variety of reasons. More liberal access to this type of abortion has dramatically reduced the incidence of death related to illegal abortion.

- The term **fetal death** refers to loss of the fetus after the eighth week of pregnancy. **Stillbirth** refers to the delivery of an infant who is lifeless.

Immaturity is a leading cause of death in the newborn. After the 20th week of pregnancy, the fetus is considered **viable**, that is, able to live outside the uterus. A fetus expelled before the 24th week or before reaching a weight of 1,000 grams (2.2 pounds) has little more than a 50% chance of survival; one born at a point closer to the full 40 weeks stands a much better chance of living. However, increasing numbers of immature infants are being saved because of advances in neonatal intensive care.

Hospitals use the Apgar score to assess a newborn's health and predict survival. Five features are rated as 0, 1, or 2 at 1 minute and 5 minutes after delivery. The maximum possible score on each test is 10. Infants with low scores require medical attention and have lower survival rates.

PASSport to Success Visit **thePoint** or see the Student Resource CD in the back of this book for the Apgar scoring system.

CHECKPOINT 24-10 ➤ What does the term *viable* mean with reference to a fetus?

The Mammary Glands and Lactation

The **mammary glands**, or breasts, of the female are accessories of the reproductive system. They provide nourishment for the baby after its birth. The mammary glands are similar in construction to the sweat glands. Each gland is divided into a number of lobes composed of glandular tissue and fat, and each lobe is further subdivided. Secretions from the lobes are conveyed through **lactiferous** (lak-TIF-er-us) **ducts**, all of which converge at the papilla (nipple) (Fig. 24-7).

The mammary glands begin developing during puberty, but they do not become functional until the end of a pregnancy. Placental lactogen (hPL) helps to prepare the breasts for lactation, and the hormone **prolactin** (PRL), produced by the anterior pituitary gland, stimulates the mammary glands' secretory cells. The first mammary gland secretion is a thin liquid called **colostrum** (ko-LOS-trum). It is nutritious but has a somewhat different composition from milk. Milk secretion begins within a few days following birth and can continue for several years as long as milk is frequently removed by the suckling baby or by pumping. Stimulation of the breast by the suckling infant causes oxytocin release from the posterior pituitary. This hormone causes the milk ducts to contract, resulting in the ejection, or *letdown*, of milk.

The newborn baby's digestive tract is not ready for the usual adult mixed diet. Mother's milk is more desirable for the young infant than milk from other animals for several reasons, some of which are listed below:

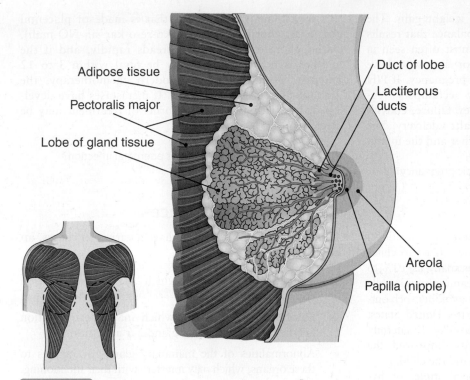

Figure 24-7 **Section of the breast (mammary gland).** [**ZOOMING IN** ➤ What muscle underlies the breast?]

- Infections that may be transmitted by foods exposed to the outside air are avoided by nursing.

- Both breast milk and colostrum contain maternal antibodies that help protect the baby against pathogens.

- The proportions of various nutrients and other substances in human milk are perfectly suited to the human infant. Substitutes are not exact imitations of human milk. Nutrients are present in more desirable amounts if the mother's diet is well balanced.

- The psychological and emotional benefits of nursing are of infinite value to both the mother and the infant.

CHECKPOINT 24-11 ➤ What is lactation?

Disorders of Pregnancy, Childbirth, and Lactation

A pregnancy that develops in a location outside the uterine cavity is said to be an **ectopic** (ek-TOP-ik) **pregnancy** (Fig. 24-8). The most common type is the tubal ectopic pregnancy, in which the embryo begins to grow in the oviduct. This structure cannot expand to contain the growing embryo and may rupture. Ectopic pregnancy may threaten the mother's life if it does not receive prompt surgical treatment.

In **placenta previa** (PRE-ve-ah) the placenta, which is usually attached to the superior part of the uterus, instead becomes attached at or near the internal opening of the cervix. The normal cervical softening and dilation that occur in later pregnancy separate part of the placenta from

its attachment. The result is painless bleeding and interference with the fetal oxygen supply.

Sometimes the placenta separates from the uterine wall prematurely, often after the 20th week of pregnancy, causing hemorrhage. This disorder, known as **abruptio placentae** (ab-RUP-she-o plah-SEN-te), or *placental abruption*, occurs most often in multigravidas (mul-te-GRAV-ih-dahz), meaning women who have had more than one pregnancy or are older than 35 years of age. Placental abruption is a common cause of bleeding during the second half of pregnancy and may require termination of pregnancy to save the mother's life.

Pregnancy-Induced Hypertension

A serious disorder that can develop in the latter part of pregnancy is **pregnancy-induced hypertension** (**PIH**), also called *preeclampsia* (pre-eh-KLAMP-se-ah) or *toxemia of pregnancy*. Signs include hypertension, protein in the urine (pro-

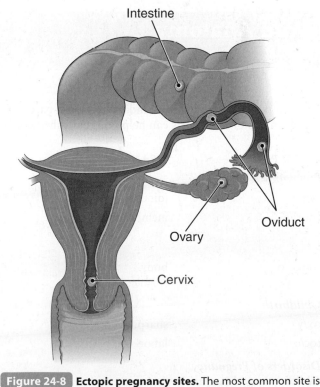

Figure 24-8 **Ectopic pregnancy sites.** The most common site is the oviduct, in which case it is a tubal ectopic pregnancy. (Reprinted with permission from Cohen BJ. *Medical Terminology*, 5th ed. Philadelphia: Lippincott Williams & Wilkins, 2008.)

24

teinuria), general edema, and sudden weight gain. The cause of this disorder is a hormone imbalance that results in constriction of blood vessels. It is most often seen in women whose nutritional state is poor and who have received little or no health care during pregnancy. If PIH remains untreated, it may lead to **eclampsia** (eh-KLAMP-se-ah) with the onset of kidney failure, convulsions, and coma during pregnancy or after delivery. The result may be the death of both the mother and the infant.

CHECKPOINT 24-12 ➤ What is an ectopic pregnancy?

Postpartum Disorders

Childbirth-related deaths are often due to infections. **Puerperal** (pu-ER-per-al) **infections**, those related to childbirth, were once the cause of death in as many as 10% to 12% of women going through labor. Cleanliness and sterile techniques have improved the chances of avoiding such outcomes of pregnancies. Nevertheless, in the United States, puerperal infection still develops in about 6% of maternity patients. Antibiotics have dramatically improved the chances of recovery for both the mother and the child.

A **hydatidiform** (hi-dah-TID-ih-form) **mole**, or hydatid mole, is a benign overgrowth of placental tissue. The placenta dilates and resembles grapelike cysts. The growth may invade the uterine wall, causing it to rupture.

A very malignant tumor that is made of placental tissue is **choriocarcinoma** (ko-re-o-kar-sih-NO-mah). Although rare, this tumor spreads rapidly, and if the mother is not treated, it may be fatal within 3 to 12 months. With the use of modern chemotherapy, the outlook for cure is very good. If metastases have developed, irradiation and other forms of treatment may be necessary.

CHECKPOINT 24-13 ➤ What is puerperal infection?

Lactation Disturbances

Disturbances in lactation may have a variety of causes, including the following:

- Malnutrition or anemia, which may prevent lactation entirely.
- Emotional disturbances, which may affect lactation (as they may affect other glandular activities).
- Abnormalities of the mammary glands or injuries to these organs, which may interfere with their functioning.
- **Mastitis** (mas-TI-tis), or "inflammation of the breast," which is caused by infection. Antibiotic treatment usually allows for the continuation of nursing.

Word Anatomy

Medical terms are built from standardized word parts (prefixes, roots, and suffixes). Learning the meanings of these parts can help you remember words and interpret unfamiliar terms.

WORD PART	MEANING	EXAMPLE
Pregnancy		
zyg/o	joined	An ovum and spermatozoon join to form a *zygote*.
chori/o	membrane, chorion	Human *chorionic* gonadotropin is produced by the outermost cells (chorion) of the embryo and acts on the corpus luteum in the ovary.
somat/o	body	Human chorionic *somatomammotropin* controls nutrients for the body and acts on the mammary glands (mamm/o).
Childbirth		
ox/y	sharp, acute	*Oxytocin* is a hormone that stimulates labor.
toc/o	labor	See preceding example.
Disorders of Pregnancy, Childbirth, and Lactation		
ecto-	outside, external	An *ectopic* pregnancy occurs outside of the uterine cavity.

Summary

I. **PREGNANCY (GESTATION)—LASTS ABOUT 38 WEEKS**
   A. Fertilization and the start of pregnancy
      1. Fertilization occurs in oviduct
      2. Zygote (fertilized egg)—formed by fusion of egg and sperm nuclei
         a. Divides rapidly
         b. Travels to uterus
         c. Implants in lining and becomes embryo
   B. The placenta
      1. Formed by tissue around embryo and in lining of uterus
      2. Functions
         a. Nourishment
         b. Gas exchange
         c. Removal of waste
         d. Production of hormones
      3. Umbilical cord—connects fetus to placenta
         a. Umbilical vein—carries blood high in oxygen
         b. Umbilical arteries (2)—carry blood low in oxygen
      4. Fetal circulation—bypasses lungs
         a. Ductus venosus—carries blood from umbilical vein to inferior vena cava
         b. Foramen ovale—hole in atrial septum that allows blood to flow from right to left atrium
         c. Ductus arteriosus—connects pulmonary artery to descending aorta
      5. Placental hormones
         a. Human chorionic gonadotropin (hCG)—maintains corpus luteum for 11 to 12 weeks
         b. Progesterone—maintains endometrium; limits uterine contractions; prepares breasts for lactation
         c. Estrogen—enlarges uterus and breasts
         d. Human placental lactogen (hPL)—stimulates lactation; regulates nutrients
         e. Relaxin—relaxes birth canal
   C. Development of the embryo
      1. First 8 weeks
      2. All body systems begin to develop
   D. The fetus
      1. Third month to birth
      2. Amniotic sac
         a. Surrounds fetus
         b. Contains fluid to cushion and protect fetus
   E. The mother
      1. Increased demands on heart, lungs, kidneys
      2. Increased nutritional needs
      3. Ultrasound used to monitor pregnancy and delivery

II. **CHILDBIRTH**
   A. Initiated by changes in uterus, placenta, fetus
   B. Four stages of labor
      1. Contractions
      2. Delivery of baby
      3. Expulsion of afterbirth
      4. Contraction of uterus
   C. Cesarean section
      1. Incision to remove fetus
   D. Multiple births
      1. Fraternal twins formed from two different ova
      2. Identical twins develop from a single zygote
      3. Larger multiples follow either pattern or a combination
      4. Increased by fertility drugs
   E. Termination of pregnancy
      1. Immature (premature) infant—born before organ systems mature
      2. Preterm—born before 37th week or weighing less than 2,500 grams
      3. Abortion—loss of fetus before 20th week or weighing less than 500 grams; spontaneous or induced
      4. Fetal death—loss of fetus after 8 weeks of pregnancy

III. **MAMMARY GLANDS AND LACTATION**
   A. Lactation—secretion of milk
      1. Colostrum—first mammary secretion
   B. Hormones
      1. hPL—prepares breasts for lactation
      2. Prolactin—stimulates secretory cells
      3. Oxytocin—promotes letdown (ejection) of milk
   C. Advantages of breastfeeding
      1. Reduces infections
      2. Transfers antibodies
      3. Provides best form of nutrition
      4. Emotional satisfaction

IV. **DISORDERS OF PREGNANCY, CHILDBIRTH, AND LACTATION**
   A. Pregnancy disorders
      1. Ectopic pregnancy—pregnancy outside of uterus, commonly in oviduct
      2. Placenta previa—improper attachment of placenta to uterus
      3. Placental abruption—separation of placenta from uterus
      4. Pregnancy-induced hypertension (PIH)
         a. Also called preeclampsia, toxemia of pregnancy
         b. Eclampsia—results from untreated PIH

24

B. Postpartum disorders
1. Puerperal infection
2. Hydatidiform mole—benign overgrowth of placenta
3. Choriocarcinoma—malignant tumor of placental tissue

C. Lactation disturbances
1. Possible causes
    a. Malnutrition
    b. Emotional disturbances
    c. Abnormalities of mammary glands
    d. Mastitis—inflammation of the breast

Questions for Study and Review

BUILDING UNDERSTANDING

Fill in the blanks

1. Fetal skin is protected by a cheeselike material called_____.

2. The first mammary secretion is called _____.

3. Sound waves can be used to safely monitor pregnancy with a technique called _____.

4. A pregnancy that develops in a location outside the uterine cavity is said to be a(n) _____ pregnancy.

5. Inflammation of the breast as a result of infection is named_____.

Matching > Match each numbered item with the most closely related lettered item.

___ 6. A placental hormone that stimulates the ovaries to secrete progesterone and estrogen

___ 7. A placental hormone that regulates maternal blood nutrient levels

___ 8. A placental hormone that softens the cervix, which widens the birth canal

___ 9. A pituitary hormone that stimulates uterine contractions

___ 10. A pituitary hormone that stimulates maternal milk production

a. human placental lactogen

b. prolactin

c. oxytocin

d. relaxin

e. human chorionic gonadotropin

Multiple choice

___ 11. For a few days after implantation, the embryo is nourished by the
    a. endometrium
    b. placenta
    c. yolk sac
    d. umbilical cord

___ 12. By what month can the sex of the fetus be accurately determined?
    a. second
    b. third
    c. fourth
    d. fifth

___ 13. The total period of pregnancy, from fertilization to birth, is about
    a. 37 weeks
    b. 38 weeks
    c. 39 weeks
    d. 40 weeks

___ 14. With regard to identical twins, which of the following statements is incorrect?
    a. they develop from a single zygote
    b. they each have their own placenta
    c. they are always the same sex
    d. they carry the same inherited traits

___ 15. The earliest that a fetus could survive outside of the uterus is after the
    a. 20th week
    b. 24th week
    c. 28th week
    d. 30th week

UNDERSTANDING CONCEPTS

16. Distinguish among the following: zygote, embryo, and fetus.
17. Explain the role of the placenta in fetal development.
18. Is blood in the umbilical arteries relatively high or low in oxygen? In the umbilical vein?
19. Describe some of the changes that take place in the mother's body during pregnancy.
20. What is the major event of each of the four stages of parturition?
21. List several reasons why breast milk is best for baby.

22. What is a cesarean section? List several reasons why it may be required.
23. Compare and contrast the following disease-related terms:
    a. fetal death and still birth
    b. spontaneous abortion and induced abortion
    c. placenta previa and abruptio placentae
    d. pregnancy-induced hypertension and eclampsia
    e. hydatidiform mole and choriocarcinoma

CONCEPTUAL THINKING

24. Why is the risk of miscarriage highest at week 12 of pregnancy?
25. Although it is strongly suggested that a woman not drink alcohol during her entire pregnancy, why is this advice particularly important during the first trimester?

26. In Sue's case, breast feeding helped Sue complete the fourth stage of labor. Explain the physiological mechanism responsible for this.

24

CHAPTER 25

Heredity and Hereditary Diseases

Learning Outcomes

After careful study of this chapter, you should be able to:

1. Briefly describe the mechanism of gene function
2. Explain the difference between dominant and recessive genes
3. Compare *phenotype* and *genotype* and give examples of each
4. Describe what is meant by a *carrier* of a genetic trait
5. Define *meiosis* and explain its function in reproduction
6. Explain how sex is determined in humans
7. Describe what is meant by the term *sex-linked* and list several sex-linked traits
8. List several factors that may influence the expression of a gene
9. Define *mutation*
10. Differentiate among congenital, genetic, and hereditary disorders and give several examples of each
11. List several factors that may cause genetic disorders
12. Define *karyotype* and explain how karyotypes are used in genetic counseling
13. Briefly describe several methods used to treat genetic disorders
14. Show how word parts are used to build words related to heredity (see Word Anatomy at the end of the chapter)

Selected Key Terms

The following terms and other boldface terms in the chapter are defined in the Glossary

allele
amniocentesis
autosome
carrier
chromosome
congenital
dominant
gene
genetic
genotype
heredity
heterozygous
homozygous
karyotype
meiosis
mutagen
mutation
pedigree
phenotype
progeny
recessive
sex-linked
trait

Disease in Context

▶ Ben's Second Case: The Genetics of Cystic Fibrosis

When 2-year-old Ben was diagnosed with cystic fibrosis (CF), his parents, Alison and David, were shocked to discover that he had inherited the genetic disease from them. At first, their attention was focused only on Ben and the treatment he would need. Later, they also began to wonder how they had given him the disease and whether or not other children they might have would be at risk. So they made an appointment with a genetic counselor.

Ms. Clarkson explained, "All of a person's traits are inherited from his or her parents in the form of genes, discrete units of DNA carried on chromosomes in the egg and sperm cells. CF is caused by a change, or mutation, in a gene located on chromosome number 7. This gene codes for a chloride ion channel that is important in manufacturing sweat, digestive fluids, and mucus." "But how come Ben has cystic fibrosis, and he inherited it from us, but we don't have any signs of the disease?" Alison asked, perplexed.

"Well," Ms. Clarkson continued, "a genetic disease can arise from a spontaneous mutation, but more likely, you and David are carriers of the CF gene."

"Meaning...?" said David.

"Meaning," replied the counselor, "that all genetic traits are determined by pairs of genes, called alleles. If even one of these alleles is a so-called dominant gene, it will always be expressed. A person with a dominant disease gene will show the disease and you know it's there. However, most genetic diseases, including CF, are caused by recessive genes. These can be masked by a dominant allele, so you need two copies of the gene to show the disease. You and Alison are disease free, but you each carry one CF gene that was passed on to Ben."

"Does this mean all of our children will be sick with CF?" Alison wondered. "Should we stop here with our family?"

"Not necessarily" answered Ms. Clarkson. "We could do a family study to look for evidence of CF in your relatives, and there is a lab test done on blood or saliva to identify carriers, but we can assume at this point that both you and David carry the CF gene. That said, there's a one in four chance that any of your children will have CF. The 25% risk is constant with each birth, whether you've had a child with CF or not. There is a prenatal test that can identify CF in a fetus, and you can choose to make family decisions based on those results. But that's a subject for future discussions. Right now, you have to concentrate on Ben and his care."

In this chapter, we will learn more about heredity and hereditary diseases. Later, we'll see what treatment options are available for Ben.

We are often struck by the resemblance of a baby to one or both of its parents, yet rarely do we stop to consider *how* various traits are transmitted from parents to offspring. This subject—heredity—has fascinated humans for thousands of years. The *Old Testament* contains numerous references to heredity (although, of course, the word was unknown in biblical times). It was not until the 19th century, however, that methodical investigation into heredity was begun. At that time, an Austrian monk, Gregor Mendel, discovered through his experiments with garden peas that there was a precise pattern in the appearance of differences among parents and their **progeny** (PROJ-eh-ne), their offspring or descendents. Mendel's most important contribution to the understanding of heredity was the demonstration that there are independent units of heredity in the cells. Later, these independent units were given the name **genes**.

Genes and Chromosomes

Genes are actually segments of DNA (deoxyribonucleic acid) contained in the threadlike chromosomes within the nucleus of each cell. Genes govern the cell by controlling the manufacture of proteins, especially enzymes, which are necessary for all the chemical reactions that occur within the cell. Other proteins regulated by genes are those used for structural materials, hormones, and growth factors.

When body cells divide by the process of mitosis, the DNA that makes up the chromosomes is replicated and distributed to the daughter cells, so that each daughter cell gets exactly the same kind and number of chromosomes as were in the original cell. Each chromosome (aside from the Y chromosome, which determines male sex) may carry thousands of genes, and each gene carries the code for a specific trait (characteristic). These traits constitute the physical, biochemical, and physiologic make-up of every cell in the body. (See Box 25-1 to learn about the Human Genome Project.)

In humans, every cell except the gametes (sex cells) contains 46 chromosomes. The chromosomes exist in pairs. One member of each pair was received at the time of fertilization from the offspring's father, and one was received from the mother. The paired chromosomes, except for the pair that determines sex, are alike in size and appearance. Thus, each body cell has one pair of sex chromosomes and 22 pairs (44 chromosomes) that are not involved in sex determination and are known as **autosomes** (AW-to-somes).

The paired autosomes carry genes for the same traits at exactly the same sites on each. Any form of a gene that appears at a specific site on a chromosome is called an **allele** (al-LELE). In humans and other organisms with two sets of chromosomes (diploid organisms), the alleles for each trait exist in pairs.

CHECKPOINT 25-1 ➤ What is a gene? What is a gene made of?

Dominant and Recessive Genes

Another of Mendel's discoveries was that genes can be either dominant or recessive. A **dominant** gene is one that expresses its effect in the cell regardless of whether its allele on the matching chromosome is the same as or different from the dominant gene. The gene need be received

---

Box 25-1 Hot Topics

The Human Genome Project: Reading the Book of Life

Packed tightly in nearly every one of your body cells (except the red blood cells) is a complete copy of your genome—the genetic instructions that direct all of your cellular activities. Written in the language of DNA, these instructions consist of genes parceled into 46 chromosomes that code for proteins. In 1990, a consortium of scientists from around the world set out to crack the genetic code and read the human genome, our "book of life." This monumental task, called the Human Genome Project, was completed in 2003 and succeeded in mapping the entire human genome—3 billion DNA base pairs arranged into about 30,000 genes. Now, scientists can pinpoint the exact location and chemical code of every gene in the body.

The human genome was decoded using a technique called sequencing. Samples of human DNA were fragmented into smaller pieces and then inserted into bacteria. As the bacteria multiplied, they produced more and more copies of the human DNA fragments, which the scientists extracted. The DNA copies were loaded into a sequencing machine capable of "reading" the string of DNA nucleotides that composed each fragment. Then, using computers, the scientists put all of the sequences from the fragments back together to get the entire human genome.

Now, scientists hope to use all these pages of the book of life to revolutionize the treatment of human disease. The information obtained from the Human Genome Project may lead to improved disease diagnosis, new drug treatments, and even gene therapy.

from only one parent to be expressed in the offspring. When the matching genes for a trait are different, the alleles are described as **heterozygous** (het-er-o-ZI-gus), or hybrid.

The effect of a **recessive** gene is not evident unless its paired allele on the matching chromosome is also recessive. Thus, a recessive trait appears only if the recessive genes for that trait are received from both parents. For example, the gene for brown eyes is dominant over the gene for blue eyes, which is recessive. Blue eyes appear in the offspring only if genes for blue eyes are received from both parents. When both the genes for a trait are the same, that is, both dominant or both recessive, the alleles are said to be **homozygous** (ho-mo-ZI-gus), or purebred. A recessive trait only appears if a person's genes are homozygous for that trait.

Any characteristic that can be observed or can be tested for is part of a person's **phenotype** (FE-no-tipe). Eye color, for example, can be seen when looking at a person. Blood type is not visible but can be determined by testing and is also a part of a person's phenotype. When someone has the recessive phenotype, his or her genetic make-up, or **genotype** (JEN-o-tipe), is obviously homozygous recessive. When a dominant phenotype appears, the person's genotype can be either homozygous dominant or heterozygous. Only genetic studies or family studies can reveal which it is.

A recessive gene is not expressed if it is present in the cell together with a dominant allele. However, the recessive gene can be passed on to offspring and may thus appear in future generations. An individual who shows no evidence of a trait but has a recessive gene for that trait is described as a **carrier** of the gene. Using genetic terminology, that person shows the dominant phenotype but has a heterozygous genotype for that trait.

CHECKPOINT 25-2 ➤ What is the difference between a dominant and a recessive gene?

Distribution of Chromosomes to Offspring

The reproductive cells (ova and spermatozoa) are produced by a special process of cell division called **meiosis** (mi-O-sis). This process divides the chromosome number in half, so that each reproductive cell has 23 chromosomes. Moreover, the division occurs in such a way that each cell receives one member of each chromosome pair that was present in the original cell. The separation occurs at random, meaning that either member of the original pair may be included in a given germ cell. Thus, the maternal and paternal sets of chromosomes get mixed up and redistributed at this time, leading to increased variety within the population. Children in a family resemble each other, but no two look exactly alike (unless they are identical twins), because they receive different combinations of maternal and paternal chromosomes.

Geneticists use a grid called a **Punnett square** to show all the combinations of genes that can result from a given

parental cross (Fig. 25-1). In these calculations, a capital letter is used for the dominant gene and the recessive gene is represented by the lower case of the same letter. For example, if *B* is the gene for the dominant trait brown eyes, then *b* would be the recessive gene for blue eyes. In the offspring, the genotype BB is homozygous dominant and the genotype Bb is heterozygous, both of which will show the dominant phenotype brown eyes. The homozygous recessive genotype bb will show the recessive phenotype blue eyes.

A Punnett square shows all the possible gene combinations of a given cross and the theoretical ratios of all the genotypes produced. Actual ratios may differ if the number of offspring is small. For example, the chances of having a male or female baby are 50-50 with each birth, but a family might have several girls before having a boy, and vice versa. The chances of seeing the theoretical ratios improve as the number of offspring increases.

CHECKPOINT 25-3 ➤ What is the process of cell division that forms the gametes?

> **PASSport to Success**
> Visit *thePoint* or see the Student Resource CD in the back of this book for a diagram of meiosis in male and female gamete formation.

Sex Determination

The two chromosomes that determine the offspring's sex, unlike the autosomes (the other 22 pairs of chromosomes), are not matched in size and appearance. The female X chromosome is larger than most other chromosomes and carries genes for other characteristics in addition to that

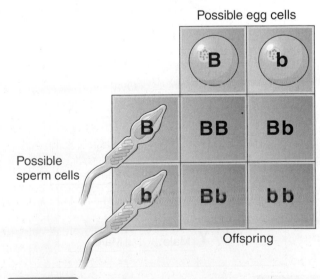

Possible egg cells

Possible sperm cells

Offspring

Figure 25-1 **A Punnett square.** Geneticists use this grid to show all the possible combinations of a given cross, in this case, Bb ×Bb. [**ZOOMING IN** ➤ What percentage of children will show the recessive phenotype blond hair?]

25

for sex. The male Y chromosome is smaller than other chromosomes and mainly determines sex. A female has two X chromosomes in each body cell; a male has one X and one Y.

By the process of meiosis, each male sperm cell receives either an X or a Y chromosome, whereas every egg cell receives only an X chromosome (Fig. 25-2). If a sperm cell with an X chromosome fertilizes an ovum, the resulting infant will be female; if a sperm with a Y chromosome fertilizes an ovum, the resulting infant will be male (see Fig. 25-2).

Sex-Linked Traits

Any trait that is carried on a sex chromosome is said to be **sex-linked**. Because the Y chromosome carries few traits aside from sex determination, most sex-linked traits are carried on the X chromosome and are best described as *X-linked*. Examples are hemophilia, certain forms of baldness, and red-green color blindness.

Sex-linked traits appear almost exclusively in males. The reason for this is that most of these traits are recessive, and if a recessive gene is located on the X chromosome in a male it cannot be masked by a matching dominant gene. (Remember that the Y chromosome with which the X chromosome pairs is very small and carries few genes.) Thus, a male who has only one recessive gene for a trait will exhibit that characteristic, whereas a female must have two recessive genes to show the trait. The female must inherit a recessive gene for that trait from each parent and be homozygous recessive in order for the trait to appear.

CHECKPOINT 25-4 ➤ What sex chromosome combination determines a female? A male?

CHECKPOINT 25-5 ➤ What term is used to describe a trait carried on a sex chromosome?

Hereditary Traits

Some observable hereditary traits are skin, eye, and hair color and facial features. Also influenced by genetics are less clearly defined traits, such as weight, body build, life span, and susceptibility to disease.

Some human traits, including the traits involved in many genetic diseases, are determined by a single pair of genes; most, however, are the result of two or more gene pairs acting together in what is termed **multifactorial inheritance**. This type of inheritance accounts for the wide range of variations within populations in such characteristics as coloration, height, and weight, all of which are determined by more than one pair of genes.

Gene Expression

The effect of a gene on a person's phenotype may be influenced by a variety of factors, including the individual's sex and the presence of other genes. For example, the genes for certain types of baldness and certain types of color blindness may be inherited by either males or females, but the traits appear mostly in males under the effects of male sex hormone.

Environment also plays a part in gene expression. One inherits a potential for a given size, for example, but one's actual size is additionally influenced by such factors as nutrition, development, and general state of health. The same is true of life span and susceptibility to diseases.

Genetic Mutation

As a rule, chromosomes replicate exactly during cell division. Occasionally, however, for reasons not yet totally understood, the genes or chromosomes change. This change may involve a single gene or whole chromosomes.

Figure 25-2 **Sex determination.** If an X chromosome from a male unites with an X chromosome from a female, the child is female (XX); if a Y chromosome from a male unites with an X chromosome from a female, the child is male (XY).

Alternatively, it may consist of chromosomal breakage, in which there is loss or rearrangement of gene fragments. Often these changes occur during cell division (mitosis or meiosis) as chromosomes come together, re-assort, and get distributed to two new cells. Such a change is termed a genetic **mutation**. Mutations may occur spontaneously or may be induced by some agent, such as ionizing radiation or chemicals, described as a **mutagen** (MU-tah-jen) or mutagenic agent.

If a mutation occurs in an ovum or a sperm cell, the altered trait will be inherited by the offspring. The vast majority of harmful mutations never are expressed because the affected fetus dies and is spontaneously aborted. Most remaining mutations are so inconsequential that they have no visible effect. Beneficial mutations, on the other hand, tend to survive and increase as a population evolves.

CHECKPOINT 25-6 ➤ What is a mutation?

Genetic Diseases

Any disorders that involve the genes may be said to be genetic, but they are not always hereditary, that is, passed from parent to offspring in the reproductive cells.

Noninherited genetic disorders may begin during maturation of the sex cells or even during development of the embryo.

Advances in genetic research have made it possible to identify the causes of many hereditary disorders and to develop genetic screening methods. In people who are "at risk" for having a child with a genetic disorder, as well as fetuses and newborns with a suspected abnormality, tests can often confirm or rule out the presence of a genetic defect.

Congenital Versus Hereditary Diseases

Before we discuss hereditary diseases, we need to distinguish them from other congenital diseases. To illustrate, let us assume that two infants are born within seconds in adjoining delivery rooms of the same hospital. It is noted that one infant has a clubfoot, a condition called **talipes** (TAL-ih-pes); the second infant has a rudimentary extra finger attached to the fifth finger of each hand, a condition called **polydactyly** (pol-e-DAK-til-e). Are both conditions hereditary? Both congenital? Is either hereditary? We can answer these questions by defining the key terms, *congenital* and *hereditary*. **Congenital** means present at the time of

Disease in Context revisited

➤ Managing Ben's Cystic Fibrosis

After learning Ben's diagnosis, his parents met with his pediatrician to discuss the treatment Ben would require to manage his cystic fibrosis. Although the doctor told them that there was no cure for cystic fibrosis yet, they were relieved to hear that there had been vast improvements in treatment in recent years. He explained that the goals of CF treatment were to minimize respiratory and digestive problems.

Therapies for respiratory problems in people with CF center on keeping the lungs clear of mucus that can block the respiratory passageways and provide an excellent growth medium for infectious organisms. Chest physical therapy, which involves pounding the chest and back with either one's hands or a machine, is the main method of removing mucus from the lungs and is repeated three to four times daily. Anti-inflammatory and mucolytic (mucus-dissolving) drugs are also useful in loosening mucus from the lungs. Unfortunately, it is difficult to remove all of the mucus, so most people with CF have per-

sistent lung infections, which require antibiotic treatment.

Management of digestive problems also centers on clearing the digestive tract of mucus, as well as ensuring adequate nutrition. Enemas and mucolytic medications are used to treat intestinal mucoid blockages. A high-calorie diet (low in fat and high in protein) improves growth and development and helps the immune system to resist lung infections. Oral pancreatic enzymes are taken before every meal to help the small intestine digest fats and proteins and absorb more vitamins.

In this case, Ben's parents learned about the genetic causes of and treatments for cystic fibrosis. It would take them some time to absorb all of this information, but they were confident that they could minimize Ben's respiratory and digestive problems. To review the respiratory system, see Chapter 18. For a review of the digestive system, see Chapter 19.

25

birth; **hereditary** means genetically transmitted or transmissible. Thus, one condition may be both congenital and hereditary; another, congenital yet not hereditary.

Hereditary conditions are usually evident at birth or soon thereafter. However, certain inherited disorders, such as adult polycystic kidney disease and Huntington disease, a nervous disorder, do not manifest themselves until about midlife (40 to 50 years of age). People with these genetic defects may pass them on to their children before they are aware of them unless genetic testing reveals their presence. In the case of our earlier examples, the clubfoot is congenital, but not hereditary, having resulted from severe distortion of the developing extremities during intrauterine growth; the extra fingers are hereditary, a familial trait that appears in another relative, a grandparent perhaps, or a parent, and that is evident at the time of birth.

CAUSES OF CONGENITAL DISORDERS Although causes of congenital deformities and birth defects often are not known, in some cases, they are known and can be avoided. For example, certain infections and toxins may be transmitted from the mother's blood by way of the placenta to the fetal circulation. Some of these cause serious developmental disorders in affected babies.

German measles (rubella) is a contagious viral infection that is ordinarily a mild disease, but if maternal infection occurs during the first 3 or 4 months of pregnancy, the fetus has a 40% chance of developing defects of the eye (cataracts), ear (deafness), brain, and heart. Infection can be prevented by appropriate immunizations.

Ionizing radiation and various toxins may damage the genes, and the disorders they produce are sometimes transmissible. Environmental agents, such as mercury and some chemicals used in industry (e.g., certain phenols and PCB), as well as some drugs, notably LSD, are known to disrupt genetic organization. (See Box 25-2, Preventing Genetic Damage.)

Intake of alcohol and cigarette smoking by a pregnant woman often cause growth retardation and low birthweight in her infant. Smaller than normal infants do not do as well as average weight babies. Some congenital brain and heart defects have been associated with a condition called **fetal alcohol syndrome**. Healthcare professionals strongly recommend total abstinence from alcohol and cigarettes during pregnancy.

Spina bifida (SPI-nah BIF-ih-dah) is incomplete closure of the spine, through which the spinal cord and its membranes may project (Fig. 25-3). The defect usually occurs in the lumbar region. If the meninges protrude (herniate), the defect is termed a meningocele (meh-NIN-gosele); if both the spinal cord and meninges protrude, it is a myelomeningocele (mi-eh-lo-meh-NIN-go-sele). In the latter case, the spinal cord ends at the point of the defect, which affects function below that point. Folic acid, a B vitamin, reduces the risk of spina bifida and other CNS defects in the fetus. Women of childbearing age should eat foods high in folic acid (green leafy vegetables, fruits, and legumes) and should take folic acid supplements even before pregnancy, as the nervous system develops early. In the United States, folic acid is added to grain products, such as bread, pasta, rice, and cereals.

CHECKPOINT 25-7 ➤ Can a disorder be congenital but not hereditary? Explain.

Box 25-2 🍎 **Health Maintenance**

Preventing Genetic Damage

It is sometimes difficult to determine whether a genetic defect is the result of a spontaneous random mutation or is related to exposure of a germ cell to an environmental toxin. Male and female sex cells are present at birth but do not become active until the reproductive years. This leaves a long time span during which toxic exposure can occur. Most of what we know about chemicals that cause mutations has been learned from environmental accidents. For example, mercury compounds have found their way into the food chain, causing neural damage to the children of parents who consumed foods containing mercury. Lead, which is toxic when ingested, as from air or water pollution, has been implicated in sperm cell abnormalities and in reduced sperm counts. Radiation accidents have been linked to increased susceptibility to certain cancers in children born after these accidents.

Meiosis is the step most prone to genetic errors. This process can be studied in males with specimens obtained from testicular biopsy. Also, samples of sperm cells, which are produced continuously in males, can be obtained easily and studied for visible defects. Advancing age in both the mother and the father is known to increase errors in meiosis. Males between 20 and 45 years of age carry the least risk of transmitting a genetic error. For females, the least risk is between ages 15 to 35 years. Because new sperm cells are produced on a 64-day cycle, men are advised to avoid conception for a few months after exposure to x-rays, cancer chemotherapy, or other chemicals capable of causing mutations.

Figure 25-3 **Spina bifida, incomplete closure of the spinal cord. (A)** Normal spinal cord. **(B)** Spina bifida with protrusion of the meninges (meningocele). **(C)** Protrusion of the spinal cord and meninges (myelomeningocele). (Reprinted with permission from Pillitteri A. *Maternal and Child Health Nursing*, 4th ed. Philadelphia: Lippincott Williams & Wilkins, 2003.)

Examples of Genetic Diseases

The best known example of a genetic disorder that is not hereditary is the most common form of **Down syndrome**, also known as **trisomy 21** because it results from an extra chromosome number 21 in each cell. This abnormality arises during formation of a sex cell. The disorder is usually recognizable at birth by the child's distinctive facial features (Fig. 25-4). Children with Down syndrome have poor muscle tone. They have lowered immunity and are also prone to heart disease, leukemia, and Alzheimer disease. Their intellectual function is impaired. However, the amount of skill they can gain depends on the severity of the disease and their family and school environments. Down syndrome is usually not inherited, although there is a hereditary form of the disorder. In most cases, both parents are normal, as are the child's siblings. The likelihood of having a baby with Down syndrome increases dramatically in women past the age of 35 years and may result from defects in either the male or female germ cells owing to age.

Most genetic diseases are **familial** or **hereditary**; that is, they are passed on from parent to child in the egg or sperm. In the case of a disorder carried by a dominant gene, only one parent needs to carry the abnormal gene to give rise to the disease. Any child who receives the defec-

Figure 25-4 **Child with Down syndrome (trisomy 21).** The typical facial features are visible in this photo. (Reprinted with permission from Pillitteri A. *Maternal and Child Health Nursing*, 4th ed. Philadelphia: Lippincott Williams & Wilkins, 2003.)

tive gene will have the disease. Any children who do not show the disease do not have the defective gene nor are they carriers. One example is **Huntington disease**, a progressive degenerative disorder associated with rapid, involuntary muscle activity and mental deterioration. The disease does not appear until about age 40 and leads to death within 15 years. There is no cure for Huntington disease, but people with the defective gene can be identified by genetic testing. Another example is **Marfan syndrome**, a connective tissue disease. People with Marfan syndrome are tall, thin, and have heart defects.

If the disease trait is carried by a recessive gene, as is the case in most inheritable disorders, a defective gene must come from each parent. Some recessively inherited diseases are described next.

In **phenylketonuria** (fen-il-ke-to-NU-re-ah) **(PKU)**, the lack of a certain enzyme prevents the proper metabolism of **phenylalanine** (fen-il-AL-ah-nin), one of the common amino acids. As a result, phenylalanine accumulates in the infant's blood and appears in the urine. If the condition remains untreated, it leads to mental retardation before the age of 2 years. Newborn infants are routinely screened for PKU.

Sickle cell disease is described in Chapter 13, where it is stated that the disease is found almost exclusively among black patients. By contrast, **cystic fibrosis** is most common in white populations; in fact, it is the most frequently inherited disease among this group. Cystic fibrosis is characterized by excessively thickened secretions in the bronchi, the intestine, and the pancreatic ducts, resulting in obstruction of these vital organs. It is associated with fre-

25

quent respiratory infections, intestinal losses, particularly of fats and fat-soluble vitamins, as well as massive salt loss. Treatment includes oral administration of pancreatic enzymes and special pulmonary exercises. Cystic fibrosis was once fatal by the time of adolescence, but now, with appropriate care, life expectancies are extending into the third decade. The gene responsible for the disease has been identified, raising hope of better diagnosis, treatment, and perhaps even correction of the defective gene that causes the disorder.

In **Tay-Sachs disease**, a certain type of fat is deposited in neurons of the CNS and retina because cellular lysosomes lack an enzyme that breaks it down. The disease occurs mainly in eastern European (Ashkenazi) Jews and generally leads to death by age four. There is no cure for Tay-Sachs, but a blood test can identify genetic carriers of the disease.

Another group of heritable muscle disorders is known collectively as the **progressive muscular atrophies**. Atrophy (AT-ro-fe) means wasting due to decrease in the size of a normally developed part. The absence of normal muscle movement in the infant proceeds within a few months to extreme weakness of the respiratory muscles, until ultimately the infant is unable to breathe adequately. Most afflicted babies die within several months. The name *floppy baby syndrome*, as the disease is commonly called, provides a vivid description of its effects.

Albinism is another recessively inherited disorder that affects the cells (melanocytes) that produce the pigment melanin. The skin and hair color are strikingly white and do not darken with age. The skin is abnormally sensitive to sunlight and may appear wrinkled. People with albinism are especially susceptible to skin cancer and to some severe visual disturbances, such as myopia (nearsightedness) and abnormal sensitivity to light (photophobia).

Fragile X syndrome is the most common cause of inherited mental retardation in both males and females. It is an X-linked recessive disorder associated with a fragile site on an arm of the X chromosome. In males, it also causes enlarged testes, hyperactivity, mitral valve malfunction, high forehead, and enlarged jaw and ears.

Other inherited disorders include **osteogenesis** (os-te-o-JEN-eh-sis) **imperfecta**, or *brittle bone disease*, in which multiple fractures may occur during and shortly after fetal life, and a disorder of skin, muscles, and bones called **neurofibromatosis** (nu-ro-fi-bro-mah-TO-sis). In the latter condition, multiple masses, often on stalks (pedunculated), grow along nerves all over the body.

More than 20 different cancers have been linked to specific gene mutations. These include cancers of the breast, ovary, and colon as well as some forms of leukemia. Note, however, that hereditary forms of cancer account for only about 1% of all cancers and that the development of cancer is complex, involving not only specific genes but also gene interactions and environmental factors.

Genetic components have been suggested in some other diseases as well, including certain forms of heart disease, diabetes mellitus, types of cleft lip and cleft palate, and perhaps Parkinson and Alzheimer disease.

CHECKPOINT 25-8 ➤ What causes phenylketonuria?

Visit *thePoint* or see the Student Resource CD in the back of this book for illustrations of some genetic diseases and a chart summarizing selected genetic disorders.

Treatment and Prevention of Genetic Diseases

The number of genetic diseases is so great (more than 4,000) that many pages of this book would be needed simply to list them all. Moreover, the list continues to grow as sophisticated research techniques and advances in biology make it clear that various diseases of previously unknown origin are genetic—some hereditary, others not. Can we identify which are inherited genetic disorders and which are due to environmental factors? Can we prevent the occurrence of any of them?

Genetic Counseling

It is possible to prevent genetic disorders in many cases and even to treat some of them. The most effective method of preventing genetic disease is through genetic counseling, a specialized field of health care. Genetic counseling centers use a team approach of medical, nursing, laboratory, and social service professionals to advise and care for clients. People who might consider genetic counseling include prospective parents over the age of 35, those who have a family history of genetic disorders, and those who are considering some form of fertility treatment.

Visit *thePoint* or see the Student Resource CD in the back of this book for a description of careers in genetic counseling.

THE FAMILY HISTORY An accurate and complete family history of both prospective parents is necessary for genetic counseling. This history should include information about relatives with respect to age, onset of a specific disease, health status, and cause of death. The families' ethnic origins may be relevant because some genetic diseases predominate in certain ethnic groups. Hospital and physician records are studied, as are photographs of family members. The ages of the prospective parents are considered as factors, as is parental or ancestral relationship (e.g., marriage between first cousins). The complete, detailed family history, or tree, is called a pedigree. Pedigrees are used to determine the pattern of inheritance of a genetic disease within a family (Fig. 25-5). They may also indicate whether

The recessive trait c is cystic fibrosis.
The dominant normal gene is C.

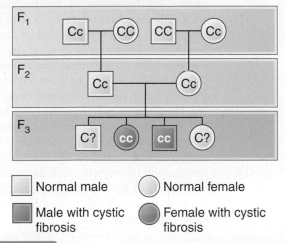

Normal male ⬜   Normal female ⬤

Male with cystic fibrosis ⬛   Female with cystic fibrosis ⬤

Figure 25-5 **A pedigree (family history) showing three generations (F₁–F₃).** The pedigree is a tool used in genetic studies and genetic counseling. In this example, one parent in each F_1 cross and both parents in the F_2 cross are normal but carry the recessive gene (c) for cystic fibrosis. For the normal children in F_3, only one gene (the dominant normal gene) is known. Note that the F_3 generation does not show strict predicted genetic ratios. Theoretically, only one in four children should be homozygous recessive (have two recessive genes. **[ZOOMING IN ➤** What are the possible genotypes of the two normal children in the F_3 generation? **]**

a given family member is a carrier of the disease. Note that in some cases, there is not enough family data to determine the genotype of all members with regard to a given trait. Also, small numbers of offspring may not show the strict genetic ratios expected from a given cross (see Fig. 25-5).

LABORATORY STUDIES One technique that enables the geneticist to study an unborn fetus is **amniocentesis** (am-ne-o-sen-TE-sis). During this procedure, a small amount of the amniotic fluid that surrounds the fetus is withdrawn (Fig. 25-6). Fetal skin cells in the amniotic fluid are removed, grown (cultured), and separated for study. The chromosomes are examined, and the amniotic fluid is analyzed for biochemical abnormalities. With these methods, almost 200 genetic diseases can be detected before birth.

Another method for obtaining fetal cells for study involves sampling of the chorionic villi through the cervix. The chorionic villi are hairlike projections

of the membrane that surrounds the embryo in early pregnancy. The method is called **chorionic villus sampling (CVS).** Samples may be taken between 8 and 10 weeks of pregnancy, and the cells obtained may be analyzed immediately. In contrast, amniocentesis cannot be done before the 14th to 16th week of pregnancy, and test results are not available for about 2 weeks.

Abnormalities in the chromosome number and some abnormalities within the chromosomes can be detected by **karyotype** (KAR-e-o-tipe) analysis. A karyotype is produced by growing cells obtained by amniocentesis or CVS in a special medium and arresting cell division at the metaphase stage. A technician uses special stains to reveal certain changes in fine structure within the chromosomes. The chromosomes, visible under the microscope, are then photographed, and the photographs are cut out and arranged in groups according to their size and form (Fig. 25-7). Abnormalities in the number or structure of the chromosomes can thereby be detected.

COUNSELING PROSPECTIVE PARENTS Armed with all the available pertinent facts, and with knowledge of genetic inheritance patterns, the counselor is equipped to inform the prospective parents of the possibility of their having genetically abnormal offspring. The couple may then use this information to make decisions about family planning. Depending on the individuals and their situation, a couple might elect to have no children, have an adoptive family, use a donor gamete, terminate a pregnancy, or accept the risk.

Figure 25-6 **Amniocentesis.** A sample of amniotic fluid is removed from the amniotic sac. Cells and fluid are tested for fetal abnormalities. (Reprinted with permission from Cohen BJ. *Medical Terminology*, 5th ed. Philadelphia: Lippincott Williams & Wilkins, 2008.)

25

A

B

CHECKPOINT **25-9** ➤ What is a pedigree and how is a pedigree used in genetic counseling?

CHECKPOINT **25-10** ➤ What is a karyotype?

Progress in Medical Treatment

The mental and physical ravages of many genetic diseases are largely preventable, provided the diseases are diagnosed and treated early in the individual's life. Some of these diseases respond well to dietary control. One such disease, called **maple syrup urine disease**, responds to very large doses of thiamin along with control of the intake of certain amino acids. The disastrous effects of **Wilson disease**, in which abnormal accumulations of copper in the tissue cause tremor, rigidity, uncontrollable stagger, and finally extensive liver damage, can be prevented by a combination of dietary and drug therapies.

Phenylketonuria is perhaps the best-known example of dietary management of inherited disease. If the disorder is undiagnosed and untreated, 98% of affected patients will be severely mentally retarded by 10 years of age. In contrast, if the condition is diagnosed and treated before the baby reaches the age of 6 months, and treatment is maintained until the age of 10 years, mental deficiency will be prevented, or at least minimized. A simple blood test for PKU is now done routinely in hospitals throughout the United States. Infants are usually screened immediately after birth, but they should be retested 24 to 48 hours after taking in protein.

Klinefelter (KLINE-fel-ter) **syndrome**, which occurs in about 1 in 600 males, is a common cause of underdevelopment of the gonads with resulting infertility. Inheritors of this disorder have abnormal sex chromosome patterns, usually an extra X chromosome. Instead of the typical male XY pattern, the cells contain an XXY combination owing to failure of the sex chromosomes to separate during cell division. Treatment of this disorder includes the use of hormones and psychotherapy.

In the future, we can anticipate greatly improved methods of screening, diagnosis, and treatment of genetic diseases. There have been reports of fetuses being treated with vitamins or hormones after prenatal diagnosis of a genetic disorder. Ahead lies the possibility of treating or correcting genetic disorders through genetic engineering—introducing genetically altered cells to produce missing factors, such as enzymes or hormones, or even correcting faulty genes in the patient's cells. Researchers have already made some attempts to supplement failed genes with healthy ones.

For the present, it is important to educate the public about the availability of screening methods for both parents and offspring. People should also be made aware of the damaging effects of radiation, drugs, and other toxic substances on the genes. Because so many congenital disorders are associated with environmental factors, public education and better health habits will probably yield greater overall benefits than genetic manipulations.

Word Anatomy

Medical terms are built from standardized word parts (prefixes, roots, and suffixes). Learning the meanings of these parts can help you remember words and interpret unfamiliar terms.

WORD PART	MEANING	EXAMPLE
Genes and Chromosomes		
chrom/o	color	*Chromosomes* color darkly with stains.
aut/o-	self	*Autosomes* are all the chromosomes aside from the two that determine sex.
heter/o	other, different	*Heterozygous* paired genes (alleles) are different from each other.
homo-	same	*Homozygous* paired genes (alleles) are the same.
phen/o	to show	Traits that can be observed or tested for make up a person's *phenotype*.
Hereditary Traits		
multi-	many	*Multifactorial* traits are determined by multiple pairs of genes.
Genetic Diseases		
dactyl/o	digit (finger or toe)	In *polydactyly* there is an extra finger on each hand.
con-	with	A *congenital* defect is present at the time of birth.
-cele	swelling	In spina bifida, the meninges can protrude through the spine as a *meningocele*.
Treatment and Prevention of Genetic Diseases		
-centesis	tapping, perforation	*Amniocentesis* is a tap of the amniotic fluid.
kary/o	nucleus	A *karyotype* is an analysis of the chromosomes contained in the nucleus of a cell.

Summary

I. **GENES AND CHROMOSOMES**
  A. Genes
    1. Hereditary units
    2. Segments of DNA
    3. Control manufacture of proteins (e.g., enzymes, hormones)
  B. Chromosomes
    1. Threadlike bodies in nucleus; 46 in humans
    2. Composed of genes
    3. 22 pairs autosomes (non-sex chromosomes)
    4. 1 pair sex chromosomes
  C. Dominant and recessive genes
    1. Dominant gene—always expressed
      a. May be heterozygous (two genes different)

      b. May be homozygous dominant (two genes the same)
    2. Recessive gene—expressed only if homozygous recessive (received from both parents)
      a. Carrier—person with recessive gene that is not apparent but can be passed to offspring
      b. Phenotype—characteristic that can be seen or tested for
      c. Genotype—genetic make-up
  D. Distribution of chromosomes to offspring
    1. Meiosis
      a. Cell division that forms sex cells with 23 chromosomes

25

b.   Each cell receives one of each chromosome pair

c.   Punnett square shows results of crosses

E.   Sex determination

1.   X chromosome larger and carries other traits

2.   Y smaller and carries mainly gene for sex determination

3.   Female cells have XX; male cells have XY

F.   Sex-linked traits

1.   Traits carried on sex chromosome (usually X)

2.   Sex-linked traits appear mostly in males

a.   Passed from mother to son on X chromosome

b.   If recessive, not masked by dominant gene on Y

c.   Examples—hemophilia, baldness, red-green color blindness

II.   **HEREDITARY TRAITS**

A.   Genes determine physical, biochemical, and physiologic characteristics of every cell

1.   Some traits determined by single gene pairs

2.   Most determined by multifactorial inheritance

a.   Involves multiple gene pairs

b.   Produces a range of variations in a population

c.   Examples—height, weight, coloration, susceptibility to disease

B.   Gene expression

1.   Factors

a.   Sex

b.   Presence of other genes

c.   Environment

C.   Genetic mutation

1.   Change in genes or chromosomes

2.   May be passed to offspring if occurs in germ cells

3.   Mutagenic agents

a.   Factors causing mutation

b.   Examples—ionizing radiation, chemicals

III.   **GENETIC DISEASES**—disorders involving genes

A.   Congenital versus hereditary diseases

1.   Congenital disorders

a.   Present at birth

b.   May or may not be hereditary

2.   Hereditary (familial) disorders

a.   Passed from parent to offspring in sex cells

3.   Causes—infections, toxins, ionizing radiation, alcohol, smoking

a.   Examples—defects caused by rubella, fetal alcohol syndrome, spina bifida

B.   Examples of genetic diseases

1.   Down syndrome—results from extra chromosome 21 (trisomy 21)

2.   Dominant inheritance—Huntington disease, Marfan sundrome

3.   Recessive inheritance—PKU (phenylketonuria), cystic fibrosis, sickle cell anemia, Tay-Sachs disease, progressive muscular atrophies, albinism, osteogenesis imperfecta, neurofibromatosis

IV.   **TREATMENT AND PREVENTION OF GENETIC DISEASES**

A.   Genetic counseling

1.   Pedigree—family history

2.   Laboratory studies

a.   Amniocentesis—withdrawal of amniotic fluid for study at 14 to 16 weeks of pregnancy

b.   Chorionic villus sampling—done at 8 to 10 weeks of pregnancy

c.   Karyotype—analysis of chromosomes

3.   Counseling the prospective parents

B.   Progress in medical treatment

1.   Dietary control—maple syrup urine disease, Wilson disease, PKU

2.   Hormone therapy—Klinefelter disease

3.   Fetal therapy

4.   Correction of faulty genes—experimental

Questions for Study and Review

BUILDING UNDERSTANDING

Fill in the blanks

1. The basic unit of heredity is a(n) _____ .

2. Chromosomes not involved in sex determination are known as _____ .

3. Any trait that is carried on a sex chromosome is said to be _____ .

4. Change in a gene or chromosome is called _____ .

5. Incomplete closure of the spine results in a disorder called _____ .

Matching > Match each numbered item with the most closely related lettered item.

___ **6.** A gene that is always expressed if present

___ **7.** A gene that is not always expressed if present

___ **8.** Term for paired genes for a trait that are the same

___ **9.** Term for paired genes for a trait that are different

a. dominant

b. recessive

c. homozygous

d. heterozygous

Multiple choice

___ **10.** The genetic code is composed of
  a. deoxyribonucleic acid
  b. ribonucleic acid
  c. protein
  d. nuclear membrane

___ **11.** Genes govern the cell by controlling the manufacture of
  a. carbohydrates
  b. lipids
  c. proteins
  d. electrolytes

___ **12.** Paired genes for a given trait are known as
  a. chromosomes
  b. ribosomes
  c. nucleotides
  d. alleles

___ **13.** A condition characterized by extra fingers or toes is called
  a. talipes
  b. polydactyly
  c. osteogenesis imperfecta
  d. neurofibromatosis

___ **14.** A complete detailed family history can be obtained by doing
  a. chorionic villus sampling
  b. amniocentesis
  c. a karyotype
  d. a pedigree

UNDERSTANDING CONCEPTS

15. How many chromosomes are there in a human body cell? In a human gamete?

16. Dana has one dominant allele for brown eyes (*B*) and one recessive allele for blue eyes. What is Dana's genotype? What is her phenotype?

17. Describe the process of meiosis and explain how it results in genetic variation.

18. Explain the great variation in the color of skin and hair in humans.

19. Describe how a mutagenic agent can produce genetic variation.

20. What is the difference between a congenital disease and a hereditary disease? List some congenital and hereditary diseases.

21. What is PKU and how should this disease be treated?

22. Compare and contrast amniocentesis and chorionic villus sampling. List some diseases that can be diagnosed using these techniques.

23. What is the most common inheritable disease among black people? Among white people? What are the symptoms of these two diseases?

CONCEPTUAL THINKING

24. If mitosis were used to produce gametes, what consequences would this have on the offspring's genotype, phenotype, and chromosome number?

25. Jason and Nicole are expecting their first child and are wondering what their child's eye color might be. Jason has blue eyes (a recessive trait) and Nicole has brown eyes (a dominant trait). Both of Jason's parents have blue eyes. One of Nicole's parents has brown eyes, the other

has blue eyes. What are Jason's and Nicole's genotype and phenotype? What are the possible genotypes and phenotypes of their children?

26. In the case story, Ben's parents were both carriers of the cystic fibrosis trait. Using a Punnett square, calculate the possible genotypic and phenotypic combinations for their offspring.

25

Glossary

A

abdominopelvic (ab-dom-ih-no-PEL-vik) Pertaining to the abdomen and pelvis.

abduction (ab-DUK-shun) Movement away from the midline.

abortifacient (ah-bor-tih-FA-shent) Agent that induces an abortion.

abortion (ah-BOR-shun) Loss of an embryo or fetus before the 20th week of pregnancy.

abscess (AB-ses) Area of tissue breakdown; a localized space in the body containing pus and liquefied tissue.

absorption (ab-SORP-shun) Transfer of digested nutrients from the digestive tract into the circulation.

accommodation (ah-kom-o-DA-shun) Coordinated changes in the lens of the eye that enable one to focus on near and far objects.

acetylcholine (as-e-til-KO-lene) (**ACh**) Neurotransmitter; released at synapses within the nervous system and at the neuromuscular junction.

acid (AH-sid) Substance that can donate a hydrogen ion to another substance.

acid-fast stain Procedure used to color cells for viewing under the microscope.

acidosis (as-ih-DO-sis) Condition that results from a decrease in the pH of body fluids.

acne (AK-ne) Disease of the sebaceous glands.

acquired immunodeficiency syndrome (**AIDS**) Viral disease that attacks the immune system, specifically the T-helper lymphocytes with CD4 receptors.

acromegaly (ak-ro-MEG-ah-le) Condition caused by oversecretion of growth hormone in adults; there is overgrowth of some bones and involvement of multiple body systems.

acrosome (AK-ro-some) Caplike structure over the head of the sperm cell that helps the sperm to penetrate the ovum.

ACTH See adrenocorticotropic hormone.

actin (AK-tin) One of the two contractile proteins in muscle cells, the other being myosin.

action potential Sudden change in the electrical charge on a cell membrane, which then spreads along the membrane; nerve impulse.

active transport Movement of a substance into or out of a cell in an opposite direction to the way in which it would normally flow by diffusion; active transport requires energy and transporters.

acupuncture (AK-u-punk-chur) Ancient Chinese method of inserting thin needles into the body at specific points to relieve pain or promote healing.

acute (ah-KUTE) Referring to a severe but short-lived disease or condition.

Addison disease Condition caused by hypofunction of the adrenal cortex.

adduction (ad-DUK-shun) Movement toward the midline.

adenoids (Ad-eh-noyds) Popular name for pharygeal tonsil located in the nasopharynx.

adenosine triphosphate (ah-DEN-o-sene tri-FOS-fate) (**ATP**) Energy-storing compound found in all cells.

ADH See antidiuretic hormone.

adhesion (ad-HE-zhun) Holding together of two surfaces or parts; band of connective tissue between parts that are normally separate; molecular attraction between contacting bodies.

adipose (AD-ih-pose) Referring to fats or a type of connective tissue that stores fat.

adrenal (ah-DRE-nal) **gland** Endocrine gland located above the kidney; suprarenal gland.

adrenaline (ah-DREN-ah-lin) See epinephrine.

adrenergic (ad-ren ER-jik) An activity or structure that responds to epinephrine (adrenaline).

adrenocorticotropic (ah-dre-no-kor-tih-ko-TRO-pik) **hormone** (**ACTH**) Hormone produced by the pituitary that stimulates the adrenal cortex.

aerobic (air-O-bik) Requiring oxygen.

afferent (AF-fer-ent) Carrying toward a given point, such as a sensory neuron that carries nerve impulses toward the central nervous system.

agglutination (ah-glu-tih-NA-shun) Clumping of cells due to an antigen–antibody reaction.

agranulocyte (a-GRAN-u-lo-site) Leukocyte without visible granules in the cytoplasm when stained; lymphocyte or monocyte.

AIDS See acquired immunodeficiency syndrome.

albinism (AL-bih-nizm) A hereditary disorder that affects melanin production.

albumin (al-BU-min) Protein in blood plasma and other body fluids; helps maintain the osmotic pressure of the blood.

albuminuria (al-bu-mih-NU-re-ah) Presence of albumin in the urine, usually as a result of a kidney disorder.

aldosterone (al-DOS-ter-one) Hormone released by the adrenal cortex that promotes sodium and water reabsorption in the kidneys.

alkali (AL-kah-li) Substance that can accept a hydrogen ion (H^+); substance that donates a hydroxide ion (OH^-); a base.

alkalosis (al-kah-LO-sis) Condition that results from an increase in the pH of body fluids.

allele (al-LELE) One member of the gene pair that controls a given trait.

allergen (AL-er-jen) Substance that causes hypersensitivity; substance that induces allergy.

allergy (AL-er-je) Tendency to react unfavorably to a certain substance that is normally harmless to most people; hypersensitivity.

alopecia (al-o-PE-she-ah) Baldness.

alveolus (al-VE-o-lus) Small sac or pouch; usually a tiny air sac in the lungs through which gases are exchanged between the outside air and the blood; tooth socket; pl., alveoli.

Alzheimer (ALZ-hi-mer) **disease** Unexplained degeneration of the cerebral cortex and hippocampus with intellectual impairment, mood changes, and confusion.

amblyopia (am-ble-O-pe-ah) Vision loss in a healthy eye because it cannot work properly with the other eye.

amino (ah-ME-no) **acid** Building block of protein.

amniocentesis (am-ne-o-sen-TE-sis) Removal of fluid and cells from the amniotic sac for prenatal diagnostic tests.

amniotic (am-ne-OT-ik) Pertaining to the sac that surrounds and cushions the developing fetus or to the fluid that fills that sac.

amniotic (am-ne-OT-ik) **sac** Fluid-filled sac that surrounds and cushions the developing fetus.

amphiarthrosis (am-fe-ar-THRO-sis) Slightly movable joint.

amyotrophic (ah-mi-o-TROF-ik) **lateral sclerosis** (**ALS**) Disorder of the nervous system in which motor neurons are destroyed.

anabolism (ah-NAB-o-lizm) Metabolic building of simple compounds into more complex substances needed by the body.

anaerobic (an-air-O-bik) Not requiring oxygen.

analgesic (an-al-JE-zik) Relieving pain; a pain-relieving agent that does not cause loss of consciousness.

anaphase (AN-ah-faze) The third stage of mitosis in which chromosomes separate to opposite sides of the cell.

anaphylaxis (an-ah-fih-LAK-sis) Severe, life-threatening allergic response.

anastomosis (ah-nas-to-MO-sis) Communication between two structures, such as blood vessels.

anatomy (ah-NAT-o-me) Study of body structure.

anemia (ah-NE-me-ah) Abnormally low level of hemoglobin or red cells in the blood, resulting in inadequate delivery of oxygen to the tissues.

androgen (AN-dro-jen) Any male sex hormone.

anesthesia (an-es-THE-ze-ah) Loss of sensation, particularly of pain; drug with this effect is an anesthetic.

aneurysm (AN-u-rizm) Bulging sac in the wall of a vessel.

angiotensin (an-je-o-TEN-sin) Substance formed in the blood by the action of the renal enzyme renin; it increases blood pressure by causing vascular constriction and stimulating the release of aldosterone from the adrenal cortex.

angina (an-JI-nah) Severe choking pain; disease or condition producing such pain. Angina pectoris is suffocating pain in the chest, usually caused by lack of oxygen supply to the heart muscle.

angioplasty (AN-je-o-plas-te) Use of a balloon inserted with a catheter to open a blocked vessel.

anion (AN-i-on) Negatively charged particle (ion).

anorexia (an-o-REK-se-ah) Chronic loss of appetite. Anorexia nervosa is a psychological condition in which a person may become seriously, even fatally, weakened from lack of food.

anoxia (ah-NOK-se-ah) See hypoxia.

ANP See atrial natriuretic peptide.

ANS See autonomic nervous system.

antagonist (an-TAG-o-nist) Muscle that has an action opposite that of a given movement; substance that opposes the action of another substance.

anterior (an-TE-re-or) Toward the front or belly surface; ventral.

anthelmintic (ant-hel-MIN-tik) Agent that acts against worms; vermicide; vermifuge.

antibiotic (an-te-bi-OT-ik) Substance produced by living cells that kills or arrests the growth of bacteria.

antibody (AN-te-bod-e) (**Ab**) Substance produced in response to a specific antigen; immunoglobulin.

antidiuretic (an-ti-di-u-RET-ik) **hormone** (**ADH**) Hormone released from the posterior pituitary gland that increases water reabsorption in the kidneys, thus decreasing the urinary output.

antigen (AN-te-jen) (**Ag**) Foreign substance that produces an immune response.

antineoplastic (an-ti-ne-o-PLAS-tik) Acting against a neoplasm (tumor).

antioxidant (an-te-OX-ih-dant) Substances in the diet that protect against harmful free radicals.

antipyretic (an-ti-pi-RET-ik) Drug that reduces fever.

antiseptic (an-tih-SEP-tik) Substance that prevents pathogens from multiplying but does not necessarily kill them.

antiserum (an-te-SE-rum) Serum containing antibodies that may be given to provide passive immunity; immune serum.

antitoxin (an-te-TOKS-in) Antibody that neutralizes a toxin.

antivenin (an-te-VEN-in) Antibody that neutralizes a snake venom.

anus (A-nus) Inferior opening of the digestive tract.

aorta (a-OR-tah) The largest artery; carries blood out of the heart's left ventricle.

apex (A-peks) Pointed region of a cone-shaped structure.

aphasia (ah-FA-ze-ah) Loss or defect in language communication; loss of the ability to speak or write is expressive aphasia; loss of understanding of written or spoken language is receptive aphasia.

apnea (AP-ne-ah) Temporary cessation of breathing.

apocrine (AP-o-krin) Referring to a gland that releases some cellular material along with its secretions.

aponeurosis (ap-o-nu-RO-sis) Broad sheet of fibrous connective tissue that attaches muscle to bone or to other muscle.

appendicular (ap-en-DIK-u-lar) **skeleton** Part of the skeleton that includes the bones of the upper extremities, lower extremities, shoulder girdle, and hips.

appendix (ah-PEN-diks) Fingerlike tube of lymphatic tissue attached to the first portion of the large intestine; vermiform (wormlike) appendix.

aqueous (A-kwe-us) Pertaining to water; an aqueous solution is one in which water is the solvent.

aqueous (A-kwe-us) **humor** Watery fluid that fills much of the eyeball anterior to the lens.

arachnoid (ah-RAK-noyd) Middle layer of the meninges.

areolar (ah-RE-o-lar) Referring to loose connective tissue, any small space, or to an areola, a circular area of marked color.

arrector pili (ah-REK-tor PI-li) Muscle attached to a hair follicle that raises the hair.

arrhythmia (ah-RITH-me-ah) Abnormal rhythm of the heartbeat; dysrhythmia.

arteriole (ar-TE-re-ole) Vessel between a small artery and a capillary.

arteriosclerosis (ar-te-re-o-skle-RO-sis) Hardening of the arteries.

artery (AR-ter-e) Vessel that carries blood away from the heart.

arthritis (arth-RI-tis) Inflammation of the joints.

arthrocentesis (ar-thro-sen-TE-sis) Puncture of a joint to withdraw fluid.

arthroscope (AR-thro-skope) Instrument for examining the interior of the knee and surgically repairing the knee.

articular (ar-TIK-u-lar) Pertaining to a joint.

ascites (ah-SI-teze) Abnormal collection of fluid in the abdominal cavity.

asepsis (a-SEP-sis) Condition in which no pathogens are present; adj., aseptic.

asthma (AZ-mah) Allergy-induced inflammation and constriction of the air passageways.

astigmatism (ah-STIG-mah-tizm) Visual defect due to an irregularity in the curvature of the cornea or the lens.

ataxia (ah-TAK-se-ah) Lack of muscular coordination; irregular muscular action.

atelectasis (at-e-LEK-tah-sis) Incomplete lung expansion; collapsed lung.

atherosclerosis (ath-er-o-skleh-RO-sis) Hardening of the arteries due to the deposit of yellowish, fatlike material in the lining of these vessels.

atom (AT-om) Smallest subunit of a chemical element.

atomic number The number of protons in the nucleus of an element's atoms; a number characteristic of each element.

atopic dermatitis (ah-TOP-ik der-mah-TI-tis) Skin condition that may involve redness, blisters, pimples, scaling, and crusting; eczema.

ATP See adenosine triphosphate.

atrial natriuretic (na-tre-u-RET-ik) **peptide** (**ANP**) Hormone produced by the atria of the heart that lowers blood pressure.

atrioventricular (a-tre-o-ven-TRIK-u-lar) (**AV**) node Part of the heart's conduction system.

atrium (A-tre-um) One of the heart's two upper chambers; adj., atrial.

atrophy (AT-ro-fe) Wasting or decrease in size of a part.

attenuated (ah-TEN-u-a-ted) Weakened.

autoclave Instrument used to sterilize material with steam under pressure.

autoimmunity (aw-to-ih-MU-nih-te) Abnormal reactivity to one's own tissues.

autologous (aw-TOL-o-gus) Related to self, such as blood or tissue taken from one's own body.

autonomic (aw-to-NOM-ik) **nervous system** (**ANS**) The part of the nervous system that controls smooth muscle, cardiac muscle, and glands; the visceral or involuntary nervous system.

autosome (AW-to-some) A chromosome not involved in sex determination. There are 44 autosomes (22 pairs) in humans.

AV node See atrioventricular node.

axial (AK-se-al) **skeleton** The part of the skeleton that includes the skull, spinal column, ribs, and sternum.

axilla (ak-SIL-ah) Hollow beneath the arm where it joins the body; armpit.

axon (AK-son) Fiber of a neuron that conducts impulses away from the cell body.

B

bacillus (bah-SIL-us) Rod-shaped bacterium; pl., bacilli (bah-SIL-i).

bacterium (bak-TE-re-um) Type of microorganism; pl., bacteria (bak-TE-re-ah).

bacteriostasis (bak-te-re-o-STA-sis) Condition in which bacterial growth is inhibited but the organisms are not killed.

band cell Immature neutrophil.

baroreceptor (bar-o-re-SEP-ter) Receptor that responds to pressure, such as those in vessel walls that respond to stretching and help regulate blood pressure; a type of mechanoreceptor.

basal ganglia (BA-sal GANG-le-ah) Gray masses in the lower part of the forebrain that aid in muscle coordination.

base Substance that can accept a hydrogen ion (H^+); substance that donates a hydroxide ion (OH^-); an alkali.

basophil (BA-so-fil) Granular white blood cell that shows large, dark blue cytoplasmic granules when stained with basic stain.

B cell Agranular white blood cell that gives rise to antibody-producing plasma cells in response to an antigen; B lymphocyte.

Bell palsy Facial paralysis caused by damage to the facial nerve (VII), usually on one side of the face.

benign (be-NINE) Denoting a mild condition, favorable for recovery, or a tumor that does not metastasize (spread).

bicarbonate ion (bi-KAR-bon-ate I-on) Ion formed from carbonic acid along with hydrogen ion.

bile Substance produced in the liver that emulsifies fats.

bilirubin (BIL-ih-ru-bin) Pigment derived from the breakdown of hemoglobin and found in bile.

biofeedback (bi-o-FEED-bak) A method for controlling involuntary responses by means of electronic devices that monitor changes and feed information back to a person.

biopsy (BI-op-se) Removal of tissue or other material from the living body for examination, usually under the microscope.

blood urea nitrogen (BUN) Amount of nitrogen from urea in the blood; test to evaluate kidney function.

bolus (BO-lus) A concentrated mass; the portion of food that is moved to the back of the mouth and swallowed.

Bowman capsule Enlarged portion of the nephron that contains the glomerulus; glomerular capsule.

bone Hard connective tissue that makes up most of the skeleton, or any structure composed of this type of tissue.

bradycardia (brad-e-KAR-de-ah) Heart rate of less than 60 beats per minute.

brain The central controlling area of the central nervous system (CNS).

brain stem Portion of the brain that connects the cerebrum with the spinal cord; contains the midbrain, pons, and medulla oblongata.

Broca (bro-KAH) **area** Area of the cerebral cortex concerned with motor control of speech.

bronchiole (BRONG-ke-ole) Microscopic branch of a bronchus.

bronchoscope (BRONG-ko-skope) Endoscope for examination of the bronchi and removal of small objects from the bronchi.

bronchus (BRONG-kus) Large air passageway in the lung; pl., bronchi (BRONG-ki).

buffer (BUF-er) Substance that prevents sharp changes in the pH of a solution.

bulbourethral (bul-bo-u-RE-thral) **gland** Gland that secretes mucus to lubricate the urethra and tip of penis during sexual stimulation; Cowper gland.

bulimia (bu-LIM-e-ah) Eating disorder also known as binge–purge syndrome.

bulk transport Movement of large amounts of material through a cell's plasma membrane.

bulla (BUL-ah) Vesicle.

BUN See blood urea nitrogen.

bursa (BER-sah) Small, fluid-filled sac found in an area subject to stress around bones and joints; pl., bursae (BER-se).

bursitis (ber-SI-tis) Inflammation of a bursa.

C

calcitonin (kal-sih-TO-nin) Hormone from the thyroid gland that lowers blood calcium levels and promotes deposit of calcium in bones; thyrocalcitonin.

calcitriol (kal-sih-TRI-ol) The active form of vitamin D; dihydroxycholecalciferol (di-hi-drok-se-ko-le-kal-SIF-eh-rol).

calculus (KAL-ku-lus) Stone, such as a urinary stone; pl., calculi (KAL-ku-li).

calyx (KA-liks) Cuplike extension of the renal pelvis that collects urine; pl., calyces (KA-lih-seze).

cancellous (KAN-sel-us) Referring to spongy bone tissue.

cancer (KAN-ser) Tumor that spreads to other tissues; a malignant neoplasm.

capillary (CAP-ih-lar-e) Microscopic vessel through which exchanges take place between the blood and the tissues.

carbohydrate (kar-bo-HI-drate) Simple sugar or compound made from simple sugars linked together, such as starch or glycogen.

carbon Element that is the basis of organic chemistry.

carbon dioxide (di-OX-ide) (CO_2) Gaseous waste product of cellular metabolism.

carbonic acid (kar-BON ik) Acid formed when carbon dioxide dissolves in water; carbonic acid then separates into hydrogen ion and bicarbonate ion.

carbonic anhydrase (an-HI-drase) Enzyme that catalyzes the interconversion of carbon dioxide with bicarbonate ion and hydrogen ion.

carcinogen (kar-SIN-o-jen) Cancer-causing substance.

carcinoma (kar-sih-NO-mah) Malignant growth of epithelial cells; a form of cancer.

cardiac (KAR-de-ak) Pertaining to the heart.

cardiopulmonary resuscitation (CPR) Method to restore heartbeat and breathing by mouth-to-mouth resuscitation and closed chest cardiac massage.

cardiovascular system (kar-de-o-VAS-ku-lar) System consisting of the heart and blood vessels that transports blood throughout the body.

caries (KA-reze) Tooth decay.

carotenemia (kar-o-te-NE-me-ah) Yellowish skin color caused by eating excessive amounts of carrots and other deeply colored vegetables.

carrier Individual who has a gene that is not expressed but that can be passed to offspring.

cartilage (KAR-tih-lij) Type of hard connective tissue found at the ends of bones, the tip of the nose, larynx, trachea, and the embryonic skeleton.

CAT See computed tomography.

catabolism (kah-TAB-o-lizm) Metabolic breakdown of substances into simpler substances; includes the digestion of food and the oxidation of nutrient molecules for energy.

catalyst (KAT-ah-list) Substance that speeds the rate of a chemical reaction.

cataract (KAT-ah-rakt) Opacity of the eye's lens or lens capsule.

catheter (KATH-eh-ter) Tube that can be inserted into a vessel or cavity; may be used to remove fluid, such as urine or blood; v., catheterize.

cation (KAT-i-on) Positively charged particle (ion).

caudal (KAWD-al) Toward or nearer to the sacral region of the spinal column.

CCK See cholecystokinin.

cecum (SE-kum) Small pouch at the beginning of the large intestine.

cell Basic unit of life.

cell membrane Outer covering of a cell; regulates what enters and leaves cell; plasma membrane.

cellular respiration Series of reactions by which nutrients are oxidized for energy within the cell.

central nervous system (CNS) Part of the nervous system that includes the brain and spinal cord.

centrifuge (SEN-trih-fuje) An instrument that separates materials in a mixture based on density.

centriole (SEN-tre-ole) Rod-shaped body near the nucleus of a cell; functions in cell division.

cerebellum (ser-eh-BEL-um) Small section of the brain located under the cerebral hemispheres; functions in coordination, balance, and muscle tone.

cerebral (SER-e-bral) **cortex** Very thin outer layer of gray matter on the surface of the cerebral hemispheres.

cerebral palsy (PAWL-ze) Disorder caused by brain damage occurring before or during the birth process.

cerebrospinal (ser-e-bro-SPI-nal) **fluid** (CSF) Fluid that circulates in and around the brain and spinal cord.

cerebrovascular (ser-e-bro-VAS-ku-lar) **accident** (CVA) Condition involving obstruction of blood flow to brain tissue or bleeding into brain tissue, usually as a result of hypertension or atherosclerosis; stroke.

cerebrum (SER-e-brum) Largest part of the brain; composed of two cerebral hemispheres.

cerumen (seh-RU-men) Earwax; adj., ceruminous (seh-RU-min-us).

cervix (SER-vix) Constricted portion of an organ or part, such as the lower portion of the uterus; neck; adj., cervical.

chemistry (KEM-is-tre) Study of the composition and properties of matter.

chemoreceptor (ke-mo-re-SEP-tor) Receptor that responds to chemicals in body fluids.

chemotherapy (ke-mo-THER-ah-pe) Treatment of a disease by administration of a chemical agent.

Cheyne-Stokes (CHANE-stokes) **respiration** Rhythmic variation in the depth of respiratory movements alternating with periods of apnea due to depression of the breathing centers.

chlamydia (klah-MID-e-ah) Type of very small bacterium that can exist only within a living cell; members of this group cause inclusion conjunctivitis, trachoma, sexually transmitted infections, and respiratory diseases.

cholecystokinin (ko-le-sis-to-KI-nin) (CCK) Duodenal hormone that stimulates release of pancreatic enzymes and bile from the gallbladder.

cholelithiasis (ko-le-lih-THI-ah-sis) Gallstones.

cholesterol (ko-LES-ter-ol) Organic fatlike compound found in animal fat, bile, blood, myelin, liver, and other parts of the body.

cholinergic (ko-lin-ER-jik) Activity or structure that responds to acetylcholine.

chondrocyte (KON-dro-site) Cell that produces cartilage.

chordae tendineae (KOR-de ten-DIN-e-e) Fibrous threads that stabilize the heart's AV valve flaps.

choriocarcinoma (ko-re-o-kar-sih-NO-mah) Very malignant tumor made of placental tissue.

choroid (KO-royd) Pigmented middle layer of the eye.

choroid plexus (KO-royd PLEKS-us) Vascular network in the brain's ventricles that forms cerebrospinal fluid.

chromosome (KRO-mo-some) Dark-staining, threadlike body in a cell's nucleus; contains genes that determine hereditary traits.

chronic (KRON-ik) Referring to a disease that develops slowly, persists over a long time, or is recurring.

chyle (kile) Milky-appearing fluid absorbed into the lymphatic system from the small intestine. It consists of lymph and droplets of digested fat.

chyme (kime) Mixture of partially digested food, water, and digestive juices that forms in the stomach.

cicatrix (SIK-ah-trix) Scar.

cilia (SIL-e-ah) Hairs or hairlike processes, such as eyelashes or microscopic extensions from a cell's surface; sing., cilium.

ciliary (SIL-e-ar-e) **muscle** Eye muscle that controls the shape of the lens.

circumduction (ser-kum-DUK-shun) Circular movement at a joint.

circumcision (sir-kum-SIJ-un) Surgery to remove the foreskin of the penis.

cirrhosis (sih-RO-sis) Chronic disease, usually of the liver, in which active cells are replaced by inactive scar tissue.

cisterna chyli (sis-TER-nah KI-li) First part of the thoracic lymph duct, which is enlarged to form a temporary storage area.

CK See creatine kinase.

clitoris (KLIT-o-ris) Small organ of great sensitivity in the external genitalia of the female.

CNS See central nervous system.

coagulation (ko-ag-u-LA-shun) Clotting, as of blood.

coccus (KOK-us) Round bacterium; pl., cocci (KOK-si).

cochlea (KOK-le-ah) Coiled portion of the inner ear that contains the organ of hearing.

colic (KOL-ik) Spasm of visceral muscle.

collagen (KOL-ah-jen) Flexible white protein that gives strength and resilience to connective tissue, such as bone and cartilage.

colloid (kol-OYD) Mixture in which suspended particles do not dissolve but remain distributed in the solvent because of their small size (e.g., cytoplasm); colloidal suspension.

colon (KO-lon) Main portion of the large intestine.

colostrum (ko-LOS-trum) Secretion of the mammary glands released prior to secretion of milk.

communicable (kom-MU-nih-kabl) Capable of being transmitted from one person to another, such as disease; contagious.

complement (KOM-ple-ment) Group of blood proteins that helps antibodies to destroy foreign cells.

compliance (kom-PLI-ans) The ease with which the lungs and thorax can be expanded.

compound Substance composed of two or more chemical elements.

computed tomography (to-MOG-rah-fe) **(CT)** Imaging method in which multiple radiographic views taken from different angles are analyzed by computer to show an area cross-section; used to detect tumors and other abnormalities; also called computed axial tomography (CAT).

concha (KON-ka) Shell-like bone in the nasal cavity; pl., conchae (KON-ke).

concussion (kon-CUSH-on) Injury resulting from a violent blow or shock.

condyle (KON-dile) Rounded projection, as on a bone.

cone Receptor cell in the eye's retina; used for vision in bright light.

congenital (con-JEN-ih-tal) Present at birth.

conjunctiva (kon-junk-TI-vah) Membrane that lines the eyelid and covers the anterior part of the sclera (white of the eye).

constipation (kon-stih-PA-shun) Infrequency of or difficulty with defecation.

contraception (con-trah-SEP-shun) Prevention of an ovum's fertilization or implantation of a fertilized ovum; birth control.

convergence (kon-VER-jens) The centering of both eyes on the same visual field.

convulsion (kon-VUL-shun) Series of muscle spasms; seizure.

Cooley anemia Severe form of β thalassemia, a hereditary blood disorder that impairs hemoglobin formation.

cornea (KOR-ne-ah) Clear portion of the sclera that covers the anterior of the eye.

coronary (KOR-on-ar-e) Referring to the heart or to the arteries supplying blood to the heart.

coronary thrombosis (throm-BO-sis) Formation of a blood clot in a vessel of the heart.

corpus callosum (kal-O-sum) Thick bundle of myelinated nerve cell fibers, deep within the brain, that carries nerve impulses from one cerebral hemisphere to the other.

corpus luteum (LU-te-um) Yellow body formed from ovarian follicle after ovulation; produces progesterone.

cortex (KOR-tex) Outer layer of an organ, such as the brain, kidney, or adrenal gland.

coryza (ko-RI-zah) Nasal discharge; acute coryza is the common cold.

countercurrent mechanism Mechanism for concentrating urine as it flows through the distal nephron.

covalent (KO-va-lent) **bond** Chemical bond formed by the sharing of electrons between atoms.

CPR See cardiopulmonary resuscitation.

cranial (KRA-ne-al) Pertaining to the cranium, the part of the skull that encloses the brain; toward the head or nearer to the head.

creatine (KRE-ah-tin) **phosphate** Compound in muscle tissue that stores energy in high energy bonds.

creatinine (kre-AT-ih-nin) Nitrogenous waste product eliminated in urine.

creatine kinase (CK) (KRE-ah-tin KI-nase) Enzyme in muscle cells that is released in increased amounts when muscle tissue is damaged; the form specific to cardiac muscle cells is creatine kinase MB (CK-MB).

crenation (kre-NA-shun) Shrinking of a cell, as when placed in a hypertonic solution.

crista (KRIS-tah) Receptor for the sense of dynamic equilibrium; pl., cristae.

croup (krupe) Loud barking cough associated with upper respiratory infection in children.

cryoprecipitate (kri-o-pre-SIP-ih-tate) Precipitate formed when plasma is frozen and then thawed.

cryptorchidism (kript-OR-kid-izm) Failure of the testis to descend into the scrotum; undescended testicle.

CSF See cerebrospinal fluid.

CT See computed tomography.

Cushing syndrome Condition caused by overactivity of the adrenal cortex.

cutaneous (ku-TA-ne-us) Referring to the skin.

cuticle (KU-tih-kl) Extension of the stratum corneum that seals the space between the nail plate and the skin above the nail root.

cyanosis (si-ah-NO-sis) Bluish discoloration of the skin and mucous membranes resulting from insufficient oxygen in the blood.

cystic (SIS-tik) **duct** Duct that carries bile into and out of the gallbladder.

cystic fibrosis (SIS-tik fi-BRO-sis) Hereditary disease involving thickened secretions and electrolyte imbalances.

cystitis (sis-TI-tis) Inflammation of the urinary bladder.

cytology (si-TOL-o-je) Study of cells.

cytoplasm (SI-to-plazm) Substance that fills the cell, consisting of a liquid cytosol and organelles.

cytosol (SI-to-sol) Liquid portion of the cytoplasm, consisting of nutrients, minerals, enzymes and other materials in water.

D

deamination (de-am-ih-NA-shun) Removal of amino groups from proteins in metabolism.

decubitus (de-KU-bih-tus) Lying down.

defecation (def-eh-KA-shun) Act of eliminating undigested waste from the digestive tract.

degeneration (de-jen-er-A-shun) Breakdown, as from age, injury, or disease.

deglutition (deg-lu-TISH-un) Act of swallowing.

dehydration (de-hi-DRA-shun) Excessive loss of body fluid.

dementia (de-MEN-she-ah) Gradual and usually irreversible loss of intellectual function.

denaturation (de-nah-tu-RA-shun) Change in structure of a protein, such as an enzyme, so that it can no longer function.

dendrite (DEN-drite) Neuron fiber that conducts impulses toward the cell body.

deoxyribonucleic (de-OK-se-ri-bo-nu-kle-ik) **acid (DNA)** Genetic material of the cell; makes up the chromosomes in the cell's nucleus.

depolarization (de-po-lar-ih-ZA-shun) Sudden reversal of the charge on a cell membrane.

dermal papillae (pah-PIL-le) Extensions of the dermis that project up into the epidermis; they contain blood vessels that supply the epidermis.

dermatitis (der-mah-TI-tis) Inflammation of the skin.

dermatome (DER-mah-tome) A region of the skin supplied by a single spinal nerve.

dermatosis (der-mah-to-sis) Any skin disease.

dermis (DER-mis) True skin; deeper part of the skin.

dextrose (DEK-strose) Glucose, a simple sugar.

diabetes insipidus (in-SIP-ih-dus) Condition due to insufficient ADH secretion by the posterior pituitary; there is excessive water loss.

diabetes mellitus (di-ah-BE-teze mel-LI-tus) Disease of insufficient insulin in which excess glucose is found in blood and urine; characterized by abnormal metabolism of glucose, protein, and fat.

diagnosis (di-ag-NO-sis) Identification of an illness.

dialysis (di-AL-ih-sis) Method for separating molecules in solution based on differences in their ability to pass through a semipermeable membrane; method for removing nitrogenous waste products from the body, as by hemodialysis or peritoneal dialysis.

diaphragm (DI-ah-fram) Dome-shaped muscle under the lungs that flattens during inhalation; separating membrane or structure.

diaphysis (di-AF-ih-sis) Shaft of a long bone.

diarrhea (di-ah-RE-ah) Abnormally frequent watery bowel movements.

diarthrosis (di-ar-THRO-sis) Freely movable joint; synovial joint.

diastole (di-AS-to-le) Relaxation phase of the cardiac cycle; adj., diastolic (di-as-TOL-ik).

diencephalon (di-en-SEF-ah-lon) Region of the brain between the cerebral hemispheres and the midbrain; contains the thalamus, hypothalamus, and pituitary gland.

diffusion (dih-FU-zhun) Movement of molecules from a region where they are in higher concentration to a region where they are in lower concentration.

digestion (di-JEST-yun) Process of breaking down food into absorbable particles.

digestive system (di-JES-tiv) The system involved in taking in nutrients, converting them to a form the body can use, and absorbing them into the circulation.

dihydroxycholecalciferol (di-hi-drok-se-ko-le-kal-SIF-eh-rol) The active form of vitamin D.

dilation (di-LA-shun) Widening of a part, such as the pupil of the eye, a blood vessel, or the uterine cervix; dilatation.

disaccharide (di-SAK-ah-ride) Compound formed of two simple sugars linked together, such as sucrose and lactose.

disease Illness; abnormal state in which part or all of the body does not function properly.

disinfection (dis-in-FEK-shun) Killing of pathogens but not necessarily harmless microbes.

dissect (dis-sekt) To cut apart or separate tissues for study.

distal (DIS-tal) Farther from a structure's origin or from a given reference point.

diverticulosis (di-ver-tik-u-LO-sis) Presence of diverticuli (small pouches) in the intestinal wall.

DNA See deoxyribonucleic acid.

dominant (DOM-ih-nant) Referring to a gene that is always expressed if present.

dopamine (DO-pah-mene) A neurotranmitter.

dorsal (DOR-sal) Toward the back; posterior.

dorsiflexion (dor-sih-FLEK-shun) Bending the foot upward at the ankle.

Down syndrome A congenital disorder usually due to an extra chromosome 21; trisomy 21.

duct Tube or vessel.

ductus arteriosus (DUK-tus ar-te-re-O-sus) Small vessel in the fetus that carries blood from the pulmonary artery to the descending aorta.

ductus deferens (DEF-er-enz) Tube that carries sperm cells from the testis to the urethra; vas deferens.

ductus venosus (ve-NO-sus) Small vessel in the fetus that carries blood from the umbilical vein to the inferior vena cava.

duodenum (du-o-DE-num) First portion of the small intestine.

dura mater (DU-rah MA-ter) Outermost layer of the meninges.

dysmenorrhea (dis-men-o-RE-ah) Painful or difficult menstruation.

dyspnea (disp-NE-ah) Difficult or labored breathing.

E

eccrine (EK-rin) Referring to sweat glands that regulate body temperature and vent directly to the surface of the skin through a pore.

ECG See electrocardiograph.

echocardiograph (ek-o-KAR-de-o-graf) Instrument to study the heart by means of ultrasound; the record produced is an echocardiogram.

eclampsia (eh-KLAMP-se-ah) Serious and sometimes fatal condition involving convulsions, liver damage, and kidney failure that can develop from pregnancy-induced hypertension.

ectopic (ek-TOP-ik) Out of a normal place, as a pregnancy or heartbeat.

eczema (EK-ze-mah) See atopic dermatitis.

edema (eh-DE-mah) Accumulation of fluid in the tissue spaces.

EEG See electroencephalograph.

effector (ef-FEK-tor) Muscle or gland that responds to a stimulus; effector organ.

efferent (EF-fer-ent) Carrying away from a given point, such as a motor neuron that carries nerve impulses away from the central nervous system.

effusion (eh-FU-zhun) Escape of fluid into a cavity or space; the fluid itself.

ejaculation (e-jak-u-LA-shun) Expulsion of semen through the urethra.

EKG See electrocardiograph.

electrocardiograph (e-lek-tro-KAR-de-o-graf) **(ECG, EKG)** Instrument to study the heart's electrical activity; record made is an electrocardiogram.

electroencephalograph '(e-lek-tro-en-SEF-ah-lo-graf) **(EEG)** Instrument used to study the brain's electrical activity; record made is an electroencephalogram.

electrolyte (e-LEK-tro-lite) Compound that separates into ions in solution; substance that conducts an electrical current in solution.

electron (e-LEK-tron) Negatively charged particle located in an energy level outside an atom's nucleus.

electrophoresis (e-lek-tro-fo-RE-sis) Separation of components in a mixture by passing an electrical current through it; components separate on the basis of their charge.

element (EL-eh-ment) One of the substances from which all matter is made; substance that cannot be decomposed into a simpler substance.

elephantiasis (el-eh-fan-TI-ah-sis) Enlargement of the extremities due to blockage of lymph flow by small filariae (fi-LA-re-e) worms.

embolism (EM-bo-lizm) The condition of having an embolus (obstruction in the circulation).

embolus (EM-bo-lus) Blood clot or other obstruction in the circulation.

embryo (EM-bre-o) Developing offspring during the first 2 months of pregnancy.

emesis (EM-eh-sis) Vomiting.

emphysema (em-fih-SE-mah) Pulmonary disease characterized by dilation and destruction of the alveoli.

emulsify (e-MUL-sih-fi) To break up fats into small particles; n., emulsification.

endarterectomy (end-ar-ter-EK-to-me) Procedure to remove plaque associated with atherosclerosis from a vessel's lining.

endocardium (en-do-KAR-de-um) Membrane that lines the heart chambers and covers the valves.

endocrine (EN-do-krin) Referring to a gland that secretes directly into the bloodstream.

endocrine system The system composed of glands that secrete hormones.

endocytosis (en-do-si-TO-sis) Movement of large amounts of material into a cell (e.g., phagocytosis and pinocytosis).

endolymph (EN-do-limf) Fluid that fills the membranous labyrinth of the inner ear.

endomysium (en-do-MIS-e-um) Connective tissue around an individual muscle fiber.

endometrium (en-do-ME-tre-um) Lining of the uterus.

endoplasmic reticulum (en-do-PLAS-mik re-TIK-u-lum) **(ER)** Network of membranes in the cellular cytoplasm; may be smooth or rough based on absence or presence of ribosomes.

end-organ Modified ending on a dendrite that functions as a sensory receptor.

endorphin (en-DOR-fin) Pain-relieving substance released naturally from the brain.

endosteum (en-DOS-te-um) Thin membrane that lines a bone's marrow cavity.

endothelium (en-do-THE-le-um) Epithelium that lines the heart, blood vessels, and lymphatic vessels.

enucleation (e-nu-kle-A-shun) Removal of the eyeball.

enzyme (EN-zime) Organic catalyst; speeds the rate of a reaction but is not changed in the reaction.

eosinophil (e-o-SIN-o-fil) Granular white blood cell that shows beadlike, bright pink cytoplasmic granules when stained with acid stain; acidophil.

epicardium (ep-ih-KAR-de-um) Membrane that forms the heart wall's outermost layer and is continuous with the lining of the fibrous pericardium; visceral pericardium.

epicondyle (ep-ih-KON-dile) Small projection on a bone above a condyle.

epidemic (ep-ih-DEM-ik) Occurrence of a disease among many people in a given region at the same time.

epidermis (ep-ih-DER-mis) Outermost layer of the skin.

epididymis (ep-ih-DID-ih-mis) Coiled tube on the surface of the testis in which sperm cells are stored and in which they mature.

epigastric (ep-ih-GAS-trik) Pertaining to the region just inferior to the sternum (breastbone).

epiglottis (ep-e-GLOT-is) Leaf-shaped cartilage that covers the larynx during swallowing.

epilepsy (EP-ih-lep-se) Chronic neurologic disorder involving abnormal electrical activity of the brain; characterized by seizures of varying severity.

epimysium (ep-ih-MIS-e-um) Sheath of fibrous connective tissue that encloses a muscle.

epinephrine (ep-ih-NEF-rin) Neurotransmitter and hormone; released from neurons of the sympathetic nervous system and from the adrenal medulla; adrenaline.

epiphysis (eh-PIF-ih-sis) End of a long bone; adj., epiphyseal (ep-ih-FIZ-e-al).

episiotomy (eh-piz-e-OT-o-me) Cutting of the perineum between the vaginal opening and the anus to reduce tissue tearing in childbirth.

epistaxis (ep-e-STAK-sis) Nosebleed.

epithelium (ep-ih-THE-le-um) One of the four main types of tissue; forms glands, covers surfaces, and lines cavities; adj., epithelial.

EPO See erythropoietin.

equilibrium (e-kwih-LIB-re-um) Sense of balance.

ER See endoplasmic reticulum.

eruption (e-RUP-shun) Raised skin lesion; rash.

erythema (er-eh-THE-mah) Redness of the skin.

erythrocyte (eh-RITH-ro-site) Red blood cell.

erythropoietin (EPO) (eh-rith-ro-POY-eh-tin) Hormone released from the kidney that stimulates red blood cell production in the red bone marrow.

esophagus (eh-SOF-ah-gus) Muscular tube that carries food from the throat to the stomach.

estrogen (ES-tro-jen) Group of female sex hormones that promotes development of the uterine lining and maintains secondary sex characteristics.

etiology (e-te-OL-o-je) Study of a disease's cause or the theory of its origin.

eustachian (u-STA-shun) **tube** Tube that connects the middle ear cavity to the throat; auditory tube.

eversion (e-VER-zhun) Turning outward, with reference to movement of the foot.

excitability In cells, the ability to transmit an electrical current along the plasma membrane.

excoriation (eks-ko-re-A-shun) Scratch into the skin.

excretion (eks-KRE-shun) Removal and elimination of metabolic waste products from the blood.

exfoliation (eks-fo-le-A-shun) Loss of cells from the surface of tissue, such as the skin.

exhalation (eks-hah-LA-shun) Expulsion of air from the lungs; expiration.

exocrine (EK-so-krin) Referring to a gland that secretes through a duct.

exocytosis (eks-o-si-TO-sis) Movement of large amounts of material out of the cell using vesicles.

exophthalmos (ek-sof-THAL-mos) Protrusion (bulging) of the eyes, commonly seen in Graves disease.

extension (eks-TEN-shun) Motion that increases the angle at a joint.

extracellular (EK-strah-sel-u-lar) Outside the cell.

extremity (ek-STREM-ih-te) Limb; an arm or leg.

exudate (EKS-u-date) Any fluid or semisolid that oozes out of tissue, particularly as a result of injury or inflammation.

F

facilitated diffusion Movement of material across the plasma membrane as it would normally flow by diffusion but using transporters to speed movement.

fallopian (fah-LO-pe-an) **tube** See oviduct.

fascia (FASH-e-ah) Band or sheet of fibrous connective tissue.

fascicle (FAS-ih-kl) Small bundle, as of muscle cells or nerve cell fibers.

fat Type of lipid composed of glycerol and fatty acids; triglyceride.

febrile (FEB-ril) Pertaining to fever.

fecalith (FE-kah-lith) Hardened piece of fecal material that may cause obstruction.

feces (FE-seze) Waste material discharged from the large intestine; excrement; stool.

feedback Return of information into a system, so that it can be used to regulate that system.

fertilization (fer-til-ih-ZA-shun) Union of an ovum and a spermatozoon.

fetus (FE-tus) Developing offspring from the third month of pregnancy until birth.

fever (FE-ver) Abnormally high body temperature.

fibrillation (fih-brih-LA-shun) Very rapid, uncoordinated beating of the heart.

fibrin (FI-brin) Blood protein that forms a blood clot.

fibrinogen (fi-BRIN-o-jen) Plasma protein that is converted to fibrin in blood clotting.

filtration (fil-TRA-shun) Movement of material through a semipermeable membrane under mechanical force.

fimbriae (FIM-bre-e) Fringelike extensions of the oviduct that sweep a released ovum into the oviduct.

fissure (FISH-ure) Deep groove.

flaccid (FLAK-sid) Flabby, limp, soft.

flagellum (flah-JEL-lum) Long whiplike extension from a cell used for locomotion; pl., flagella.

flatus (FLA-tus) Gas in the digestive tract; condition of having gas is flatulence (FLAT-u-lens).

flexion (FLEK-shun) Bending motion that decreases the angle between bones at a joint.

follicle (FOL-ih-kl) Sac or cavity, such as the ovarian follicle or hair follicle.

follicle-stimulating hormone (FSH) Hormone produced by the anterior pituitary that stimulates development of ova in the ovary and spermatozoa in the testes.

fontanel (fon-tah-NEL) Membranous area in the infant skull where bone has not yet formed; also spelled fontanelle; "soft spot."

foramen (fo-RA-men) Opening or passageway, as into or through a bone; pl., foramina (fo-RAM-in-ah).

foramen magnum Large opening in the skull's occipital bone through which the spinal cord passes to join the brain.

foramen ovale (o-VA-le) Small hole in the fetal atrial septum that allows blood to pass directly from the right atrium to the left atrium.

formed elements Cells and cell fragments in the blood.

fornix (FOR-niks) A recess or archlike structure.

fossa (FOS-sah) Hollow or depression, as in a bone; pl., fossae (FOS-se).

fovea (FO-ve-ah) Small pit or cup-shaped depression in a surface; the fovea centralis near the center of the retina is the point of sharpest vision.

fragile (FRAH-jil) **X syndrome** Hereditary form of mental retardation; x-linked recessive disorder that appears in both males and females.

frontal (FRONT-al) Describing a plane that divides a structure into anterior and posterior parts.

FSH See follicle-stimulating hormone.

fulcrum (FUL-krum) Pivot point in a lever system; joint in the skeletal system.

fundus (FUN-dus) The deepest portion of an organ, such as the eye or the uterus.

fungus (FUN-gus) Type of plantlike microorganism; yeast or mold; pl., fungi (FUN-ji).

G

gallbladder (GAWL-blad-er) Muscular sac on the inferior surface of the liver that stores bile.

gamete (GAM-ete) Reproductive cell; ovum or spermatozoon.

gamma globulin (GLOB-u-lin) Protein fraction in the blood plasma that contains antibodies.

ganglion (GANG-le-on) Collection of nerve cell bodies located outside the central nervous system.

gangrene (GANG-grene) Death of tissue accompanied by bacterial invasion and putrefaction.

gastric-inhibitory peptide (GIP) Duodenal hormone that inhibits release of gastric juice and stimulates insulin release from the pancreas.

gastrin (GAS-trin) Hormone released from the stomach that stimulates stomach activity.

gastrointestinal (gas-tro-in-TES-tih-nal) **(GI)** Pertaining to the stomach and intestine or the digestive tract as a whole.

gene Hereditary factor; portion of the DNA on a chromosome.

genetic (jeh-NET-ik) Pertaining to the genes or heredity.

genitalia (jen-ih-TA-le-ah) Reproductive organs, both external and internal.

genotype (JEN-o-tipe) Genetic make-up of an organism.

gestation (jes-TA-shun) Period of development from conception to birth.

GH See growth hormone.

GI See gastrointestinal.

gigantism (ji-GAN-tizm) Excessive growth due to oversecretion of growth hormone in childhood.

gingiva (JIN-jih-vah) Tissue around the teeth; gum.

glans Enlarged distal portion of the penis.

glaucoma (glaw-KO-mah) Disorder involving increased fluid pressure within the eye.

glial cells (GLI-al) Cells that support and protect the nervous system; neuroglia.

glioma (gli-O-mah) Tumor of neuroglial tissue.

glomerular (glo-MER-u-lar) **filtrate** Fluid and dissolved materials that leave the blood and enter the kidney nephron through the glomerular (Bowman) capsule.

glomerulonephritis (glo-mer-u-lo-nef-RI-tis) Kidney disease often resulting from antibodies to a streptococcal infection.

glomerulus (glo-MER-u-lus) Cluster of capillaries in the nephron's glomerular (Bowman) capsule.

glottis (GLOT-is) Space between the vocal cords.

glucagon (GLU-kah-gon) Hormone from the pancreatic islets that raises blood glucose level.

glucocorticoid (glu-ko-KOR-tih-koyd) Steroid hormone from the adrenal cortex that raises nutrients in the blood during times of stress, e.g., cortisol.

glucose (GLU-kose) Simple sugar; main energy source for the cells; dextrose.

glycemic (gli-SE-mik) **effect** Measure of how rapidly a food raises the blood glucose level and stimulates release of insulin.

glycogen (GLI-ko-jen) Compound built from glucose molecules that is stored for energy in liver and muscles.

glycolysis (gli-KOL-ih-sis) First, anaerobic phase of the metabolic breakdown of glucose for energy.

glycosuria (gli-ko-SU-re-ah) Presence of glucose in the urine.

goblet cell Single-celled gland that secretes mucus.

goiter (GOY-ter) Enlargement of the thyroid gland.

Golgi (GOL-je) **apparatus** System of cellular membranes that formulates special substances; also called Golgi complex.

gonad (GO-nad) Sex gland; ovary or testis.

gonadotropin (gon-ah-do-TRO-pin) Hormone that acts on a reproductive gland (ovary or testis) e.g., FSH, LH.

gout Type of arthritis caused by a metabolic disturbance.

Graafian (GRAF-e-an) **follicle** See ovarian follicle.

gram (g) Basic unit of weight in the metric system.

gram stain Procedure used to color microorganisms for viewing under the microscope.

granulocyte (GRAN-u-lo-site) Leukocyte with visible granules in the cytoplasm when stained.

Graves disease Common form of hyperthyroidism.

gray matter Nervous tissue composed of unmyelinated fibers and cell bodies.

greater vestibular (ves-TIB-u-lar) **gland** Gland that secretes mucus into the vagina; Bartholin gland.

growth hormone (GH) Hormone produced by anterior pituitary that promotes tissue growth; somatotropin.

gustation (gus-TA-shun) Sense of taste; adj., gustatory.

gyrus (JI-rus) Raised area of the cerebral cortex; pl., gyri (JI-ri).

H

Haversian (ha-VER-shan) **canal** Channel in the center of an osteon (Haversian system), a subunit of compact bone.

Haversian system See osteon.

hay fever Seasonal allergy often due to pollen.

heart (hart) Organ that pumps blood through the cardiovascular system.

helminth (HEL-minth) Worm.

hemapheresis (hem-ah-fer-E-sis) Return of blood components to a donor following separation and removal of desired components.

hematocrit (he-MAT-o-krit) **(Hct)** Volume percentage of red blood cells in whole blood; packed cell volume.

hematoma (he-mah-TO-mah) Tumor or swelling filled with blood.

hematuria (hem-ah-TU-re-ah) Blood in the urine.

hemocytometer (he-mo-si-TOM-eh-ter) Device used to count blood cells under the microscope.

hemodialysis (he-mo-di-AL-ih-sis) Removal of impurities from the blood by their passage through a semipermeable membrane in a fluid bath.

hemoglobin (he-mo-GLO-bin) **(Hb)** Iron-containing protein in red blood cells that binds oxygen.

hemolysis (he-MOL-ih-sis) Rupture of red blood cells; v., hemolyze (HE-mo-lize).

hemolytic (he-mo-LIT-ik) **disease of the newborn** (HDN) Condition that results from Rh incompatibility between a mother and her fetus; erythroblastosis fetalis.

hemophilia (he-mo-FIL-e-ah) Hereditary bleeding disorder associated with a lack of clotting factors in the blood.

hemopoiesis (he-mo-poy-E-sis) Production of blood cells; hematopoiesis.

hemorrhage (HEM-eh-rij) Loss of blood.

hemorrhoids (HEM-o-royds) Varicose veins in the rectum.

hemostasis (he-mo-STA-sis) Stoppage of bleeding.

hemothorax (he-mo-THOR-aks) Accumulation of blood in the pleural space.

heparin (HEP-ah-rin) Substance that prevents blood clotting; anticoagulant.

hepatitis (hep-ah-TI-tis) Inflammation of the liver.

heredity (he-RED-ih-te) Transmission of characteristics from parent to offspring by means of the genes; the genetic makeup of the individual.

hereditary (he-RED-ih-tar-e) Transmitted or transmissible through the genes; familial.

hernia (HER-ne-ah) Protrusion of an organ or tissue through the wall of the cavity in which it is normally enclosed.

heterozygous (het-er-o-ZI-gus) Having unmatched alleles for a given trait; hybrid.

hilum (HI-lum) Indented region of an organ where vessels and nerves enter or leave.

hippocampus (hip-o-KAM-pus) Sea horse–shaped region of the limbic system that functions in learning and formation of long-term memory.

histamine (HIS-tah-mene) Substance released from tissues during an antigen–antibody reaction.

histology (his-TOL-o-je) Study of tissues.

HIV See human immunodeficiency virus.

Hodgkin disease Chronic malignant disease of lymphoid tissue.

homeostasis (ho-me-o-STA-sis) State of balance within the body; maintenance of body conditions within set limits.

homozygous (ho-mo-ZI-gus) Having identical alleles for a given trait; purebred.

hormone Secretion of an endocrine gland; chemical messenger that has specific regulatory effects on certain other cells.

host An organism in or on which a parasite lives.

human chorionic gonadotropin (ko-re-ON-ik gon-ah-do-TRO-pin) **(hCG)** Hormone produced by embryonic cells soon after implantation that maintains the corpus luteum.

human immunodeficiency virus (HIV) Virus that causes AIDS.

human placental lactogen (hPL) Hormone produced by the placenta that prepares the breasts for lactation and maintains nutrient levels in maternal blood.

humoral (HU-mor-al) Pertaining to body fluids, such as immunity based on antibodies circulating in the blood.

Huntington disease Progressive degenerative disorder carried by a dominant gene.

hyaline (HI-ah-lin) Clear, glasslike; referring to a type of cartilage.

hydatidiform (hi-dah-TID-ih-form) **mole** Benign overgrowth of placental tissue.

hydrocephalus (hi-dro-SEF-ah-lus) Abnormal accumulation of CSF within the brain.

hydrolysis (hi-DROL-ih-sis) Splitting of large molecules by the addition of water, as in digestion.

hydrophilic (hi-dro-FIL-ik) Mixing with or dissolving in water, such as salts; literally "water-loving."

hydrophobic (hi-dro-FO-bik) Repelling and not dissolving in water, such as fats; literally "water-fearing."

hymen Fold of membrane near the opening of the vaginal canal.

hypercapnia (hi-per-KAP-ne-ah) Increased level of carbon dioxide in the blood.

hyperglycemia (hi-per-gli-SE-me-ah) Abnormal increase in the amount of glucose in the blood.

hyperopia (hi-per-O-pe-ah) Farsightedness.

hyperpnea (hi-PERP-ne-ah) Abnormal increase in the depth and rate of breathing.

hypersensitivity (hi-per-SEN-sih-tiv-ih-te) Exaggerated reaction of the immune system to a substance that is normally harmless to most people; allergy.

hypertension (hi-per-TEN-shun) High blood pressure.

hypertonic (hi-per-TON-ik) Describing a solution that is more concentrated than the fluids within a cell.

hypertrophy (hy-PER-tro-fe) Enlargement or overgrowth of an organ or part.

hyperventilation (hi-per-ven-tih-LA-shun) Increased amount of air entering the alveoli of the lungs due to deep and rapid respiration.

hypocapnia (hi-po-KAP-ne-ah) Decreased level of carbon dioxide in the blood.

hypochondriac (hi-po-KON-dre-ak) Pertaining to a region just inferior to the ribs.

hypogastric (hi-po-GAS-trik) Pertaining to an area inferior to the stomach or the most inferior midline region of the abdomen.

hypoglycemia (hi-po-gli-SE-me-ah) Abnormal decrease in the amount of glucose in the blood.

hypophysis (hi-POF-ih-sis) Pituitary gland.

hypopnea (hi-POP-ne-ah) Decrease in the rate and depth of breathing.

hypospadias (hi-po-SPA-de-as) Opening of the urethra on the undersurface of the penis.

hypotension (hi-po-TEN-shun) Low blood pressure.

hypothalamus (hi-po-THAL-ah-mus) Region of the brain that controls the pituitary and maintains homeostasis.

hypothermia (hi-po-THER-me-ah) Abnormally low body temperature.

hypotonic (hi-po-TON-ik) Describing a solution that is less concentrated than the fluids within a cell.

hypoventilation (hi-po-ven-tih-LA-shun) Insufficient amount of air entering the alveoli.

hypoxemia (hi-pok-SE-me-ah) Lower than normal concentration of oxygen in arterial blood.

hypoxia (hi-POK-se-ah) Lower than normal level of oxygen in the tissues.

hysterectomy (his-ter-EK-to-me) Surgical removal of the uterus.

I

iatrogenic (i-at-ro-JEN-ik) Resulting from the adverse effects of treatment.

idiopathic (id-e-o-PATH-ik) Describing a disease without known cause.

ileum (IL-e-um) Third portion of the small intestine.

ileus (IL-e-us) Intestinal obstruction caused by lack of peristalsis or by muscle contraction.

iliac (IL-e-ak) Pertaining to the ilium, the upper portion of the hipbone.

immunity (ih-MU-nih-te) Power of an individual to resist or overcome the effects of a particular disease or other harmful agent.

immunization (ih-mu-nih-ZA-shun) Use of a vaccine to produce immunity; vaccination.

immunodeficiency (im-u-no-de-FISH-en-se) Any failure of the immune system.

immunoglobulin (im-mu-no-GLOB-u-lin) **(Ig)** See antibody.

immunotherapy (im-mu-no-THER-a-pe) Stimulation of the immune system to fight disease, such as cancer.

impetigo (im-peh-TI-go) Acute, contagious staphylococcal or streptococcal skin infection.

implantation (im-plan-TA-shun) Embedding of a fertilized ovum into the uterine lining.

incidence (IN-sih-dense) In epidemiology, the number of new disease cases appearing in a particular population during a specific time period.

infarct (IN-farkt) Area of tissue damaged from lack of blood supply caused by a vessel blockage.

infection (in-FEK-shun) Invasion by pathogens.

infectious mononucleosis (mon-o-nu-kle-O-sis) Acute viral infection associated with enlargement of the lymph nodes.

inferior (in-FE-re-or) Below or lower.

inferior vena cava (VE-nah KA-vah) Large vein that drains the lower body and empties into the heart's right atrium.

infertility (in-fer-TIL-ih-te) Decreased ability to reproduce.

inflammation (in-flah-MA-shun) Response of tissues to injury; characterized by heat, redness, swelling, and pain.

influenza (in-flu-EN-zah) Acute contagious viral disease of the upper respiratory tract.

infundibulum (in-fun-DIB-u-lum) Stalk that connects the pituitary gland to the brain's hypothalamus.

ingestion (in-JES-chun) The intake of food.

inguinal (IN-gwih-nal) Pertaining to the groin region or the region of the inguinal canal.

inhalation (in-hah-LA-shun) Drawing of air into the lungs; inspiration.

insertion (in-SER-shun) Muscle attachment connected to a movable part.

insulin (IN-su-lin) Hormone from the pancreatic islets that lowers blood glucose level.

integument (in-TEG-u-ment) Skin; adj., integumentary.

integumentary system The skin and all its associated structures.

intercalated (in-TER-cah-la-ted) **disk** A modified plasma membrane in cardiac tissue that allows rapid transfer of electrical impulses between cells.

intercellular (in-ter-SEL-u-lar) Between cells.

intercostal (in-ter-KOS-tal) Between the ribs.

interferon (in-ter-FERE-on) **(IFN)** Group of substances released from virus-infected cells that prevent spread of infection to other cells; also nonspecifically boost the immune system.

interleukin (in-ter-LU-kin) Substance released by a T cell or macrophage that stimulates other cells of the immune system.

interneuron (in-ter-NU-ron) Nerve cell that transmits impulses within the central nervous system.

interphase (IN-ter-faze) Stage in a cell's life between one mitosis and the next when the cell is not dividing.

interstitial (in-ter-STISH-al) Between; pertaining to an organ's spaces or structures between active tissues.

intestine (in-TES-tin) Organ of the digestive tract between the stomach and the anus, consisting of the small and large intestine.

intracellular (in-trah-SEL-u-lar) Within a cell.

intussusception (in-tuh-suh-SEP-shun) Slipping of a part of the intestine into a part below it.

inversion (in-VER-zhun) Turning inward, with reference to movement of the foot.

ion (I-on) Charged particle formed when an electrolyte goes into solution.

ionic bond Chemical bond formed by the exchange of electrons between atoms.

iris (I-ris) Circular colored region of the eye around the pupil.

ischemia (is-KE-me-ah) Lack of blood supply to an area.

islets (I-lets) Groups of cells in the pancreas that produce hormones; islets of Langerhans (LAHNG-er-hanz).

isometric (i-so-MET-rik) **contraction** Muscle contraction in which there is no change in muscle length but an increase in muscle tension, as in pushing against an immovable force.

isotonic (i-so-TON-ik) Describing a solution that has the same concentration as the fluid within a cell.

isotonic contraction Muscle contraction in which the tone within the muscle remains the same but the muscle shortens to produce movement.

isotope (I-so-tope) Form of an element that has the same atomic number as another form of that element but a different atomic weight; isotopes differ in their numbers of neutrons.

isthmus (IS-mus) Narrow band, such as the band that connects the two lobes of the thyroid gland.

J

jaundice (JAWN-dis) Yellowish skin discoloration that is usually due to the presence of bile in the blood.

jejunum (je-JU-num) Second portion of the small intestine.

joint Area of junction between two or more bones; articulation.

juxtaglomerular (juks-tah-glo-MER-u-lar) **(JG) apparatus** Structure in the kidney composed of cells of the afferent arteriole and distal convoluted tubule that secretes the enzyme renin when blood pressure decreases below a certain level.

K

karyotype (KAR-e-o-tipe) Picture of the chromosomes arranged according to size and form.

keloid (KE-loyd) Mass or raised area that results from excess production of scar tissue.

keratin (KER-ah-tin) Protein that thickens and protects the skin; makes up hair and nails.

ketoacidosis (ke-to-as-ih-DO-sis) Acidosis that results from accumulation of ketone bodies in the blood.

kidney (KID-ne) Organ of excretion.

kilocalorie (kil-o-KAL-o-re) Measure of the energy content of food; technically, the amount of heat needed to raise l kg of water 1° centigrade.

kinesthesia (kin-es-THE-ze-ah) Sense of body movement.

Klinefelter (KLINE-fel-ter) **syndrome** Genetic disorder involving abnormal sex chromosomes, usually an extra X chromosome.

Kupffer (KOOP-fer) **cells** Macrophages in the liver that help to fight infection.

Kussmaul (KOOS-mowl) **respiration** Deep, rapid respiration characteristic of acidosis (overly acidic body fluids) as seen in uncontrolled diabetes.

kwashiorkor (kwash-e-OR-kor) Severe protein and energy malnutrition seen in children after weaning.

kyphosis (ki-FO-sis) Exaggerated lumbar curve of the spine.

L

labium (LA-be-um) Lip; pl., labia (LA-be-ah).

labyrinth (LAB-ih-rinth) Inner ear, named for its complex shape.

laceration (las-er-A-shun) Rough, jagged skin wound.

lacrimal (LAK-rih-mal) Referring to tears or the tear glands.

lacrimal apparatus lacrimal (tear) gland and its associated ducts.

lactation (lak-TA-shun) Secretion of milk.

lacteal (LAK-te-al) Lymphatic capillary that drains digested fats from the villi of the small intestine.

lactic (LAK-tik) **acid** Organic acid that accumulates in muscle cells functioning without oxygen.

laryngeal (lah-RIN-je-al) **pharynx** Lowest portion of the pharynx, opening into the larynx and esophagus.

larynx (LAR-inks) Structure between the pharynx and trachea that contains the vocal cords; voice box.

laser (LA-zer) Device that produces a very intense light beam.

lateral (LAT-er-al) Farther from the midline; toward the side.

lens Biconvex structure of the eye that changes in thickness to accommodate for near and far vision; crystalline lens.

leptin (LEP-tin) Hormone produced by adipocytes that aids in weight control by decreasing food intake and increasing energy expenditure.

lesion (LE-zhun) Wound or local injury.

leukemia (lu-KE-me-ah) Malignant blood disease characterized by abnormal development of white blood cells.

leukocyte (LU-ko-site) White blood cell.

leukocytosis (lu-ko-si-TO-sis) Increase in the number of white cells in the blood, such as during infection.

leukopenia (lu-ko-PE-ne-ah) Deficiency of leukocytes in the blood.

leukoplakia (lu-ko-PLA-ke-ah) Thickened white patches on the oral mucous membranes, often due to smoking.

LH See luteinizing hormone.

ligament (LIG-ah-ment) Band of connective tissue that connects a bone to another bone; thickened portion or fold of the peritoneum that supports an organ or attaches it to another organ.

limbic (LIM- bik) **system** Area between the brain's cerebrum and diencephalon that is involved in emotional states and behavior.

lipid (LIP-id) Type of organic compound, one example of which is a fat.

liter (LE-ter) **(L)** Basic unit of volume in the metric system; 1,000 mL; 1.06 qt.

lithotripsy (LITH-o-trip-se) Use of external shock waves to shatter stones (calculi).

liver (LIV-er) Large gland inferior to the diaphragm in the superior right abdomen; has many functions, including bile secretion, detoxification, storage, and interconversion of nutrients.

loop of Henle (HEN-le) Hairpin shaped segment of the renal tubule between the proximal and distal convoluted tubules; nephron loop.

lordosis (lor-DO-sis) Exaggerated lumbar curve of the spine.

lumbar (LUM-bar) Pertaining to the region of the spine between the thoracic vertebrae and the sacrum.

lumen (LU-men) Central opening of an organ or vessel.

lung Organ of respiration.

lunula (LU-nu-la) Pale half-moon shaped area at the proximal end of the nail.

lupus erythematosus (LU-pus er-ih-the-mah-TO-sis) Chronic inflammatory autoimmune disease that involves the skin and sometimes other organs.

luteinizing (LU-te-in-i-zing) **hormone (LH)** Hormone produced by the anterior pituitary that induces ovulation and formation of the corpus luteum in females; in males, it stimulates cells in the testes to produce testosterone.

lymph (limf) Fluid in the lymphatic system.

lymph node Mass of lymphoid tissue along the path of a lymphatic vessel that filters lymph and harbors white blood cells active in immunity.

lymphadenitis (lim-fad-en-I-tis) Inflammation of lymph nodes.

lymphadenopathy (lim-fad-en-OP-ah-the) Any disorder of lymph nodes.

lymphangitis (lim-fan-JI-tis) Inflammation of lymphatic vessels.

lymphatic duct (lim-FAH-tic) Vessel of the lymphatic system.

lymphatic system System consisting of the lymphatic vessels and lymphoid tissue; involved in immunity, digestion, and fluid balance.

lymphedema (lim-feh-DE-mah) Edema due to obstruction of lymph flow.

lymphocyte (LIM-fo-site) Agranular white blood cell that functions in immunity.

lymphoma (lim-FO-mah) Any tumor, benign or malignant, that occurs in lymphoid tissue.

lysosome (LI-so-some) Cell organelle that contains digestive enzymes.

M

macrophage (MAK-ro-faj) Large phagocytic cell that develops from a monocyte; presents antigen to lymphocytes in immune response.

macula (MAK-u-lah) Spot; flat, discolored spot on the skin, such as a freckle or measles lesion; also called macule; small yellow spot in the eye's retina that contains the fovea, the point of sharpest vision; receptor for the sense of static equilibrium.

magnetic resonance imaging (MRI) Method for studying tissue based on nuclear movement after exposure to radio waves in a powerful magnetic field.

major histocompatibility complex (MHC) Group of genes that codes for specific proteins (antigens) on cellular surfaces; these antigens are important in cross-matching for tissue transplantation; they are also important in immune reactions.

malignant (mah-LIG-nant) Describing a tumor that spreads; describing a disorder that tends to become worse and cause death.

malnutrition (mal-nu-TRISH-un) State resulting from lack of food, lack of an essential dietary component, or faulty use of food in the diet.

MALT Mucosal-associated lymphoid tissue; tissue in the mucous membranes that helps fight infection.

mammary (MAM-er-e) gland Breast.

mammogram (MAM-o-gram) Radiographic study of the breast.

maple syrup urine disease Recessive hereditary disease that affects amino acid metabolism and, among other symptoms, produces the smell of maple syrup in urine and on the body.

marasmus (mah-RAZ-mus) Severe malnutrition in infants.

mast cell White blood cell related to a basophil that is present in tissues; active in inflammatory and allergic reactions.

mastectomy (mas-TEK-to-me) Removal of the breast; mammectomy.

mastication (mas-tih-KA-shun) Act of chewing.

mastitis (mas-TI-tis) Inflammation of the breast.

matrix (MA-triks) The nonliving background material in a tissue; the intercellular material.

meatus (me-A-tus) Short channel or passageway, as in a bone.

medial (ME-de-al) Nearer the midline of the body.

mediastinum (me-de-as-TI-num) Region between the lungs and the organs and vessels it contains.

medulla (meh-DUL-lah) Inner region of an organ; marrow.

medullary (MED-u-lar-e) cavity Channel at the center of a long bone that contains bone marrow.

medulla oblongata (ob-long-GAH-tah) Part of the brain stem that connects the brain to the spinal cord.

megakaryocyte (meg-ah-KAR-e-o-site) Very large cell that gives rise to blood platelets.

meibomian (mi-BO-me-an) gland Gland that produces a secretion that lubricates the eyelashes.

meiosis (mi-O-sis) Process of cell division that halves the chromosome number in the formation of the reproductive cells.

melanin (MEL-ah-nin) Dark pigment found in skin, hair, parts of the eye, and certain parts of the brain.

melanocyte (MEL-ah-no-site) Cell that produces melanin.

melanoma (mel-ah-NO-mah) Malignant tumor of melanocytes.

melatonin (mel-ah-TO-nin) Hormone produced by the pineal gland.

membrane Thin sheet of tissue.

Mendelian (men-DE-le-en) laws Principles of heredity discovered by an Austrian monk named Gregor Mendel.

meninges (men-IN-jeze) Three layers of fibrous membranes that cover the brain and spinal cord.

menopause (MEN-o-pawz) Time during which menstruation ceases.

menses (MEN-seze) Monthly flow of blood from the female reproductive tract.

menstruation (men-stru-A-shun) The period of menstrual flow.

mesentery (MES-en-ter-e) Membranous peritoneal ligament that attaches the small intestine to the dorsal abdominal wall.

mesocolon (mes-o-KO-lon) Peritoneal ligament that attaches the colon to the dorsal abdominal wall.

mesothelium (mes-o-THE-le-um) Epithelial tissue found in serous membranes.

metabolic rate Rate at which energy is released from nutrients in the cells.

metabolic syndrome Condition related to type 2 diabetes mellitus with insulin resistance, obesity, hyperglycemia, high blood pressure, and metabolic disturbances; also called syndrome X.

metabolism (meh-TAB-o-lizm) All the physical and chemical processes by which an organism is maintained.

metaphase (MET-ah-faze) Second stage of mitosis, during which the chromosomes line up across the equator of the cell.

metarteriole (met-ar-TE-re-ole) Small vessel that connects the arterial system directly with the venous system in a blood shunt; thoroughfare channel.

metastasis (meh-TAS-tah-sis) Spread of tumor cells; pl., metastases (meh-TAS-tah-seze).

meter (ME-ter) (m) Basic unit of length in the metric system; 1.1 yards.

MHC See Major histocompatibility complex.

microbiology (mi-kro-bi-OL-o-je) Study of microscopic organisms.

micrometer (MI-kro-me-ter) (μm) 1/1,000th of a millimeter; micron; an instrument for measuring through a microscope (pronounced mi-KROM-eh-ter).

microorganism (mi-kro-OR-gan-izm) Microscopic organism.

microscope (MI-kro-skope) Magnifying instrument used to examine cells and other structures not visible with the naked eye; exam-ples are the compound light microscope, transmission electron microscope (TEM) and scanning electron microscope (SEM).

microvilli (mi-kro-VIL-li) Small projections of the plasma membrane that increase surface area; sing., microvillus.

micturition (mik-tu-RISH-un) Act of urination; voiding of the urinary bladder.

midbrain Upper portion of the brainstem.

mineral (MIN-er-al) Inorganic substance; in the diet, an element needed in small amounts for health.

mineralocorticoid (min-er-al-o-KOR-tih-koyd) Steroid hormone from the adrenal cortex that regulates electrolyte balance, e.g. aldosterone.

mitochondria (mi-to-KON-dre-ah) Cell organelles that manufacture ATP with the energy released from the oxidation of nutrients; sing., mitochondrion.

mitosis (mi-TO-sis) Type of cell division that produces two daughter cells exactly like the parent cell.

mitral (MI-tral) valve Valve between the heart's left atrium and left ventricle; left AV valve; bicuspid valve.

mixture Blend of two or more substances.

molecule (MOL-eh-kule) Particle formed by chemical bonding of two or more atoms; smallest subunit of a compound.

monocyte (MON-o-site) Phagocytic agranular white blood cell.

monosaccharide (mon-o-SAK-ah-ride) Simple sugar; basic unit of carbohydrates.

mortality (mor-TAL-ih-te) rate Percentage of a population that dies from a given disease within a given time period.

motor (MO-tor) Describing structures or activities involved in transmitting impulses away from the central nervous system; efferent.

motor end plate Region of a muscle cell membrane that receives nervous stimulation.

motor unit Group consisting of a single neuron and all the muscle fibers it stimulates.

mouth Proximal opening of the digestive tract where food is ingested, chewed, mixed with saliva, and swallowed.

MRI See magnetic resonance imaging.

mucosa (mu-KO-sah) Lining membrane that produces mucus; mucous membrane.

mucus (MU-kus) Thick protective fluid secreted by mucous membranes and glands; adj., mucous.

multiple (SKLE-ro-SIS) sclerosis Disease that affects the myelin sheath around axons leading to neuron degeneration.

murmur Abnormal heart sound.

muscle (MUS-l) Tissue that contracts to produce movement; includes skeletal, smooth, and cardiac types; adj., muscular.

muscular (MUS-ku-lar) system The system of skeletal muscles that moves the skeleton, supports and protects the organs, and maintains posture.

mutagen (MU-tah-jen) Agent that causes mutation; adj., mutagenic (mu-tah-JEN-ik).

mutation (mu-TA-shun) Change in a gene or a chromosome.

myalgia (mi-AL-je-ah) Muscular pain.

mycology (mi-KOL-o-je) Study of fungi (yeasts and molds).

myelin (MI-el-in) Fatty material that covers and insulates the axons of some neurons.

myocardium (mi-o-KAR-de-um) Middle layer of the heart wall; heart muscle.

myoglobin (MI-o-glo-bin) Compound that stores oxygen in muscle cells.

myoma (mi-O-mah) Usually benign tumor of the uterus; fibroma; fibroid.

myometrium (mi-o-ME-tre-um) Muscular layer of the uterus.

myopia (mi-O-pe-ah) Nearsightedness.

myosin (MI-o-sin) One of the two contractile proteins in muscle cells, the other being actin.

myxedema (mik-seh-DE-mah) Condition that results from hypothyroidism in adults.

N

narcotic (nar-KOT-ik) Drug that acts on the CNS to alter perception and response to pain.

nasopharynx (na-zo-FAR-inks) Upper portion of the pharynx located posterior to the nasal cavity.

natural killer (NK) cell Type of lymphocyte that can nonspecifically destroy abnormal cells.

naturopathy (na-chur-OP-a-the) Philosophy of helping people to heal themselves by developing healthy lifestyles.

nausea (NAW-ze-ah) Unpleasant sensation due to disturbance in the upper GI tract that may precede vomiting.

necrosis (neh-KRO-sis) Tissue death.

negative feedback Self-regulating system in which the result of an action is the control over that action; a method for keeping body conditions within a normal range and maintaining homeostasis.

neoplasm (NE-o-plazm) Abnormal growth of cells; tumor; adj., neoplastic.

nephron (NEF-ron) Microscopic functional unit of the kidney.

nephron loop Hairpin shaped segment of the renal tubule between the proximal and distal convoluted tubules; loop of Henle.

nerve Bundle of neuron fibers outside the central nervous system.

nerve impulse Electrical charge that spreads along the membrane of a neuron; action potential.

nervous system (NER-vus) The system that transports information in the body by means of electrical impulses.

neuralgia (nu-RAL-je-ah) Pain in a nerve.

neurilemma (nu-rih-LEM-mah) Thin sheath that covers certain peripheral axons; aids in axon regeneration.

neuritis (nu-RI-tis) Inflammation of a nerve, with pain, tenderness, and loss of sensation.

neuroglia (nu-ROG-le-ah) Supporting and protective cells of the nervous system; glial cells.

neuromuscular junction Point at which a nerve fiber contacts a muscle cell.

neuron (NU-ron) Conducting cell of the nervous system.

neurotransmitter (nu-ro-TRANS-mit-er) Chemical released from the ending of an axon that enables a nerve impulse to cross a synapse.

neutron (NU-tron) Noncharged particle in an atom's nucleus.

neutrophil (NU-tro-fil) Phagocytic granular white blood cell; polymorph; poly; PMN; seg.

nevus (NE-vus) Mole or birthmark.

nitrogen (NI-tro-jen) Chemical element found in all proteins.

node Small mass of tissue, such as a lymph node; space between cells in the myelin sheath.

norepinephrine (nor-epi-ih-NEF-rin) Neurotransmitter similar to epinephrine; noradrenaline.

normal saline Isotonic or physiologic salt solution.

nosocomial (nos-o-KO-me-al) Acquired in a hospital, as an infection.

nucleic acid (nu-KLE-ik) Complex organic substance composed of nucleotides that makes up DNA and RNA.

nucleolus (nu-KLE-o-lus) Small unit within the nucleus that assembles ribosomes.

nucleotide (NU-kle-o-tide) Building block of DNA and RNA.

nucleus (NU-kle-us) Largest cellular organelle, containing the DNA, which directs all cell activities; group of neurons in the central nervous system; in chemistry, the central part of an atom.

O

obstipation (ob-stih-PA-shun) Extreme constipation.

occlusion (ok-LU-zhun) Closing, as of a vessel.

olfaction (ol-FAK-shun) Sense of smell; adj., olfactory.

omentum (o-MEN-tum) Portion of the peritoneum; greater omentum extends over the anterior abdomen; lesser omentum extends between the stomach and liver.

oncology (on-KOL-o-je) Study of tumors.

ophthalmic (of-THAL-mik) Pertaining to the eye.

ophthalmoscope (of-THAL-mo-skope) Instrument for examining the posterior (fundus) of the eye.

opportunistic (op-por-tu-NIS-tik) Describing an infection that takes hold because a host has been compromised (weakened) by disease.

organ (OR-gan) Body part containing two or more tissues functioning together for specific purposes.

organelle (or-gan-EL) Specialized subdivision within a cell.

organic (or-GAN-ik) Referring to the complex compounds found in living things that contain carbon, and usually hydrogen, and oxygen.

organism (OR-gan-izm) Individual plant or animal; any organized living thing.

organ of Corti (KOR-te) Receptor for hearing located in the cochlea of the internal ear.

origin (OR-ih-jin) Source; beginning; muscle attachment connected to a nonmoving part.

oropharynx (o-ro-FAR-inks) Middle portion of the pharynx, located behind the mouth.

orthopnea (or-THOP-ne-ah) Difficulty in breathing that is relieved by sitting in an upright position.

osmosis (os-MO-sis) Diffusion of water through a semipermeable membrane.

osmotic (os-MOT-ik) **pressure** Tendency of a solution to draw water into it; directly related to a solution's concentration.

osseus (OS-e-us) Pertaining to bone tissue.

ossicle (OS-ih-kl) One of three small bones of the middle ear: malleus, incus, or stapes.

ossification (os-ih-fih-KA-shun) Process of bone formation.

osteoblast (OS-te-o-blast) Bone-forming cell.

osteoclast (OS-te-o-clast) Cell that breaks down bone.

osteocyte (OS-te-o-site) Mature bone cell; maintains bone but does not produce new bone tissue.

osteon (OS-te-on) Subunit of compact bone, consisting of concentric rings of bone tissue around a central channel; haversian system.

osteopenia (os-te-o-PE-ne-ah) Reduction in bone density to below average levels.

osteoporosis (os-te-o-po-RO-sis) Abnormal loss of bone tissue with tendency to fracture.

otoliths (O-to-liths) Crystals that add weight to fluids in the inner ear and function in the sense of static equilibrium.

ovarian follicle (o-VA-re-an FOL-ih-kl) Cluster of cells in which the ovum develops within the ovary; Graafian follicle.

ovary (O-vah-re) Female reproductive gland.

oviduct (O-vih-dukt) Tube that carries ova from the ovaries to the uterus; fallopian tube, uterine tube.

ovulation (ov-u-LA-shun) Release of a mature ovum from an ovarian follicle.

ovum (O-vum) Female reproductive cell or gamete; pl., ova.

oxidation (ok-sih-DA-shun) Chemical breakdown of nutrients for energy.

oxygen (OK-sih-jen) (O_2) The gas needed to break down nutrients completely for energy within the cell.

oxygen debt Amount of oxygen needed to reverse the effects produced in muscles functioning without oxygen.

oxytocin (ok-se-TO-sin) Hormone from the posterior pituitary that causes uterine contraction and milk ejection ("letdown") from the breasts.

P

pacemaker Sinoatrial (SA) node of the heart; group of cells or artificial device that sets the rate of heart contractions.

palate (PAL-at) Roof of the oral cavity; anterior portion is hard palate, posterior portion is soft palate.

pallor (PAL-or) Paleness of the skin.

pancreas (PAN-kre-as) Large, elongated gland behind the stomach; produces digestive enzymes and hormones (e.g., insulin).

pandemic (pan-DEM-ik) Disease that is prevalent throughout an entire country, continent, or the world.

Papanicolaou (pap-ah-nik-o-LAH-o) **test** Histologic test for cervical cancer; Pap test or smear.

papilla (pah-PIL-ah) Small nipplelike projection or elevation.

papillary muscles (PAP-ih-lar-e) Columnar muscles in the heart's ventricular walls that anchor and pull on the chordae tendineae to prevent the valve flaps from everting when the ventricles contract.

papule (PAP-ule) Firm, raised lesion of the skin.

paracentesis (par-eh-sen-TE-sis) Puncture of the abdominal cavity, usually to remove a fluid accumulation, such as ascites; abdominocentesis.

parasite (PAR-ah-site) Organism that lives on or within another (the host) at the other's expense.

parasympathetic nervous system Craniosacral division of the autonomic nervous system; generally reverses the fight-or-flight (stress) response.

parathyroid (par-ah-THI-royd) **gland** Any of four to six small glands embedded in the capsule enclosing the thyroid gland; produces parathyroid hormone, which raises the blood calcium level by causing calcium release from bones.

parietal (pah-RI-eh-tal) Pertaining to the wall of a space or cavity.

Parkinson disease Progressive neurologic condition characterized by tremors, rigidity of limbs and joints, slow movement, and impaired balance.

parturition (par-tu-RISH-un) Childbirth; labor.

pathogen (PATH-o-jen) Disease-causing organism; adj., pathogenic (path-o-JEN-ik).

pathology (pah-THOL-o-je) Study of disease.

pathophysiology (path-o-fiz-e-OL-o-je) Study of the physiologic basis of disease.

pedigree (PED-ih-gre) Family history; used in the study of heredity; family tree.

pelvic inflammatory disease (PID) Ascending infection that involves the pelvic organs; common causes are gonorrhea and chlamydia.

pelvis (PEL-vis) Basinlike structure, such as the lower portion of the abdomen or the upper flared portion of the ureter (renal pelvis).

pemphigus (PEM-fih-gus) An autoimmune skin disease with blistering of the skin.

penis (PE-nis) Male organ of urination and sexual intercourse.

perforating canal Channel across a long bone that contains blood vessels and nerves; Volkmann canal.

pericardium (per-ih-KAR-de-um) Fibrous sac lined with serous membrane that encloses the heart.

perichondrium (per-ih-KON-dre-um) Layer of connective tissue that covers cartilage.

perilymph (PER-e-limf) Fluid that fills the inner ear's bony labyrinth.

perimysium (per-ih-MIS-e-um) Connective tissue around a fascicle of muscle tissue.

perineum (per-ih-NE-um) Pelvic floor; external region between the anus and genital organs.

periosteum (per-e-OS-te-um) Connective tissue membrane covering a bone.

peripheral (peh-RIF-er-al) Located away from a center or central structure.

peripheral nervous system (PNS) All the nerves and nervous tissue outside the central nervous system.

peripheral neuritis (peh-RIF-er-al nu-RI-tis) Degeneration of nerves supplying the distal extremities; polyneuritis.

peristalsis (per-ih-STAL-sis) Wavelike movements in the wall of an organ or duct that propel its contents forward.

peritoneum (per-ih-to-NE-um) Serous membrane that lines the abdominal cavity and forms outer layer of abdominal organs; forms supporting ligaments for some organs.

peritonitis (per-ih-to-NI-tis) Inflammation of the peritoneum.

peroxisome (per-OK-sih-some) Cell organelle that enzymatically destroys harmful substances produced in metabolism.

Peyer (PI-er) **patches** Clusters of lymphatic nodules in the mucous membranes lining the distal portion of the small intestine.

pH Symbol indicating hydrogen ion (H^+) concentration; scale that measures the relative acidity and alkalinity (basicity) of a solution.

phagocyte (FAG-o-site) Cell capable of engulfing large particles, such as foreign matter or cellular debris, through the plasma membrane.

phagocytosis (fag-o-si-TO-sis) Engulfing of large particles through the plasma membrane.

pharynx (FAR-inks) Throat; passageway between the mouth and esophagus.

phenotype (FE-no-tipe) All the characteristics of an organism that can be seen or tested for.

phenylketonuria (fen-il-ke-to-NU-re-ah) **(PKU)** Hereditary metabolic disorder involving inability to metabolize the amino acid phenylalanine.

phimosis (fi-MO-sis) Tightness of the foreskin.

phlebitis (fleh-BI-tis) Inflammation of a vein.

phospholipid (fos-fo-LIP-id) Complex lipid containing phosphorus.

phrenic (FREN-ik) Pertaining to the diaphragm.

phrenic nerve Nerve that activates the diaphragm.

physiology (fiz-e-OL-o-je) Study of the function of living organisms.

pia mater (PI-ah MA-ter) Innermost layer of the meninges.

PID See pelvic inflammatory disease.

pineal (PIN-e-al) **gland** Gland in the brain that is regulated by light; involved in sleep–wake cycles.

pinna (PIN-nah) Outer projecting portion of the ear; auricle.

pinocytosis (pi-no-si-TO-sis) Intake of small particles and droplets by the plasma membrane of a cell.

pituitary (pih-TU-ih-tar-e) **gland** Endocrine gland located under and controlled by the hypothalamus; releases hormones that control other glands; hypophysis.

placenta (plah-SEN-tah) Structure that nourishes and maintains the developing fetus during pregnancy.

plaque (PLAK) A patch or flat area; fatty material that deposits in vessel linings in atherosclerosis.

plasma (PLAZ-mah) Liquid portion of the blood.

plasma cell Cell derived from a B cell that produces antibodies.

plasma membrane Outer covering of a cell; regulates what enters and leaves cell; cell membrane.

plasmapheresis (plas-mah-fer-E-sis) Separation and removal of plasma from a blood donation and return of the formed elements to the donor.

platelet (PLATE-let) Cell fragment that forms a plug to stop bleeding and acts in blood clotting; thrombocyte.

pleura (PLU-rah) Serous membrane that lines the chest cavity and covers the lungs.

pleurisy (PLUR-ih-se) Inflammation of the pleura; pleuritis.

plexus (PLEK-sus) Network of vessels or nerves.

pneumonia (nu-MO-ne-ah) Inflammation of the lungs, commonly due to infection; pneumonitis.

pneumothorax (nu-mo-THO-raks) Accumulation of air in the pleural space.

PNS See peripheral nervous system.

poliomyelitis (po-le-o-mi-eh-LI-tis) (polio) Viral disease of the nervous system that occurs most commonly in children.

polycythemia (pol-e-si-THE-me-ah) Increase in the number of red cells in the blood.

polydipsia (pol-e-DIP-se-ah) Excessive thirst.

polyp (POL-ip) Protruding growth, often grapelike, from a mucous membrane.

polysaccharide (pol-e-SAK-ah-ride) Compound formed from many simple sugars linked together, such as starch and glycogen.

pons (ponz) Area of the brain between the midbrain and medulla; connects the cerebellum with the rest of the central nervous system.

portal system Venous system that carries blood to a second capillary bed through which it circulates before returning to the heart.

positive feedback A substance or condition that acts within a system to promote more of the same activity.

positron emission tomography (to-MOG-rah-fe) **(PET)** Imaging method that uses a radioactive substance to show activity in an organ.

posterior (pos-TE-re-or) Toward the back; dorsal.

potential (po-TEN-shal) An electrical charge, as on the neuron plasma membrane.

precipitation (pre-sip-ih-TA-shun) Clumping of small particles as a result of an antigen–antibody reaction; seen as a cloudiness.

preeclampsia (pre-eh-KLAMP-se-ah) See pregnancy induced hypertension.

pregnancy (PREG-nan-se) Period during which an embryo or fetus is developing in the body.

pregnancy-induced hypertension (PIH) Hypertension, proteinuria, and edema associated with a hormone imbalance in the latter part of pregnancy; if untreated, may lead to eclampsia; preeclampsia, toxemia of pregnancy.

prepuce (PRE-puse) Loose fold of skin that covers the glans penis; foreskin.

presbycusis (pres-be-KU-sis) Slowly progressive hearing loss that often accompanies aging.

presbyopia (pres-be-O-pe-ah) Loss of visual accommodation that occurs with age, leading to farsightedness.

prevalence (PREV-ah-lens) In epidemiology, the overall frequency of a disease in a given group.

prime mover Muscle that performs a given movement; agonist.

prion (PRI-on) An infectious protein particle that causes progressive neurodegenerative disease.

PRL see prolactin.

progeny (PROJ-eh-ne) Offspring, descendent.

progesterone (pro-JES-ter-one) Hormone produced by the corpus luteum and placenta; maintains the uterine lining for pregnancy.

prognosis (prog-NO-sis) Prediction of the probable outcome of a disease based on the condition of the patient and knowledge about the disease.

prolactin (pro-LAK-tin) Hormone from the anterior pituitary that stimulates milk production in the breasts; PRL.

prone Face down or palm down.

prophase (PRO-faze) First stage of mitosis, during which the chromosomes become visible and the organelles disappear.

prophylaxis (pro-fih-LAK-sis) Prevention of disease.

proprioceptor (pro-pre-o-SEP-tor) Sensory receptor that aids in judging body position and changes in position; located in muscles, tendons, and joints.

prostaglandin (pros-tah-GLAN-din) Any of a group of hormones produced by many cells; these hormones have a variety of effects.

prostate (PROS-tate) **gland** Gland that surrounds the urethra below the bladder and contributes secretions to the semen.

protein (PRO-tene) Organic compound made of amino acids; contains nitrogen in addition to carbon, hydrogen, and oxygen (some contain sulfur or phosphorus).

prothrombin (pro-THROM-bin) Clotting factor; converted to thrombin during blood clotting.

prothrombinase (pro-THROM-bih-nase) Blood clotting factor that converts prothrombin to thrombin.

proton (PRO-ton) Positively charged particle in an atom's nucleus.

protozoon (pro-to-ZO-on) Animal-like microorganism; pl., protozoa.

proximal (PROK-sih-mal) Nearer to point of origin or to a reference point.

pruritis (pru-RI-tis) Intense itching of the skin.

psoriasis (so-RI-ah-sis) Chronic skin disease with red, flat areas covered with silvery scales.

ptosis (TO-sis) Dropping down of a part.

puerperal (pu-ER-per-al) Related to childbirth.

pulmonary circuit Pathway that carries blood from the heart to the lungs for oxygenation and then returns the blood to the heart.

pulse Wave of increased pressure in the vessels produced by heart contraction.

pupil (PU-pil) Opening in the center of the eye through which light enters.

Purkinje (pur-KIN-je) **fibers** Part of the heart's conduction system; conduction myofibers.

pus Mixture of bacteria and leukocytes formed in response to infection.

pustule (PUS-tule) Vesicle filled with pus.

pyelonephritis (pi-eh-lo-neh-FRI-tis) Inflammation of the liver, calyces, and renal pelvis, often due to bacterial infection.

pylorus (pi-LOR-us) Distal region of the stomach that leads to the pyloric sphincter.

pyrogen (PI-ro-jen) Substance that produces fever.

pyruvic (pi-RU-vik) **acid** Intermediate product in the breakdown of glucose for energy.

R

radioactivity (ra-de-o-ak-TIV-ih-te) Emission of atomic particles from an element.

radiography (ra-de-og-rah-fe) Production of an image by passage of x-rays through the body onto sensitized film; record produced is a radiograph.

rash Surface skin lesion.

receptor (re-SEP-tor) Specialized cell or ending of a sensory neuron that can be excited by a stimulus. A site in the cell membrane to which a special substance (e.g., hormone, antibody) may attach.

recessive (re-SES-iv) Referring to a gene that is not expressed if a dominant gene for the same trait is present.

reflex (RE-fleks) Simple, rapid, automatic response involving few neurons.

reflex arc (ark) Pathway through the nervous system from stimulus to response, commonly involves a receptor, sensory neuron, central neuron(s), motor neuron, and effector.

refraction (re-FRAK-shun) Bending of light rays as they pass from one medium to another of a different density.

relaxin (re-LAKS-in) Placental hormone that softens the cervix and relaxes the pelvic joints.

renin (RE-nin) Enzyme released from the kidney's juxtaglomerular apparatus that indirectly increases blood pressure by activating angiotensin.

repolarization (re-po-lar-ih-ZA-shun) Sudden return to the original charge on a cell membrane following depolarization.

resorption (re-SORP-shun) Loss of substance, such as that of bone or a tooth.

respiration (res-pih-RA-shun) Process by which oxygen is obtained from the environment and delivered to the cells.

respiratory system System consisting of the lungs and breathing passages involved in exchange of oxygen and carbon dioxide between the outside air and the blood.

reticular (reh-TIK-u-lar) **formation** Network in the limbic system that governs wakefulness and sleep.

reticuloendothelial (reh-tik-u-lo-en-do-THE-le-al) **system** Protective system consisting of highly phagocytic cells in body fluids and tissues, such as the spleen, lymph nodes, bone marrow, and liver.

retina (RET-ih-nah) Innermost layer of the eye; contains light-sensitive cells (rods and cones).

retroperitoneal (ret-ro-per-ih-to-NE-al) Behind the peritoneum, as are the kidneys, pancreas, and abdominal aorta.

retrovirus (RET-ro-vi-rus) Virus that has RNA as the genetic material and copies the RNA into DNA to replicate in the host cells (e.g., HIV).

reverse transcriptase (tran-SKRIP-tase) Enzyme needed for transcribing RNA into DNA in a retrovirus.

Rh factor A red cell antigen; D antigen.

rheumatoid (RU-mah-toyd) **arthritis** Disease of connective tissue that affects the joints.

rhodopsin (ro-DOP-sin) Light-sensitive pigment in the rods of the eye; visual purple.

rib One of the slender curved bones that make up most of the thorax; costa; adj., costal.

ribonucleic (RI-bo-nu-kle-ik) **acid (RNA)** Substance needed for protein manufacture in the cell.

ribosome (RI-bo-some) Small body in the cell's cytoplasm that is a site of protein manufacture.

rickets (RIK-ets) Softening of bone (osteomalacia) in children, usually caused by a deficiency of vitamin D.

Rickettsia (rih-KET-se-ah) Extremely small oval to rod-shaped bacterium that can grow only within a living cell.

RNA See ribonucleic acid.

rod Receptor cell in the retina of the eye; used for vision in dim light.

roentgenogram (rent-GEN-o-gram) Image produced by means of x-rays; radiograph.

rotation (ro-TA-shun) Twisting or turning of a bone on its own axis.

rugae (RU-je) Folds in the lining of an organ, such as the stomach or urinary bladder; sing., ruga (RU-gah).

rule of nines Method for estimating the extent of a burn based on multiples of nine.

S

SA node See sinoatrial node.

saliva (sah-LI-vah) Secretion of the salivary glands; moistens food and contains an enzyme that digests starch.

salt Compound formed by reaction between an acid and a base (e.g. NaCl, table salt).

saltatory (SAL-tah-to-re) **conduction** Transmission of an electrical impulse from node to node along a myelinated fiber; faster than continuous conduction along the entire membrane.

sagittal (SAJ-ih-tal) Describing a plane that divides a structure into right and left portions.

sarcoma (sar-KO-mah) Malignant tumor of connective tissue; a form of cancer.

sarcoplasmic reticulum (sar-ko-PLAS-mik re-TIK-u-lum) **(SR)** Intracellular membrane in muscle cells that is equivalent to the endoplasmic reticulum (ER) in other cells; stores calcium needed for muscle contraction.

saturated fat Fat that has more hydrogen atoms and fewer double bonds between carbons than do unsaturated fats.

scar Fibrous connective tissue that replaces normal tissues destroyed by injury or disease; cicatrix.

Schwann (shvahn) **cell** Cell in the nervous system that produces the myelin sheath around peripheral axons.

sclera (SKLE-rah) Outermost layer of the eye; made of tough connective tissue; "white" of the eye.

scleroderma (skle-ro-DER-mah) An autoimmune disease associated with overproduction of collagen.

scoliosis (sko-le-O-sis) Lateral curvature of the spine.

scrotum (SKRO-tum) Sac in which testes are suspended.

sebaceous (seh-BA-chus) Pertaining to sebum; an oily substance secreted by skin glands.

sebum (SE-bum) Oily secretion that lubricates the skin; adj., sebaceous (se-BA-shus).

secretin (se-KRE-tin) Hormone from the duodenum that stimulates pancreatic release of water and bicarbonate.

seizure (SE-zhur) Series of muscle spasms; convulsion.

selectively permeable Describing a membrane that regulates what can pass through (e.g., a cell's plasma membrane).

sella turcica (SEL-ah TUR-sih-ka) Saddlelike depression in the floor of the skull that holds the pituitary gland.

semen (SE-men) Mixture of sperm cells and secretions from several glands of the male reproductive tract.

semicircular canal Bony canal in the internal ear that contains receptors for the sense of dynamic equilibrium; there are three semicircular canals in each ear.

semilunar (sem-e-LU-nar) Shaped like a half-moon, such as the flaps of the pulmonary and aortic valves.

seminal vesicle (VES-ih-kl) Gland that contributes secretions to the semen.

seminiferous (seh-mih-NIF-er-us) **tubules** Tubules in which sperm cells develop in the testis.

semipermeable (sem-e-PER-me-ah-bl) Capable of being penetrated by some substances and not others.

sensory (SEN-so-re) Describing cells or activities involved in transmitting impulses toward the central nervous system; afferent.

sensory adaptation Gradual loss of sensation when sensory receptors are exposed to continuous stimulation.

sensory receptor Part of the nervous system that detects a stimulus.

sepsis (SEP-sis) Presence of pathogenic microorganisms or their toxins in the bloodstream or other tissues; adj., septic.

septicemia (sep-tih-SE-me-ah) Presence of pathogenic organisms or their toxins in the bloodstream; blood poisoning.

septum (SEP-tum) Dividing wall, as between the chambers of the heart or the nasal cavities.

serosa (se-RO-sah) Serous membrane; epithelial membrane that secretes a thin, watery fluid.

Sertoli cells See sustentacular cells.

serum (SE-rum) Liquid portion of blood without clotting factors; thin, watery fluid; adj., serous (SE-rus).

sex-linked Referring to a gene carried on a sex chromosome, usually the X chromosome.

sexually transmitted infection (STI) Communicable disease acquired through sexual relations; sexually transmitted disease (STD); venereal disease (VD).

shingles Viral infection that follows the nerve pathways; caused by the same virus that causes chicken pox; herpes zoster.

shock Pertaining to the circulation: a life-threatening condition in which there is inadequate blood flow to the tissues.

sickle cell disease Hereditary disease in which abnormal hemoglobin causes red blood cells to change shape (sickle) when they release oxygen.

sign Manifestation of a disease as noted by an observer.

sinoatrial (si-no-A-tre-al) **(SA) node** Tissue in the right atrium's upper wall that sets the rate of heart contractions; the heart's pacemaker.

sinus (SI-nus) Cavity or channel, such as the paranasal sinuses in the skull bones.

sinus rhythm Normal heart rhythm originating at the SA node.

sinusoid (SI-nus-oyd) Enlarged capillary that serves as a blood channel.

skeletal (SKEL-eh-tal) **system** The body system that includes the bones and joints.

skeleton (SKEL-eh-ton) Bony framework of the body; adj., skeletal.

skull Bony framework of the head.

solute (SOL-ute) Substance that is dissolved in another substance (the solvent).

solution (so-LU-shun) Homogeneous mixture of one substance dissolved in another; the components in a mixture are evenly distributed and cannot be distinguished from each other.

solvent (SOL-vent) Substance in which another substance (the solute) is dissolved.

somatic (so-MAT-ik) **nervous system** Division of the nervous system that controls voluntary activities and stimulates skeletal muscle.

somatotropin (so-mah-to-TRO-pin) Growth hormone.

spasm Sudden and involuntary muscular contraction.

specific gravity The weight of a substance as compared to the weight of an equal volume of pure water.

spermatic (sper-MAT-ik) **cord** Cord that extends through the inguinal canal and suspends the testis; contains blood vessels, nerves, and ductus deferens.

spermatozoon (sper-mah-to-ZO-on) Male reproductive cell or gamete; pl., spermatozoa; sperm cell.

sphincter (SFINK-ter) Muscular ring that regulates the size of an opening.

sphygmomanometer (sfig-mo-mah-NOM-eh-ter) Device used to measure blood pressure; blood pressure apparatus or cuff.

spina bifida (SPI-nah BIF-ih-dah) Incomplete closure of the spine.

spinal cord Nervous tissue contained in the spinal column; major relay area between the brain and the peripheral nervous system.

spirillum (spi-RIL-um) Corkscrew or spiral-shaped bacterium; pl., spirilla.

spirochete (SPI-ro-kete) Spiral-shaped microorganism that moves in a waving and twisting motion.

spirometer (spi-ROM-eh-ter) Instrument for recording lung volumes; tracing is a spirogram.

spleen Lymphoid organ in the upper left region of the abdomen.

spore Resistant form of bacterium; reproductive cell in lower plants.

squamous (SKWA-mus) Flat and irregular, as in squamous epithelium.

SR See sarcoplasmic reticulum.

staging A procedure for evaluating the extent of tumor spread.

stain (stane) Dye that aids in viewing structures under the microscope.

staphylococcus (staf-ih-lo-KOK-us) Round bacterium found in a cluster resembling a bunch of grapes; pl., staphylococci (staf-ih-lo-KOK-si).

stasis (STA-sis) Stoppage in the normal flow of fluids, such as blood, lymph, urine, or contents of the digestive tract.

stem cell Cell that has the potential to develop into different types of cells.

stenosis (sten-O-sis) Narrowing of a duct or canal.

stent Small tube inserted into a vessel to keep it open.

sterility Complete inability to reproduce.

sterilization (ster-ih-li-ZA-shun) Process of killing every living microorganism on or in an object; procedure that makes an individual incapable of reproduction.

steroid (STE-royd) Category of lipids that includes the hormones of the sex glands and the adrenal cortex.

stethoscope (STETH-o-skope) Instrument for conveying sounds from the patient's body to the examiner's ears.

STI See sexually transmitted infection.

stimulus (STIM-u-lus) Change in the external or internal environment that produces a response.

stomach (STUM-ak) Organ of the digestive tract that stores food, mixes it with digestive juices, and moves it into the small intestine.

strabismus (strah-BIZ-mus) Deviation of the eye resulting from lack of eyeball muscle coordination.

stratified In multiple layers (strata).

stratum (STRA-tum) A layer; pl., strata.

stratum basale (bas-A-le) Deepest layer of the epidermis; layer that produces new epidermal cells; stratum germinativum.

stratum corneum (KOR-ne-um) The thick uppermost layer of the epidermis.

striations (stri-A-shuns) Stripes or bands, as seen in skeletal muscle and cardiac muscle.

stricture (STRICK-ture) Narrowing of a part.

stroke Damage to the brain due to lack of oxygen; usually caused by a blood clot in a vessel (thrombus) or rupture of a vessel; cerebrovascular accident (CVA).

subacute (sub-a-KUTE) Not as severe as an acute infection nor as long-lasting as a chronic disorder.

subcutaneous (sub-ku-TA-ne-us) Under the skin.

submucosa (sub-mu-KO-sah) Layer of connective tissue beneath the mucosa.

substrate Substance on which an enzyme works.

sudoriferous (su-do-RIF-er-us) Producing sweat; referring to the sweat glands.

sulcus (SUL-kus) Shallow groove, as between convolutions of the cerebral cortex; pl., sulci (SUL-si).

superior (su-PE-re-or) Above; in a higher position.

superior vena cava (VE-nah KA-vah) Large vein that drains the upper part of the body and empties into the heart's right atrium.

supine (SU-pine) Face up or palm up.

surfactant (sur-FAK-tant) Substance in the alveoli that prevents their collapse by reducing surface tension of the contained fluids.

suspension (sus-PEN-shun) Heterogeneous mixture that will separate unless shaken.

suspensory ligaments Filaments attached to the ciliary muscle of the eye that hold the lens in place.

sustentacular (sus-ten-TAK-u-lar) **cells** Cells in the seminiferous tubules that aid in development of spermatozoa; Sertoli cells.

suture (SU-chur) Type of joint in which bone surfaces are closely united, as in the skull; stitch used in surgery to bring parts together or to stitch parts together in surgery.

sympathetic nervous system Thoracolumbar division of the autonomic nervous system; stimulates a fight-or-flight (stress) response.

symptom (SIMP-tom) Evidence of disease noted by the patient; such evidence noted by an examiner is called a sign or an objective symptom.

synapse (SIN-aps) Junction between two neurons or between a neuron and an effector.

synarthrosis (sin-ar-THRO-sis) Immovable joint.

syndrome (SIN-drome) Group of symptoms characteristic of a disorder.

synergist (SIN-er-jist) Substance or structure that enhances the work of another. A muscle that works with a prime mover to produce a given movement.

synovial (sin-O-ve-al) Pertaining to a thick lubricating fluid found in joints, bursae, and tendon sheaths; pertaining to a freely movable (diarthrotic) joint.

system (SIS-tem) Group of organs functioning together for the same general purposes.

systemic (sis-TEM-ik) Referring to a generalized infection or condition.

systemic circuit Pathway that carries blood to all tissues of the body except the lungs.

systole (SIS-to-le) Contraction phase of the cardiac cycle; adj., systolic (sis-TOL-ik).

T

tachycardia (tak-e-KAR-de-ah) Heart rate more than 100 beats per minute.

tachypnea (tak-IP-ne-ah) Excessive rate of respiration.

tactile (TAK-til) Pertaining to the sense of touch.

target tissue Tissue that is capable of responding to a specific hormone.

Tay-Sachs disease Hereditary disease affecting fat metabolism.

T cell Lymphocyte active in immunity that matures in the thymus gland; destroys foreign cells directly; T lymphocyte.

tectorial (tek-TO-re-al) **membrane** Part of the hearing apparatus; generates nerve impulses as cilia move against it in response to sound waves.

telophase (TEL-o-faze) Final stage of mitosis, during which new nuclei form and the cell contents usually divide.

tendinitis (ten-din-I-tis) Inflammation of a tendon.

tendon (TEN-don) Cord of fibrous connective tissue that attaches a muscle to a bone.

teniae (TEN-e-e) **coli** Bands of smooth muscle in the wall of the large intestine.

testis (TES-tis) Male reproductive gland; pl., testes (TES-teze).

testosterone (tes-TOS-ter-one) Male sex hormone produced in the testes; promotes sperm cell development and maintains secondary sex characteristics.

tetanus (TET-an-us) Constant contraction of a muscle; infectious disease caused by a bacterium (*Clostridium tetani*); lockjaw.

tetany (TET-an-e) Muscle spasms due to low blood calcium, as in parathyroid deficiency.

thalassemia (thal-ah-SE-me-ah) Hereditary blood disorder that impairs hemoglobin production; the two forms are alpha (α) and beta (β).

thalamus (THAL-ah-mus) Region of the brain located in the diencephalon; chief relay center for sensory impulses traveling to the cerebral cortex.

therapy (THER-ah-pe) Treatment.

thoracentesis (thor-a-sen-TE-sis) Puncture of the chest for aspiration of fluid in the pleural space.

thorax (THO-raks) Chest; adj., thoracic (tho-RAS-ik).

thrombocyte (THROM-bo-site) Blood platelet; cell fragment that participates in clotting.

thrombocytopenia (throm-bo-si-to-PE-ne-ah) Deficiency of platelets in the blood.

thrombolytic (throm-bo-LIT-ik) Dissolving blood clots.

thrombosis (throm-BO-sis) Condition of having a thrombus (blood clot in a vessel).

thrombus (THROM-bus) Blood clot within a vessel.

thymosin (THI-mo-sin) Hormone produced by the thymus gland.

thymus (THI-mus) Endocrine gland in the upper portion of the chest; stimulates development of T cells.

thyroid (THI-royd) Endocrine gland in the neck.

thyroiditis (thi-royd-I-tis) Inflammation of the thyroid gland.

thyroid-stimulating hormone (TSH) Hormone produced by the anterior pituitary that stimulates the thyroid gland; thyrotropin.

thyroxine (thi-ROK-sin) Hormone produced by the thyroid gland; increases metabolic rate and needed for normal growth; T_4.

tinea (TIN-e-ah) Common term for fungal skin infection.

tissue Group of similar cells that performs a specialized function.

tonicity (to-NIS-ih-te) The osmotic concentration or osmotic pressure of a solution. The effect that a solution will have on osmosis.

tonsil (TON-sil) Mass of lymphoid tissue in the region of the pharynx.

tonus (TO-nus) Partially contracted state of muscle; also, tone.

toxemia (tok-SE-me-ah) General toxic condition in which poisonous bacterial substances are absorbed into the bloodstream; presence of harmful substances in the blood as a result of abnormal metabolism.

toxin (TOK-sin) Poison.

toxoid (TOK-soyd) Altered toxin used to produce active immunity.

trachea (TRA-ke-ah) Tube that extends from the larynx to the bronchi; windpipe.

tracheostomy (tra-ke-OS-to-me) Surgical opening into the trachea for the introduction of a tube through which a person may breathe.

trachoma (trah-KO-mah) Acute eye infection caused by chlamydia.

tract Bundle of neuron fibers within the central nervous system.

trait Characteristic.

transfusion (trans-FU-zhun) Introduction of blood or blood components directly into the bloodstream.

transplantation (trans-plan-TA-shun) The grafting to a recipient of an organ or tissue from an animal or other human to replace an injured or incompetent body part.

transverse Describing a plane that divides a structure into superior and inferior parts.

trauma (TRAW-mah) Injury or wound.

tricuspid (tri-KUS-pid) **valve** Valve between the heart's right atrium and right ventricle.

trigeminal neuralgia (tri-JEM-ih-nal nu-RAL-je-ah) Severe spasmodic pain affecting the fifth cranial nerve; tic douloureux (tik du-lu-RU).

triglyceride (tri-GLIS-er-ide) Simple fat composed of glycerol and three fatty acids.

trigone (TRI-gone) Triangular-shaped region in the floor of the bladder that remains stable as the bladder fills.

triiodothyronine (tri-i-o-do-THI-ro-nin) Thyroid hormone that functions with thyroxine to raise cellular metabolism; T_3.

tropomyosin (tro-po-MI-o-sin) Protein that works with troponin to regulate contraction in skeletal muscle.

troponin (tro-PO-nin) Protein that works with tropomyosin to regulate contraction in skeletal muscle.

TSH See thyroid-stimulating hormone.

tuberculosis (tu-ber-ku-LO-sis) **(TB)** Infectious disease, often of the lung, caused by the bacillus *Mycobacterium tuberculosis*.

tumor (TU-mor) Abnormal growth or neoplasm.

tympanic (tim-PAN-ik) **membrane** Membrane between the external and middle ear that transmits sound waves to the bones of the middle ear; eardrum.

U

ulcer (UL-ser) Sore or lesion associated with death and disintegration of tissue.

ultrasound (UL-trah-sound) Very high frequency sound waves.

umbilical (um-BIL-ih-kal) **cord** Structure that connects the fetus with the placenta; contains vessels that carry blood between the fetus and placenta.

umbilicus (um-BIL-ih-kus) Small scar on the abdomen that marks the former attachment of the umbilical cord to the fetus; navel.

universal solvent Term used for water because it dissolves more substances than any other solvent.

unsaturated fat Fat that has fewer hydrogen atoms and more double bonds between carbons than do saturated fats.

urea (u-RE-ah) Nitrogenous waste product excreted in the urine; end product of protein metabolism.

uremia (u-RE-me-ah) Accumulation of nitrogenous waste products in the blood.

ureter (U-re-ter) Tube that carries urine from the kidney to the urinary bladder.

urethra (u-RE-thrah) Tube that carries urine from the urinary bladder to the outside of the body.

urinalysis (u-rin-AL-ih-sis) Laboratory examination of urine's physical and chemical properties.

urinary bladder Hollow organ that stores urine until it is eliminated.

urinary (U-rin-ar-e) **system** The system involved in elimination of soluble waste, water balance, and regulation of body fluids.

urination (u-rin-A-shun) Voiding of urine; micturition.

urine (U-rin) Liquid waste excreted by the kidneys.

urticaria (ur-tih-KA-re-ah) Hives; allergic skin reaction with elevated red patches (wheals).

uterus (U-ter-us) Muscular, pear-shaped organ in the female pelvis within which the fetus develops during pregnancy; adj., uterine.

uvea (U-ve-ah) Middle coat of the eye, including the choroid, iris, and ciliary body; vascular and pigmented structures of the eye.

uvula (U-vu-lah) Soft, fleshy, V-shaped mass that hangs from the soft palate.

V

vaccination (vak-sin-A-shun) Administration of a vaccine to protect against a specific disease; immunization.

vaccine (vak-SENE) Substance used to produce active immunity; usually, a suspension of attenuated or killed pathogens or some component of a pathogen given by inoculation to prevent a specific disease.

vagina (vah-JI-nah) Distal part of the birth canal that opens to the outside of the body; female organ of sexual intercourse.

valence (VA-lens) The combining power of an atom; the number of electrons lost or gained by atoms of an element in chemical reactions.

valve Structure that prevents fluid from flowing backward, as in the heart, veins, and lymphatic vessels.

varicose (VAR-ih-kose) Pertaining to an enlarged and twisted vessel, as in varicose vein.

vas deferens (DEF-er-enz) Tube that carries sperm cells from the testis to the urethra; ductus deferens.

vascular (VAS-ku-lar) Pertaining to blood vessels.

vasectomy (vah-SEK-to-me) Surgical removal of part or all of the ductus (vas) deferens; usually done on both sides to produce sterility.

vasoconstriction (vas-o-kon-STRIK-shun) Decrease in a blood vessel's diameter.

vasodilation (vas-o-di-LA-shun) Increase in a blood vessel's diameter.

VD Venereal disease; see sexually transmitted infection.

vector (VEK-tor) An insect or other animal that transmits a disease-causing organism from one host to another.

vein (vane) Vessel that carries blood toward the heart.

vena cava (VE-nah KA-vah) Large vein that carries blood into the heart's right atrium; superior vena cava or inferior vena cava.

venereal (ve-NE-re-al) **disease** (**VD**) Infectious disease acquired through sexual activity; sexually transmitted infection (STI).

venous sinus (VE-nus SI-nus) Large channel that drains deoxygenated blood.

ventilation (ven-tih-LA-shun) Movement of air into and out of the lungs.

ventral (VEN-tral) Toward the front or belly surface; anterior.

ventricle (VEN-trih-kl) Cavity or chamber; one of the heart's two lower chambers; one of the brain's four chambers in which cerebrospinal fluid is produced; adj., ventricular (ven-TRIK-u-lar).

venule (VEN-ule) Vessel between a capillary and a vein.

vernix caseosa (VEr-niks ka-se-O-sah) Cheeselike sebaceous secretion that covers a newborn.

vertebra (VER-teh-brah) A bone of the spinal column; pl., vertebrae (VER-teh-bre).

verruca (veh-RU-kah) Wart.

vesicle (VES-ih-kl) Small sac or blister filled with fluid.

vesicular transport Use of vesicles to move large amounts of material through the plasma membrane of a cell.

vestibular apparatus (ves-TIB-u-lar) Part of the inner ear concerned with equilibrium; consists of the semicircular canals and vestibule.

vestibule (VES-tih-bule) Part of the internal ear that contains receptors for the sense of static equilibrium; any space at the entrance to a canal or organ.

vibrio (VIB-re-o) Slight curved or comma-shaped bacterium; pl., vibrios.

villi (VIL-li) Small fingerlike projections from the surface of a membrane; projections in the lining of the small intestine through which digested food is absorbed; sing., villus.

viroid (VI-royd) Infectious agent composed of RNA with no protein. Viroids are intracellular parasites linked so far only to diseases in plants.

virulence (VIR-u-lens) Power of an organism to overcome a host's defenses.

virus (VI-rus) Extremely small infectious agent that can reproduce only within a living cell.

viscera (VIS-er-ah) Organs in the ventral body cavities, especially the abdominal organs; adj., visceral.

viscosity (vis-KOS-ih-te) Thickness, as of the blood or other fluid.

vitamin (VI-tah-min) Organic compound needed in small amounts for health.

vitreous (VIT-re-us) **body** Soft, jellylike substance that fills the eyeball and holds the shape of the eye; vitreous humor.

vocal cords Folds of mucous membrane in the larynx used in producing speech.

Volkmann canal See perforating canal.

volvulus (VOL-vu-lus) Twisting of the intestine.

von Willebrand disease Hereditary blood clotting disorder in which there is a shortage of von Willebrand factor.

W

Wernicke (VER-nih-ke) **area** Portion of the cerebral cortex concerned with speech recognition and the meaning of words.

white matter Nervous tissue composed of myelinated fibers.

Wilson disease Recessive hereditary disease associated with a defect in copper metabolism and accumulation of copper in the liver, brain, or other tissues.

X

x-ray Ray or radiation of extremely short wavelength that can penetrate opaque substances and affect photographic plates and fluorescent screens.

Z

zygote (ZI-gote) Fertilized ovum; cell formed by the union of a sperm and an egg.

Glossary of Word Parts

Use of Word Parts in Medical Terminology

Medical terminology, the special language of the health occupations, is based on an understanding of a few relatively basic elements. These elements—roots, prefixes, and suffixes—form the foundation of almost all medical terms. A useful way to familiarize yourself with each term is to learn to pronounce it correctly and say it aloud several times. Soon it will become an integral part of your vocabulary.

The foundation of a word is the word root. Examples of word roots are *abdomin*, referring to the belly region; and *aden*, pertaining to a gland. A word root is often followed by a vowel to facilitate pronunciation, as in *abdomino* and *adeno*. We then refer to it as a "combining form."

A prefix is a part of a word that precedes the word root and changes its meaning. For example, the prefix *mal* in malnutrition means "abnormal." A suffix, or word ending, is a part that follows the word root and adds to or changes its meaning. The suffix *-rhea* means "profuse flow" or "discharge," as in diarrhea, a condition characterized by excessive discharge of liquid stools.

Many medical words are compound words; that is, they are made up of more than one root or combining form. Examples of such compound words are *erythrocyte* (red blood cell) and *hydrocele* (fluid-containing sac), and many more difficult words, such as *sternoclavicular* (indicating relations to both the sternum and the clavicle).

A general knowledge of language structure and spelling rules is also helpful in mastering medical terminology. For example, adjectives include words that end in *-al*, as in sternal (the noun is sternum), and words that end in *-ous*, as in mucous (the noun is mucus).

The following list includes some of the most commonly used word roots, prefixes, and suffixes, as well as examples of their use. Prefixes are followed by a hyphen; suffixes are preceded by a hyphen; and word roots have no hyphen. Commonly used combining vowels are added following a slash.

Word Parts

a-, an- absent, deficient, lack of: *aphasia, atrophy, anemia, anuria*
ab- away from: *abduction, aboral*
abdomin/o belly or abdominal area: *abdominocentesis, abdominoscopy*
acous, acus hearing, sound: *acoustic, presbyacusis*
acr/o- end, extremity: *acromegaly, acromion*
actin/o, actin/i relation to raylike structures or, more commonly, to light or roentgen (x-) rays, or some other type of radiation: *actiniform, actinodermatitis*
ad- (sometimes converted to *ac-, af-, ag-, ap-, as-, at-,*) toward, added to, near: *adrenal, accretion, agglomerated, afferent*
aden/o gland: *adenectomy, adenitis, adenocarcinoma*
aer/o air, gas: *aerobic, aerate*
-agogue inducing, leading, stimulating: *cholagogue, galactagogue*
-al pertaining to, resembling: *skeletal, surgical, ileal*
alb/i- white: *albinism, albiduria*
alge, alg/o, alges/i pain: *algetic, algophobia, analgesic*
-algia pain, painful condition: *myalgia, neuralgia*
amb/i- both, on two sides: *ambidexterity, ambivalent*
ambly- dimness, dullness: *amblyopia*
amphi on both sides, around, double: *amphiarthrosis, amphibian*
amyl/o starch: *amylase, amyloid*
an- absent, deficient, lack of: *anaerobic, anoxia, anemic*
ana- upward, back, again, excessive: *anatomy, anastomosis, anabolism*
andr/o male: *androgen, androgenous*
angi/o vessel: *angiogram, angiotensin*
ant/i- against; to prevent, suppress, or destroy: *antarthritic, antibiotic, anticoagulant*
ante- before, ahead of: *antenatal, antepartum*
anter/o- position ahead of or in front of (i.e., anterior to) another part: *anterolateral, anteroventral*
-apheresis take away, withdraw: *hemapheresis, plasmapheresis*
ap/o- separation, derivation from: *apocrine, apoptosis, apophysis*
aqu/e water: *aqueous, aquatic, aqueduct*
-ar pertaining to, resembling: *muscular, nuclear*

arthr/o joint or articulation: *arthrolysis, arthrostomy, arthritis*
-ary pertaining to, resembling: *salivary, dietary, urinary*
-ase enzyme: *lipase, protease*
-asis *See –sis*
atel/o- imperfect: *atelectasis*
ather/o gruel: *athersclerosis, atheroma*
audi/o sound, hearing: *audiogenic, audiometry, audiovisual*
aut/o- self: *autistic, autodigestion, autoimmune*

bar/o pressure: *baroreceptor, barometer*
bas/o- alkaline: *basic, basophilic*
bi- two, twice: *bifurcate, bisexual*
bil/i bile: *biliary, bilirubin*
bio- life, living organism: *biopsy, antibiotic*
blast/o, -blast early stage of a cell, immature cell: *blastula, blastophore, erythroblast*
bleph, blephar/o eyelid, eyelash: *blepharism, blepharitis, blepharospasm*
brachi, brachi/o arm: *brachial, brachiocephalic, brachiotomy*
brachy- short: *brachydactylia, brachyesophagus*
brady- slow: *bradycardia*
bronch/o-, bronch/i bronchus: *bronchiectasis, bronchoscope*
bucc cheek: *buccal*

capn/o carbon dioxide: *hypocapnia, hypercapnia*
carcin/o cancer: *carcinogenic, carcinoma*
cardi/o, cardi/a heart: *carditis, cardiac, cardiologist*
cata- down: *catabolism, catalyst*
-cele swelling; enlarged space or cavity: *cystocele, meningocele, rectocele*
celi/o abdomen: *celiac, celiocentesis*
centi- relating to 100 (used in naming units of measurements): *centigrade, centimeter*
-centesis perforation, tapping: *aminocentesis, paracentesis*
cephal/o head: *cephalalgia, cephalopelvic*

cerebr/o brain: *cerobrospinal, cerebrum*
cervi neck: *cervical, cervix*
cheil/o lips; brim or edge: *cheilitis, cheilosis*
chem/o, chem/i chemistry, chemical: *chemotherapy, chemocautery, chemoreceptor*
chir/o, cheir/o hand: *cheiralgia, cheiromegaly, chiropractic*
chol/e, chol/o bile, gall: *chologogue, cholecyst, cholelith*
cholecyst/o gallbladder: *cholecystitis, cholecystokinin*
chondr/o, chondri/o cartilage: *chondric, chondrocyte, chondroma*
chori/o membrane: *chorion, choroid, choriocarcinoma*
chrom/o, chromat/o color: *chromosome, chromatin, chromophilic*
-cid, -cide to cut, kill or destroy: *bactericidal, germicide, suicide*
circum- around, surrounding: *circumorbital, circumrenal, circumduction*
-clast break: *osteoclast*
clav/o, cleid/o clavicle: *cleidomastoid, subclavian*
co- with, together: *cofactor, cohesion, coinfection*
colp/o vagina: *colpectasia, colposcope, colpotomy*
con- with: *concentric, concentrate, conduct*
contra- opposed, against: *contraindication, contralateral*
corne/o horny: *corneum, cornified, cornea*
cortic/o cortex: *cortical, corticotropic, cortisone*
cost/a, cost/o- ribs: *intercostal, costosternal*
counter- against, opposite to: *counteract, counterirritation, countertraction*
crani/o skull: *cranium, craniotomy*
cry/o- cold: *cryalgesia, cryogenic, cryotherapy*
crypt/o- hidden, concealed: *cryptic, cryptogenic, cryptorchidism*
-cusis hearing: *acusis, presbyacusis*
cut- skin: *subcutaneous*
cyan/o- blue: *cyanosis, cyanogen*
cyst/i, cyst/o sac, bladder: *cystitis, cystoscope*
cyt/o, -cyte cell: *cytology, cytoplasm, osteocyte*

dactyl/o digits (usually fingers, but sometimes toes): *dactylitis, polydactyly*
de- remove: *detoxify, dehydration*
dendr tree: *dendrite*
dent/o, dent/i tooth: *dentition, dentin, dentifrice*
derm/o, dermat/o skin: *dermatitis, dermatology, dermatosis*
di- twice, double: *dimorphism, dibasic, dihybrid*
dipl/o- double: *diplopia, diplococcus*
dia- through, between, across, apart: *diaphragm, diaphysis*
dis- apart, away from: *disarticulation, distal*
dors/i, dors/o- back (in the human, this combining form is the same as poster/o-): *dorsal, dorsiflexion, dorso-nuchal*
dys- disordered, difficult, painful: *dysentery, dysphagia, dyspnea*

e- out: *enucleation, evisceration, ejection*
-ectasis expansion, dilation, stretching: *angiectasis, bronchiectasis*
ecto- outside, external: *ectoderm, ectogenous*
-ectomy surgical removal or destruction by other means: *appendectomy, thyroidectomy*
edem swelling: *edema*
-emia condition of blood: *glycemia, hyperemia*
encephal/o brain: *encephalitis, encephalogram*
end/o- in, within, innermost: *endarterial, endocardium, endothelium*
enter/o intestine: *enteritis, enterocolitis*
epi- on, upon: *epicardium, epidermis*
equi- equal: *equidistant, equivalent, equilibrium*
erg/o work: *ergonomic, energy, synergy*
eryth-, erythr/o red: *erythema, erythrocyte*
-esthesia sensation: *anesthesia, paresthesia*
eu- well, normal, good: *euphoria, eupnea*
ex/o- outside, out of, away from: *excretion, exocrine, exophthalmic*
extra- beyond, outside of, in addition to: *extracellular, extrasystole, extravasation*

fasci fibrous connective tissue layers: *fascia, fascitis, fascicle*
fer, -ferent to bear, to carry: *afferent, efferent, transfer*
fibr/o threadlike structures, fibers: *fibrillation, fibroblast, fibrositis*

gastr/o stomach: *gastritis, gastroenterostomy*
-gen an agent that produces or originates: *allergen, pathogen, fibrinogen*
-genic produced from, producing: *neurogenic, pyogenic, psychogenic*

genit/o organs of reproduction: *genitoplasty, genitourinary*
gen/o- a relationship to reproduction or sex: *genealogy, generate, genetic, genotype*
-geny manner of origin, development or production: *ontogeny, progeny*
gest/o gestation, pregnancy: *progesterone, gestagen*
glio, -glia gluey material; specifically, the support tissue of the central nervous system: *glioma, neuroglia*
gloss/o tongue: *glossitis, glossopharyngeal*
glyc/o- relating to sugar, glucose, sweet: *glycemia, glycosuria*
gnath/o related to the jaw: *prognathic, gnathoplasty*
gnos to perceive, recognize: *agnostic, prognosis, diagnosis*
gon seed, knee: *gonad, gonarthritis*
-gram record, that which is recorded: *electrocardiogram, electroencephalogram*
graph/o, -graph instrument for recording, record, writing: *electrocardiograph, electroencephalograph, micrograph*
-graphy process of recording data: *photography, radiography*
gyn/o, gyne, gynec/o female, woman: *gynecology, gynecomastia, gynoplasty*
gyr/o circle: *gyroscope, gyrus, gyration*

hema, hemo, hemat/o blood: *hematoma, hematuria, hemorrhage*
hemi- one half: *hemisphere, heminephrectomy, hemiplegia*
hepat/o liver: *hepatitis, hepatogenous*
heter/o- other, different: *heterogenous, heterosexual, heterochromia*
hist/o, histi/o tissue: *histology, histiocyte*
homeo-, homo- unchanging, the same: *homeostasis, homosexual*
hydr/o water: *hydrolysis, hydrocephalus*
hyper- above, over, excessive: *hyperesthesia, hyperglycemia, hypertrophy*
hypo- deficient, below, beneath: *hypochondrium, hypodermic, hypogastrium*
hyster/o uterus: *hysterectomy*

-ia state of, condition of: *myopia, hypochondria, ischemia*
-iatrics, -trics medical specialty: *pediatrics, obstetrics*
iatr/o physician, medicine: *iatrogenic*
-ic pertaining to, resembling: *metric, psychiatric, geriatric*
idio- self, one's own, separate, distinct: *idiopathic, idiosyncrasy*
-ile pertaining to, resembling: *febrile, virile*
im-, in- in, into, lacking: *implantation, infiltration, inanimate*
infra- below, inferior: *infraspinous, infracortical*
insul/o pancreatic islet, island: *insulin, insulation, insulinoma*
inter- between: *intercostal, interstitial*
intra- within a part or structure: *intracranial, intracellular, intraocular*
isch suppression: *ischemia*
-ism state of: *alcoholism, hyperthyroidism*
iso- same, equal: *isotonic, isometric*
-ist one who specializes in a field of study: *cardiologist, gastroenterologist*
-itis inflammation: *dermatitis, keratitis, neuritis*

juxta- next to: *juxtaglomerular, juxtaposition*

kary/o nucleus: *karyotype, karyoplasm*
kerat/o cornea of the eye, certain horny tissues: *keratin, keratitis, keratoplasty*
kine movement: *kinetic, kinesiology, kinesthesia*

lacri- tear: *lacrimal*
lact/o milk: *lactation, lactogenic*
laryng/o larynx: *laryngeal, laryngectomy, laryngitis*
later/o- side: *lateral*
-lemma sheath: *neurilemma, sarcolemma*
leuk/o- (also written as *leuc-, leuco-*) white, colorless: *leukocyte, leukoplakia*
lip/o lipid, fat: *lipase, lipoma*
lig- bind: *ligament, ligature*
lingu/o tongue: *lingual, linguadental*
lith/o stone (calculus): *lithiasis, lithotripsy*
-logy study of: *physiology, gynecology*
lute/o yellow: *macula lutea, corpus luteum*
lymph/o lymph, lymphatic system, lymphocyte: *lymphoid, lymphedema*
lyso-, -lysis, -lytic: loosening, dissolving, separating: *hemolysis, paralysis, lysosome*

macr/o- large, abnormal length: *macrophage, macroblast.* **See also** -mega, mega/o-

mal- bad, diseased, disordered, abnormal: *malnutrition, malocclusion, malunion*

malac/o, -malacia softening: *malacoma, osteomalacia*

mamm/o breast, mammary gland: *mammogram, mammoplasty, mammal*

man/o pressure: *manometer, sphygmomanometer*

mast/o breast: *mastectomy, mastitis*

meg/a-, megal/o, -megaly unusually or excessively large: *megacolon, megaloblast, splenomegaly, megakaryocyte*

melan/o dark, black: *melanin, melanocyte, melanoma*

men/o physiologic uterine bleeding, menses: *menstrual, menorrhagia, menopause*

mening/o membranes covering the brain and spinal cord: *meningitis, meningocele*

mes/a, mes/o- middle, midline: *mesencephalon, mesoderm*

meta- change, beyond, after, over, near: *metabolism, metacarpal, metaplasia*

-meter, metr/o measure: *hemocytometer, sphygmomanometer, spirometer, isometric*

metr/o uterus: *endometrium, metroptosis, metrorrhagia*

micro- very small: *microscope, microbiology, microsurgery, micrometer*

mon/o- single, one: *monocyte, mononucleosis*

morph/o shape, form: *morphogenesis, morphology*

multi- many: *multiple, multifactorial, multipara*

my/o muscle: *myenteron, myocardium, myometrium*

myc/o, mycet/o fungus: *mycid, mycete, mycology, mycosis, mycelium*

myel/o marrow (often used in reference to the spinal cord): *myeloid, myeloblast, osteomyelitis, poliomyelitis*

myring/o tympanic membrane: *myringotomy, myringitis*

myx/o mucus: *myxoma, myxovirus*

narc/o stupor: *narcosis, narcolepsy, narcotic*

nas/o nose: *nasopharynx, paranasal*

natri sodium: *hyponatremia, natriuretic*

necr/o death, corpse: *necrosis*

neo- new: *neoplasm, neonatal*

neph, nephr/o kidney: *nephrectomy, nephron*

neur/o, neur/i nerve, nervous tissue: *neuron, neuralgia, neuroma*

neutr/o neutral: *neutrophil, neutropenia*

noct/i night: *noctambulation, nocturia, noctiphobia*

ocul/o eye: *oculist, oculomotor, oculomycosis*

odont/o tooth, teeth: *odontalgia, orthodontics*

-odynia pain, tenderness: *myodynia, neurodynia*

-oid like, resembling: *lymphoid, myeloid*

olig/o- few, a deficiency: *oligospermia, oliguria*

-oma tumor, swelling: *hematoma, sarcoma*

-one ending for steroid hormone: *testosterone, progesterone*

onych/o nails: *paronychia, onychoma*

oo, ovum, egg: *oocyte, oogenesis,* (do not confuse with oophor-)

oophor/o ovary: *oophorectomy, oophoritis, oophorocystectomy.* **See also** ovar-

ophthalm/o eye: *ophthalmia, ophthalmologist, ophthalmoscope*

-opia disorder of the eye or vision: *heterotropia, myopia, hyperopia*

or/o mouth: *oropharynx, oral*

orchi/o, orchid/o testis: *orchitis, cryptorchidism*

orth/o- straight, normal: *orthopedics, orthopnea, orthosis*

-ory pertaining to, resembling: *respiratory, circulatory*

oscill/o to swing to and fro: *oscilloscope*

osmo- osmosis: *osmoreceptor, osmotic*

oss/i, osse/o, oste/o bone, bone tissue: *osseous, ossicle, osteocyte, osteomyelitis*

ot/o ear: *otalgia, otitis, otomycosis*

-ous pertaining to, resembling: *fibrous, venous, androgynous*

ov/o egg, ovum: *oviduct, ovulation*

ovar, ovari/o ovary: *ovariectomy.* **See also** oophor

ox-, -oxia pertaining to oxygen: *hypoxemia, hypoxia, anoxia*

oxy sharp, acute: *oxygen, oxytocia*

pan- all: *pandemic, panacea*

papill/o nipple: *papilloma, papillary*

para- near, beyond, apart from, beside: *paramedical, parametrium, parathyroid, parasagittal*

pariet/o wall: *parietal*

path/o, -pathy disease, abnormal condition: *pathogen, pathology, neuropathy*

ped/o, pedia child, foot: *pedophobia, pediatrician, pedialgia*

-penia lack of: *leukopenia, thrombocytopenia*

per- through, excessively: *percutaneous, perfusion*

peri- around: *pericardium, perichondrium*

-pexy fixation: *nephropexy, proctopexy*

phag/o to eat, to ingest: *phagocyte, phagosome*

-phagia, -phagy eating, swallowing: *aphagia, dysphagia*

-phasia speech, ability to talk: *aphasia, dysphasia*

phen/o to show: *phenotype*

-phil, -philic to like, have an affinity for: *eosinophilia, hemophilia, hydrophilic*

phleb/o vein: *phlebitis, phlebotomy*

-phobia fear, dread, abnormal aversion: *phobic, acrophobia, hydrophobia*

phot/o light: *photoreceptor, photophobia*

phren/o diaphragm: *phrenic, phrenicotomy*

physi/o natural, physical: *physiology, physician*

pil/e, pil/i, pil/o hair, resembling hair: *pileous, piliation, pilonidal*

pin/o to drink: *pinocytosis*

-plasty molding, surgical formation: *cystoplasty, gastroplasty, kineplasty*

-plegia stroke, paralysis: *paraplegia, hemiplegia*

pleur/o side, rib, pleura: *pleurisy, pleurotomy*

-pnea air, breathing: *dyspnea, eupnea*

pneum/o, pneumat/o air, gas, respiration: *pneumothorax, pneumograph, pneumatocele*

pneumon/o lung: *pneumonia, pneumonectomy*

pod/o foot: *podiatry, pododynia*

-poiesis making, forming: *erythropoiesis, hematopoiesis*

polio- gray: *polioencephalitis, poliomyelitis*

poly- many: *polyarthritis, polycystic, polycythemia*

post- behind, after, following: *postnatal, postocular, postpartum*

pre- before, ahead of: *precancerous, preclinical, prenatal*

presby- old age: *presbycusis, presbyopia*

pro- before, in front of, in favor of: *prodromal, prosencephalon, prolapse, prothrombin*

proct/o rectum: *proctitis, proctocele, proctologist*

propri/o own: *proprioception*

pseud/o false: *pseudoarthrosis, pseudostratified, pseudopod*

psych/o mind: *psychosomatic, psychotherapy*

-ptosis downward displacement, falling, prolapse: *blepharoptosis, enteroptosis, nephroptosis*

pulm/o, pulmon/o lung: *pulmonic, pulmonology*

py/o pus: *pyuria, pyogenic, pyorrhea*

pyel/o renal pelvis: *pyelitis, pyelogram, pyelonephrosis*

pyr/o fire, fever: *pyrogen, antipyretic, pyromania*

quadr/i- four: *quadriceps, quadriplegic*

rachi/o spine: *rachicentesis, rachischisis*

radio- emission of rays or radiation: *radioactive, radiography, radiology*

re- again, back: *reabsorption, reaction, regenerate*

rect/o rectum: *rectal, rectouterine*

ren/o kidney: *renal, renopathy*

reticul/o network: *reticulum, reticular*

retro- backward, located behind: *retrocecal, retroperitoneal*

rhin/o nose: *rhinitis, rhinoplasty*

-rhage, -rhagia* bursting forth, excessive flow: *hemorrhage, menorrhagia*

-rhaphy* suturing or sewing up a gap or defect in a part: *herniorrhaphy, gastrorrhaphy, cystorrhaphy*

-rhea* flow, discharge: *diarrhea, gonorrhea, seborrhea*

sacchar/o sugar: *monosaccharide, polysaccharide*

salping/o tube: *salpingitis, salpingoscopy*

sarc/o flesh: *sarcolemma, sarcoplasm, sarcomere*

scler/o hard, hardness: *scleroderma, sclerosis*

scoli/o- twisted, crooked: *scoliosis, scoliosometer*

* When a suffix beginning with *rh* is added to a word root, the *r* is doubled.

-scope instrument used to look into or examine a part: *bronchoscope, endoscope, arthroscope*

semi- partial, half: *semipermeable, semicoma*

semin/o semen, seed: *seminiferous, seminal*

sep, septic poison, rot, decay: *sepsis, septicemia*

sin/o sinus: *sinusitis, sinusoid, sinoatrial*

-sis condition or process, usually abnormal: *dermatosis, osteoporosis*

soma-, somat/o, -some body: *somatic, somatotype, somatotropin*

son/o sound: *sonogram, sonography*

sphygm/o pulse: *sphygmomanometer*

spir/o breathing: *spirometer, inspiration, expiration*

splanchn/o- internal organs: *splanchnic, splanchnoptosis*

splen/o spleen: *splenectomy, splenic*

staphyl/o grapelike cluster: *staphylococcus*

stat, -stasis stand, stoppage, remain at rest: *hemostasis, static, homeostasis*

sten/o- contracted, narrowed: *stenosis*

sthen/o, -sthenia, -sthenic strength: *asthenic, calisthenics, neurasthenia*

steth/o chest: *stethoscope*

stoma, stomat/o mouth: *stomatitis*

-stomy surgical creation of an opening into a hollow organ or an opening between two organs: *colostomy, tracheostomy, gastroenterostomy*

strept/o chain: *streptococcus, streptobacillus*

sub- under, below, near, almost: *subclavian, subcutaneous, subluxation*

super- over, above, excessive: *superego, supernatant, superficial*

supra- above, over, superior: *supranasal, suprarenal*

sym-, syn- with, together: *symphysis, synapse*

syring/o fistula, tube, cavity: *syringectomy, syringomyelia*

tach/o-, tachy- rapid: *tachycardia, tachypnea*

tars/o eyelid, foot: *tarsitis, tarsoplasty, tarsoptosis*

-taxia, -taxis order, arrangement: *ataxia, chemotaxis, thermotaxis*

tel/o end: *telophase, telomere*

tens- stretch, pull: *extension, tensor*

test/o testis: *testosterone, testicular*

tetr/a four: *tetralogy, tetraplegia*

therm/o-, -thermy heat: *thermalgesia, thermocautery, diathermy, thermometer*

thromb/o blood clot: *thrombosis, thrombocyte*

toc/o labor: *eutocia, dystocia, oxytocin*

tom/o, -tomy incision of, cutting: *anatomy, phlebotomy, laparotomy*

ton/o tone, tension: *tonicity, tonic*

tox, toxic/o poison: *toxin, cytotoxic, toxemia, toxicology*

trache/o trachea, windpipe: *tracheal, tracheitis, tracheotomy*

trans- across, through, beyond: *transorbital, transpiration, transplant, transport*

tri- three: *triad, triceps*

trich/o hair: *trichiasis, trichosis, trichology*

troph/o, -trophic, -trophy nutrition, nurture: *atrophic, hypertrophy*

trop/o, -tropin, -tropic turning toward, acting on, influencing, changing: *thyrotropin, adrenocorticotropic, gonadotropic*

tympan/o drum: *tympanic, tympanum*

ultra- beyond or excessive: *ultrasound, ultraviolent, ultrastructure*

uni- one: *unilateral, uniovular, unicellular*

-uria urine: *glycosuria, hematuria, pyuria*

ur/o urine, urinary tract: *urology, urogenital*

vas/o vessel, duct: *vascular, vasectomy, vasodilation*

viscer/o internal organs, viscera: *visceral, visceroptosis*

vitre/o glasslike: *vitreous*

xer/o dryness: *xeroderma, xerophthalmia, xerosis*

-y condition of: *tetany, atony, dysentery*

zyg/o joined: *zygote, heterozygous, monozygotic*

Appendices

Metric Measurements

Appendix 1-1 Metric Measurements

Unit	Abbreviation	Metric Equivalent	U.S. Equivalent
Units of length			
Kilometer	km	1,000 meters	0.62 miles; 1.6 km/mile
Meter*	m	100 cm; 1,000 mm	39.4 inches; 1.1 yards
Centimeter	cm	1/100 m; 0.01 m	0.39 inches; 2.5 cm/inch
Millimeter	mm	1/1,000 m; 0.001 m	0.039 inches; 25 mm/inch
Micrometer	μm	1/1,000 mm; 0.001 mm	
Units of Weight			
Kilogram	kg	1,000 g	2.2 lb
Gram*	g	1,000 mg	0.035 oz.; 28.5 g/oz
Milligram	mg	1/1,000 g; 0.001 g	
Microgram	μg	1/1,000 mg; 0.001 mg	
Units of volume			
Liter*	L	1,000 mL	1.06 qt
Deciliter	dL	1/10 L; 0.1 L	
Milliliter	mL	1/1,000 L; 0.001 L	0.034 oz.; 29.4 mL/oz
Microliter	μL, mcL	1/1,000 mL; 0.001 mL	

* Basic unit.

Celsius–Fahrenheit Temperature Conversion Scale

Celsius to Fahrenheit

Use the following formula to convert Celsius readings to Fahrenheit readings:

$$°F = 9/5°C + 32$$

For example, if the Celsius reading is 37°

$$°F = (9/5 × 37) + 32$$

$$= 66.6 + 32$$

98.6°F (normal body temperature)

Fahrenheit to Celsius

Use the following formula to convert Fahrenheit readings to Celsius readings:

$$°C = 5/9 (°F - 32)$$

For example, if the Fahrenheit reading is 68°

$$°C = 5/9 (68 - 32)$$

$$= 5/9 × 36$$

20°C (a nice spring day)

temperature
conversion
scale

Periodic Table of the Elements

The periodic table lists the chemical elements according to their atomic numbers. The boxes in the table have information about the elements, as shown by the example at the top of the chart. The upper number in each box is the atomic number, which represents the number of protons in the nucleus of the atom. Under the name of the element is its chemical symbol, an abbreviation of its modern or Latin name. The Latin names of four common elements are shown below the chart. The bottom number in each box gives the atomic weight (mass) of that element's atoms compared with the weight of carbon atoms. Atomic weight is the sum of the weights of the protons and neutrons in the nucleus.

All the elements in a column share similar chemical properties based on the number of electrons in their outermost energy levels. Those in column VIII are non-reactive (inert) and are referred to as the noble gases. The 26 elements found in the body are color coded according to quantity (see totals above the chart). Carbon, hydrogen, oxygen, and nitrogen make up 96% of body weight. The first three of these are present in all carbohydrates, lipids, proteins, and nucleic acids. Nitrogen is an additional component of all proteins. Nine other elements make up almost all the rest of body weight. The remaining 13 elements are present in very small amounts and are referred to as trace elements. Although needed in very small quantities, they are essential for good health, as they are parts of enzymes and other compounds used in metabolism.

PERIODIC TABLE OF THE ELEMENTS

Notation:

6	Atomic number
Carbon	Name
C	Symbol
12.01	Atomic weight

- 96% of body weight
- 3.9% of body weight
- 0.1% of body weight

I																	VIII
1 Hydrogen **H** 1.01	II											III	IV	V	VI	VII	2 Helium **He** 4.00
3 Lithium **Li** 6.94	4 Beryllium **Be** 9.01											5 Boron **B** 10.81	6 Carbon **C** 12.01	7 Nitrogen **N** 14.01	8 Oxygen **O** 16.00	9 Fluorine **F** 19.00	10 Neon **Ne** 20.18
11 Sodium **Na** 22.99	12 Magnesium **Mg** 24.31											13 Aluminum **Al** 26.98	14 Silicon **Si** 28.09	15 Phosphorus **P** 30.97	16 Sulfur **S** 32.07	17 Chlorine **Cl** 35.45	18 Argon **Ar** 39.95
19 Potassium **K** 39.10	20 Calcium **Ca** 40.08	21 Scandium **Sc** 44.96	22 Titanium **Ti** 47.88	23 Vanadium **V** 50.94	24 Chromium **Cr** 52.00	25 Manganese **Mn** 54.94	26 Iron **Fe** 55.85	27 Cobalt **Co** 58.93	28 Nickel **Ni** 58.69	29 Copper **Cu** 63.55	30 Zinc **Zn** 65.39	31 Gallium **Ga** 69.72	32 Germanium **Ge** 72.59	33 Arsenic **As** 74.92	34 Selenium **Se** 78.96	35 Bromine **Br** 79.90	36 Krypton **Kr** 83.80
37 Rubidium **Rb** 85.47	38 Strontium **Sr** 87.62	39 Yttrium **Y** 88.91	40 Zirconium **Zr** 91.22	41 Niobium **Nb** 92.91	42 Molybdenum **Mo** 95.94	43 Technetium **Tc** (98)	44 Ruthenium **Ru** 101.1	45 Rhodium **Rh** 102.9	46 Palladium **Pd** 106.4	47 Silver **Ag** 107.9	48 Cadmium **Cd** 112.4	49 Indium **In** 114.8	50 Tin **Sn** 118.7	51 Antimony **Sb** 121.8	52 Tellurium **Te** 127.6	53 Iodine **I** 126.9	54 Xenon **Xe** 131.3
55 Cesium **Cs** 132.91	56 Barium **Ba** 137.34		72 Hafnium **Hf** 178.5	73 Tantalum **Ta** 180.9	74 Tungsten **W** 183.9	75 Rhenium **Re** 186.2	76 Osmium **Os** 190.2	77 Iridium **Ir** 192.2	78 Platinum **Pt** 195.1	79 Gold **Au** 196.9	80 Mercury **Hg** 200.6	81 Thallium **Tl** 204.4	82 Lead **Pb** 207.2	83 Bismuth **Bi** 209.0	84 Polonium **Po** (210)	85 Astatine **At** (210)	86 Radon **Rn** (222)
87 Francium **Fr** (223)	88 Radium **Ra** (226)		104 Rutherfordium **Rf** (257)	105 Dubnium **Db** (260)	106 Seaborgium **Sg** (263)	107 Bohrium **Bh** (262)	108 Hassium **Hs** (265)	109 Meitnerium **Mt** (267)	110 Darmstadtium **Ds** (271)	111 Unnamed (272)	112 Unnamed (277)						

57-71 Lanthanides

57 Lanthanum **La** 138.9	58 Cerium **Ce** 140.1	59 Praseodymium **Pr** 140.9	60 Neodymium **Nd** 144.2	61 Promethium **Pm** (145)	62 Samarium **Sm** (150.4)	63 Europium **Eu** 152.0	64 Gadolinium **Gd** 157.3	65 Terbium **Tb** 158.9	66 Dysprosium **Dy** 162.5	67 Holmium **Ho** 164.9	68 Erbium **Er** 167.3	69 Thulium **Tm** 168.9	70 Ytterbium **Yb** 173.0	71 Lutetium **Lu** 175.0

89-103 Actinides

89 Actinium **Ac** (227)	90 Thorium **Th** 232.0	91 Protactinium **Pa** (231)	92 Uranium **U** (238)	93 Neptunium **Np** (237)	94 Plutonium **Pu** (244)	95 Americium **Am** (243)	96 Curium **Cm** (247)	97 Berkelium **Bk** (247)	98 Californium **Cf** (251)	99 Einsteinium **Es** (254)	100 Fermium **Fm** (257)	101 Mendelevium **Md** (256)	102 Nobelium **No** (259)	103 Lawrencium **Lr** (257)

Name	Latin name	Symbol
Copper	*cuprium*	Cu
Iron	*ferrum*	Fe
Potassium	*kalium*	K
Sodium	*natrium*	Na

APPENDIX 4

Tests

Appendix 4-1	Routine Urinalysis

Test	Normal Value	Clinical Significance
General characteristics and measurements		
Color	Pale yellow to amber	Color change can be due to concentration or dilution, drugs, metabolic or inflammatory disorders
Odor	Slightly aromatic	Foul odor typical of urinary tract infection, fruity odor in uncontrolled diabetes mellitus
Appearance (clarity)	Clear to slightly hazy	Cloudy urine occurs with infection or after refrigeration; may indicate presence of bacteria, cells, mucus, or crystals
Specific gravity	1.003–1.030 (first morning catch; routine is random)	Decreased in diabetes insipidus, acute renal failure, water intoxication; increased in liver disorders, heart failure, dehydration
pH	4.5–8.0	Acid urine accompanies acidosis, fever, high protein diet; alkaline urine in urinary tract infection, metabolic alkalosis, vegetarian diet
Chemical determinations		
Glucose	Negative	Glucose present in uncontrolled diabetes mellitus, steroid excess
Ketones	Negative	Present in diabetes mellitus and in starvation
Protein	Negative	Present in kidney disorders, such as glomerulonephritis, acute kidney failure
Bilirubin	Negative	Breakdown product of hemoglobin; present in liver disease or in bile blockage
Urobilinogen	0.2–1.0 Ehrlich units /dL	Breakdown product of bilirubin; increased in hemolytic anemias and in liver disease; remains negative in bile obstruction
Blood (occult)	Negative	Detects small amounts of blood cells, hemoglobin, or myoglobin; present in severe trauma, metabolic disorders, bladder infections
Nitrite	Negative	Product of bacterial breakdown of urine; positive result suggests urinary tract infection and needs to be followed up with a culture of the urine
Microscopic		
Red blood cells	0–3 per high-power field	Increased because of bleeding within the urinary tract from trauma, tumors, inflammation, or damage within the kidney
White blood cells	0–4 per high-power field	Increased by kidney or bladder infection
Renal epithelial cells	Occasional	Increased number indicates damage to kidney tubules
Casts	None	Hyaline casts normal; large number of abnormal casts indicates inflammation or a systemic disorder
Crystals	Present	Most are normal; may be acid or alkaline
Bacteria	Few	Increased in urinary tract infection or contamination from infected genitalia
Others		Any yeasts, parasites, mucus, spermatozoa, or other microscopic findings would be reported here

Appendix 4-2   Complete Blood Count

Test	Normal Value*	Clinical Significance
Red blood cell (RBC) count	Men: 4.2–5.4 million/μL Women: 3.6–5.0 million/μL	Decreased in anemia; increased in dehydration, polycythemia
Hemoglobin (Hb)	Men: 13.5–17.5 g/dL Women: 12–16 g/dL	Decreased in anemia, hemorrhage, and hemolytic reactions; increased in dehydration, heart and lung disease
Hematocrit (Hct) or packed cell volume (PCV)	Men: 40%–50% Women: 37%–47%	Decreased in anemia; increased in polycythemia, dehydration These values, calculated from the RBC count, Hb, and Hct, give information valuable in the diagnosis and classification of anemia
Red blood cell (RBC) indices (examples)		
Mean corpuscular volume (MCV)	87–103 μL/red cell	Measures the average size or volume of each RBC: small size (microcytic) in iron-deficiency anemia; large size (macrocytic) typical of pernicious anemia
Mean corpuscular hemoglobin (MCH)	26–34 pg/red cell	Measures the weight of hemoglobin per RBC; useful in differentiating types of anemia in a severely anemic patient
Mean corpuscular hemoglobin concentration (MCHC)	31–37 g/dL	Defines the volume of hemoglobin per RBC; used to determine the color or concentration of hemoglobin per RBC
White blood cell (WBC) count	5,000–10,000μL	Increased in leukemia and in response to infection, inflammation, and dehydration; decreased in bone marrow suppression
Platelets	150,000–350,000/μL	Increased in many malignant disorders; decreased in disseminated intravascular coagulation (DIC) or toxic drug effects; spontaneous bleeding may occur at platelet counts below 20,000 μL
Differential (Peripheral blood smear)		A stained slide of the blood is needed to perform the differential. The percentages of the different WBCs are estimated, and the slide is microscopically checked for abnormal characteristics in WBCs, RBCs, and platelets
WBCs		
Segmented neutrophils (SEGs, POLYs)	40%–74%	Increased in bacterial infections; low numbers leave person very susceptible to infection
Immature neutrophils (BANDs)	0%–3%	Increased when neutrophil count increases
Lymphocytes (LYMPHs)	20%–40%	Increased in viral infections; low numbers leave person dangerously susceptible to infection
Monocytes (MONOs)	2%–6%	Increased in specific infections
Eosinophils (EOs)	1%–4%	Increased in allergic disorders
Basophils (BASOs)	0.5%–1%	Increased in allergic disorders

*Values vary depending on instrumentation and type of test.

Appendix 4-3   Blood Chemistry Tests

Test	Normal Value	Clinical Significance
Basic panel: An overview of electrolytes, waste product management, and metabolism		
Blood urea nitrogen (BUN)	7–18 mg/dL	Increased in renal disease and dehydration; decreased in liver damage and malnutrition
Carbon dioxide (CO_2) (includes bicarbonate)	23–30 mmol/L	Useful to evaluate acid-base balance by measuring total carbon dioxide in the blood: Elevated in vomiting and pulmonary disease; decreased in diabetic acidosis, acute renal failure, and hyperventilation
Chloride (Cl)	98–106 mEq/L	Increased in dehydration, hyperventilation, and congestive heart failure; decreased in vomiting, diarrhea, and fever
Creatinine	0.6–1.2 mg/dL	Produced at a constant rate and excreted by the kidney; increased in kidney disease
Glucose	Fasting: 70–110 mg/dL Random: 85–125 mg/dL	Increased in diabetes and severe illness; decreased in insulin overdose or hypoglycemia
Potassium (K)	3.5–5 mEq/L	Increased in renal failure, extensive cell damage, and acidosis; decreased in vomiting, diarrhea, and excess administration of diuretics or IV fluids
Sodium (Na)	101–111 mEq/L or 135–148 mEq/L (depending on test)	Increased in dehydration and diabetes insipidus; decreased in overload of IV fluids, burns, diarrhea, or vomiting
Additional blood chemistry tests		
Alanine aminotransferase (ALT)	10–40 U/L	Used to diagnose and monitor treatment of liver disease and to monitor the effects of drugs on the liver; increased in myocardial infarction
Albumin	3.8–5.0 g/dL	Albumin holds water in blood; decreased in liver disease and kidney disease
Albumin-globulin ratio (A/G ratio)	Greater than 1	Low A/G ratio signifies a tendency for edema because globulin is less effective than albumin at holding water in the blood
Alkaline phosphatase (ALP)	20–70 U/L (varies by method)	Enzyme of bone metabolism; increased in liver disease and metastatic bone disease
Amylase	21–160 U/L	Used to diagnose and monitor treatment of acute pancreatitis and to detect salivary gland inflammation
Aspartate aminotransferase (AST)	0–41 U/L (varies)	Enzyme present in tissues with high metabolic activity; increased in myocardial infarction and liver disease
Bilirubin, total	0.2–1.0 mg/dL	Breakdown product of hemoglobin from red blood cells; increased when excessive red blood cells are being destroyed or in liver disease
Calcium (Ca)	8.8–10.0 mg/dL	Increased in excess parathyroid hormone production and in cancer; decreased in alkalosis, elevated phosphate in renal failure, and excess IV fluids
Cholesterol	120–220 mg/dL desirable range	Screening test used to evaluate risk of heart disease; levels of 200 mg/dL or above indicate increased risk of heart disease and warrant further investigation
Creatine kinase (CK)	Men: 38–174 U/L Women: 96–140 U/L	Elevated enzyme level indicates myocardial infarction or damage to skeletal muscle. When elevated, specific fractions (isoenzymes) are tested for
Gamma-glutamyl transferase (GGT)	Men: 6–26 U/L Women: 4–18 U/L	Used to diagnose liver disease and to test for chronic alcoholism
Globulins	2.3–3.5 g/dL	Proteins active in immunity; help albumin keep water in blood
Iron, serum (Fe)	Men: 75–175 µg/dL Women: 65–165 µg/dL	Decreased in iron deficiency and anemia; increased in hemolytic conditions
High-density lipoproteins (HDLs)	Men: 30–70 mg/dL Women: 30–85 mg/dL	Used to evaluate the risk of heart disease

(continued)

Appendix 4-3   Blood Chemistry Tests (continued)

Test	Normal Value	Clinical Significance
Lactic dehydrogenase (LDH or LD)	95–200 U/L (Normal ranges vary greatly)	Enzyme released in many kinds of tissue damage, including myocardial infarction, pulmonary infarction, and liver disease
Lipase	4–24 U/L (varies with test)	Enzyme used to diagnose pancreatitis
Low-density lipoproteins (LDLs)	80–140 mg/dL	Used to evaluate the risk of heart disease
Magnesium (Mg)	1.3–2.1 mEq/L	Vital in neuromuscular function; decreased levels may occur in malnutrition, alcoholism, pancreatitis, diarrhea
Phosphorus (P) (inorganic)	2.7–4.5 mg/dL	Evaluated in response to calcium; main store is in bone: elevated in kidney disease; decreased in excess parathyroid hormone
Protein, total	6–8 g/dL	Increased in dehydration, multiple myeloma; decreased in kidney disease, liver disease, poor nutrition, severe burns, excessive bleeding
Serum glutamic oxalacetic transaminase (SGOT)		See Aspartate aminotransferase (AST)
Serum glutamic pyruvic transaminase (SGPT)		See Alanine aminotransferase (ALT)
Thyroxin (T_4)	5–12.5 μg/dL (varies)	Screening test of thyroid function; increased in hyperthyroidism; decreased in myxedema and hypothyroidism
Thyroid-stimulating hormone (TSH)	0.5–6 mIU/L	Produced by pituitary to promote thyroid gland function; elevated when thyroid gland is not functioning
Triiodothyronine (T_3)	120–195 mg/dL	Elevated in specific types of hyperthyroidism
Triglycerides	Men: 40–160 mg/dL Women: 35–135 mg/dL	An indication of ability to metabolize fats; increased triglycerides and cholesterol indicate high risk of atherosclerosis
Uric acid	Men: 3.5–7.2 mg/dL Women: 2.6–6.0 mg/dL	Produced by breakdown of ingested purines in food and nucleic acids; elevated in kidney disease, gout, and leukemia

APPENDIX 5 Diseases

Appendix 5-1   Bacterial Diseases

Organism	Disease and Description
Cocci	
Neisseria gonorrhoeae (gonococcus)	Gonorrhea. Acute inflammation of mucous membranes of the reproductive and urinary tracts (with possible spread to the peritoneum in the female). Systemic infection may cause gonococcal arthritis and endocarditis. Organism also causes ophthalmia neonatorum, an eye inflammation of the newborn.
Neisseria meningitidis (meningococcus)	Epidemic meningitis. Inflammation of the membranes covering brain and spinal cord. A vaccine is available for use in high-risk populations.
Staphylococcus aureus and other staphylococci	Boils, carbuncles, impetigo, osteomyelitis, staphylococcal pneumonia, cystitis, pyelonephritis, empyema, septicemia, toxic shock, and food poisoning. Strains resistant to antibiotics are a cause of infections originating in hospitals, such as wound infections.
Streptococcus pneumoniae	Pneumonia; inflammation of the alveoli, bronchioles, and bronchi; middle ear infections; meningitis. May be prevented by use of polyvalent pneumococcal vaccine.
Streptococcus pyogenes, Streptococcus hemolyticus, and other streptococci	Septicemia, septic sore throat, scarlet fever, puerperal sepsis, erysipelas, streptococcal pneumonia, rheumatic fever, subacute bacterial endocarditis, acute glomerulonephritis.
Bacilli	
Bordetella pertussis	Pertussis (whooping cough). Severe infection of the trachea and bronchi. The "whoop" is caused by the effort to recover breath after coughing. All children should be immunized against pertussis.
Brucella abortus (and others)	Brucellosis, or undulant fever. Disease of animals such as cattle and goats transmitted to humans through unpasteurized dairy products or undercooked meat. Acute phase of fever and weight loss; chronic disease with abscess formation and depression.
Clostridium botulinum	Botulism. Very severe poisoning caused by eating food in which the organism has been allowed to grow and excrete its toxin. Causes muscle paralysis and may result in death from asphyxiation. Infant botulism results from ingestion of spores. It causes respiratory problems and flaccid paralysis, which usually respond to treatment.
Clostridium perfringens	Gas gangrene. Acute wound infection. Organisms cause death of tissues accompanied by the generation of gas within them.
Clostridium tetani	Tetanus. Acute, often fatal poisoning caused by introduction of the organism into deep wounds. Characterized by severe muscular spasms. Also called *lockjaw*.
Corynebacterium diphtheriae	Diphtheria. Acute throat inflammation with the formation of a leathery membranelike growth (pseudomembrane) that can obstruct air passages and cause death by asphyxiation. Toxin produced by this organism can damage heart, nerves, kidneys, and other organs. Disease preventable by appropriate vaccination.
Escherichia coli, Proteus spp., and other colon bacilli	Normal inhabitants of the colon, and usually harmless there. Cause of local and systemic infections, food poisoning, diarrhea (especially in children), septicemia, and septic shock. *E. coli* is a common hospital-acquired infection.

(continued)

Appendix 5-1 Bacterial Diseases (*continued*)

Organism	Disease and Description
Francisella tularensis	Tularemia, or deer fly fever. Transmitted by contact with an infected animal or by a tick or fly bite. Symptoms are fever, ulceration of the skin, and enlarged lymph nodes.
Haemophilus influenzae type b (Hib)	Severe infections in children under 3 years of age. Causes meningitis, also epiglottitis, septicemia, pneumonia, pericarditis, and septic arthritis. Preschool vaccinations are routine.
Helicobacter pylori	Acute inflammation of the stomach (gastritis), ulcers of the stomach's pyloric area and the duodenum.
Legionella pneumophila	Legionnaires disease (pneumonia). Seen in localized epidemics; may be transmitted by air conditioning towers and by contaminated soil at excavation sites. Not spread person to person. Characterized by high fever, vomiting, diarrhea, cough, and bradycardia. Mild form of the disease called Pontiac fever.
Mycobacterium leprae (Hansen bacillus)	Leprosy. Chronic illness in which hard swellings occur under the skin, particularly of the face, causing a distorted appearance. In one form of leprosy, the nerves are affected, resulting in loss of sensation in the extremities.
Mycobacterium tuberculosis (tubercle bacillus)	Tuberculosis. Infectious disease in which the organism causes primary lesions called *tubercles*. These break down into cheeselike masses of tissue, a process known as *caseation*. Any body organ can be infected, but in adults, the usual site is the lungs. Still one of the most widespread diseases in the world, tuberculosis is treated with chemotherapy; strains of the bacillus have developed resistance to drugs.
Pseudomonas aeruginosa	Common organism is a frequent cause of wound and urinary infections in debilitated hospitalized patients. Often found in solutions that have been standing for long periods.
Salmonella typhi (and others)	Salmonellosis occurs as enterocolitis, bacteremia, localized infection, or typhoid. Depending on type, presenting symptoms may be fever, diarrhea, or abscesses; complications include intestinal perforation and endocarditis. Carried in water, milk, meat, and other food.
Shigella dysenteriae (and others)	Serious bacillary dysentery. Acute intestinal infection with diarrhea (sometimes bloody); may cause dehydration with electrolyte imbalance or septicemia. Transmitted through fecal-oral route or other poor sanitation.
Yersinia pestis	Plague, the "black death" of the Middle Ages. Transmitted to humans by fleas from infected rodents. Symptoms of the most common form are swollen, infected lymph nodes, or *buboes*. Another form may cause pneumonia. All forms may lead to a rapidly fatal septicemia.
Curved rods	
Vibrio	
Vibrio cholerae	Cholera. Acute intestinal infection characterized by prolonged vomiting and diarrhea, leading to severe dehydration, electrolyte imbalance, and in some cases, death.
Spirochetes	
Borrelia burgdorferi	Lyme disease, transmitted by the extremely small deer tick. Usually starts with a bulls-eye rash followed by flulike symptoms, at which time antibiotics are effective. May progress to neurologic problems and joint inflammation.
Borrelia recurrentis (and others)	Relapsing fever. Generalized infection in which attacks of fever alternate with periods of apparent recovery. Organisms spread by lice, ticks, and other insects.
Treponema pallidum	Syphilis. Infectious disease transmitted mainly by sexual intercourse. Untreated syphilis is seen in the following three stages: primary—formation of primary lesion (chancre); secondary—skin eruptions and infectious patches on mucous membranes; tertiary—development of generalized lesions (gummas) and destruction of tissues resulting in aneurysm, heart disease, and degenerative changes in brain, spinal cord, ganglia, and meninges. Also a cause of intrauterine fetal death or stillbirth.
Treponema vincentii	Vincent disease (trench mouth). Infection of the mouth and throat accompanied by formation of a pseudomembrane, with ulceration.

(*continued*)

Appendix 5-1   Bacterial Diseases (continued)

Organism	Disease and Description
Other bacteria	
(Note: The following organisms are smaller than other bacteria and vary in shape. Like viruses, they grow within cells, but they differ from viruses in that they are affected by antibiotics.)	
Chlamydia oculogenitalis	Inclusion conjunctivitis, acute eye infection. Carried in genital organs; transmitted during birth or through water in inadequately chlorinated swimming pools.
Chlamydia psittaci	Psittacosis, also called ornithosis. Disease transmitted by various birds, including parrots, ducks, geese, and turkeys. Primary symptoms are chills, headache, and fever, more severe in older people. The duration may be from 2 to 3 weeks, often with a long convalescence. Antibiotic drugs are effective remedies.
Chlamydia trachomatis	Sexually transmitted infection causing pelvic inflammatory disease and other reproductive tract infections. Also causes inclusion conjunctivitis, an acute eye infection, and trachoma, a chronic infection that is a common cause of blindness in underdeveloped areas of the world. Infection of the conjunctiva and cornea characterized by redness, pain, and lacrimation. Antibiotic therapy is effective if begun before there is scarring. The same organism causes lymphogranuloma venereum (LGV), a sexually transmitted infection characterized by swelling of inguinal lymph nodes and accompanied by signs of general infection
Coxiella burnetti	Q fever. Infection transmitted from cattle, sheep, and goats to humans by contaminated dust and also carried by arthropods. Symptoms are fever, headache, chills, and pneumonitis. This disorder is almost never fatal.
Rickettsia prowazekii	Epidemic typhus. Transmitted to humans by lice; associated with poor hygiene and war. Main symptoms are headache, hypotension, delirium, and a red rash. Frequently fatal in older people.
Rickettsia rickettsii	Rocky Mountain spotted fever. Tick-borne disease occurring throughout the United States. Symptoms are fever, muscle aches, and a rash that may progress to gangrene over bony prominences. The disease is rarely fatal.
Rickettsia typhi	Endemic or murine typhus. A milder disease transmitted to humans from rats by fleas. Symptoms are fever, rash, headache, and cough. The disease is rarely fatal.

Appendix 5-2   Viral Diseases

Organism	Disease and Description
Common cold viruses	Common cold (coryza), viral infection of the upper respiratory tract. A wide variety of organisms may be involved. May lead to complications, such as pneumonia and influenza.
Cytomegalovirus (CMV)	Common mild salivary gland infection. In an immunosuppressed person may cause infection of the retina, lung, and liver, GI tract ulceration, and brain inflammation. Causes severe fetal or neonatal damage.
Encephalitis viruses	Encephalitis, which usually refers to any brain inflammation accompanied by degenerative tissue changes. Encephalitis has many causes besides viruses. Viral forms of encephalitis include Western and Eastern epidemic, equine, St. Louis, Japanese B, and others. Some are known to be transmitted from birds and other animals to humans by insects, principally mosquitoes
Epstein-Barr virus (EBV)	Mononucleosis, a highly infectious disease spread by saliva. Common among teenagers and young adults. There is fever, sore throat, marked fatigue, and enlargement of the spleen and lymph nodes. Infects B lymphocytes (mononuclear leukocytes) causing them to multiply. Virus remains latent for life after infection. EBV also causes Burkitt lymphoma, a malignant B lymphocyte tumor common in parts of Africa.
Hantavirus	Hantavirus pulmonary syndrome (HPS) with high mortality rate. Spread through inhalation of virus from dried urine of infected rodents.

(continued)

Appendix 5-2   Viral Diseases (continued)

Organism	Disease and Description
Hepatitis viruses	Liver inflammation. Varieties A through E are recognized.
Hepatitis A virus (HAV)	Transmitted by fecal contamination. Does not become chronic or produce carrier state. Infection provides lifelong immunity. Vaccine is available.
Hepatitis B virus (HBV)	Transmitted by direct exchange of blood and body fluids. Can cause rapidly fatal disease or develop into chronic disease and carrier state. Risk of progress to liver cancer. Vaccine is available.
Hepatitis C virus (HCV)	Spread through blood exchange (usually transfusions before 1992 when screening began) or shared needles. May become chronic and lead to cirrhosis, liver failure, liver cancer. Antiviral drugs may limit infection.
Hepatitis D virus (HDV)	Spread by blood exchange and occurs as coinfection with hepatitis B. Responsible for half of rapidly fatal liver failure cases and also a high rate of chronic disease that progresses to death.
Hepatitis E virus (HEV)	Transmitted by fecal contamination and occurs in epidemics in Middle East and Asia. Resembles hepatitis A. Can be fatal in pregnant women.
Herpes simplex virus type 1	Cold sores or fever blisters that appear around the mouth and nose of people with colds or other illnesses accompanied by fever.
Herpes simplex virus type 2	Genital herpes. Acute inflammatory disease of the genitalia, often recurring. A very common sexually transmitted infection.
Human immunodeficiency virus (HIV)	Acquired immunodeficiency syndrome (AIDS). Disease that infects T cells of the immune system and is usually fatal if untreatd. Diagnosed by antibody tests, decline in specific (CD4) cells, and presenting disease, including *Candida albicans* infection, *Pneumocystis jirovici* pneumonia (PCP), Kaposi sarcoma, persistent swelling of lymph nodes (lymphadenopathy), chronic diarrhea, and wasting. Spread by contact with contaminated body fluids and by transplacental route.
Human papillomavirus (HPV)	Genital warts (condylomata acuminata). Sexually transmitted warts of the genital and perianal area in men and women. Associated with cervical dysplasia and cancer. A vaccine against the most prevalent strains is available.
Influenza virus	Epidemic viral infection, marked by chills, fever, muscular pains, and prostration. The most serious complication is bronchopneumonia caused by *Haemophilus influenzae* (a bacillus) or streptococci.
Mumps virus	Epidemic parotitis. Acute inflammation with swelling of the parotid salivary glands. Mumps can have many complications, such as orchitis (inflammation of the testes) in young men and meningitis in young children.
Pneumonia viruses	Lung infections caused by a number of different viruses, such as the influenza and parainfluenza viruses, adenoviruses, and varicella viruses.
Poliovirus	Poliomyelitis (polio). Acute viral infection that may attack the anterior horns of the spinal cord, resulting in paralysis of certain voluntary muscles. Most countries have eliminated polio through vaccination programs.
Rhabdovirus	Rabies. An acute, fatal disease transmitted to humans through the saliva of an infected animal. Rabies is characterized by violent muscular spasms induced by the slightest sensations. Because the swallowing of water causes throat spasms, the disease is also call hydrophobia ("fear of water"). The final stage of paralysis ends in death. Rabies vaccines are available for humans and animals.
Rotavirus	Attacks lining of small intestine causing severe diarrhea in children. A new vaccine was approved in 2006.
Rubella virus	Rubella or German measles. A less severe form of measles, but especially dangerous during the first 3 months of pregnancy because the disease organism can cause heart defects, deafness, mental deficiency, and other permanent damage in the fetus.
Rubeola virus	Measles. An acute respiratory inflammation followed by fever and a generalized skin rash. Patients are prone to the development of dangerous complications, such as bronchopneumonia and other secondary infections caused by staphylococci and streptococci.
SARS virus	Highly infectious respiratory disease called severe acute respiratory syndrome (SARS). Emerged in China early in 2003 and spread to other countries before it was isolated and identified as a viral infection. Believed to have spread from small mammals to humans.

(continued)

Appendix 5-2   Viral Diseases (continued)

Organism	Disease and Description
Varicella zoster	Chickenpox (varicella). A usually mild infection, almost completely confined to children, characterized by blisterlike skin eruptions. Vaccine now available.
	Shingles (herpes zoster). A very painful eruption of skin blisters that follows the course of certain peripheral nerves. These blisters eventually dry up and form scabs that resemble shingles. Vaccine now available for people 60 years and older.

Appendix 5-3   Prion Diseases

Agent	Disease
(Note: Prions are infectious agents that contain protein but no nucleic acid. They cause slow, spongy degeneration of brain tissue, known as spongiform encephalitis, in humans and animals.)	
Chronic wasting disease agent	Chronic wasting disease in deer and elk.
Creutzfeldt-Jakob agent	Creutzfeldt-Jacob disease (CJD), a spongiform encephalopathy in humans.
Kuru agent	Kuru spongiform encephalopathy in humans.
Mad cow agent	Mad cow spongiform encephalopathy, or bovine spongiform encephalopathy (BSE) in cows and humans.
Scrapie agent	Scrapie spongiform encephalopathy in sheep.

Appendix 5-4   Fungal Diseases

Disease/Organism	Description
Actinomycosis	"Lumpy jaw" in cattle and humans. The organisms cause the formation of large tissue masses, which are often accompanied by abscesses. The lungs and liver may be involved.
Blastomycosis (*Blastomyces dermatitidis*)	General term for any infection caused by a yeastlike organism. There may be skin tumors and lesions in the lungs, bones, liver, spleen, and kidneys.
Candidiasis (*Candida albicans*)	Infection that can involve the skin and mucous membranes. May cause diaper rash, infection of the nail beds, and infection of the mucous membranes of the mouth (thrush), throat, and vagina.
Coccidioidomycosis (*Coccidioides immitis*)	Systemic fungal disease also called *San Joaquin Valley fever*. Because it often attacks the lungs, it may be mistaken for tuberculosis.
Histoplasmosis (*Histoplasma capsulatum*)	Variety of disorders, ranging from mild respiratory symptoms or enlargement of liver, spleen, and lymph nodes to cavities in the lungs with symptoms similar to those of tuberculosis.
Pneumocystis jiroveci (formerly carinii)	Pneumonia (PCP). Opportunistic infection in people with a depressed immune system. Invades lungs and causes a foamy exudate to collect in alveoli.

Ringworm
  Tinea capitis
  Tinea corporis
  Tinea pedis
	Common fungal skin infections, many of which cause blisters and scaling with discoloration of the affected areas. All are caused by similar organisms from a group of fungi called *dermatophytes*. They are easily transmitted by person to person contact or by contaminated articles.

Appendix 5-5   Protozoal Diseases

Organism	Disease And Description
Amebae	
Entamoeba histolytica	Amebic dysentery. Severe ulceration of the wall of the large intestine caused by amebae. Acute diarrhea may be an important symptom. This organism also may cause liver abscesses.
Ciliates	
Balantidium coli	Gastrointestinal disturbances and ulcers of the colon.
Flagellates	
Giardia lamblia	Gastrointestinal disturbances.
Leishmania donovani (and others)	Kala-azar. In this disease, there is enlargement of the liver and spleen as well as skin lesions.
Trichomonas vaginalis	Inflammation and discharge from the vagina. In males, it involves the urethra and causes painful urination.
Trypanosoma	African sleeping sickness. Disease begins with a high fever, followed by invasion of the brain and spinal cord by the organisms. Usually, the disease ends with continued drowsiness, coma, and death.
Sporozoa (apicomplexans)	
Cryptosporidium	Cramps and diarrhea that can be long term and severe in people with a weakened immune system, such as those with AIDS. Spread in water and by personal contact in close quarters.
Plasmodium; varieties include *vivax, falciparum, malariae*	Malaria. Characterized by recurrent attacks of chills followed by high fever. Severe malarial attacks can be fatal because of kidney failure, cerebral disorders, and other complications.
Toxoplasma gondii	Toxoplasmosis. Common infectious disease transmitted by cats and raw meat. Mild forms cause fever and lymph node enlargement. May cause fatal encephalitis in immunosuppressed patients. Infection of a pregnant woman is a cause of fetal stillbirth or congenital damage.

Answers to Chapter Checkpoint and Zooming In Questions

Chapter 1

Answers to Checkpoint Questions

1-1 Study of body structure is anatomy; study of body function is physiology.

1-2 The breakdown phase of metabolism is catabolism; the building phase of metabolism is anabolism.

1-3 Negative feedback systems are primarily used to maintain homeostasis.

1-4 The three planes in which the body can be cut are sagittal, frontal (coronal), and transverse (horizontal). The midsagittal plane divides the body into two equal halves.

1-5 The posterior cavity is the dorsal cavity; the anterior cavity is the ventral cavity.

1-6 The three central regions of the abdomen are the epigastric, umbilical, and hypogastric regions; the three left and right lateral regions of the abdomen are the hypochondriac, lumbar, and iliac (inguinal) regions.

1-7 The basic unit of length in the metric system is the meter; of weight, the gram; of volume, the liter.

Answers to Zooming In Questions

1-7 The figures are standing in the anatomic position.

1-8 The transverse (horizontal) plane divides the body into superior and inferior parts. The frontal (coronal) plane divides the body into anterior and posterior parts.

1-11 The ventral cavity contains the diaphragm.

Chapter 2

Answers to Checkpoint Questions

2-1 Atoms are subunits of elements.

2-2 Three types of particles found in atoms are protons, neutrons, and electrons.

2-3 Molecules are units composed of two or more atoms. They are the subunits of compounds.

2-4 Water is the most abundant compound in the body.

2-5 In a solution, the components dissolve and remain evenly distributed (the mixture is homogeneous); in a suspension, the particles settle out unless the mixture is shaken (the mixture is heterogeneous).

2-6 When an electrolyte goes into solution, it separates into charged particles called ions (cations and anions).

2-7 A covalent bond is formed by the sharing of electrons.

2-8 A value of 7.0 is neutral on the pH scale. An acid measures lower than 7.0; a base measures higher than 7.0.

2-9 A buffer is a substance that maintains a steady pH of a solution.

2-10 Isotopes that break down to give off radiation are termed radioactive.

2-11 Organic compounds are found in living things.

2-12 The element carbon is the basis of organic chemistry.

2-13 The three main categories of organic compounds are carbohydrates, lipids, and proteins.

2-14 A catalyst is a compound that speeds up the rate of a chemical reaction.

Answers to Zooming In Questions

2-1 The number of protons is equal to the number of electrons. There are eight protons and eight electrons.

2-2 Two hydrogen atoms bond with an oxygen atom to form water.

2-4 Two electrons are needed to complete the energy level of each hydrogen atom.

2-5 The amount of hydroxide ion (OH^-) in a solution decreases when the amount of hydrogen ion (H^+) increases.

2-7 Monosaccharides are the building blocks of disaccharides and polysaccharides.

2-8 There are three carbon atoms in glycerol.

2-9 The amino group of an amino acid contains nitrogen.

2-10 The shape of the enzyme after the reaction is the same as it was before the reaction.

Chapter 3

Answers to Checkpoint Questions

3-1 The cell shows organization, metabolism, responsiveness, homeostasis, growth, and reproduction.

3-2 Three types of microscopes are the compound light microscope, transmission electron microscope (TEM), and scanning electron microscope (SEM).

3-3 The main substance of the plasma membrane is a bilayer of phospholipids. Three types of materials found within the membrane are cholesterol, proteins, and carbohydrates (glycoproteins and glycolipids).

3-4 The cell organelles are specialized structures that perform different tasks.

3-5 The nucleus is called the control center of the cell because it contains the chromosomes, hereditary units that control all cellular activities.

3-6 The two types of organelles used for movement are the cilia, which are small and hairlike, and the flagellum, which is long and whiplike.

3-7 Nucleotides are the building blocks of nucleic acids.

3-8 DNA codes for proteins in the cell.

3-9 The three main types of RNA active in protein synthesis are messenger RNA (mRNA), ribosomal RNA (rRNA) and transfer RNA (tRNA).

3-10 Before mitosis can occur, the DNA must replicate (double). The replication occurs during interphase.

3-11 The four stages of mitosis are prophase, metaphase, anaphase, and telophase.

3-12 Diffusion, osmosis, filtration, and facilitated diffusion do not require cellular energy; active transport, endocytosis (phagocytosis and pinocytosis), and exocytosis require cellular energy.

3-13 An isotonic solution is the same concentration as the fluid within the cell; a hypotonic solution is less concentrated; a hypertonic solution is more concentrated.

Answers to Zooming In Questions

3-1 The transmission electron microscope (TEM) shows the most internal structure (B). The scanning electron microscope (SEM) shows the cilia in three dimensions (C).

3-2 Ribosomes attached to the ER make it look rough. Cytosol is the liquid part of the cytoplasm.

3-3 Two layers make up the main substance of the plasma membrane.

3-4 Epithelial cells (B) would best cover a large surface area because they are flat.

3-6 The nucleotides pair up so that there is one large nucleotide and one smaller nucleotide in each pair.

3-9 If the original cell has 46 chromosomes, each daughter cell will have 46 chromosomes after mitosis.

3-11 If diffusion were occurring in the body, the net would be the plasma membrane.

3-12 If the solute could pass through the membrane, the solute and solvent molecules would equalize on the two sides of the membrane, and the fluid level would be the same on both sides.

3-13 If the concentration of solute was increased on side B of this system, the osmotic pressure would increase.

3-15 An increase in the number of transporters would increase the rate of facilitated diffusion. A decrease in the number of transporters would decrease the rate of facilitated diffusion.

3-16 A lysosome would likely help to destroy a particle taken in by phagocytosis.

3-18 If lost blood were replaced with pure water, red blood cells would swell because the blood would become hypotonic to the cells.

Chapter 4

Answers to Checkpoint Questions

4-1 The three basic shapes of epithelium are squamous (flat and irregular), cuboidal (square), and columnar (long and narrow).

4-2 Exocrine glands secrete through ducts; endocrine glands do not have ducts and secrete directly into surrounding tissue and the bloodstream.

4-3 The intercellular material in connective tissue is the matrix.

4-4 The main type of fiber in connective tissue is composed of collagen.

4-5 Circulating connective tissues are blood and lymph. Generalized connective tissues are loose (areolar, adipose) and dense, as found in membranes, capsules, ligaments, and tendons. Structural connective tissues are cartilage and bone.

4-6 The three types of muscle tissue are skeletal (voluntary), cardiac, and smooth (visceral) muscle.

4-7 The basic cellular unit of the nervous system is the neuron and it carries nerve impulses.

4-8 The nonconducting support cells of the nervous system are neuroglia (glial cells).

4-9 The three types of epithelial membranes are the cutaneous membrane (skin), serous membranes, and mucous membranes.

4-10 A benign tumor does not spread; a malignant tumor spreads (metastasizes) to other tissues.

4-11 The three standard approaches to treatment of cancer are surgery, radiation, and chemotherapy.

Answers to Zooming In Questions

4-1 The epithelial cells are in a single layer.

4-5 Areolar connective tissue has the most fibers; adipose tissue is modified for storage.

Chapter 5

Answers to Checkpoint Questions

5-1 Disease is an abnormality of the structure or function of a part, organ, or system.

5-2 A predisposing cause of disease is a factor that may not in itself give rise to a disease but that increases the probability of a person's becoming ill.

5-3 The two medical sciences that are involved in study of disease are pathology (study of disease) and physiology (study of function).

5-4 A communicable disease is one that can be transmitted from one person to another.

5-5 A diagnosis is the identification of an illness based on signs and symptoms.

5-6 A parasite is an organism that lives on or within a host and at the host's expense.

5-7 A pathogen is any disease-causing organism.

5-8 The skin, respiratory tract, digestive, urinary and reproductive systems are portals of entry and exit for microorganisms.

5-9 Microbiology includes the study of bacteria, viruses, fungi, protozoa, and algae.

5-10 The term normal flora refers to the microorganisms that normally live in or on the body.

5-11 Resistant forms of bacteria are called endospores.

5-12 The three basic shapes of bacteria are cocci (round), bacilli (rod-shaped), and curved rods, including vibrios, spirilla, and spirochetes.

5-13 Viruses are smaller than bacteria, are not cellular, and have no enzyme system. They contain only DNA or RNA, not both.

5-14 The protozoa are most animal-like.

5-15 Helminthology is the study of worms.

5-16 Three levels of asepsis are sterilization, disinfection, and antisepsis.

5-17 Handwashing is the single most important measure for preventing the spread of infection.

5-18 An antibiotic is a substance produced by living cells that has the power to kill or arrest the growth of bacteria.

5-19 Stains are used to color cells so that they can be examined under the microscope.

Answers to Zooming In Questions

5-3 Streptococci are the cells shown in Figure 5-3D.

5-5 Flagella indicate that the cells in A are capable of movement.

5-9 The term intracellular means that the parasites are inside cells. Vectors transmit disease organisms from one host to another.

5-10 Skeletal (striated) muscle tissue is shown in B.

Chapter 6
Answers to Checkpoint Questions

6-1 The skin and all its associated structures make up the integumentary system.

6-2 The superficial layer of the skin is the epidermis; the deeper layer is the dermis.

6-3 The subcutaneous layer is composed of loose connective tissue and adipose (fat) tissue.

6-4 The sebaceous glands produce an oily secretion called sebum.

6-5 The sweat glands are the sudoriferous glands.

6-6 Each hair develops within a sheath called the hair follicle.

6-7 Temperature is regulated through the skin by dilation (widening) and constriction (narrowing) of blood vessels and by evaporation of perspiration from the body surface.

6-8 Melanin, hemoglobin, and carotene impart color to the skin.

6-9 A lesion is any wound or local damage to tissue.

6-10 Epithelial and connective tissues repair themselves most easily.

6-11 Dermatosis is any skin disease; dermatitis is inflammation of the skin.

6-12 Melanoma is a cancer of the skin's pigment-producing cells.

6-13 Some viruses that affect the skin are herpes simplex virus, herpes zoster virus, and papillomavirus.

6-14 A fungus causes a tinea or ringworm infection.

6-15 Some autoimmune disorders that involve the skin are pemphigus, lupus erythematosus, and scleroderma.

Answers to Zooming In Questions

6-4 The sebaceous glands and apocrine sweat glands secrete to the outside through the hair follicles. The sweat glands are made of simple cuboidal epithelium.

6-6 Blue color is associated with cyanosis. Yellow color is associated with jaundice.

Chapter 7
Answers to Checkpoint Questions

7-1 The shaft of the long bone is the diaphysis; the end of a long bone is the epiphysis.

7-2 Compact bone makes up the main shaft of long bones and the outer layer of other bones; spongy (cancellous) bone makes up the ends of the long bones and the center of other bones.

7-3 The cells found in bone are osteoblasts, which build bone tissue, osteocytes, which maintain bone, and osteoclasts, which break down (resorb) bone.

7-4 Calcium compounds are deposited in the matrix of bone to harden it.

7-5 The epiphyseal plates are the secondary growth centers of a long bone.

7-6 The markings on bones help to form joints, serve as points for muscle attachments, and allow passage of nerves and blood vessels.

7-7 The skeleton of the trunk consists of the vertebral column and the bones of the thorax, which are the ribs and the sternum.

7-8 The five regions of the vertebral column are the cervical vertebrae, thoracic vertebrae, lumbar vertebrae, sacrum, and coccyx.

7-9 The appendicular skeleton consists of bones of the shoulder girdle, hip, and extremities.

7-10 The three types of joints classified according to the material between the adjoining bones are fibrous, cartilaginous, and synovial.

7-11 A synovial joint or diarthrosis is the most freely movable type of joint.

7-12 Arthritis is the most common type of joint disorder.

Answers to Zooming In Questions

7-5 A suture is the type of joint between bones of the skull.

7-6 The maxilla and palatine bones make up each side of the hard palate.

7-7 A foramen is a hole.

7-9 The anterior fontanel is the largest fontanel.

7-10 The cervical and lumbar vertebrae form a convex curve; the thoracic and sacral vertebrae form a concave curve.

7-14 The costal cartilages attach to the ribs.

7-15 The prefix *supra* means above; the prefix *infra* means below.

7-17 The radius is the lateral bone of the forearm.

7-19 The olecranon of the ulna forms the bony prominence of the elbow.

7-21 The ischium is nicknamed the "sit bone."

7-24 The tibia is the medial bone of the leg.

7-25 The calcaneus is the heel bone.

Chapter 8

Answers to Checkpoint Questions

8-1 The three types of muscle are smooth muscle, cardiac muscle, and skeletal muscle.

8-2 The three main functions of skeletal muscle are movement of the skeleton, maintenance of posture, and generation of heat.

8-3 The neuromuscular junction is the special synapse where a nerve cell makes contact with a muscle cell.

8-4 Acetylcholine (ACh) is the neurotransmitter involved in the stimulation of skeletal muscle cells.

8-5 Excitability and contractility are the two properties of muscle cells that are needed for response to a stimulus.

8-6 Actin and myosin are the filaments that interact to produce muscle contraction.

8-7 Calcium is needed to allow actin and myosin to interact.

8-8 ATP is the compound produced by the oxidation of nutrients that supplies the energy for muscle cell contraction.

8-9 Lactic acid is produced when muscles work without oxygen, causing muscle fatigue.

8-10 A muscle's attachment to a less movable part of the skeleton is the origin; a muscle's attachment to a movable part of the skeleton is the insertion.

8-11 The muscle that produces a movement is called the prime mover; the muscle that produces an opposite movement is the antagonist.

8-12 The action of most muscles is represented by a third-class lever in which the fulcrum is behind the point of effort and the weight.

8-13 The diaphragm is the muscle most important in breathing.

8-14 The muscles of the abdominal wall are strengthened by having the muscle fibers run in different directions.

Answers to Zooming In Questions

8-1 The endomysium is the innermost layer of connective tissue in a skeletal muscle. Perimysium surrounds a fascicle of muscle fibers.

8-5 The actin and myosin filaments do not change in length as muscle contracts, they simply overlap more.

8-7 Contraction of the biceps brachii produces flexion at the elbow.

8-11 The frontalis, temporalis, nasalis, and zygomaticus are named for the bones they are near.

Chapter 9

Answers to Checkpoint Questions

9-1 Structurally, the nervous system can be divided into a central and a peripheral nervous system.

9-2 The somatic nervous system is voluntary and controls skeletal muscle; the autonomic (visceral) nervous system is involuntary and controls involuntary muscles and glands.

9-3 The fiber of the neuron that carries impulses toward the cell body is the dendrite; the fiber that carries impulses away from the cell body is the axon.

9-4 Myelinated fibers are white, and unmyelinated tissues are gray.

9-5 Sensory (afferent) nerves convey impulses toward the CNS; motor (efferent) nerves convey impulses away from the CNS.

9-6 Neuroglia (glial cells) are the nonconducting cells of the nervous system that protect, nourish, and support the neurons.

9-7 In an action potential, depolarization is the stage when the charge on the membrane reverses; repolarization is when the charge returns to the resting state.

9-8 Sodium ion (Na^+) and potassium ion (K^+) are the two ions involved in the generation of an action potential.

9-9 Neurotransmitters are the chemicals used to carry information across the synaptic cleft.

9-10 In the spinal cord, an H-shaped section of gray matter is located internally, and the white matter is located around it. The gray matter extends in two pairs of columns called dorsal and ventral horns.

9-11 The tracts in the white matter of the spinal cord carry impulses to and from the brain. Ascending tracts conduct toward the brain; descending tracts conduct away from the brain.

9-12 A reflex arc is a pathway through the nervous system from a stimulus to an effector.

9-13 There are 31 pairs of spinal nerves.

9-14 There are two neurons in each motor pathway of the autonomic nervous system.

9-15 The sympathetic system stimulates a stress response, and the parasympathetic system reverses it.

Answers to Zooming In Questions

9-2 The neuron shown is a motor neuron.

9-11 No. The spinal cord is not as long as the spinal column. There are seven cervical vertebrae and eight cervical spinal nerves.

9-13 The reflex arc shown is a somatic reflex arc. An interneuron is located between the sensory and motor neurons in the CNS.

9-14 There are two neurons in this spinal reflex. Acetylcholine is the neurotransmitter released at the synapse shown by number 5, as this is a somatic reflex arc involving skeletal muscle.

9-15 The sacral spinal nerves (S1) carry impulses from the skin of the toes. The cervical spinal nerves (C6,7,8) carry impulses from the skin of the anterior hand and fingers.

9-16 The parasympathetic division of the autonomic nervous system has ganglia closer to the effector organ than does the sympathetic system.

Chapter 10
Answers to Checkpoint Questions

10-1 The main divisions of the brain are the cerebrum, diencephalon, brain stem, and cerebellum.

10-2 The three layers of the meninges are the dura mater, arachnoid, and pia mater.

10-3 CSF is produced in the ventricles of the brain. The two lateral ventricles are in the cerebral hemispheres, the third ventricle is in the diencephalon, and the fourth is between the brain stem and the cerebellum.

10-4 The frontal, parietal, temporal and occipital are the four surface lobes of each cerebral hemisphere.

10-5 The cerebral cortex is the outer layer of gray matter of the cerebral hemispheres where higher functions occur.

10-6 The thalamus of the diencephalon directs sensory input to the cerebral cortex; the hypothalamus helps to maintain homeostasis.

10-7 The three subdivisions of the brain stem are the midbrain, pons, and medulla oblongata.

10-8 The cerebellum aids in coordination of voluntary muscles, maintenance of balance, and maintenance of muscle tone.

10-9 Stroke is the common term for cerebrovascular accident.

10-10 Neuroglia are commonly involved in brain tumors.

10-11 There are 12 pairs of cranial nerves.

10-12 A mixed nerve has both sensory and motor fibers.

Answers to Zooming In Questions

10-3 Dural (venous) sinuses are located in the space where the dura mater divides into two layers.

10-4 The fourth ventricle is continuous with the central canal of the spinal cord.

10-5 The lateral ventricles are the largest ventricles.

10-6 The central sulcus separates the frontal from the parietal lobe.

10-7 Folding provides the cortex with increased surface area.

10-8 The primary sensory area (cortex) is posterior to the central sulcus. The primary motor area (cortex) is anterior to the central sulcus.

10-10 The pituitary gland is attached to the hypothalamus of the brain.

Chapter 11
Answers to Checkpoint Questions

11-1 Structures that protect the eye include the skull bones, eyelid, eyelash, eyebrow, conjunctiva, and lacrimal gland.

11-2 The sclera, choroid, and retina are the tunics (coats) of the eyeball.

11-3 The structures that refract light as it passes through the eye are the cornea, aqueous humor, lens, and vitreous body.

11-4 The rods and cones are the receptor cells of the retina.

11-5 The extrinsic eye muscles pull on the eyeball so that both eyes center on one visual field, a process known as convergence.

11-6 The iris adjusts the size of the pupil to regulate the amount of light that enters the eye.

11-7 The ciliary muscle adjusts the thickness of the lens to accommodate for near vision.

11-8 Cranial nerve II is the optic nerve. It carries impulses from the retinal rods and cones to the brain.

11-9 Hyperopia, myopia, and astigmatism are some errors of refraction.

11-10 The ossicles of the middle ear are three small bones, the malleus, incus, and stapes, that transmit sound waves from the tympanic membrane to the inner ear.

11-11 The organ of hearing is the organ of Corti located in the cochlear duct within the cochlea.

11-12 The receptors for equilibrium are located in the vestibule and semicircular canals.

11-13 Static equilibrium and dynamic equilibrium are the two forms of equilibrium.

11-14 The senses of taste and smell are the special senses that respond to chemical stimuli.

11-15 The general senses are touch, pressure, temperature, position (proprioception), and pain.

11-16 Proprioceptors are the receptors that respond to change in position. They are located in muscles, tendons, and joints.

Answers to Zooming In Questions

11-6 Location and direction of fibers are characteristics used in naming the extrinsic eye muscles.

11-7 The circular muscles of the iris contract to make the pupil smaller; the radial muscles contract to make the pupil larger.

11-8 The suspensory ligaments of the ciliary muscle hold the lens in place.

11-10 The oculomotor nerve (III) moves the eye.

11-16 The cilia on the receptor cells bend when the fluid around them moves.

Chapter 12

Answers to Checkpoint Questions

12-1 Hormones are chemicals that have specific regulatory effects on certain cells or organs in the body. Some of their effects are to regulate growth, metabolism, reproduction, and behavior.

12-2 Negative feedback is the main method used to regulate the secretion of hormones.

12-3 The hypothalamus controls the pituitary.

12-4 The anterior pituitary produces growth hormone (GH), thyroid-stimulating hormone (TSH), adrenocorticotropic hormone (ACTH), prolactin (PRL) follicle stimulating hormone (FSH) and luteinizing hormone (LH).

12-5 The posterior pituitary releases antidiuretic hormone (ADH) and oxytocin.

12-6 Thyroid hormones increase the metabolic rate in cells.

12-7 The mineral calcium is regulated by calcitonin and parathyroid hormone (PTH).

12-8 Epinephrine (adrenaline) is the main hormone from the adrenal medulla.

12-9 Glucocorticoids, mineralocorticoids, and sex hormones are released by the adrenal cortex.

12-10 Cortisol raises glucose levels in the blood.

12-11 Insulin and glucagon are the two hormones produced by the pancreatic islets to regulate glucose levels.

12-12 Insulin is low or ineffective in cases of diabetes mellitus.

12-13 Secondary sex characteristics are features associated with gender other than reproductive activity.

12-14 The stomach, small intestine, kidney, brain, heart and placenta are some organs other than endocrine glands that produce hormones.

12-15 Epinephrine, norepinephrine, ACTH, cortisol, growth hormone, thyroid hormones, sex hormones, and insulin are some hormones released in time of stress.

Answers to Zooming In Questions

12-3 The infundibulum connects the hypothalamus and the pituitary gland.

12-4 The larynx is superior to the thyroid; the trachea is inferior to the thyroid.

12-7 The outer region of the adrenal is the cortex; the inner region is the medulla.

Chapter 13

Answers to Checkpoint Questions

13-1 Some substances transported in blood are oxygen, carbon dioxide, nutrients, electrolytes, vitamins, hormones, urea, and toxins.

13-2 7.35 to 7.45 is the pH range of the blood.

13-3 The two main components of the blood are the liquid portion or plasma, and the formed elements, which include the cells and cell fragments.

13-4 Protein is the most abundant type of substance in plasma aside from water.

13-5 Blood cells form in the red bone marrow.

13-6 Hematopoietic stem cells give rise to all blood cells.

13-7 The main function of hemoglobin is to carry oxygen in the blood.

13-8 Neutrophils, eosinophils, and basophils are the granular leukocytes. Lymphocytes and monocytes are the agranular leukocytes.

13-9 The main function of leukocytes is to destroy pathogens.

13-10 The blood platelets are essential to blood coagulation (clotting).

13-11 When fibrinogen converts to fibrin a blood clot forms.

13-12 A, B, AB and O are the four ABO blood type groups.

13-13 The blood antigens most often involved in incompatibility reactions are the A antigen, B antigen, and Rh antigen.

13-14 Blood is commonly separated into its component parts by a centrifuge.

13-15 Anemia is an abnormally low level of red cells or hemoglobin in the blood.

13-16 Leukemia is a cancer of the tissues that produce white cells, resulting in an excess number of white cells in the blood.

13-17 Platelets are low in cases of thrombocytopenia.

13-18 The hematocrit is the percentage of red cell volume in whole blood.

Answers to Zooming In Questions

13-2 Erythrocytes (red blood cells) are the most numerous cells in the blood.

13-3 Erythrocytes are described as biconcave because they have an inward depression on both sides.

13-4 The granulocytes have segmented nuclei. Monocytes are the largest in size. Lymphocytes are the smallest in size.

13-6 Simple squamous epithelium makes up the capillary wall.

13-8 Fibrin in the blood forms a clot.

13-9 No. To test for Rh antigen, you have to use anti-Rh serum. The two types of antigens are independent.

13-10 A neutrophil is in the upper left corner of the picture. Platelets are the small dark bodies between the cells.

Chapter 14

Answers to Checkpoint Questions

14-1 The innermost layer of the heart is the endocardium, the middle is the myocardium, and the outermost is the epicardium.

14-2 The pericardium is the sac that encloses the heart.

14-3 The upper chamber on each side of the heart is the atrium; each lower chamber is the ventricle.

14-4 Valves direct the flow of blood through the heart.

14-5 The coronary circulation is the blood supply to the myocardium.

14-6 The contraction phase of the cardiac cycle is systole; the relaxation phase is diastole.

14-7 Cardiac output is determined by the stroke volume, the volume of blood ejected from the ventricle with each beat, and by the heart rate, the number of times the heart beats per minute.

14-8 The small mass of tissue that starts the heartbeat is the sinoatrial (SA) node.

14-9 The autonomic nervous system is the main influence on the rate and strength of heart contractions.

14-10 A heart murmur is an abnormal heart sound.

14-11 Congenital heart disease is a defect present at birth.

14-12 Rheumatic fever is caused by certain streptococci.

14-13 Atherosclerosis commonly causes narrowing of the coronary vessels.

14-14 ECG and EKG stand for electrocardiography.

14-15 Coronary angioplasty is the technique used to open a restricted coronary artery with a balloon catheter.

Answers to Zooming In Questions

14-1 The left lung is smaller than the right lung because the heart is located more toward the left of the thorax.

14-2 The left ventricle has the thickest wall.

14-4 The aorta carries blood into the systemic circuit.

14-5 The myocardium is the thickest layer of the heart wall.

14-6 The right AV valve has three cusps; the left AV valve has two.

14-10 The AV (tricuspid and mitral) valves close when the ventricles contract, and the semilunar (pulmonary and aortic) valves open.

14-11 The internodal pathways connect the SA and AV nodes.

14-12 The SA and AV nodes are affected by the autonomic nervous system.

14-16 The cardiac cycle shown in the diagram is 0.8 seconds.

Chapter 15

Answers to Checkpoint Questions

15-1 The five types of blood vessels are arteries, arterioles, capillaries, venules, and veins

15-2 The pulmonary circuit carries blood from the heart to the lungs and back to the heart; the systemic circuit carries blood to and from all remaining tissues in the body.

15-3 Smooth muscle makes up the middle layer of arteries and veins. Smooth muscle is involuntary muscle controlled by the autonomic nervous system.

15-4 There is one cell layer in the wall of a capillary.

15-5 The aorta is divided into the ascending aorta, aortic arch, thoracic aorta, and abdominal aorta.

15-6 The common iliac arteries are formed by the final division of the abdominal aorta.

15-7 The brachiocephalic artery supplies the arm and head on the right side.

15-8 An anastomosis is a communication between two vessels.

15-9 Superficial means near the surface.

15-10 The superior vena cava and inferior vena cava drain the systemic circuit and empty into the right atrium.

15-11 A venous sinus is a large channel that drains deoxygenated blood.

15-12 The hepatic portal system takes blood from the abdominal organs to the liver.

15-13 As materials diffuse across the capillary wall, blood pressure helps to push materials out of the capillaries, and the blood osmotic pressure helps to draw materials into the capillaries.

15-14 Vasodilation and vasoconstriction are the two type of vasomotor changes.

15-15 Vasomotor activities are regulated in the medulla of the brain stem.

15-16 The pulse is the wave of pressure that begins at the heart and travels along the arteries.

15-17 Blood pressure is the force exerted by blood against the walls of the vessels.

15-18 Systolic and diastolic blood pressure are measured.

15-19 Hypertension is high blood pressure, and hypotension is low blood pressure.

15-20 Circulatory shock is inadequate blood flow to the tissues.

Answers to Zooming In Questions

15-1 Pulmonary capillaries pick up oxygen. Systemic capillaries release oxygen.

15-2 Veins have valves to control blood flow.

15-3 The artery has a thicker wall than the vein.

15-4 There is one brachiocephalic artery.

15-8 There are two brachiocephalic veins.

15-10 The hepatic veins drain into the inferior vena cava.

15-12 The proximal valve is closer to the heart.

Chapter 16

Answers to Checkpoint Questions

16-1 The lymphatic system drains excess fluid and proteins from the tissues, protects against pathogens, and absorbs fats from the small intestine.

16-2 The lymphatic capillaries are more permeable than blood capillaries and begin blindly. They are closed at one end and do not bridge two vessels.

16-3 The two main lymphatic vessels are the right lymphatic duct and the thoracic duct.

16-4 The lymph nodes filter lymph. They also have lymphocytes and monocytes to fight infection.

16-5 The spleen filters blood.

16-6 T cells of the immune system develop in the thymus.

16-7 Tonsils are located in the vicinity of the pharynx (throat).

16-8 Lymphadenopathy is any disease of the lymph nodes.

16-9 Lymphoma is any tumor of lymphoid tissue. Two examples of malignant lymphoma are Hodgkin disease and nonHodgkin lymphoma.

Answers to Zooming In Questions

16-1 A vein receives lymph collected from the body.

16-5 An afferent vessel carries lymph into a node. An efferent vessel carries lymph out of a node.

Chapter 17

Answers to Checkpoint Questions

17-1 Factors that influence the occurrence of infection include access to preferred body tissues, the portal of entry, virulence, dose, and the individual's predisposition to infection.

17-2 The unbroken skin and mucous membranes constitute the first line of defense against the invasion of pathogens.

17-3 Some nonspecific factors that help to control infection are chemical and mechanical barriers, phagocytosis, natural killer cells, inflammation, fever, and interferon.

17-4 Innate immunity is inherited in a person's genetic material; adaptive immunity is acquired during an individual's lifetime.

17-5 An antigen is any foreign substance, usually a protein, that induces an immune response.

17-6 Four types of T cells are cytotoxic, helper, regulatory, and memory.

17-7 An antibody is a substance produced in response to an antigen.

17-8 Plasma cells, derived from B cells, produce antibodies.

17-9 Complement is a group of proteins in the blood that sometimes is required for the destruction of foreign cells.

17-10 The active form of natural adaptive immunity comes from contact with a disease organism; the passive form comes from the passage of antibodies from a mother to her fetus through the placenta, colostrum, or breast milk.

17-11 Bacterial diseases for which there are vaccines include smallpox, whooping cough (pertussis), diphtheria, tetanus, *Haemophilus influenzae* type b (Hib), and pneumococcus.

17-12 Viral diseases for which there are vaccines include poliomyelitis, measles (rubeola), mumps, rubella (German measles), hepatitis A and B, chicken pox (varicella), influenza, rotavirus, human papilloma virus (HPV), and rabies.

17-13 An immune serum is an antiserum prepared in an animal; immune sera can be used in emergencies to provide passive immunization.

17-14 Disorders of the immune system include allergy, autoimmunity, and immune deficiency diseases.

17-15 The tendency of every organism to destroy foreign substances is the greatest obstacle to transplantation of tissues from one individual to another.

Answers to Zooming In Questions

17-2 Digestive enzymes are contained in the lysosome that joins the phagocytic vesicle.

17-3 Plasma cells and memory cells develop from activated B cells.

Chapter 18

Answers to Checkpoint Questions

18-1 The three phases of respiration are pulmonary ventilation, external exchange of gases, and internal exchange of gases.

18-2 As air passes over the nasal mucosa, it is filtered, warmed, and moistened.

18-3 The scientific name for the throat is pharynx, for the voice box is larynx, and for the windpipe is trachea.

18-4 The three regions of the pharynx are the nasopharynx, oropharynx, and laryngeal pharynx.

18-5 The cells that line the respiratory passageways have cilia to filter impurities and to move fluids.

18-6 Gas exchange in the lungs occurs in the alveoli.

18-7 The pleura is the membrane that encloses the lung.

18-8 The two phases of breathing are inhalation, which is active, and exhalation, which is passive.

18-9 Diffusion is the movement of molecules from an area in which they are in higher concentration to an area where they are in lower concentration.

18-10 Hemoglobin is the substance in red blood cells that carries almost all of the oxygen in the blood.

18-11 The main form in which carbon dioxide is carried in the blood is as bicarbonate ion.

18-12 The medulla of the brain stem sets the basic pattern of respiration.

18-13 The phrenic nerve is the motor nerve that controls the diaphragm.

18-14 Carbon dioxide is the main chemical controller of respiration.

18-15 COPD is chronic obstructive pulmonary disease. Chronic bronchitis and emphysema are commonly involved in COPD.

Answers to Zooming In Questions

18-2 The heart is located in the medial depression of the left lung.

18-4 The epiglottis is named for its position above the glottis.

18-7 The external and internal intercostals are the muscles between the ribs.

18-8 Gas pressure decreases as the volume of its container increases.

18-9 Residual volume can not be measured with a spirometer.

18-14 The esophagus is posterior to the trachea.

Chapter 19
Answers to Checkpoint Questions

19-1 Food must be broken down by digestion into particles small enough to pass through the plasma membrane.

19-2 The digestive tract has a wall composed of a mucous membrane (mucosa), a submucosa, smooth muscle, and a serous membrane (serosa).

19-3 The peritoneum is the large serous membrane that lines the abdominopelvic cavity and covers the organs it contains.

19-4 There are 20 baby teeth, which are also called deciduous teeth.

19-5 Proteins are digested in the stomach.

19-6 The three divisions of the small intestine are the duodenum, jejunum, and ileum.

19-7 Most digestion takes place in the small intestine under the effects of digestive juices from the small intestine and the accessory organs. Most absorption of digested food and water also occurs in the small intestine.

19-8 The divisions of the large intestine are the cecum, ascending colon, transverse colon, descending colon, sigmoid colon, and rectum.

19-9 The large intestine reabsorbs some water and stores, forms, and eliminates the stool. It also houses bacteria that provide some vitamins.

19-10 The salivary glands are the parotid, submandibular (submaxillary), and sublingual.

19-11 The gallbladder stores bile.

19-12 Bile emulsifies fats.

19-13 The pancreas produces the most complete digestive secretions.

19-14 Absorption is the movement of digested nutrients into the circulation.

19-15 The two types of control over the digestive process are nervous control and hormonal control.

19-16 Hunger is the desire for food that can be satisfied by the ingestion of a filling meal. Appetite is a desire for food that is unrelated to a need for food.

19-17 Caries, gingivitis, and periodontitis are common diseases of the mouth and teeth.

19-18 Crohn disease and ulcerative colitis are inflammatory bowel diseases.

19-19 Hepatitis is inflammation of the liver.

Answers to Zooming In Questions

19-1 Smooth muscle (circular and longitudinal) is between the submucosa and the serous membrane in the digestive tract wall.

19-3 The mesentery is the part of the peritoneum around the small intestine.

19-4 The salivary glands are the accessory organs that secrete into the mouth.

19-7 The oblique muscle layer is an additional muscle layer in the stomach as compared to the rest of the digestive tract.

19-8 The ileum of the small intestine joins the cecum.

19-10 The accessory organs shown secrete into the duodenum.

Chapter 20
Answers to Checkpoint Questions

20-1 The two phases of metabolism are catabolism, the breakdown phase of metabolism, and anabolism, the building phase of metabolism.

20-2 Cellular respiration is the series of reactions that releases energy from nutrients in the cell.

20-3 Glucose is the main energy source for the cells.

20-4 An essential amino acid or fatty acid cannot be made metabolically and must be taken in as part of the diet.

20-5 Minerals are chemical elements, and vitamins are complex organic substances.

20-6 The normal range of blood glucose is 85 to 125 mg/dL

20-7 Typical recommendations are 55% to 60% carbohydrate; 30% or less fat; 15% to 20% protein.

20-8 Some factors that affect heat production are exercise, hormone production, food intake, and age.

20-9 The hypothalamus of the brain is responsible for regulating body temperature.

20-10 Normal body temperature is 36.2°C to 37.6°C (97°F to 100°F).

20-11 Heat cramps, heat exhaustion, and heat stroke are brought on by excessive heat.

20-12 Hypothermia is excessively low body temperature.

Answers to Zooming In Questions

20-1 Pyruvic acid produces lactic acid under anaerobic conditions; it produces CO_2 and H_2O under aerobic conditions.

20-4 The BMI is 24 (77 ÷ 3.2 = 24).

Chapter 21

Answers to Checkpoint Questions

21-1 Body fluids are grouped into intracellular fluid and extracellular fluid.

21-2 Water is lost from the body through the kidneys, the skin, the lungs, and the intestinal tract.

21-3 The control center for the sense of thirst is located in the hypothalamus of the brain.

21-4 Sodium is the main cation in extracellular fluid. Potassium is the main cation in intracellular fluid.

21-5 Chloride is the main anion in extracellular fluid.

21-6 Some electrolytes are lost through the feces and sweat. The kidneys have the main job of balancing electrolytes. Several hormones, such as aldosterone, parathyroid hormone, and calcitonin, are also involved.

21-7 The acid–base balance of body fluids is maintained by buffer systems, respiration, and kidney function.

21-8 Abnormally low pH of body fluids results in acidosis; abnormally high pH of body fluids results in alkalosis.

21-9 Edema is the accumulation of excessive fluid in the intercellular spaces.

Answers to Zooming In Questions

21-1 Water is lost through the skin, lungs, kidneys, and intestine.

Chapter 22

Answers to Checkpoint Questions

22-1 Systems other than the urinary system that eliminate waste include the digestive, respiratory, and integumentary systems.

22-2 The urinary system consists of two kidneys, two ureters, the bladder, and the urethra.

22-3 The retroperitoneal space is posterior to the peritoneum.

22-4 The renal artery supplies blood to the kidney, and the renal vein drains blood from the kidney.

22-5 The outer region of the kidney is the renal cortex; the inner region is the renal medulla.

22-6 The nephron is the functional unit of the kidney.

22-7 The glomerulus is the coil of capillaries in the glomerular (Bowman) capsule.

22-8 Glomerular filtration is the movement of materials under pressure from the blood into the glomerular capsule of the nephron.

22-9 The four processes involved in the formation of urine are glomerular filtration, tubular reabsorption, tubular secretion, and the countercurrent mechanism for concentrating the urine.

22-10 The JG apparatus produces renin when blood pressure falls too low for the kidneys to function effectively. The signal for renin production is low volume or low sodium in the filtrate leaving the nephron.

22-11 The ureter carries urine from the kidney to the bladder.

22-12 The urethra carries urine from the bladder to the outside.

22-13 Acute kidney disorders arise suddenly, usually as a result of infection. Chronic conditions arise slowly and are often progressive, with gradual loss of kidney functions.

22-14 The scientific name for stones is calculi.

22-15 Inflammation of the bladder is cystitis.

Answers to Zooming In Questions

22-1 The renal artery supplies blood to the kidney. The renal vein drains blood from the kidney.

22-2 The aorta supplies blood to the renal artery. The inferior vena cava receives blood from the renal vein.

22-3 The outer region of the kidney is the renal cortex. The inner region of the kidney is the renal medulla.

22-4 The proximal convoluted tubule is closer to the glomerular capsule. The distal convoluted tubule is farther away from the glomerular capsule.

22-6 The afferent arteriole has a wider diameter than the efferent arteriole.

22-9 The juxtaglomerular apparatus is made up of cells from the afferent arteriole and the distal convoluted tubule.

22-10 The urethra passes through the prostate gland in the male.

Chapter 23

Answers to Checkpoint Questions

23-1 Meiosis is the process of cell division that halves the chromosome number in a cell to produce a gamete.

23-2 The testis is the male gonad. Testosterone is the main male sex hormone.

23-3 The spermatozoon, or sperm cell, is the male sex cell (gamete).

23-4 The main subdivisions of the sperm cell are the head, midpiece, and tail (flagellum).

23-5 Sperm cells leave the seminiferous tubules within the testis and then travel through the epididymis, ductus (vas) deferens, ejaculatory duct, and urethra.

23-6 Glands that contribute secretions to the semen, aside from the testes, are the seminal vesicles, prostate, and bulbourethral glands.

23-7 Follicle-stimulating hormone (FSH) and luteinizing hormone (LH) are the pituitary hormones that regulate male and female reproduction.

23-8 Infectious diseases of the reproductive tract include chlamydial and gonococcal infections, genital herpes, syphilis, *E. coli* infections, mumps.

23-9 The ovary is the female gonad.

23-10 The ovum (egg cell) is the female gamete.

23-11 The ovarian (graafian) follicle surrounds the egg as it ripens.

23-12 Ovulation is the process of releasing an egg cell from the ovary.

23-13 The follicle becomes the corpus luteum after ovulation

23-14 The fetus develops in the uterus.

23-15 The two hormones produced in the ovaries are estrogen and progesterone.

23-16 Menopause is the period during which menstruation ceases.

23-17 Contraception is the use of artificial methods to prevent fertilization of the ovum or implantation of the fertilized ovum.

Answers to Zooming In Questions

23-1 The four glands that empty secretions into the urethra are the testes, seminal vesicles, prostate, and bulbourethral glands.

23-2 The ductus (vas) deferens receives secretions from the epididymis.

23-4 Mitochondria are the organelles that provide energy for sperm cell motility.

23-5 The corpus spongiosum of the penis contains the urethra.

23-8 The fundus of the uterus is the deepest part.

23-10 The endometrium is most highly developed in the second part of the menstrual cycle.

23-11 The opening of the urethra is anterior to the opening of the vagina.

23-13 LH shows the greatest increase at the time of ovulation.

Chapter 24

Answers to Checkpoint Questions

24-1 A zygote is formed by the union of an ovum and a spermatozoon.

24-2 The placenta nourishes the developing fetus.

24-3 The umbilical cord carries blood between the fetus and the placenta.

24-4 Fetal circulation is adapted to bypass the lungs

24-5 The heartbeat first appears during the fourth week of embryonic development.

24-6 The amniotic sac is the fluid-filled sac that holds the fetus.

24-7 The approximate length of pregnancy in days is 266.

24-8 Parturition is the process of labor and delivery.

24-9 A cesarean section is an incision made in the abdominal wall and the uterine wall for delivery of a fetus.

24-10 The term viable with reference to a fetus means able to live outside the uterus.

24-11 Lactation is the secretion of milk from the mammary glands.

24-12 An ectopic pregnancy is one that develops in a location outside the uterine cavity.

24-13 Puerperal infection is an infection that is related to childbirth.

Answers to Zooming In Questions

24-1 The ovum is fertilized in the oviduct (fallopian, uterine) tube.

24-2 The purple color signifies a mixture of oxygenated and unoxygenated blood.

24-5 The umbilical cord connects the fetus to the placenta.

24-7 The pectoralis major underlies the breast.

Chapter 25

Answers to Checkpoint Questions

25-1 A gene is an independent unit of heredity. Each is a segment of DNA contained in a chromosome.

25-2 A dominant gene is always expressed, regardless of the gene on the matching chromosome. A recessive gene is only expressed if the gene on the matching chromosome is also recessive.

25-3   Meiosis is the process of cell division that forms the gametes.

25-4   The sex chromosome combination that determines a female is XX; a male is XY.

25-5   A trait carried on a sex chromosome is described as sex-linked.

25-6   A mutation is a change in a cell's genetic material (a gene or chromosome).

25-7   A congenital disease is present at birth. A hereditary disease is genetically transmitted or transmissible. A disorder may occur during development and be present at birth but not be inherited through the genes.

25-8   Phenylketonuria is caused by a hereditary lack of an enzyme needed for phenylalanine metabolism.

25-9   A pedigree is a complete, detailed family history. It is used to determine the inheritance pattern of a genetic disease within a family.

25-10 A karyotype is a picture of the chromosomes cut out and arranged in groups according to size and form.

Answers to Zooming In Questions

25-1   25% of children will show the recessive phenotype blond hair. 50% of children will be heterozygous.

25-5   The possible genotypes of the two normal children in the F3 generation are CC or Cc.

25-7   There are 44 autosomes shown in B.

Dissection Atlas

Axial skeleton
Head

1	Frontal bone
4	Orbit
5	Nasal cavity
6	Maxilla
7	Zygomatic bone
8	Mandible

Trunk and thorax
Vertebral column

12	Sacrum
13	Coccyx
14	Intervertebral discs

Thorax

15	Sternum
16	Ribs
17	Coastal cartilate
18	Infrasternal angle

Appendicular skeleton
Upper limb and shoulder girdle

19	Clavicle
22	Radius
23	Ulna
24	Carpal bones
25	Metacarpal bones
26	Phalanges of the hand

Lower limb and pelvis

28	Pubix
30	Symphysis pubix
31	Femur
32	Tibia
33	Fibula
34	Patella
35	Tarsal bones
36	Metatarsal bones
37	Phalanges of the foot

Figure A7-1 **Skeleton of a female adult (anterior aspect).** (Reprinted with permission from Rohen JW, Yokochi C, Lütjen-Drecoll E. *Color Atlas of Anatomy*, 6th ed. Stuttgart, New York: Schattauer, 2006.)

Axial skeleton
Head

2	Occipital bone
3	Parietal bone
8	Mandible

Trunk and thorax
Vertebral column

9	Cervical vertebrae
10	Thoracic vertebrae
11	Lumbar vertebrae
12	Sacrum
13	Coccyx

Thorax

| 16 | Ribs |

Appendicular skeleton
Upper limb and shoulder girdle

20	Scapula
21	Humerus
22	Radius
23	Ulna

Lower limb and pelvis

27	Ilium
29	Ischium
30	Symphysis pubix
31	Femur
32	Tibia
33	Fibula
38	Calcaneus

Figure A7-2 **Skeleton of a female adult (posterior aspect).** (Reprinted with permission from Rohen JW, Yokochi C, Lütjen-Drecoll E. *Color Atlas of Anatomy,* 6th ed. Stuttgart, New York: Schattauer, 2006.)

1	Internal jugular vein
2	Common carotid artery
3	Vertebral artery
4	Ascending aorta
5	Descending aorta
6	Inferior vena cava
7	Celiac trunk
8	Superior mesenteric artery
9	Renal vein
10	Common iliac artery
11	Larynx
12	Trachea
13	Left subclavian artery
14	Left axillary vein
15	Pulmonary veins
16	Diaphragm
17	Suprarenal gland
18	Kidney
19	Ureter
20	Inferior mesenteric artery
21	Femoral vein

Figure A7-3 **Major vessels of the trunk.** The position of the heart is indicated by the dotted line. (Reprinted with permission from Rohen JW, Yokochi C, Lütjen-Drecoll E. *Color Atlas of Anatomy*, 6th ed. Stuttgart, New York: Schattauer, 2006.)

1	Cricothyroid muscle
2	Right internal jugular vein
3	Vagus nerve
4	Right common carotid artery
5	Right subclavian vein
6	Right brachiocephalic vein
7	Superior vena cava
8	Upper lobe of right lung
9	Right auricle
10	Middle lobe of right lung
11	Oblique fissure of right lung
12	Lower lobe of right lung
13	Diaphragm
14	Falciform ligament
15	Costal margin
16	Transverse colon
17	Thyroid gland
18	Trachea
19	Left internal jugular vein
20	Left cephalic vein
21	Left brachiocephalic vein
22	Pericardium (cut edge)
23	Upper lobe of left lung
24	Right ventricle
25	Left ventricle
26	Anerior interventricular sulcus
27	Lower lobe of left lung
28	Xiphoid process
29	Liver
30	Stomach

Figure A7-4 **Positions of thoracic organs.** The anterior thoracic wall has been removed. Arrow: horizontal fissure of the right lung. (Reprinted with permission from Rohen JW, Yokochi C, Lütjen-Drecoll E. *Color Atlas of Anatomy*, 6th ed. Stuttgart, New York: Schattauer, 2006.)

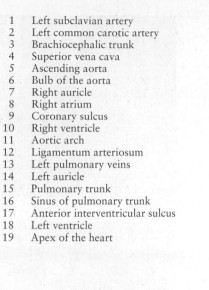

1	Left subclavian artery
2	Left common carotic artery
3	Brachiocephalic trunk
4	Superior vena cava
5	Ascending aorta
6	Bulb of the aorta
7	Right auricle
8	Right atrium
9	Coronary sulcus
10	Right ventricle
11	Aortic arch
12	Ligamentum arteriosum
13	Left pulmonary veins
14	Left auricle
15	Pulmonary trunk
16	Sinus of pulmonary trunk
17	Anterior interventricular sulcus
18	Left ventricle
19	Apex of the heart

Figure A7-5　**Heart of a 30-year-old woman (anterior aspect).** (Reprinted with permission from Rohen JW, Yokochi C, Lütjen-Drecoll E. *Color Atlas of Anatomy*, 6th ed. Stuttgart, New York: Schattauer, 2006.)

1	Internal jugular vein and right common carotid artery
2	Right and left brachio-cephalic vein
3	Aortic arch
4	Superior vena cava
5	Foramen ovale
6	Inferior vena cava
7	Ductus venosus
8	Liver
9	Umbilical vein
10	Small intestine
11	Umbilical artery
12	Urachus
13	Trachea and left internal jugular vein
14	Left pulmonary artery
15	Ductus arteriosus (Botalli)
16	Right ventricle
17	Hepatic arteries (red) and portal vein (blue)
18	Stomach
19	Urinary bladder

Figure A7-6　**Thoracic and abdominal regions in the newborn (anterior aspect).** The right atrium has been opened to show the foramen ovale. The left lobe of the liver has been removed. (Reprinted with permission from Rohen JW, Yokochi C, Lütjen-Drecoll E. *Color Atlas of Anatomy*, 6th ed. Stuttgart, New York: Schattauer, 2006.)

1   Thyroid gland
2   Upper lobe of right lung
3   Middle lobe of right lung
4   Heart
5   Diaphragm
6   Round ligament of liver
    (ligamentum teres)
7   Transverse colon
8   Cecum
9   Small intestine (ileum)
10 Thymus
11 Upper lobe of left lung
12 Lower lobe of left lung
13 Pericardium (cut edge)
14 Liver (left lobe)
15 Stomach
16 Greater omentum
17 Small intestine (jejunum)
18 Sigmoid colon

Figure A7-7 **Abdominal organs in situ.** The greater omentum has been partly removed or reflected. (Reprinted with permission from Rohen JW, Yokochi C, Lütjen-Drecoll E. *Color Atlas of Anatomy*, 6th ed. Stuttgart, New York: Schattauer, 2006.)

1   Diaphragm
2   Hepatic veins
3   Inferior vena cava
4   Common hepatic artery
5   Suprarenal gland
6   Celiac trunk
7   Right renal vein
8   Kidney
9   Abdominal aorta
10 Subcostal nerve
11 Iliohypogastric nerve
12 Central tendon of di-
    aphragm
13 Inferior phrenic artery
14 Cardiac part of stomach
15 Spleen
16 Splenic artery
17 Superior renal artery
18 Superior mesenteric artery
19 Inferior mesenteric artery
20 Inferior mesenteric artery
21 Ureter

Figure A7-8 **Retroperitoneal organs, kidneys, and suprarenal glands in situ (anterior aspect).** Red, arteries; blue, veins. (Reprinted with permission from Rohen JW, Yokochi C, Lütjen-Drecoll E. *Color Atlas of Anatomy*, 6th ed. Stuttgart, New York: Schattauer, 2006.)

1	Ureter
2	Seminal vesicle
3	Prostate gland
6	Bulb of penis
8	Epididymis
9	Testis
10	Urinary bladder
12	Ductus deferens
13	Corpus cavernosum of penis
14	Corpus spongiosum of penis
15	Glans penis
16	Ampulla of rectum
17	Levator ani muscle
18	Anal canal and external anal sphincter muscle
19	Spermatic cord (cut)

Figure A7-9 **Male genital organs in situ (right lateral aspect).** (Reprinted with permission from Rohen JW, Yokochi C, Lütjen-Drecoll E. *Color Atlas of Anatomy*, 6th ed. Stuttgart, New York: Schattauer, 2006.)

1	Body of fifth lumbar vertebra, suspensory ligament of ovary, and sacral promontory
2	Ureter
3	Medial umbilical ligament (remnant of umbilical artery) (cut)
4	Infundibulum of uterine tube
5	Ampulla of uterine tube
6	Ovary
7	Uterine artery
8	Uterine tube
9	Rectum
10	Levator ani muscle (pelvic diaphragm – cut edge)
11	External anal sphincter muscle
12	Anus (probe)
13	Internal iliac artery
14	Remnant of urachus (median umbilical ligament)
15	Uterus
16	Round ligament of uterus
17	Urinary bladder
18	Vagina
19	Clitoris
20	Labium minus
21	External orifice of urethra (red probe)
22	Vaginal orifice (green probe)
26	External iliac artery
31	Greater vestibular gland and bulb of the vestibule

Figure A7-10 **Female internal genital organs in situ.** Right half of the pelvis and sacrum have been removed. (Reprinted with permission from Rohen JW, Yokochi C, Lütjen-Drecoll E. *Color Atlas of Anatomy*, 6th ed. Stuttgart, New York: Schattauer, 2006.)

Index

Page numbers in *italics* denote figures; page numbers followed by *t* denote tables; and page numbers followed by *B* denote boxes.